T0260517

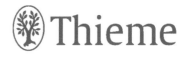

Neuroscience for Dentistry

Barbara J. O'Kane, MS, PhD
Professor
Department of Oral Biology
Creighton University School of Dentistry
Omaha, Nebraska, USA

Laura C. Barritt, PhD
Professor and Chair
Department of Oral Biology
Creighton University School of Dentistry
Omaha, Nebraska, USA

566 illustrations

Thieme
New York • Stuttgart • Delhi • Rio de Janeiro

Library of Congress Cataloging-in-Publication Data
is available from the publisher.

Illustrations by Voll M and Wesker K. From:
Schuenke M, Schulte E, Schumacher U, THIEME Atlas of Anatomy.

© 2022. Thieme. All rights reserved.

Thieme Medical Publishers, Inc.
333 Seventh Avenue, 18th Floor,
New York, NY 10001, USA
www.thieme.com
+1 800 782 3488,
customerservice@thieme.com

Cover design: © Thieme
Cover Image source: © Thieme/Andrew J. Rekito
Typesetting by Thomson Digital, India

Printed in Germany by Beltz Grafische Betriebe   5 4 3 2 1

ISBN: 978-1-62623-781-0

Also available as an e-book:
eISBN (PDF): 978-1-62623-782-7
eISBN (epub): 978-1-63853-520-1

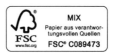

To my children and grandchildren, especially the girls.....#s♀em.

Barbara J. O'Kane, MS, PhD

To my husband, Steve, for his patience and support.
To my family for their encouragement.
And in memory of my father.

Laura C. Barritt, PhD

Contents

Preface

Practicing dentists are concerned with neural mechanisms controlling orofacial pain, masticatory function, taste, and proprioceptive input to the temporomandibular joint (TMJ) and teeth. As a result, one of the primary objectives of a dental neuroscience course should be to instruct the motor, sensory, and autonomic innervation of the head and neck pathways as well as the fundamentals of the biology and management of orofacial pain.

Most neuroscience textbooks provide excellent content coverage but do not focus on head and neck neuroscience from a dental medicine perspective and, although suitable for most health care students, the content does not adequately target dental students. The lack of specific dental information in neuroscience textbooks requires instructors, students, and practitioners to integrate information from multiple sources in order to develop a clear and comprehensive understanding of the orofacial region. Because of this, we set out to create a textbook that emphasizes the importance of the orofacial region and presents dental applicable information in the context of fundamental neuroscience.

Neuroscience for Dentistry is a unique textbook that integrates fundamental concepts of general neuroscience with essential information on the neural mechanisms involved in the orofacial region and orofacial pain pathways. The text is arranged in two sections. Part I provides a concise overview of general neuroanatomy and targets all health science students enrolled in a first-year neuroscience course. Part II focuses specifically on the neural mechanisms that regulate mastication, speech, swallowing, as well as proprioceptive input from the muscles, joints, and periodontal ligament. Detailed information on the cranial nerves is provided, with specific emphasis on orofacial pain pathways, pain modulation, and pain control. The focus on orofacial neuroscience and orofacial pain is a distinctive attribute of *Neuroscience for Dentistry* and it addresses the fundamental need for a neuroscience textbook that is tailored to dental students, students of dental hygiene, and residents in oral maxillofacial surgery.

Although the textbook is written for dental students, it can also be used to teach neuroanatomy to other health science students or serve as a reference for dental practitioners and residents. To facilitate multidisciplinary use, the text is structured so that individual units and selected chapters can be used independently.

Key features of *Neuroscience for Dentistry* include:
* Presentation of essential concepts of general and orofacial neuroanatomy through concise, high-yield descriptions and illustrations.
* Schematics, charts, and tables to augment the concepts presented in the text.
* Each chapter provides an introductory overview of chapter content and learning objectives.
* National board style questions at the end of each chapter emphasize board-relevant information and allow for self-study.
* Relevant clinical correlations are integrated throughout the textbook to emphasize the relationship between basic neuroscience and clinical disorders.

Barbara J. O'Kane, MS, PhD
Laura C. Barritt, PhD

Acknowledgments

This book would not have been possible without the help of many dedicated individuals. We offer special thanks to our talented colleagues, Drs. Margaret A. Jergenson and Gilbert M. Willett, for providing their expertise and contributing the chapters on Neurophysiology, Temporomandibular Joint, and Local Anesthesia: Intraoral Injections. We are grateful to the many colleagues and students who gave insightful feedback, suggestions, and honest critique of the chapters. Additionally, we thank our editors for their guidance and support. We also acknowledge Thieme's group of medical illustrators who created new art to complement the existing illustrations from Thieme's extensive collection. Many of the images that enhance the chapters of this book are from the award-winning three-volume *Thieme Atlas of Anatomy* and Gilroy's *Anatomy: An Essential Textbook* with illustrations by Markus Voll and Karl Wesker.

Barbara J. O'Kane, MS, PhD
Laura C. Barritt, PhD

Contributors

Margaret A. Jergenson, DDS
Professor
Department of Oral Biology
Creighton University School of Dentistry
Omaha, Nebraska, USA

Gilbert M. Willett, PT, MS, PhD
Associate Professor
Department of Oral Biology
Creighton University School of Dentistry
Omaha, Nebraska, USA

Part A

Basic Neuroscience

Unit I
Central Nervous System

1 Organization of the Nervous System

1.1 Overview of the Nervous System

The nervous system is anatomically divided into the **central nervous system** (**CNS**) and the **peripheral nervous system** (**PNS**). The CNS is made up of the **brain** and **spinal cord**. The PNS consists of both cranial and spinal nerves that act as conduits for information travelling between the body and the CNS. The PNS can be functionally subdivided into **sensory** and **motor** components. The motor division of the PNS is subdivided into the **somatic** nervous system that primarily controls voluntary activities and the **visceral efferent nervous system** that primarily controls **involuntary** activities. The **visceral motor system** is also called the **autonomic nervous system** (**ANS**). It has two branches: the **sympathetic nervous system** and **parasympathetic system** (▶ Fig. 1.1).

1.2 The Central Nervous System

- The CNS is composed of the brain and spinal cord (▶ Fig. 1.2).
- The brain can be divided into the following major structures: **cerebrum**, **brainstem**, and **cerebellum** (▶ Fig. 1.3).
  - The cerebrum is made up of two **cerebral hemispheres**, each containing several **lobes**.
  - The **midbrain**, **pons**, and **medulla** make up the brainstem.

- The cerebellum has lobes and hemispheres as well as a midline structure known as the **vermis**.
- The brain resides in the **cranium** while the spinal cord is contained within the **vertebral column**.
- The function of the CNS is to process and coordinate information that is received from the body and then direct the appropriate responses necessary for the maintenance of normal activity.
- The CNS is composed of neurons (▶ Fig. 1.4a, b), which transmit impulses and neuroglial cells (▶ Fig. 1.4c), which perform a more supportive function in maintaining homeostasis. Neuroglia do not transmit impulses
- The gray and white matter of the CNS is largely made up of the cell bodies of neurons and the myelinated axons of neurons, respectively (▶ Fig. 1.5).

1.3 The Peripheral Nervous System

- The PNS is made up of 12 cranial nerves (▶ Fig. 1.6a) and 31 pairs of spinal nerves (▶ Fig. 1.6b).
- The main function of the PNS is to connect the CNS to the rest of the body. **Sensory receptors**, which are specialized structures in the periphery, detect stimuli (e.g., heat, pain, touch) which are transmitted to the CNS via peripheral nerves.
- The PNS can be functionally divided into sensory and motor divisions (▶ Fig. 1.1).
  - The sensory division is also called the **afferent** division. It carries sensory information picked up by the receptors in the periphery and takes it into the CNS.

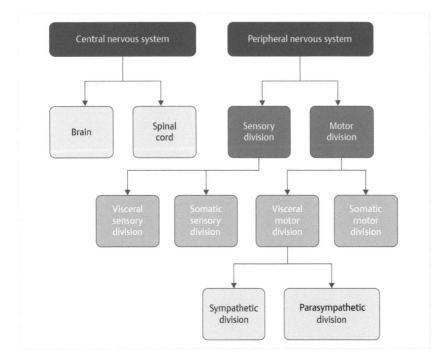

Fig. 1.1 The nervous system is divided into the central (CNS) and peripheral (PNS) nervous systems. The CNS consists of the brain and spinal cord, which constitute a functional unit. The PNS consists of the nerves emerging from the brain and spinal cord (cranial and spinal nerves, respectively).

○ The motor division is referred to as the **efferent** division. It carries signals from the CNS to its targets such as muscles, viscera, and glands.

• The sensory and motor divisions of the PNS are further subdivided into somatic and visceral components (▶ Fig. 1.1).

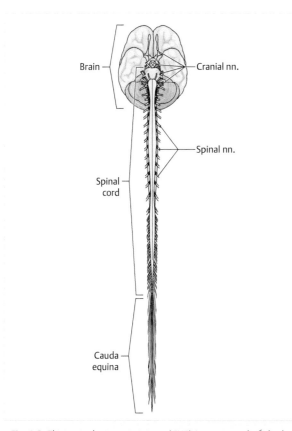

Fig. 1.2 The central nervous system (CNS) is composed of the brain and spinal cord. (Reproduced with permission from Gilroy AM, MacPherson BR. Atlas of Anatomy. Third Edition. © Thieme 2016. Illustrations by Markus Voll and Karl Wesker.)

○ The somatic afferent (sensory) division carries sensory information produced in somatic structures such as skin, muscles, bones, and joints.

○ The visceral afferent (sensory) division carries sensory information generated in viscera such as the heart, lungs, and gastrointestinal tract.

○ The somatic efferent (motor) division carries signals from the CNS to somatic structures. The result is contraction of muscles that are under voluntary control as well as those muscles that are involved in **somatic reflexes**.

○ The visceral efferent (motor) division, or the ANS, carries impulses to glands, cardiac muscle, and smooth muscle.

• The visceral motor arm of the PNS (ANS) has two components: the sympathetic nervous system and the parasympathetic system (▶ Fig. 1.1).

○ The sympathetic nervous system is referred to as the "**fight or flight**" response and is associated with situations that are perceived as potentially harmful to the body.

○ The parasympathetic system is called the "**rest and digest**" response because it returns the body back to the homeostatic state.

• Nerves of the PNS can carry either motor or sensory information but the majority carry both types and therefore are called **mixed nerves** (▶ Fig. 1.7).

○ Mixed spinal nerves are formed by the joining of a dorsal root (sensory fibers) and a ventral root (motor fibers).

 – The dorsal root exits the spinal cord from the dorsal aspect of the gray matter, the **dorsal horn** which carries sensory information. Sensory cell bodies are located in the **dorsal root ganglion** (**DRG**).

 – The ventral root exits the spinal cord from the ventral aspect and carries motor information. The cell bodies for the ventral root are located in the ventral aspect of the gray matter known as the **ventral horn**.

 – The dorsal root and ventral root join together just distal to the DRG to form a **mixed spinal nerve**.

○ Cranial nerves emerge from **nuclei** or collections of neuronal cell bodies in the brain, and can be sensory, motor, or both (mixed).

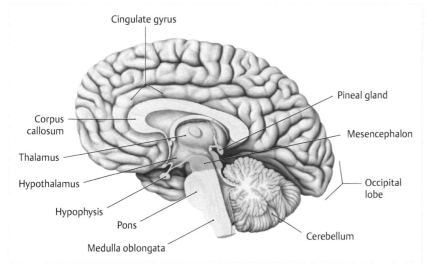

Fig. 1.3 Midsagittal section of adult brain showing the right hemisphere. (Reproduced with permission from Schuenke M, Schulte E, Schumacher U. THIEME Atlas of Anatomy Third Edition, Vol 3. © Thieme 2020. Illustrations by Markus Voll and Karl Wesker.)

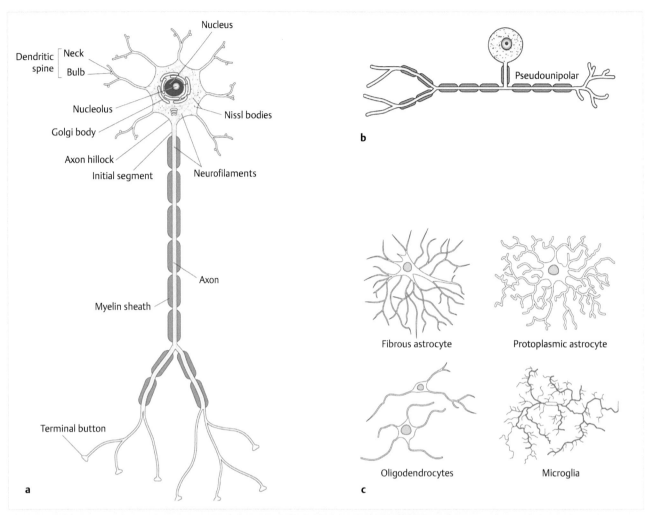

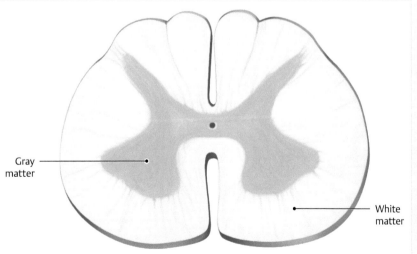

Fig. 1.4 **(a)** Structure of a neuron (multipolar). **(b)** Pseudounipolar (sensory) neuron. **(c)** Neuroglial cells found in the central nervous system. (Reproduced with permission from Michael J, Sircar S. Fundamentals of Medical Physiology. © Thieme 2011.)

Fig. 1.5 Gray and white matter in the spinal cord as seen in cross section. (Reproduced with permission from Schuenke M, Schulte E, Schumacher U. THIEME Atlas of Anatomy Third Edition, Vol 1. © Thieme 2020. Illustrations by Markus Voll and Karl Wesker.)

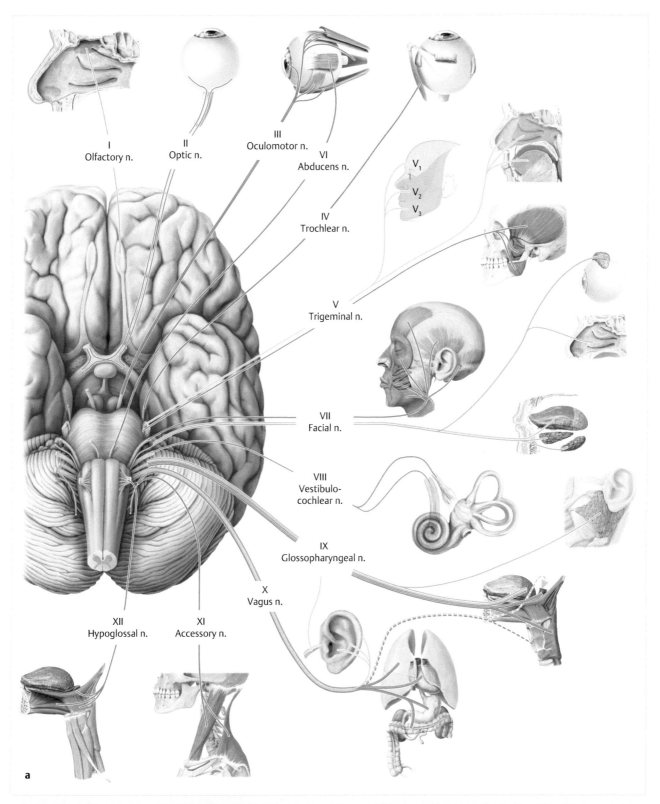

I
Olfactory n.

II
Optic n.

III
Oculomotor n.

VI
Abducens n.

IV
Trochlear n.

V₁

V₂

V₃

V
Trigeminal n.

VII
Facial n.

VIII
Vestibulo-
cochlear n.

IX
Glossopharyngeal n.

X
Vagus n.

XII
Hypoglossal n.

XI
Accessory n.

a

Fig. 1.6 (a) Cranial nerves from inferior (basal) view. The 12 pairs of cranial nerves (CN) are numbered according to the order of their emergence from the brainstem. Note: The sensory and motor fibers of the cranial nerves enter and exit the brainstem together (in contrast to spinal nerves, whose sensory and motor fibers enter and leave through posterior and anterior roots, respectively).

(Continued)

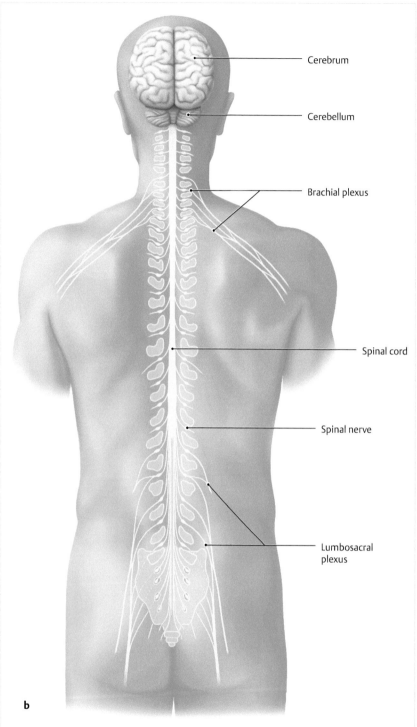

Cerebrum

Cerebellum

Brachial plexus

Spinal cord

Spinal nerve

Lumbosacral plexus

b

Fig. 1.6 (*Continued*) **(b)** Spinal nerves: 31 pairs of nerves emerge from the spinal cord. Spinal nerves contain both sensory and motor fibers that emerge from the spinal cord as separate roots and unite to form the mixed nerve. In certain regions, the spinal nerves may combine to form plexuses (e.g., cervical, brachial, or lumbosacral). (Reproduced with permission from Schuenke M, Schulte E, Schumacher U. THIEME Atlas of Anatomy Third Edition, Vol 1. © Thieme 2020. Illustrations by Markus Voll and Karl Wesker.)

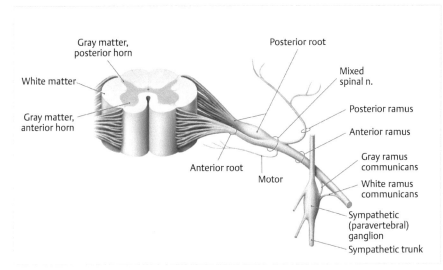

Fig. 1.7 Spinal cord segment. The spinal cord consists of 31 segments, each innervating a specific area of the skin (a dermatome) of the head, trunk, or limbs. Afferent (sensory) posterior rootlets and efferent (motor) anterior rootlets form the posterior and anterior roots of the spinal nerve for that segment. The two roots fuse to form a mixed (motor and sensory) spinal nerve that exits the intervertebral foramen and immediately thereafter divides into an anterior and posterior ramus. (Reproduced with permission from Schuenke M, Schulte E, Schumacher U. THIEME Atlas of Anatomy Third Edition, Vol 3. © Thieme 2020. Illustrations by Markus Voll and Karl Wesker.)

Questions and Answers

1. Which of the following divisions of the nervous system carries signals from the periphery into the CNS?
   a) Motor
   b) Sensory
   c) Efferent
   d) Sympathetic

Level 1: Easy

   Answer B: The sensory division carries information into the CNS. (**A**) Motor division carries information from CNS to target. (**C**) Motor information is carried on efferent fibers. (**D**) The sympathetic division is part of the ANS and is motor/efferent

2. The targets of the sensory somatic afferent division of the nervous system include which of the following?
   a) Skin
   b) GI tract
   c) Glands
   d) Smooth muscle

Level 2: Moderate

   Answer A: Skin is innervated by the somatic afferent division. (**B**) Viscera are innervated by visceral afferent division. (**C**) Glands are innervated by the visceral afferent division. (**D**) Smooth muscle is innervated by the visceral afferent division.

3. The sympathetic nervous system can be described as:
   a) Part of the PNS
   b) Visceral motor division
   c) Part of the ANS
   d) Visceral efferent division
   e) All of the above are correct

Level 2: Moderate

   Answer E: The sympathetic nervous system can be described as all of the above.

4. The CNS is composed of which of the following structures?
   a) Brain
   b) Spinal nerves
   c) Cranial nerves
   d) Ganglia

Level 1: Easy

   Answer A: The CNS is composed of the brain and spinal cord. (**B**) Spinal nerves, (**C**) Cranial nerves, and (**D**) Ganglia are all part of the PNS.

5. Mixed spinal nerves consist of which of the following?
   a) Sensory fibers
   b) Motor fibers
   c) Dorsal root
   d) Ventral root
   e) All of the above are correct

Level 2: Moderate

   Answer E: All of the structures listed make up a mixed spinal nerve.

2 Development of the Nervous System

Learning Objectives

1. Compare the marginal layer of the neural tube to the mantle layer.
2. Describe the neural crest derivatives that may be associated with the somatic sensory nervous system; the derivatives associated with the autonomic nervous system; and the derivatives associated with the adrenal gland and skin.
3. Describe the adult derivatives of the secondary vesicles.
4. Compare the function and location of the alar and basal plate in the spinal cord.
5. Explain the potential outcome that results from a failure of neural crest cells to migrate.
6. Explain the potential outcome that results from a failure of neuroblasts to migrate from the ventricular zone during cortical development.

2.1 Overview of Nervous System Development

2.1.1 Introduction

Development of the central and peripheral nervous system begins in the third week of embryonic development due to inductive signals originating from the **notochord (axial mesoderm)**. Signaling molecules secreted from the notochord induces a portion of the overlying ectoderm to differentiate into **neuroectoderm** and form the **neural plate**. This is followed by **neurulation** which is the process by which the neural plate folds inward and then fuses to form the **neural tube.** The central nervous system differentiates from the neural tube, whereas the peripheral nervous system develops from **neural crest cells** that originate from the dorsal margin of the neural tube. Failure for neurulation to occur properly leads to several pathological conditions that may impact fetal development.

2.1.2 Neural Tube Development

Primary and Secondary Neurulation

- Differential growth of the neural plate results in upward growth and inward folding of the lateral edges of the neural plate to form the **neural folds**. The center of the neural plate invaginates downward, forming the **neural groove** (▶ Fig. 2.1a, b).
- During neurulation, the dorsal margins of the neural folds begin to fuse in the midline, converting the neural groove into the neural tube. As the neural folds begin to fuse, **neural crest cells** separate from the free edge and migrate away from the neural tube (▶ Fig. 2.1c, d).
- The neural tube continues to fuse along the craniocaudal axis and becomes separated from the surface ectoderm. Two openings, known as **anterior** and **posterior neuropores**, initially remain open on the cranial (rostral) and caudal ends of the fused neural tube and then close during the fourth

week. Failure of the neural tube to fuse properly leads to neural tube defects.

- The expanded cranial portion of the neural tube gives rise to the **brain** and the caudal portion gives rise to the **spinal cord**. The lumen of the tube, known as the **neural canal,** persists and develops into the **ventricles** of the brain and **central canal** of the spinal cord.
- In the caudal end of the neural tube, a solid cell mass known as the **conus medullaris** appears on day 20. The conus medullaris forms a central cavity and then fuses with the terminal end of the neural tube to form the distal portion of the spinal cord in a process known as **secondary neurulation.**

Neural Crest Formation and Migration (▶ Table 2.1)

- **Neural crest cells** develop from the dorsal surface of the neural folds and detach as the neural tube starts to fuse. Neural crest cells migrate away from the neural tube along specific routes and populate the developing head, heart, and trunk, where they differentiate into a variety of structures (▶ Fig. 2.2).
- Defects in neural crest migration lead to a variety of developmental disorders including craniofacial abnormalities.
  - Cranial neural crest cells
    - Neural crest cells move cranially toward the head and neck and contribute to neurons of the **cranial sensory ganglia** and **autonomic ganglia** of the **peripheral nervous system**.
    - The two inner meningeal layers collectively referred to as the **leptomeninges**, consisting of **arachnoid** and **pia**, are also derived from cranial neural crest cells.

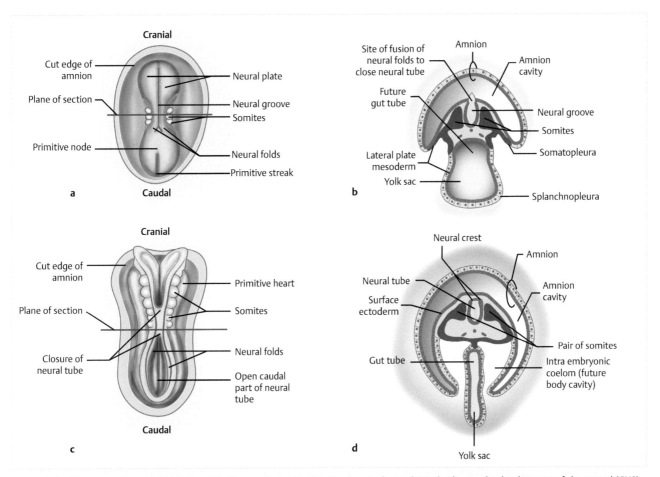

Fig. 2.1 (a–d) Process of neurulation. Schematic diagram demonstrating the stages of neurulation leading to the development of the central (CNS) and peripheral nervous system (PNS). Dorsal view of embryo (**a,c**); cross-section of embryo (**b,d**). The neural tube develops from the neural plate on the dorsal surface of the embryo. A central groove initially develops in the neural plate forming the neural groove. Neural crest cells migrate from the free edge of the groove as the neural groove fuses together, and the closed neural tube separates from the overlying ectoderm. The brain and spinal cord differentiate from the neural tube, whereas neural structures associated with PNS develop from neural crest cells.

Table 2.1 Neural crest derivatives

Cranial region	Cardiac region	Trunk/Body
• Ectomesenchyme skeletal and connective tissue of pharyngeal arches • Odontoblasts of the teeth • Cementoblasts of the teeth • Parafollicular cells of thyroid gland • Cranial sensory ganglia neurons • Autonomic ganglia neurons • Leptomeninges (pia-arachnoid)	• Cells of aorticopulmonary septum of heart	• Melanocytes of the epidermis • Spinal sensory ganglia neurons • Autonomic ganglia of body • Enteric ganglia neurons • Chromaffin cells of adrenal medulla • Schwann cells of PNS • Satellite cells of PNS

Abbreviation: PNS, peripheral nervous system.

- In addition, cranial neural crest cells combine with mesenchyme in developing pharyngeal arch region to form neural crest–derived **ectomesenchyme.** Ectomesenchyme forms the connective tissue and skeletal derivatives of the head and neck, including the dentin and cementum of the teeth.
  ○ Cardiac neural crest cells
    - Neural crest cells migrate toward the cardiac region to aid in the development and septation of the heart and great vessels.
  ○ Trunk neural crest cells

- Neural crest cells migrate caudally to the trunk (body) and give rise to neurons of the **peripheral spinal sensory ganglia (dorsal root ganglia)**, **enteric ganglia** of the gastrointestinal tract, **autonomic ganglia** of the autonomic nervous system, and **chromaffin cells** of the adrenal medulla.
- In addition, neural crest cells migrate throughout the developing embryo and differentiate into **melanocytes** associated with the epidermis of the skin and supportive **neuroglial cells**, such as **satellite** and **Schwann cells** of the peripheral nervous system.

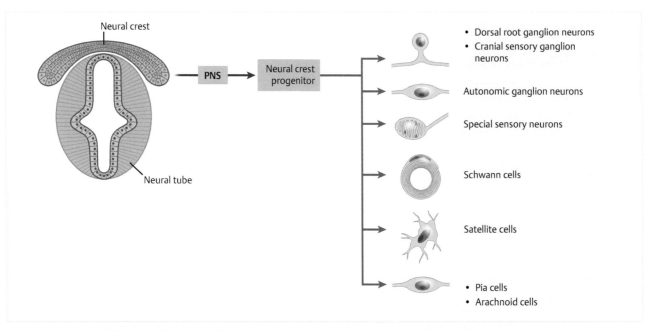

Fig. 2.2 Development of the neural crest cells. Main migratory pathways and derivatives of the neural crest cell.

Abnormalities in the proliferation, migration, and survival of neural crest cells gives rise to numerous syndromes and disorders including aorticopulmonary septal defects and craniofacial abnormalities

- **DiGeorge syndrome** is a primary immunodeficiency disease that results from abnormal neural crest cell migration to the head, neck, and cardiac region. Clinical manifestations include increased susceptibility to infection due to congenital absence of the thymus, disruption in the formation of the parathyroid gland, as well as cardiac abnormalities associated with aorticopulmonary septal defects.
- **Treacher Collins syndrome** results from a failure of neural crest cell to migrate to the region of the developing face, leading to craniofacial abnormalities involving the growth and development of the bones of the face. Patients exhibit hypoplasia of the maxilla and mandible, as well as abnormalities in the external ear.
- **Hirschsprung disease** results from abnormal migration of neural crests cell to the wall of the colon and the failure of the enteric and autonomic ganglion cells to differentiate. Patients exhibit intestinal blockage resulting from impaired peristalsis.

Cranial Sensory Placodes (▶ Fig. 2.3)

- During the fourth week of embryonic development, a series of bilateral ectodermal thickenings, known as **neurogenic placodes,** develop in a craniocaudal sequence from the region surrounding the anterior neural plate and cranial neural crest cells. The cranial placodes fall into two broad categories: **neurogenic** and **non-neurogenic placodes**.
- Neurogenic placodes give rise to neurons associated with the special sensory systems involved in smell and sight.
  - Olfactory (Nasal) placode differentiate into the bipolar neurosensory epithelial cells of the olfactory nerve (CN I) and induce the development of the olfactory bulbs.
  - Otic placodes develop into the neurosensory epithelial cells and non-neural epithelium associated with the cochlea and vestibular end organs of the inner ear and neurons of the vestibulocochlear ganglion (CV VII).
- The second group of neurogenic placodes differentiates into neurons associated with the **cranial sensory ganglia (CN V, VII, IX,** and **X)** of the developing pharyngeal arches in the head and neck region. These placodes develop from ectoderm and neural crest–derived cells and include:
  - **Trigeminal placodes** form neurons of the **trigeminal ganglion** that provide cutaneous sensory innervation to the face and jaw.
  - **Epibranchial placodes** develop in association with **CNVII, IX, X** and are associated with visceral sensory neurons of the **geniculate, petrosal,** and **nodose (inferior) ganglia,** respectively. These neurons innervate taste buds and visceral organs.
- Two additional ectodermal placodes develop but give rise to **non-neurogenic** structures:
  - **Optic (lens) placodes**—differentiate to form the **lens epithelium** of the eye. The optic placode develops in association with the **optic cup**, a neural outgrowth from the developing brain, which gives rise to the **retina.**
  - **Adenohypophyseal placode (anterior pituitary glands)**—differentiates from a thickening of ectoderm in the oral cavity known as **Rathke pouch** and forms the anterior

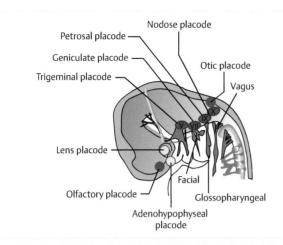

Fig. 2.3 Cranial sensory placode formation. Cranial sensory placodes develop as bilateral ectodermal thickenings and differentiate into two groups, neurogenic or non-neurogenic placodes. Neurogenic placodes give rise to special sensory neurons and neuroepithelium that mediate olfaction, hearing, and balance (*purple*). An additional group of neurogenic placodes develops from ectoderm and neural crest into the sensory neurons associated with cranial sensory ganglia (V, VII, IX, and X) (red). Non-neurogenic placodes develop from ectoderm and give rise to the optic (lens) and anterior pituitary gland (*yellow*). (Modified with permission from Greenstein B, Greenstein A. Neuroanatomy and Neurophysiology. © Thieme 2000.)

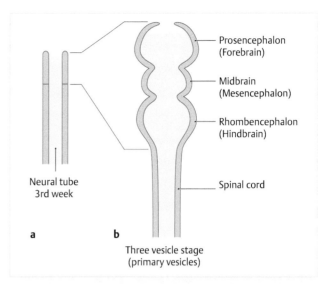

Fig. 2.4 (a,b) Primary brain vesicle formation (dorsal view, neural tube cut open). Three primary vesicles develop from the rostral end of the neural tube due to rapid cellular proliferation. The primary vesicles will give rise to the neural tissue of the forebrain, midbrain, and hindbrain. The spinal cord develops from caudal portion of the neural tube. (Reproduced with permission from Schuenke M, Schulte E, Schumacher U. THIEME Atlas of Anatomy Third Edition, Vol 3. © Thieme 2020. Illustrations by Markus Voll and Karl Wesker.)

pituitary gland. The anterior pituitary gland will fuse with the posterior lobe which differentiates from the diencephalon.

Neural Tube Morphogenesis (▶ Table 2.2)

- During the fourth and fifth week of embryonic development, rapid cellular proliferation within the walls of the neural tube results in hollow swellings, or **brain vesicles** forming in the rostral end of the neural tube. As the developing brain vesicles rapidly enlarge, folds or **flexures** form in the rostral neural tube which will enable the developing skull to accommodate the expanding brain. The developing spinal cord develops from the distal portion of the neural tube.
- **Primary Vesicle and Flexure Development of the Brain** (▶ Fig. 2.4).
  - During the fourth week of development, cranial expansion of the wall of the neural tube leads to the development of three distinct **primary brain vesicles:**
    – Prosencephalon (forebrain).
    – Mesencephalon (midbrain).
    – Rhombencephalon (hindbrain).
- At the primary vesicle stage, two curvatures, the **cephalic** and **cervical flexures,** develop in the rostral neural tube (▶ Fig. 2.5).
  - The **cephalic (mesencephalic) flexure** develops initially as a ventral fold at the level of the midbrain.
  - The second curvature, known as the **cervical flexure**, develops on the ventral surface at the junction of the hindbrain and spinal cord.
- Secondary vesicle and ventricle development of the brain.

Table 2.2 Derivatives of brain vesicles

Three primary vesicles	Five secondary vesicles	Derivatives of vesicle wall	Derivatives of cavities
Prosencephalon (forebrain)	Telencephalon	Cerebral hemispheres	Lateral ventricles
	Diencephalon	Thalamus	Third ventricle
Mesencephalon (midbrain)	Mesencephalon	Midbrain	Cerebral aqueduct
Rhombencephalon (hindbrain)	Metencephalon	Pons Cerebellum	Cranial (rostral) part fourth ventricle
	Myelencephalon	Medulla oblongata	Caudal part fourth ventricle

- During the end of the fifth week, the three primary vesicle walls continue to expand and become subdivided into **five secondary brain vesicles**. Concomitantly, the lumen of the rostral neural tube dilates to form a series of four interconnected **ventricles (cavities)** containing cerebrospinal fluid.
  - The **choroid plexus**, which is a vascular network consisting of ependymal cells, develops from the roof of each ventricle and functions in the production of cerebrospinal fluid. The ventricular system communicates with the **central canal** of the spinal cord, facilitating the circulation of **cerebrospinal fluid.**

- The five secondary brain vesicles include (▶ Fig. 2.6):
  - The prosencephalon vesicle divides into the telencephalon and diencephalon.
    - The walls of telencephalon continue to expand to form two lateral outgrowths, which become the primitive **cerebral hemispheres**. A ventral outgrowth gives rise to the **olfactory bulb.**
    - In the region of the telencephalon, the ventricle dilates and splits to form the two **lateral ventricles**.

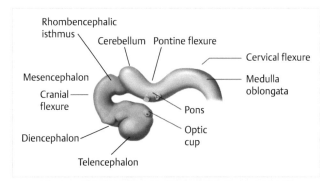

Fig. 2.5 Development of cephalic and cervical flexures. As the brain vesicles expand, the embryo folds forming two flexures: a cephalic (mesencephalic) flexure develops in the midbrain and the second flexure develops at the junction of the hindbrain and spinal cord, as the cervical flexure. (Reproduced with permission from Schuenke M, Schulte E, Schumacher U. THIEME Atlas of Anatomy Third Edition, Vol 3. © Thieme 2020. Illustrations by Markus Voll and Karl Wesker.)

- The diencephalon gives rise to bilateral outgrowths which form the optic vesicles, and a ventral evagination, known as the **infundibular stalk** and **neurohypophysis (posterior pituitary)**. A midline dilation of the lumen in the region of the diencephalon forms the **third ventricle**.
- The lateral ventricles of the telencephalon connect to the third ventricle of the diencephalon through the **interventricular foramina (of Monroe)**.
  - The mesencephalon remains unchanged, but a narrow groove, the **rhombencephalic isthmus,** develops and separates the mesencephalon from the rhombencephalon.
    - The lumen of the mesencephalon narrows to form the **cerebral aqueduct** that connects the third and fourth ventricles.
  - The rhombencephalon divides into secondary vesicles known as the **metencephalon** and **myelencephalon.**
    - The **pons** and **cerebellum** differentiate from the metencephalon, and the medulla oblongata develops from the myelencephalon.
    - As the secondary vesicles of the rhombencephalon differentiate, a third flexure, the **pontine flexure**, develops between the mesencephalic and cervical flexures and demarcates the boundary between the metencephalon and myelencephalon.
    - The folding of the rhombencephalon at the pontine flexures leads to the formation of the **fourth ventricle**.

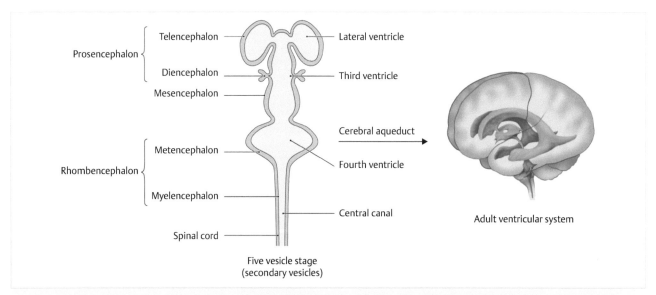

Fig. 2.6 Development of secondary brain vesicles and ventricular systems. The three primary vesicles expand and subdivide to form secondary vesicles. The forebrain differentiates into the telencephalon and diencephalon associated with the future cerebral cortex. The hindbrain differentiates into two structures: the metencephalon and myelencephalon. The metencephalon forms the pons and cerebellum. The myelencephalon differentiates into the medulla. As the vesicles differentiate, the lumen of rostral neural tube dilates to form four interconnected cavities known as ventricles that become filled with cerebrospinal fluid (CSF). (Reproduced with permission from Schuenke M, Schulte E, Schumacher U. THIEME Atlas of Anatomy Second Edition, Vol 3. © Thieme 2016. Illustrations by Markus Voll and Karl Wesker.)

Congenital hydrocephalus is a condition in which cerebrospinal fluid accumulates leading to dilation of the ventricular system. The most common cause of fluid accumulation is obstruction of CSF circulation that results from a narrowing (stenosis) of the cerebral aqueduct. This obstruction, called **aqueductal stenosis,** may occur during the formation of cerebral aqueduct within the mesencephalon.

Neural Tube Cellular Differentiation (▶ Table 2.3) (▶ Fig. 2.7a, b)

- Neuroectoderm lining the lumen of the neural tube differentiates into three layers: an internal layer called the **ventricular zone**, an intermediate layer called the **mantle zone**, and an external layer called the **marginal zone.**
- The **neuroepithelial stem cells** of the ventricular layer undergo rapid cell proliferation and give rise to **neuroblasts (neurons)**, supportive **neuroglial cells**, and the **ependymal cells** of the choroid plexus.
- Following cellular proliferation in the ventricular layer, neurons migrate to their final destinations within the brain and spinal cord and eventually become organized in a laminar arrangement as the **gray matter.**
- Axons that differentiate from these neurons become organized into groups of ascending and descending tracts and form the **white matter** of the brain and spinal cord. Nerve fibers that cross the midline from one side of the brain or spinal cord to the other are referred to as **commissures,** and function to connect the two regions.

2.2 Spinal Cord Differentiation

2.2.1 Gray Matter: Alar and Basal Plate Development (▶ Fig. 2.8a–c)

- In the spinal cord, neurons migrate from the ventricular zone and enter the mantle layer to form the gray matter. As neurons in the mantle zone grow, a longitudinal groove, known as the **sulcus limitans,** develops in the inner wall of the neural tube and divides the expanding mantle zone into dorsal and ventral regions. The neurons differentiating in the dorsal and ventral regions contribute to **sensory (afferent)** and **motor (efferent)** pathways, respectively, and become organized within the gray matter into functionally related groups of neurons known as **nuclei** and **laminae.**
- The dorsal region of the mantle zone is referred to as the **alar plate,** which eventually becomes the **dorsal (posterior) horn** of the spinal cord. The alar plate (dorsal horn) is comprised of sensory nuclei that receive sensory information from the periphery via nerve fibers that enter the spinal cord through the **dorsal roots.** The neurons developing from the alar plate form **interneurons** and **projection neurons.**
- The ventral region of the mantle zone is called the **basal plate,** which forms the **ventral (anterior) horn** of the spinal cord. The neurons of the basal plate (ventral horn) differentiate into **somatic motor neurons** that innervate skeletal muscle. Axons of the ventral horn neurons carry motor fibers and contribute to the **ventral roots** of spinal nerves.
- An additional group of neurons, which differentiate from an intermediate region between the alar and basal plates, will develop into the **autonomic preganglionic visceral motor neurons** located in the **lateral horn** of the spinal cord. These neurons are associated with the thoracolumbar (T1–L3) and sacral (S2–S4) segments of the spinal cord.

Table 2.3 Derivatives of neural tube wall: spinal cord and brainstem

	Ventricular layer Inner zone	Mantle layer Intermediate zone	Marginal layer Outer zone
Spinal cord	Immature neurons will migrate to form: • Interneurons (relay) • Projection neurons • Somatic motor neurons • Visceral motor neurons Supportive neuroglial cells will migrate to form: • Astrocytes • Oligodendrocytes • Radial glial Ependymal cells line central canal	Gray matter Neuron cell bodies associated with spinal nerves Alar plate: • Dorsal horn sensory nuclei (interneurons) Basal plate: • Ventral horn somatic motor nuclei • Lateral horn visceral motor neurons	White matter axonal tracts (fasciculi): • Ascending • Descending • Commissures
Brainstem	Immature neurons: • Interneurons • Projection neurons • Somatic motor neurons • Visceral motor neurons Supportive neuroglial cells will migrate to form: • Astrocytes • Oligodendrocytes • Radial glial Ependymal cells line fourth ventricle and choroid plexus	Gray matter Neuron cell bodies associated with cranial nerves • Alar plate—sensory nuclei • Basal plate—motor nuclei	White matter axonal tracts (fasciculi): • Ascending • Descending Commissures

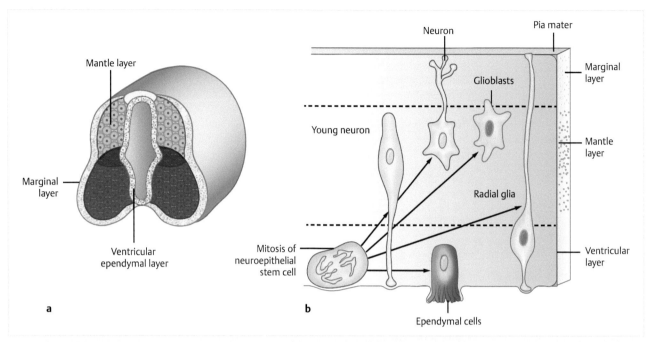

Fig. 2.7 (a,b) Cellular differentiation of neural tube. (a) Neuroectoderm forming the wall of the neural tube differentiates into three layers: an inner ventricular (ependymal) layer, a middle layer known as the mantle layer, and the outer marginal layer. (b) Each layer differentiates and gives rise to neuroglial cells, neuronal cell bodies of the gray matter, and the axons of the white matter. During development, neuroglial cells provide a structural scaffold that aids in the differentiation and migration of neurons to their final location.

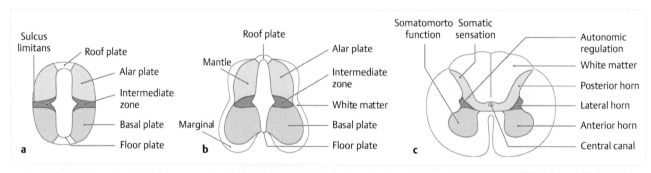

Fig. 2.8 (a–c) Schematic pictures of the developing spinal cord cut in cross-section. (a,b) The developing neural tube differentiates into paired basal and alar plates, and an unpaired roof and floor plate. Neurons that originate in the mantle layer of the basal plate of the spinal cord become the efferent (motor) neurons, while neurons arising from the alar plate develop into interneurons that receive sensory input from the body. In the developing thoracolumbar and sacral regions, a paired intermediate plate develops and differentiates into efferent neurons associated with the autonomic nervous system (ANS). The outer marginal zone develops into white matter and contains afferent and efferent axonal fibers. (c) In the adult, the white matter aggregates to form three columns (funiculi), while the basal, intermediate, and alar plates differentiate into the gray matter of the ventral, lateral, and dorsal horns (columns), respectively. (Reproduced with permission from Schuenke M, Schulte E, Schumacher U. THIEME Atlas of Anatomy Second Edition, Vol 3. © Thieme 2016. Illustrations by Markus Voll and Karl Wesker.)

- Two thin cellular regions span the midline between the alar and basal plates, forming a **roof plate** and **floor plate**, respectively. The roof and floor plates serve to connect nerve fibers crossing from one side of the neural tube to the other. The floor plate contains the **ventral white commissure**.

2.2.2 White Matter (▶ Fig. 2.9a, b)

- The white matter surrounds the gray matter in the spinal cord and brainstem.
- During development, axons from neurons in the alar and basal plates extend into the marginal zone and give rise to the white matter of the spinal cord. The nerve fibers of the white matter become organized into longitudinally arranged **columns,** referred to as **funiculi**. The funiculi consist of functionally related groups of **axonal tracts (fasciculi)** that transmit information to different levels of the spinal cord and brain. Typically, a group of tracts (fasciculi) travel together as the ascending and descending pathways that interconnect the spinal cord and brainstem to higher regions of the CNS.
- Axons originating from motor neurons in the ventral horn extend through the marginal layer and form motor fibers of the **ventral root** (▶ Fig. 2.10a).

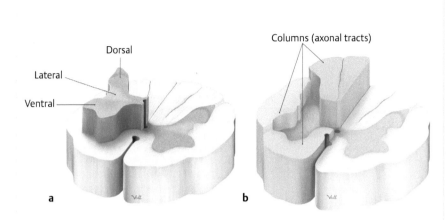

Dorsal

Lateral

Ventral

Columns (axonal tracts)

a

b

Fig. 2.9 (a,b) Gray matter of the spinal cord. Three-dimensional representation of the spinal cord, oblique anterior view from the upper left. **(a)** Gray matter showing the location of the dorsal, lateral, and ventral horns (columns). Each column consists of clusters of functionally similar nuclei, which contains neurons associated with a specific function; interneurons of the dorsal horn receive somatic sensory input; the lateral horn contains autonomic motor neurons controlling visceral functions; the ventral horn consists of somatic motor neurons controlling voluntary motor function. **(b)** White matter surrounds the gray matter and consists of several functionally related axon tracts that are organized into three columns (funiculi). (Reproduced with permission from Schuenke M, Schulte E, Schumacher U. THIEME Atlas of Anatomy Second Edition, Vol 3. © Thieme 2016. Illustrations by Markus Voll and Karl Wesker.)

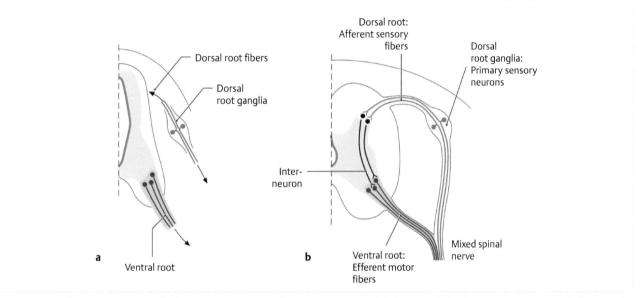

Dorsal root fibers

Dorsal root ganglia

Dorsal root: Afferent sensory fibers

Dorsal root ganglia: Primary sensory neurons

Inter- neuron

Ventral root

a

b

Ventral root: Efferent motor fibers

Mixed spinal nerve

Fig. 2.10 (a,b) Schematic showing the development of a spinal nerve. **(a)** During early development, afferent (*blue*) and efferent (*red*) axons develop separately from neuron cell bodies and migrate along specific routes to their functional target. *Arrows* indicate the route of axonal migration. Neural crests cells migrate and develop into primary afferent (sensory) neurons found in the dorsal root (spinal) sensory ganglia. A central afferent process grows toward the central nervous system (CNS) and a peripheral afferent fiber extends toward developing body. Neural crest cells also give rise to autonomic neurons associated with autonomic ganglia (not shown in diagram). Somatic α-motor neurons (lower motor, ventral horn neurons) develop in the basal plate of the spinal cord. **(b)** Interneurons (*black*) develop from the alar plate and may form functional reflex connections between sensory and motor neurons or may receive and transmit sensory input to higher levels of the brain. The dorsal and ventral nerve roots represent the part of the peripheral nerve that connects the nerve to the spinal cord or brain. Efferent motor fibers of the ventral root join the afferent sensory fibers of the dorsal root distal to dorsal root ganglion to form peripheral spinal nerves. Spinal nerves emerging from the vertebral column represent mixed peripheral nerves that carry both efferent and afferent axons. There are 31 spinal nerves numbered according to their emergence from the vertebral canal. The C1–C7 nerve roots emerge above their respective vertebrae; the C8 nerve root emerges between the C7 and T1 vertebrae. The remaining nerve roots emerge below their respective vertebrae. (Reproduced with permission from Schuenke M, Schulte E, Schumacher U. THIEME Atlas of Anatomy Second Edition, Vol 3. © Thieme 2016. Illustrations by Markus Voll and Karl Wesker.)

- Axons associated with neuron cell bodies located in the spinal sensory ganglia (dorsal root ganglia) form the primary sensory (afferent) nerve fibers of the **dorsal root** (▸ Fig. 2.10b). The nerve fibers extend from peripheral sensory receptors and pass through dorsal root ganglia, to enter the dorsal horn, where the fibers may synapse on interneurons or ascend in the marginal layer (white matter) of the spinal cord to higher regions of the CNS.
- The motor fibers of the ventral root join with sensory nerve fibers of the dorsal root distal to the dorsal root ganglia to form a **mixed spinal nerve** (▸ Fig. 2.10). The spinal nerves exit the developing vertebral column through the **intervertebral foramina**, an opening between adjacent vertebrae, and divide into **dorsal** and **ventral rami**.

2.2.3 Segmental Nerve Distribution: Myotomes and Dermatomes

- During development, the spinal cord exhibits a segmented pattern. The spinal cord gives rise to 31 pairs of spinal nerves that develop in association with bilateral swellings of mesodermal tissue known as **somites** (▸ Fig. 2.11a, b).
- The paired somites, which represent body segments, extend from the midbrain to the caudal end of spinal cord. The somites establish a segmental pattern of motor and sensory innervation and direct the differentiation of adjacent spinal nerve roots.
- Each somite pair differentiates into three segments of tissue: a **dermatome**, a **myotome**, and a **sclerotome**, that gives rise to the dermis of the skin, skeletal muscle, and vertebrae, respectively. Each spinal nerve originating from a specific spinal cord segment innervates the associated region of muscle and skin that develops from a single specific somite (▸ Fig. 2.11b).
- The groups of muscles that receive motor innervation from a single spinal nerve root are called **myotomes,** and the area of skin innervated by a single spinal sensory nerve root innervates is known as a **dermatome**. In the embryo, the motor and sensory innervation pattern exhibits an orderly arrangement, but due to the rotational growth of limbs, it becomes more complex in the adult (▸ Fig. 2.12a,b).

2.2.4 Positional Changes in Spinal Cord (▸ Fig. 2.13a–c)

- During the first trimester, the spinal cord and surrounding vertebral column grow at similar rates. The spinal cord extends the entire length of the vertebral column and each

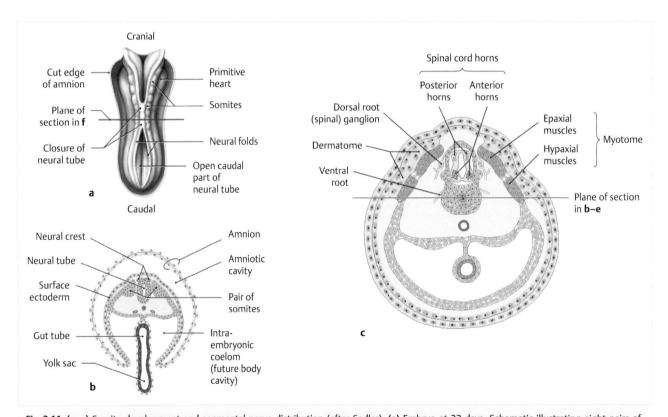

Fig. 2.11 (a–c) Somite development and segmental nerve distribution (after Sadler). **(a)** Embryo at 22 days. Schematic illustrating eight pairs of somites flanking the partially closed neural tube along the dorsal surface. **(b)** Schematic cross-section taken at the plane of section shown in **(a)**. **(c)** Schematic cross-section depicting segmented differentiation of paired somites. Paired somites, which represent specific body segments, extend from the midbrain to the caudal end of the spinal cord. Each pair of somites differentiates into a dermatome, myotome, and sclerotome segment, and directs the differentiation of the adjacent spinal nerve roots. As the paired somites and spinal nerve roots differentiate, a segmented arrangement of motor and sensory innervation becomes established. The segmented arrangement correlates with distinct innervation patterns associated with specific territories of the head, trunk, and extremities. The specific group of muscles that receives motor innervation from the same spinal motor root is known as a myotome. The area of skin transmitting cutaneous sensory input from a specific spinal sensory root is called a dermatome. (Reproduced with permission from Schuenke M, Schulte E, Schumacher U. THIEME Atlas of Anatomy Second Edition, Vol 1. © Thieme 2014. Illustrations by Markus Voll and Karl Wesker.)

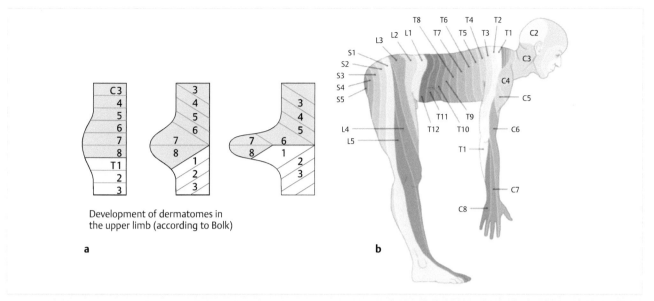

Development of dermatomes in the upper limb (according to Bolk)

a

b

Fig. 2.12 (a,b) Schematic representation of the embryonic and adult dermatome pattern. (a) A segmental pattern of innervation to the muscle (myotome) and skin (dermatomes) appears during embryonic development as each pair of spinal nerve roots differentiates along with an adjacent somite body segment. In the developing trunk, dermatomes are layered horizontally, and the corresponding nerve roots initially follow the outgrowth of the extremities. As the development continues, the limbs rotate around a longitudinal axis, which results in an oblique orientation of the dermatome pattern in the extremities. (b) In the adult, the dermatome pattern is slightly more complex than in the embryo. The dermatomes remain horizontally distributed in the trunk but follow a vertical pattern along the long axis of the limbs. In addition, the exact pattern may vary between individuals, and the innervation pattern may exhibit overlap between adjacent dermatomes. (▶ Fig. 2.12a: Modified with permission from Kahle W, Frotscher M. Color Atlas of Human Anatomy, Sixth Edition, Vol 3. © Thieme 2011. ▶ Fig. 2.12b: Reproduced with permission from Schuenke M, Schulte E, Schumacher U. THIEME Atlas of Anatomy Second Edition, Vol 3. © Thieme 2016. Illustrations by Markus Voll and Karl Wesker.)

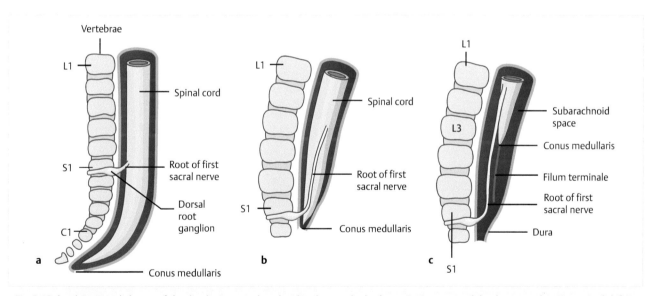

a

b

c

Fig. 2.13 (a–c) Positional change of the developing spinal cord within the vertebral column. During neonatal development, there is a rostral shift in the position of the spinal cord as a result of differential growth rates between the spinal cord and the vertebral column. (a) Third prenatal month. The spinal cord extends from the foramen magnum at the base of the skull throughout the length of the vertebral canal. The terminal part of the spinal cord, known as the conus medullaris, lies at the coccyx. (b) Rapid prenatal growth of the vertebral column causes a positional shift of the conus medullaris to ascend to the first lumbar (L1) vertebrae. (c) At the time of birth, the conus medullaris lies at the level of the L3 vertebra and is anchored to the vertebral column by the filum terminalis. In the adult, the conus medullaris lies at the L1 vertebral bodies and the spinal cord segments do not lie at the corresponding vertebral levels (not shown).

spinal nerve emerges laterally from the vertebral column at their level of origin.

- As development proceeds, the growth rate of the vertebral column exceeds that of the spinal cord, such that at the time of birth the terminal part of the spinal cord, known as the **conus medullaris**, shifts to the third lumbar vertebrae (**L3**), and does not fill the vertebral column.
- The conus medullaris becomes anchored to the vertebral coccyx by a thin layer of specialized connective tissue known as the **filum terminale**.
- The space created within the vertebral column due to differential growth rates creates a dilation of the subarachnoid space known as the **lumbar cistern**.
- In the adult, the conus medullaris reaches the level between the first and second lumbar vertebrae. The spinal nerves emerging from the terminal segments of the spinal cord (**L2–Co1**) become elongated to form the **cauda equina** (horsetail) within the lumbar cistern. The spinal nerves of the cauda equina do not lie adjacent to their corresponding vertebral level and must descend within the lumbar cistern from their segment of origin to exit the corresponding vertebral level.

2.3 Brain Differentiation

2.3.1 Brainstem Differentiation

- The **brainstem**, comprised of the **medulla, pons,** and **midbrain**, exhibits a similar developmental pattern to that of the spinal cord.
  - The neuroblasts migrate from the ventricular zone into the mantle layer and differentiate into nuclei associated with the sensory and motor columns of the alar and basal plates.
  - The marginal layer of the brainstem comprises the white matter and consists of numerous ascending and descending tracts.

- Due to the expansion of the fourth ventricle, the nuclei of the alar plate migrate to the floor of the fourth ventricle and become located lateral to the motor neurons of the basal plate (▶ Fig. 2.14a–c). This pattern continues throughout the brainstem, so that the sensory nuclei of the alar plate reside laterally, and the motor nuclei of the basal plate are medially located.
- In the brainstem, the nuclei of alar and basal regions are associated with **cranial nerves** rather than spinal nerves. Cranial nerves provide a similar function as spinal nerves; however, some cranial nerves carry special sensory input for smell, sight, sound, and taste, while others provide innervation to muscles that function in speech, swallowing, and mastication (▶ Fig. 2.15a, b).
  - Because of the functional and structural diversity in the head and neck region, cranial nerves exhibit a more complex pattern of sensory innervation.
  - The cranial nerve nuclei of the alar and basal plates become organized into seven functional columns which reflect the functional requirements of the head and neck region. None of the cranial nerves carry all seven functional modalities (▶ Fig. 2.16a–c) (▶ Table 2.4).
- CN I and II develop from the forebrain, while the cranial nerve nuclei associated with CN III through XII, originate from the brainstem.

2.3.2 Forebrain and Cerebellar Differentiation (▶ Table 2.5)

- Rostral to the brainstem, differentiation of the developing neural tube is more complex and is modified to accommodate the development of the cerebellar and cerebral cortices.

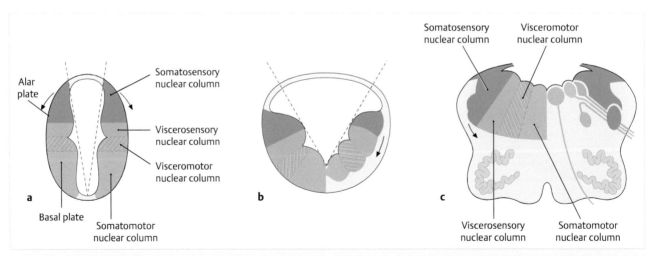

Fig. 2.14 (a–c) Brainstem development, migration of motor and sensory neurons, and establishment of cranial nerve nuclei (cross-sectional and cranial view of brainstem). **(a)** Early in embryonic development, the motor neurons reside in the ventral part of the brainstem (basal plate) and the sensory neurons lie in the dorsal part (alar plate). In the brainstem, the neurons of the alar and basal plate are associated with cranial nerves rather than spinal nerves. **(b)** As development continues and the fourth ventricle expands, the neurons in the alar plate migrate in a ventrolateral direction toward the floor of the fourth ventricle. Motor neurons of the basal plate remain ventral but migrate toward the midline. **(c)** The region of the medulla and pons from the rhombencephalon exhibit four nuclear columns that contain specific cranial nuclei. The somatomotor (*lilac*), visceromotor (*orange* and *green* stripes), viscerosensory (*light blue*), and somatosensory (*dark blue*) columns are indicated from medial to lateral. (*after His and Herrick*). (Reproduced with permission from Schuenke M, Schulte E, Schumacher U. THIEME Atlas of Anatomy Third Edition, Vol 3. © Thieme 2020. Illustrations by Markus Voll and Karl Wesker.)

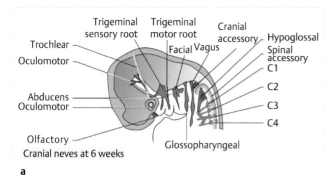

Cranial neves at 6 weeks

a

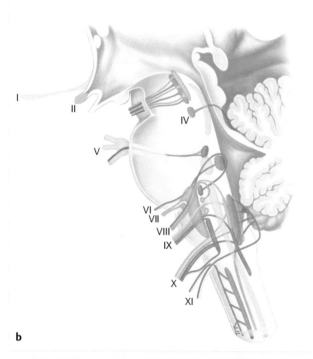

b

Fig. 2.15 (a,b) Schematic diagrams illustrating cranial nerve development and position of cranial nerve nuclei in the adult. **(a)** (Sagittal view) Schematic of developing embryo at 6 weeks showing the relative position of the 12 cranial nerves and cervical spinal nerves (C1–C4). **(b)** (Left lateral view; mid-sagittal section) Relative position of the cranial nuclei and nerves in the adult. The cranial nerves are numbered and described according to their level of emergence from the brainstem. The level of emergence does not necessarily correspond to the location of the cranial nerve nuclei associated with the cranial nerve. (▶ Fig. 2.15a: Modified with permission from Greenstein B, Greenstein A. Neuroanatomy and Neurophysiology. © Thieme 2000. ▶ Fig. 2.15b: Reproduced with permission from Schuenke M, Schulte E, Schumacher U. THIEME Atlas of Anatomy Third Edition, Vol 3. © Thieme 2020. Illustrations by Markus Voll and Karl Wesker.)

○ During development of the cerebral and cerebellar cortex, neuroblasts migrate away from the ventricular layer in the alar plate toward the pial surface to form the cortices of the gray matter in the outer marginal layer. The intermediate zone or mantle layer primarily contains axonal tracts and constitutes the white matter. The pattern of neuronal

migration results in the areas of the gray and white matter to become inverted in the developing cerebellar and cerebral cortices, such that the nuclei of the gray matter form the outer region closest to the meninges, and the white matter lies closest to the ventricles (▶ Fig. 2.17a–c).
○ During cortical development, neuronal migration results in the formation of the cortical cell layers associated with cerebellum and cerebral hemispheres.
 – The neuroblasts that differentiate first migrate to the boundary between the mantle and marginal layers to form the deepest layers of the cortex.
 – The neuroblasts that differentiate last migrate toward the pial surface to form the superficial layers of marginal zone.
○ In the region of the cerebral and cerebellar cortices, the final laminar arrangement of neurons is facilitated by supportive radial glial cells that send out cytoplasmic extensions from the ventricular zone to the marginal layer. The radial glial cells serve as scaffolding for the neurons to migrate sequentially to the superficial layers of the marginal zone.
○ In addition to neurons in the outer marginal zone of the gray matter, the cerebellum and cerebral hemispheres each contain several clusters of **deep cerebellar** and **cerebral (subcortical) nuclei**, respectively, that develop from neurons remaining close to the ventricular layer.

Clinical Correlation Box 2.4: Disorders of Neuronal Migration and Laminar Organization

Proper cortical development of the cerebellar and cerebral cortices depends on the proliferation of neurons and glial cells, cellular migration to the marginal zone, neuronal circuit formation, and the organization of neurons into cortical layers (lamination). The process of neuronal migration and lamination depends on radial glial cell differentiation.
• In the cerebral cortex, the process of neuronal migration and cortical patterning is tied to the process of cortical folding and gyri and sulci formation. Abnormalities in cortical development may result in neurological disorders such as autism, epilepsy, attention deficit disorders, schizophrenia, and cerebral palsy.
 ○ Developmental defects such as **Microcephaly,** which is associated with impaired growth of the cerebral hemispheres; **Lissencephaly,** which is a malformation characterized by the absence of gyri and sulci; and **Focal Cortical Dysplasia,** which is associated with abnormal pattering in the cortical layers, lead to cognitive dysfunction, and reflect the complexity of cortical formation.
• Defects in the development and migration of **cerebellar neurons** result in developmental delays in sensorimotor function and **sensorimotor ataxia,** which is a loss of coordinated voluntary motor function often associated with cerebellar deficits.

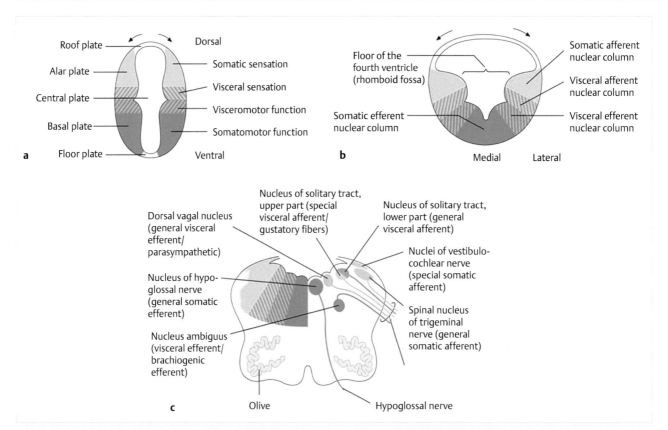

Fig. 2.16 (a–c) Arrangement of brainstem nuclear columns during embryonic development (*after Herrick*). Cross-sections through spinal cord and brainstem, superior view. The functional organization of the brainstem is determined by the location of the cranial nerve nuclei and corresponds to the pattern of neuron migration. **(a)** In the spinal cord, the motor neurons develop from the basal plate and lie in the ventral region of the cord. The sensory neurons of the spinal cord arise from the alar plate and reside in the dorsal region of the cord. **(b)** Early embryonic view of the brainstem (*arrows* indicate the migration path). In the brainstem, the cranial nerves of the alar and basal plate become organized into seven functional columns that reflect the functional requirements of the head. Sensory neurons of the alar plate migrate laterally to form sensory nuclei, while motor neurons of the basal plate migrate medially to form the motor nuclei. This results in a general mediolateral arrangement of the neurons into specific nuclear columns. **(c)** Cross-section through the medulla. The adult brainstem features a medial to lateral arrangement of four longitudinal columns of nuclei. In each column, the nuclei which have the same function are arranged in a craniocaudal pattern. The nuclei in the somatic afferent and visceral afferent column differentiate into general somatic (GSA) nuclei, general visceral afferent (GVA) nuclei, and special sensory afferent (SVA) nuclei. Similarly, the visceral efferent nuclear column differentiates into general visceral efferent (GVE) (parasympathetic) nuclei and special visceral efferent (SVE) (branchiomeric) nuclei. SVE nuclei develop in association with the skeletal muscles of the head that arise from the pharyngeal arches. In the region of the medulla, general somatic nuclei correspond to the motor nuclei of the CN XII (hypoglossal nerve). (Reproduced with permission from Schuenke M, Schulte E, Schumacher U. THIEME Atlas of Anatomy Third Edition, Vol 3. © Thieme 2020. Illustrations by Markus Voll and Karl Wesker.)

Table 2.4 Origin of cranial nerve nuclei

Brainstem region				Forebrain region	
	Medulla	Pons	Midbrain	Diencephalon	Telencephalon
CN	CN IX Glossopharyngeal	CN V	CN III	CN II	CN I
	CN X	Trigeminal	Oculomotor	Optic	Olfactory
	Vagus	CN VI	CN VI		
	CN XI	Abducens	Trochlear		
	Spinal Accessory	CN VII			
	CNXII	Facial			
	Hypoglossal	CN VIII Vestibulocochlear			

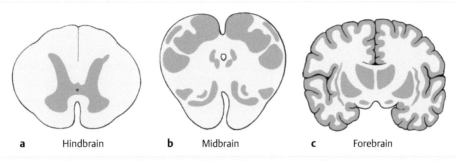

| **a** | Hindbrain | **b** | Midbrain | **c** | Forebrain |

Fig. 2.17 (a–c) Comparison of white and gray matter distribution between regions of the adult brain. Cross-sections through hindbrain **(a)**, midbrain **(b)**, and forebrain **(c)**. **(a)** During development, neural tube differentiation of the spinal cord occurs from three layers: an inner ventricular layer, a mantle layer, and an outer marginal layer. Migration and differentiation of neurons begin at the boundary between the ventricular and intermediate (mantle) layers and results in the formation of an internal layer of gray matter surrounded by an external layer of white matter. **(b)** In comparison, neural tube differentiation is more complex in the midbrain and forebrain, leading to a positional shift of the gray and white matter. **(c)** In the cerebellum and cerebrum, the three-zone configuration becomes modified to include a new layer known as the cortical plate that accommodates the development of the cerebellar and cerebral cortices. Neurons associated with the cortical plate arise from neuroblasts migrating to a superficial, outer marginal layer just below the pia to form the outer cortex of gray matter. The axons from these neurons lie in the intermediate (mantle) zone immediately internal to the cortical plate and form the subcortical white matter. In the cerebellum and cerebral cortex, an additional layer of neurons develops in close association to the ventricular system and differentiate into a deep layer of gray matter that is surrounded by the subcortical white matter. The neurons of the deep gray matter develop into the deep cerebellar nuclei and deep cortical nuclei (basal nuclei). (Modified with permission from Kahle W, Frotscher M.Color Atlas of Human Anatomy. Sixth Edition, Vol 3. © Thieme 2011.)

Table 2.5 Derivatives of neural tube wall: cerebellum and forebrain

	Ventricular layer Inner zone	Mantle layer Intermediate zone	Marginal layer Outer zone

Cerebellum	Immature neurons migrate to form:
	• Interneurons
	  ○ Basket cells
	  ○ Stellate cells
	• Projection neurons
	• Purkinje cells
	• Granular cells
	• Deep cerebellar neurons
	Supportive neuroglial cells migrate to form
	• Astrocytes
	• Oligodendrocytes
	• Radial glial
	Ependymal cells line third ventricles and choroid plexus
		White matter:
		Axonal tracts form the
		• Cerebellar peduncles
		Gray matter:
		• Deep cerebellar nuclei
			Gray matter:
			Cerebellar cortex:
			Three layers:
			• Molecular layer
			• Purkinje layer
			• Granular layer

Forebrain
Cerebral hemispheres
Diencephalon
	Immature neurons:
	• Interneurons
	• Projection neurons
	• Pyramidal cells
	• Golgi I and II cells
	Supportive neuroglial cells:
	• Astrocytes
	• Oligodendrocytes
	• Radial glial
	Ependymal cells line lateral ventricles and choroid plexus
		White matter:
		Axonal tracts:
		• Ascending
		• Descending
		• Commissures
		Gray matter:
		• Basal ganglia nuclei
		  ○ Corpus striatum (cerebral hemispheres)
		  ○ Subthalamic nuclei (diencephalon)
		  ○ Substantia nigra (midbrain)
			Gray matter:
			• Laminar arrangement of cortical neurons

2.4 Development and Derivatives of the Rhombencephalon

2.4.1 Myelencephalon: Medulla Oblongata

- In the region of myelencephalon, enlargement of the roof plate and fourth ventricle causes the sensory nuclei of alar plates to become located lateral to the motor nuclei of the basal plates (▶ Fig. 2.18a–c).
- Cranial nerves **CN IX, X, XII** develop from the medulla:
  - Neurons of the basal plate in the medulla form the motor nuclei of cranial nerves **IX, X, XI,** and **XII.**
  - Neurons of the alar plate of the medulla form the sensory neurons of cranial nerves **V, VIII, IX,** and **X,** as well as the **dorsal column nuclei** and inferior **olivary nuclei.**
- The marginal layer of the medulla, similar to that of the spinal cord, contains white matter arranged as ascending and descending axonal tracts.

2.4.2 Metencephalon: Pons and Cerebellum

Pons (▶ Fig. 2.19)

- The pons develops from the marginal layer of the basal plates of the metencephalon. The pons consists of two basic divisions: a dorsal region called the **pontine tegmentum**, which is an extension of the medulla, and a ventral region called the **basilar pons**, which serves as the pathway for nerve fibers to connect between the spinal cord, cerebral cortex, and cerebellum.
- Cranial nerve nuclei, **V, VI, VII,** and **VIII** develop at the level of the pons.

Pontine Tegmentum

- Neurons of the **basal plate** in the pontine tegmentum form the motor nuclei of cranial nerves **V, VI, VII,** and **superior salivatory nucleus.**
- Neurons of the **alar plate** of the pontine tegmentum develop into the sensory neurons of cranial nerves **V, VII,** and **VIII.**

Basilar Pons

- Pontine nuclei, which relay signals from the motor cortex to the cerebellum, develop from the alar plate.

Cerebellum (▶ Fig. 2.20)

- The cerebellum is derived from the **rhombic lips,** of the alar plate of the metencephalon. In the third month of embryonic development, the developing cerebellum gives rise to a midline structure known as the **vermis**; and two lateral growths form the **cerebellar hemispheres**.

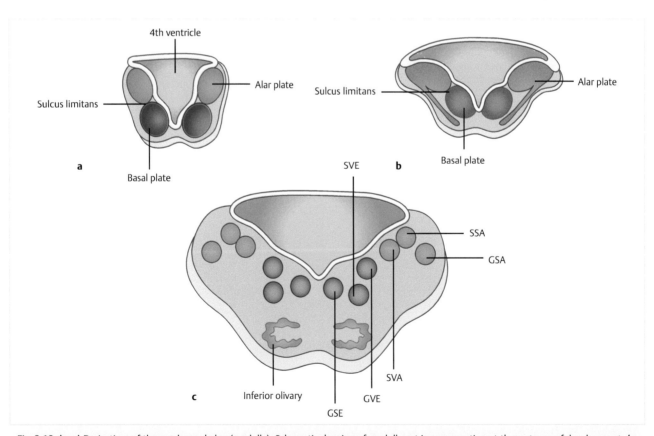

Fig. 2.18 (a–c) Derivatives of the myelencephalon (medulla). Schematic drawing of medulla cut in cross-section at three stages of development. **(a, b)** Note the expansion of the fourth ventricle during development leads to a shift in the alar and basal plates from a dorsoventral to a mediolateral position. **(c)** The motor and sensory nuclei of CN IX, X, XI, and XII develop from the medulla. The inferior olivary nucleus, which integrates sensory input and motor control from different regions of the brain, also develops in the medulla from migrating alar plate neurons.

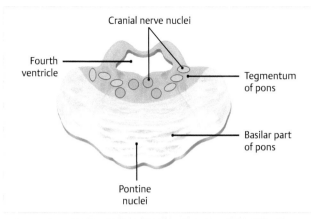

Fig. 2.19 Derivatives of the metencephalon (pons). Schematic drawing of a cross-section through the pons. The pons consists of two divisions: a dorsal region called the pontine tegmentum, which is an extension of the medulla and contains the cranial nerve nuclei, and a ventral region called the basilar pons. The region of the basilar pons is functionally comparable to cerebral peduncles in the mesencephalon (midbrain) and the pyramids in the medulla. These regions represent the ascending and descending tracts that pass from the spinal cord and brainstem to the cerebral cortex. In the pons, the basilar pons also contains the pontine nuclei that relay motor signals from the cerebral cortex to the cerebellum. Neurons migrate from the alar plate to form the sensory nuclei (*yellow*) associated with CN V, VII, and VIII, and the pontine nuclei. Motor nuclei (*blue*) of CN V, VI, and VII develop from neurons in the basal plate. (Modified with permission from Schuenke M, Schulte E, Schumacher U. THIEME Atlas of Anatomy Second Edition, Vol 3. © Thieme 2016. Illustrations by Markus Voll and Karl Wesker.)

- The cerebellar cortex, which is comprised of three cell layers; an **outer molecular layer**, a **Purkinje cell layer**, and **inner granular layer**, differentiates to form the cerebellar gray matter. The neurons of the cerebellar cortex migrate from the ventricular zone into the outer marginal zone, just below the pia mater and establish a laminar arrangement (▶ Fig. 2.20b).
  - Several neuroblasts remain close to the ventricular zone and differentiate into the **deep cerebellar nuclei.**
  - The mantle layer of the developing cerebellum forms the subcortical white matter. It consists of basket and stellate cells, along with the axons passing from the deep cerebellar nuclei to the brainstem and forebrain.

2.4.3 Development and Derivatives of the Mesencephalon (Midbrain) (▶ Fig. 2.21)

- The cranial nerve nuclei, CN IV and III, develop from the midbrain. The basal plates and floor plate of the midbrain form the **midbrain tegmentum**. The alar plates and roof plate form the **midbrain tectum.**
  - Neurons of the **basal plate** of the tegmentum form the motor nuclei of **cranial nerves III** and **IV**.
  - Neuroblasts of the **basal plate** also form the **red nuclei, substantia nigra**, and **reticular formation** of the **tegmentum**.

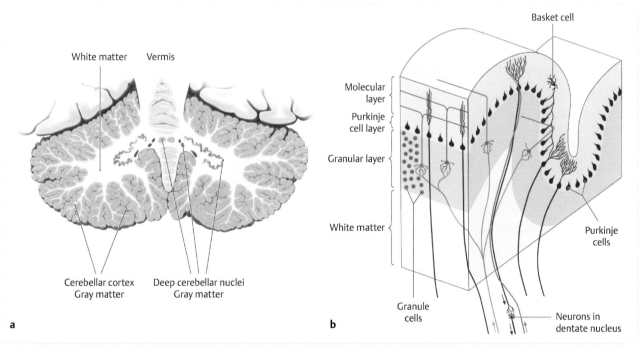

Fig. 2.20 (a,b) Derivatives of the cerebellum. **(a)** Section of the cerebellum through the superior cerebellar peduncles, viewed from behind. The vermis is flanked by two cerebellar hemispheres. Note the location of the gray matter comprising the outer cerebellar cortex and the four pairs of deep cerebellar nuclei that are embedded within the cerebellar white matter. The four deep cerebellar nuclei are noted by color, and the cortical regions have been color-coded to match the corresponding nuclei. (Fastigial nucleus: *green*; Emboliform nucleus: *blue*; Globose nuclei: *blue*; Dentate nucleus: *pink*.) **(b)** The cerebellar cortex consists of three layers: an outer molecular layer, a middle Purkinje layer, and an inner granular layer. Each layer contains different cell types and exhibits different connections which have been color-coded. (Granule cell: *blue*; Purkinje: *purple*; mossy fibers: *green*; climbing fibers: *pink*.) (Reproduced with permission from Schuenke M, Schulte E, Schumacher U. THIEME Atlas of Anatomy Second Edition, Vol 3. © Thieme 2016. Illustrations by Markus Voll and Karl Wesker.)

- ○ The alar plate and the roof plate contribute to the **tectum**, and differentiate into the sensory neurons of the **superior** and **inferior colliculi.**
- ○ The **mesencephalic nucleus of V** also develops from neurons in the alar plate and resides in the mesencephalon.
- The marginal zone of the mesencephalon enlarges to form the **cerebral peduncles (crus cerebri),** which contain the efferent fibers of the descending motor tracts passing from the cerebral cortex to the brainstem.

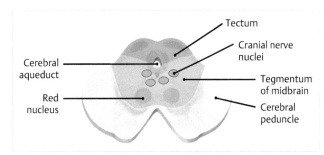

Fig. 2.21 Derivatives and structures of the mesencephalon (midbrain). A cross-section at the level of midbrain depicting the three key structural components: the tectum (roof), the tegmentum (floor), and the cerebral peduncles. The tectum lies dorsal to the cerebral aqueduct, the tegmentum, and the cerebral peduncles (crus cerebri). The neurons of the alar plate differentiate into the sensory nuclei associated with the inferior and superior colliculi of the tectum. The midbrain tegmentum contains the motor nuclei (*blue*) of CN III, and IV, the red nucleus, and the substantia nigra (not shown), which differentiated from neurons in the basal plate (not shown). The mesencephalic nucleus of V is also found in the tegmentum (not shown). The cerebral peduncles are found ventrally and contain the ascending and descending axonal tracts. (Reproduced with permission from Schuenke M, Schulte E, Schumacher U. THIEME Atlas of Anatomy Second Edition, Vol 3. © Thieme 2016. Illustrations by Markus Voll and Karl Wesker.)

2.4.4 Development and Derivatives of Prosencephalon (Forebrain) (▶ Fig. 2.22a–d)

- In comparison to the developing brainstem, forebrain (prosencephalon) development is modified to accommodate the formation of the cerebral cortex; thus, the basal plates of the prosencephalon regresses in size and the alar plates become prominent.
- In the fifth week the rostral portion of the prosencephalon expands to form the telencephalon while the caudal portion of prosencephalon forms the diencephalon.
- Rapid growth of the telencephalon results in medial displacement of the diencephalon, such that the diencephalon becomes situated below the telencephalon and above the brainstem (▶ Fig. 2.23a, b).
- The cranial nerve nuclei, **CN I** and **II**, develop as outgrowths from the prosencephalon.

Diencephalon (▶ Fig. 2.24a, b)

- During development, the third ventricle expands and divides the diencephalon vesicle into dorsal and ventral regions. The walls of the diencephalon differentiate into four regions:
- The **epithalamus** and **thalamus,** dorsally and the **subthalamus** and **hypothalamus,** ventrally.
  - ○ **Epithalamus** develops from the roof plate and the dorsal aspect of the diencephalon alar plate as the third ventricle expands.
    - The pineal gland, a small endocrine gland which regulates circadian rhythms, differentiates from the epithalamus.
    - The choroid plexus develops forms the roof of the third ventricle.

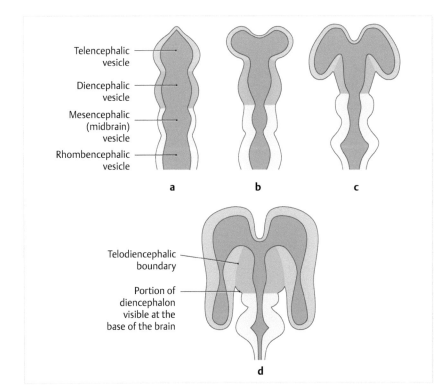

Fig. 2.22 (a–d) Development of the prosencephalon. During development, the two hemispheres of the telencephalon (*red*) expands and overgrows the diencephalon. This process shifts the boundary between the telencephalon and diencephalon until only a small area of the diencephalon can be seen at the base of the developed brain. The region of the forebrain develops in association with cranial nerve I and II. (Reproduced with permission from Schuenke M, Schulte E, Schumacher U. THIEME Atlas of Anatomy Second Edition, Vol 3. © Thieme 2016. Illustrations by Markus Voll and Karl Wesker.)

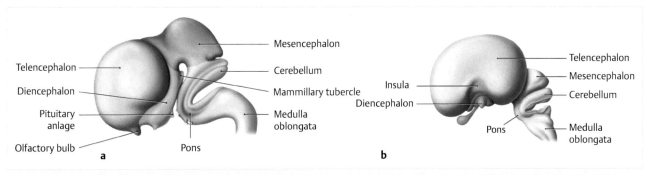

Telencephalon

Diencephalon

Pituitary anlage

Olfactory bulb

a

Mesencephalon

Cerebellum

Mammillary tubercle

Medulla oblongata

Pons

Insula

Diencephalon

Telencephalon

Mesencephalon

Cerebellum

Pons

Medulla oblongata

b

Fig. 2.23 **(a,b)** Development and growth of the telencephalon and diencephalon. **(a)** (*Lateral view; fetus end of second month prenatal development*). Early in development, the olfactory placode gives rise to the neurosensory cell of the olfactory nerve and induces the formation of the olfactory bulb from the floor of the telencephalon. A portion of the pituitary gland known as the posterior pituitary or neurohypophysis develops as an outgrowth from the floor of the diencephalon (pituitary anlage). The posterior lobe remains attached to the diencephalon via the infundibulum. The anterior lobe develops from Rathke pouch, a thickening of oral ectoderm (adenohypophyseal placode) that arises from the roof of the future oral cavity and fuses with the posterior lobe. **(b)** (*Lateral view; fetus approximately third month of prenatal development*). By this time, the telencephalon has begun to overgrow the other brain areas. The insula, shown on the surface, will become covered by the cerebral hemispheres. The optic nerve (CN II) develops as an outgrowth of the optic vesicles that develop from the diencephalon. (Reproduced with permission from Schuenke M, Schulte E, Schumacher U. THIEME Atlas of Anatomy Second Edition, Vol 1. © Thieme 2014. Illustrations by Markus Voll and Karl Wesker.)

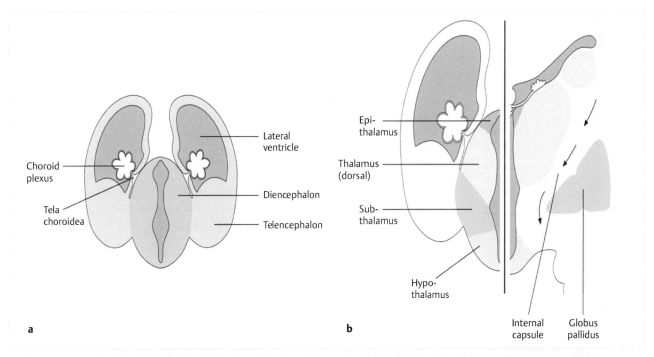

Choroid plexus

Tela choroidea

Lateral ventricle

Diencephalon

Telencephalon

a

Epi-thalamus

Thalamus (dorsal)

Sub-thalamus

Hypo-thalamus

Internal capsule

Globus pallidus

b

Fig. 2.24 Derivatives of the diencephalon. **(a)** (*Coronal section; the embryonic brain taken at the boundary between the telencephalon and the diencephalon*). The development of the telencephalon (*red*) has progressed. The lateral ventricles containing the choroid plexus have already completely overgrown the diencephalon (*blue*) from behind. The medial wall of the lateral ventricles is very thin and has not yet fused to the diencephalon. Between the telencephalon and diencephalon is a vascularized sheet of connective tissue, the tela choroidea, that contributes to the formation of the choroid plexus. The choroid plexus produces cerebrospinal fluid (CSF). **(b)** (*Coronal section showing half of the developing telencephalon and diencephalon [left] and the same structures in an adult brain [right]*). Note the lateral and third ventricles shown near the midline. The alar plate of the diencephalon differentiates into four regions: the epithalamus and thalamus develop dorsally, and the subthalamus and hypothalamus develop ventrally. A notable feature of the adult brain is the presence of the ascending and descending axonal tracts that form the internal capsule (*black arrows* show position-tracts run in both directions). The internal capsule is shown passing between the thalamus and the deep cortical gray matter (basal ganglia) of the telencephalon. The internal capsule forms the lateral boundary of the thalamus in the diencephalon. Fibers extending between the thalamus to the cortex represent the corticothalamic and thalamocortical fibers that interconnect the thalamus and cortex. The internal capsule also transmits fibers from the cortex to the brainstem, spinal cord, basal ganglia, and midbrain (not shown). The fibers in the internal capsule fan out in the cerebral cortex forming the corona radiata (not shown). (Reproduced with permission from Schuenke M, Schulte E, Schumacher U. THIEME Atlas of Anatomy Second Edition, Vol 3. © Thieme 2016. Illustrations by Markus Voll and Karl Wesker.)

- **Thalamus** develops from the alar plate into two symmetrical lobes of gray matter that contain groups of thalamic nuclei.
- Three types of thalamic nuclei differentiate from neuroblasts of the alar plate: **specific relay nuclei, association nuclei,** and **nonspecific, intralaminar nuclei.** Each of the thalamic nuclei connects to discrete regions of the cerebral cortex. **Hypothalamus** develops from the alar plate and floor plate and gives rise to:
    - The **hypothalamic nuclei** and **mammillary bodies** differentiate from the alar plate.
    - The **infundibulum** which gives rise to the **infundibular stalk** and **neurohypophysis** (posterior lobe of pituitary) develop as ventral outgrowth.
    - The neurohypophysis grows as downward extension from the diencephalon to fuse with adenohypophysis to form the **pituitary gland**.
- **Subthalamus** (**basal ganglia**) develops from the alar plate, ventral to thalamus and lateral to the hypothalamus. During development, the lateral part of the subthalamus becomes displaced into telencephalon to form the globus pallidus, a part of the basal ganglia (deep cerebral nuclei). The medial part of the subthalamus remains in the diencephalon.
- The **optic cup** develops from the diencephalon as an outgrowth, known as the **optic vesicle,** in the third week of embryonic development. The **optic cup** along with **lens placode** develops from surface ectoderm, and forms the eyes.
    - Optic vesicles arise from neuroepithelium and develop into the optic nerve (CN II), iris, ciliary bodies, and the retina.
    - Lens placodes develop from surface ectoderm and differentiate into the lens, and corneal epithelium.

Telencephalon (▶ Fig. 2.25a, b)

- The telencephalon develops as bilateral outgrowths of the lateral walls of the prosencephalon during the fifth week of embryonic development and gives rise to the right and left **cerebral hemispheres.**
    - Continued lateral expansion of each hemisphere leads to the bilateral growth of the four lobes, **frontal, parietal, occipital,** and **temporal lobes** in the 14th week of embryonic development.
    - Each hemisphere also gives rise to the **insula** (insular cortex), the **hippocampus** (hippocampal formation), the nuclei of the **limbic system**, and the **olfactory bulb**.
    - On the medial side of each hemisphere, the areas of the **hippocampus** and **insula,** become surrounded by the developing frontal, parietal, and temporal lobes and eventually, both regions become embedded, deep to the lateral fissure in the temporal lobe.
    - The **olfactory bulbs** (CNI), which are part of the olfactory system, develop as outgrowths on the ventral surface of the cerebrum. The olfactory bulbs provide direct input to the **olfactory cortex** via the **olfactory tracts**.
    - The insular cortex, hippocampal formation, and the olfactory cortex contribute to a group of anatomically interconnected nuclei and cortical structures known as the **limbic system.**
- Each cerebral hemisphere differentiates into an outer **cerebral cortex**, an inner region of **cerebral white matter,** and the **corpus striatum.** The cerebral hemispheres surround the lateral ventricles (▶ Fig. 2.26).
    - **Cerebral cortex:** The majority of the cortex is known as the **neocortex** and consists of an outer mantle layer of gray matter that develops as successive waves of neurons migrate from the ventricular layer into the outer marginal layer.
        - The pattern of neuronal migration results in the formation of six layers of interconnected neurons that form functional columns. Neurons within the cortical layers differentiate into two broad cellular groups: **pyramidal cells** (cortical projection neurons) and **granular cells** (interneurons). Each group contains

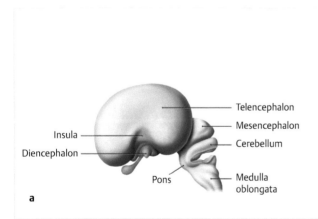
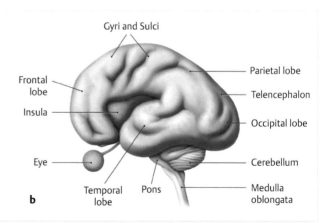

Fig. 2.25 Telencephalon development and growth of the cerebral hemispheres. **(a)** (*Lateral view; fetus third month of development*). The telencephalon develops as bilateral outgrowths of the prosencephalon and by the third month has expanded and overgrown other areas. The insula (insular cortex) is still visible on the surface but eventually becomes covered by the frontal, parietal, and temporal lobes as the cerebral hemisphere expand. **(b)** (*Lateral view; fetus approximately seventh month prenatal development*). Bilaterally, the four lobes of the cerebral hemispheres, the frontal, parietal, temporal, and occipital lobes, begin to develop by the 14th week. Due to the rapid growth of the cerebral cortex, the cortical surface folds into gyri (ridges) and sulci (grooves) and may be recognized by the eighth month. (Reproduced with permission from Schuenke M, Schulte E, Schumacher U. THIEME Atlas of Anatomy Second Edition, Vol 1. © Thieme 2014. Illustrations by Markus Voll and Karl Wesker.)

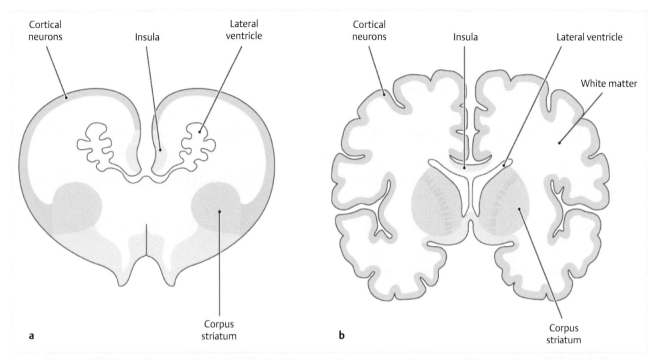

Fig. 2.26 (a,b) Derivatives of the telencephalon (cerebrum): **(a)** (*coronal section embryonic telencephalon*). The telencephalon differentiated into two cerebral hemispheres. Each cerebral hemisphere contains the cerebral cortex, cerebral white matter, basal nuclei, and the lateral ventricles. The majority of the cerebral cortex consists of an outer mantle layer of gray matter, which is also known as the neocortex and represents approximately 90% of the cortical mantle. **(b)** The insula (insular cortex) also develops from this region, but invaginates and lies deep to the frontal, parietal, and temporal lobes. The neurons of the cortical gray matter are interconnected into functional columns and distributed through six layers. The neocortex is involved in higher functions such as sensory perception, generation of motor commands, spatial reasoning, conscious thought, and in humans, language. The hippocampal formation and olfactory cortex, which are cortical components of the limbic system, also develop from the cerebral hemisphere; however, the two regions comprise the allocortex and exhibit a three-layered arrangement of cortical neurons. The hippocampal cortex lies medial to the external surface of the temporal lobe (not shown in view). The olfactory cortex develops on the ventral (inferior) surface of the frontal lobe association with olfactory nerve and bulb (not shown in view). The white matter lies internal to the outer cortical region. The corpus striatum, which represents a cluster of nuclei in the deep cortical gray matter, resides within the subcortical white matter. In the adult brain, the axonal fibers of the internal capsule pass through the corpus striatum. (Reproduced with permission from Schuenke M, Schulte E, Schumacher U. THIEME Atlas of Anatomy Second Edition, Vol 3. © Thieme 2016. Illustrations by Markus Voll and Karl Wesker.)

multiple cellular subtypes that are differentially distributed throughout the motor and sensory cortices and other cortical areas.

- Variation in the laminar organization of the neocortex exists in the region of the hippocampal formation and olfactory cortex. The developing neuroblasts in these regions become arranged into three to four neuronal cell layers and comprise the region known as the **allocortex** of the cerebral cortex.

○ **Cerebral white matter:** The white matter of cerebral hemispheres lies internal (subcortical) to the cerebral cortex and consists of three main groups of axonal fiber tracts: **association fiber tracts, commissural fiber tracts,** and **projection fiber tracts**.

- **Association fibers**, which include long (fasciculi) and short (cortical) fibers, connect cortical areas within a single hemisphere and allow the cortex to function in a coordinated manner.
- **Commissural fibers** connect the corresponding regions of the right and left hemispheres and include the corpus collosum, the anterior and posterior commissure, and fornix.

- **Projections fibers** connect the cerebral cortex to the thalamus, brainstem, and spinal cord as large ascending (afferent) and descending (efferent) tracts. Most of these ascending and descending fiber tracts pass through the **internal capsule.**
- The **internal capsule**, which develops as the cerebral hemispheres expand and fuse with diencephalon, represents a bilateral group of projection nerve fibers that connect the white matter of the cerebral hemispheres to the thalamus, midbrain, brainstem, and spinal cord. The internal capsule is continuous with the **corona radiata** above, and below, with the **cerebral peduncles (crus cerebri)** of the midbrain.
- In the adult, the fibers of the internal capsule comprise, an anterior limb, a genu (bend), and a posterior limb, that passes through the **corpus striatum**, a region of deep cortical gray matter embedded within the subcortical white matter.

○ **Corpus Striatum** (striate nucleus) refers to a group of **deep cerebral nuclei (subcortical nuclei)** that differentiate from neuroblasts originating near the ventricular zone and comprise nuclei of the mantle layer. The subcortical nuclei of the corpus striatum are also referred to as the **basal** ganglia of the forebrain, and include the **caudate nucleus, putamen, globus pallidus,** and **nucleus accumbens.**

- By the eighth month of fetal development, numerous grooves and ridges, known as **sulci** and **gyri**, respectively, develop due to rapid cortical surface growth. The extensive cortical folding occurs as a mechanism to accommodate increased surface area within the limited confines of the skull.

Clinical Correlation Box 2.5: Holoprosencephaly

Holoprosencephaly refers to a group of abnormalities associated with the malformations in the cerebral cortex and midline facial structures. It is often a lethal disorder caused by the failure of the telencephalon to divide into two cerebral hemispheres. Holoprosencephaly may vary in severity. In the least severe case the cerebral cortex has divided; however, there are midline facial abnormalities involving the nose, eyes, and palate which result from abnormal signaling between the brain and developing facial structures.

Questions and Answers

1. Failure of neural crest cells to migrate into the developing craniofacial region cause dysgenesis of each of the following structures EXCEPT one. Which one is the exception?
   a) Maxilla
   b) Thymus
   c) Parathyroid
   d) Enteric ganglia

Level 2: Moderate

Answer D: Neural crest cells migrate to three regions: the body (trunk), cardiac region, and craniofacial region. The enteric ganglion cells are neural crest-derived; however, they are not derived from cranial neural crest cells. Enteric ganglia are autonomic neurons found in the gut and differentiate from neural crest cells migrating into the trunk. The cells that migrate into the craniofacial region give rise to ectomesenchyme that forms the connective tissue/skeletal elements of the head and neck. The absence of neural crest cell migration and ectomesenchyme formation will lead to a failure of the bone of the maxilla (**A**) and the computed tomography (CT) that supports the thymus (**B**) and (**C**) parathyroid gland to develop correctly. The CT of thymus and parathyroid is required for the differentiation of the parenchymal epithelial cells to differentiate.

2. During a routine ultrasound, an expectant mother is told that her child has anencephaly and the child may not survive. You explain to your patient that this congenital defect resulted from a failure of which of the following events to occur?
   a) Anterior neuropore to close
   b) Neural crest cells to migrate
   c) Telencephalon to divide
   d) Corpus callosum to differentiate

Level 2: Moderate

Answer A: The failure of the anterior neuropores to close gives rise to anencephaly which is characterized by the absence of the brain and skull to form properly. Closure of the anterior neuropore occurs at the end of the fourth week before neural crest cell migration (**B**) and is necessary for the rostral (cranial) portion of the neural tube to develop. Failure of the cranial (rostral) portion of the neural tube to develop would impact the subsequent development of the forebrain and its developmental derivatives the (**C**) telencephalon and (**D**) corpus callosum to differentiate.

3. Which of the following events occurs as an outcome of notochord signaling during the development of the nervous system?
   a) Induction of ectoderm to form the neural plate
   b) Migration of neural crest cells from the neural plate
   c) Formation of the sulcus limitans
   d) Expansion of the neural canal to form ventricles

Level 1: Easy

Answer A: The notochord plays an integral role in the development of the neural tube by signaling to the ectoderm to form the neural plate. The migration of neural crest cells (**B**) occurs as the result of signaling from the neural tube. The formation of sulcus limitans (**C**) and the formation of the ventricular system (**D**) occur later in development and does not involve notochord signaling.

4. Each of the following develop from the alar plate of the diencephalon EXCEPT one. Which one is the exception?
   a) Pineal gland
   b) Hypothalamus
   c) Neurohypophysis
   d) Hippocampus

Level 1: Easy

Answer D: The hippocampus which is part of the limbic system develops along the medial aspect of the temporal lobe during the differentiation of the telencephalon. The remaining choices Pineal gland (**A**), hypothalamus (**B**), and neurohypophysis (**C**) are all derived from the alar plate of the diencephalon.

5. A magnetic resonance imaging (MRI) of a newborn reveals the cerebral hemispheres exhibit small irregular gyri (microgyri) due to abnormal neuronal migration. Which of the following cells aids in proper neuronal migration?
   a) Oligodendrocytes
   b) Astrocytes
   c) Radial glial cells
   d) Microglia cells

Level 2: Moderate

Answer C: Radial glial cells are a transient cell population present during the histogenesis of the neural tube and are one of the first cells to differentiate during neuroepithelial cell differentiation. Radial glial cells provide scaffolding that aids in neuronal migration. After development, most radial glia cells disappear. Failure of radial glial cells to differentiate will impact neurogenesis and neuronal migration and lead to abnormalities in the cortical gyri and sulci development; a process that is dependent on proper neuronal migration. Oligodendrocytes (**A**) myelinate axons within the CNS. Astrocytes (**B**) function in maintaining the ionic environment, and microglial cells (**D**) have phagocytic function.

3 Neurohistology

1. Describe the histological features of a neuron and relate the structure to its primary function.
2. Describe the primary function of myelin, microglial cells, and ependymal cells.
3. Explain the different types of neurons, their location, and general overview of their function.
4. Compare the different types of neuroglial cells, their location, and their function.
5. Compare the organization of white matter in the spinal cord to that of cerebral cortex.
6. Describe the organization of the cerebellar cortex.
7. Describe the histological organization of the superficial gray matter in the cerebral cortex.
8. Compare the central (CNS) and peripheral nervous system (PNS) and include the names given to a collection of nerve cell bodies; groups of nerve fibers; types of supporting cells present in each region.
9. Describe the components of a peripheral nerve and the organization of the connective tissue investing the peripheral nerve.

3.1 Classification of Cells of the Nervous System

3.1.1 Introduction

- Early in embryonic development, neuroectoderm and neural crest cells give rise to neuroepithelial stem cells of the CNS and PNS, respectively. The neuroepithelial stem cells differentiate into neuroblasts and glioblasts, which eventually give rise to two principal cell types: **nerve cells (neurons)** and **neuroglial (glial** or **glia) cells** (▶ Fig. 3.1).
- Neurons and glial cells are both found in the CNS and PNS.
  - Neurons serve as the structural and functional link between the nervous system and body. Neurons rapidly transmit information as electrical impulses and convey that information to other neurons and effector cells at specific points of contact called **synapses**.
  - Neuroglial (glial) cells are specialized non-neuronal supportive cells that provide structural integrity and the metabolic support necessary for neuronal development and function.

3.2 Neurons

3.2.1 Structural Components of Neurons

- Neurons exhibit considerable variation in shape and size; however, each neuron consists of a **cell body** and a variable number of **neurites** or **cell processes** that extend from the cell body. The cell processes are designated as **dendrites** and **axons.**

- The structural components of neurons are comparable to other cells in the body; however, neurons exhibit a regional distribution of cytoskeletal proteins and organelles between the **neuron cell body**, the **dendrites,** and the **axon** (▶ Table 3.1 and ▶ Table 3.2) (▶ Fig. 3.2, ▶ Fig. 3.3, ▶ Fig. 3.4).

3.2.2 Myelination of Axon

- Two types of neuroglial cells, **oligodendrocytes**, and **Schwann cells,** found in the CNS and PNS, respectively, surround each axon and form a protective sheath (▶ Fig. 3.5).
  - In myelinated axons, oligodendrocytes and Schwann cells deposit a lipid layer, known as myelin around the axons.
  - Myelin increases the propagation speed of the electrical impulse. The myelin sheath surrounding an axon is discontinuous, containing small gaps along the length of the axon which are devoid of myelin. These regions, called nodes of Ranvier, contain Na + ion channels and serve as sites of axonal membrane depolarization. Nodes of Ranvier permit the rapid spread of a nerve impulse to move from one node to the next through the process of **saltatory conduction**.
  - In unmyelinated axons of peripheral nerves, the plasma membrane of the neuroglial cell invests the axon as a single layer, and the nerve impulse propagates at a slower rate through continuous conduction.

The speed at which a nerve impulse may be transmitted is dependent on the myelin sheath surrounding axons in the CNS and PNS. Oligodendrocytes and Schwann cells are responsible for myelination of axons in the CNS and PNS, respectively. Demyelination of axons occurs in Multiple Sclerosis and Guillain-Barre syndrome, leading to somatic and autonomic deficits. Symptoms may manifest as weakness, numbness, and tingling, GI disturbances, cardiac arrhythmia, or ventilation problems.

- **Multiple sclerosis** is an inflammatory condition restricted to the **CNS** and is characterized by the production of autoantibodies directed against proteins in the myelin sheath. Destruction of the myelin sheath leads to scar formation in the areas of myelin damage and progressive axonal degeneration.
- In comparison, **Guillain-Barre syndrome** is associated with acute inflammatory processes in the PNS, leading to the demyelination of peripheral nerve fibers and root, with little damage to the underlying axon.

3.2.3 Axonal Transport

- **Axonal transport** is the process through which metabolic byproducts and organelles of the neuron may pass between the soma and the terminal end of the axon. The mechanism of axonal transport is essential for neuronal survival, synaptic transmission, regeneration, and neurite outgrowth (▶ Fig. 3.6).

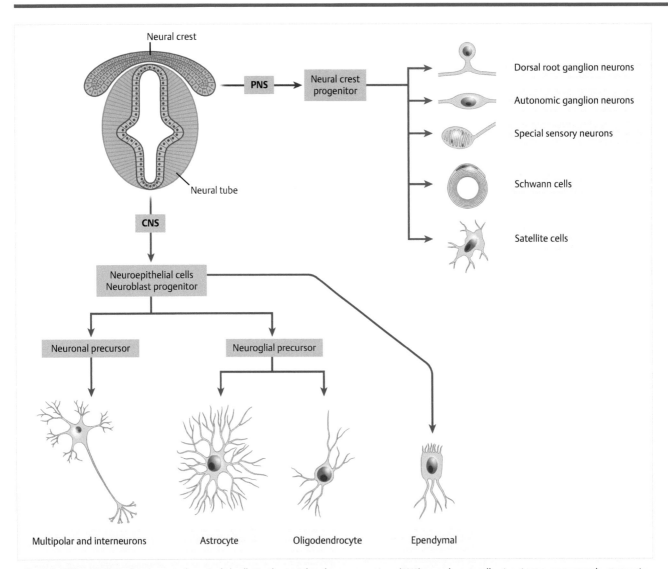

Fig. 3.1 Differentiation of neurons and neuroglial cells. In the peripheral nervous system (PNS) neural crest cells give rise to sensory and autonomic neurons and supportive neuroglial cells. In the central nervous system (CNS) neurons and neuroglial cells differentiate from the neural tube.

Table 3.1 Overview of neuron structure

Neuron cell body: nucleus and cytoplasm	
Structure and notable features	**Function**
Nucleus • Centrally located within neuron cell body • Euchromatic (light-stained) appearance indicative of high transcription **Nucleolus** Prominent, centrally located within nucleus	• Site of gene transcription • Site of ribosomal RNA synthesis
Cytoplasm (perikaryon) • Nissl substance (rER)	• Ribosomes and aggregates of rough endoplasmic reticulum synthesize proteins • Amount of Nissl substance correlates with the high levels of protein synthesis occurring in the neuron • Dispersed throughout the cell EXCEPT axon
• Residual bodies (lysosomes)	• Lysosomes are small cytoplasmic membrane-bound vesicles that serve as scavengers and degrade waste products • Accumulate in long-lived cells (i.e., neurons)
• Cytoskeleton (three types): • Microtubules • Microfilaments • Intermediate filaments (neurofilaments)	• Necessary for axonal transport of organelles, proteins, and synaptic vesicles • Important in neuronal pathfinding and neurite outgrowth following nerve fiber damage • Aid in maintaining axonal diameter and length

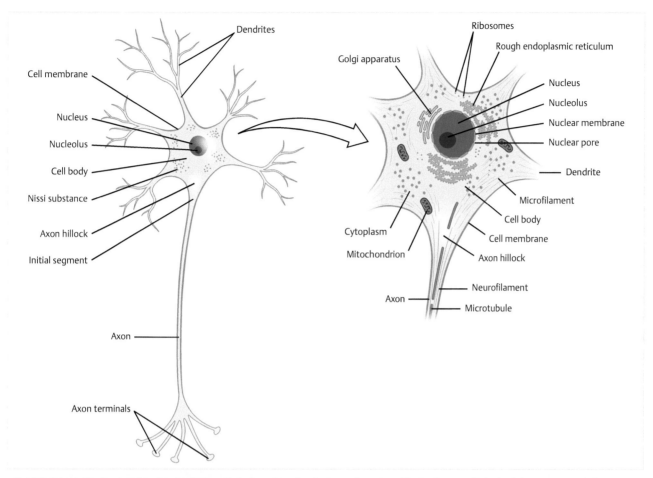

Fig. 3.2 Schematic showing the structural organelles of a neuron by electron microscopy. The nucleus, nucleolus, golgi apparatus, rough endoplasmic reticulum, mitochondria, along with microtubules and microfilaments, which are also known as neurofibrils, are depicted. The normal histological features of a neuron and the distribution of the cellular structural components may change with age and disease.

Table 3.2 Overview of neuron structure

Neurites: nerve cell processes	
Structure and notable features	**Function**
Dendrite: • Each neuron may contain one or more dendrites • Always unmyelinated (bare) cell processes • Variable length—usually short (millimeters) • Terminal ends exhibit a simple to complex branching (arborization) and serve as points of synaptic contact • May contain dendritic spines at synaptic ends to increase surface area	Receives, integrates, and transmits electrical signals from other neurons toward the cell body
Axons: • Only one axon per neuron • Myelinated or unmyelinated cell process Extent of myelination impacts speed of signal conduction • Variable length—can be very long (meters) • Exhibit branching with axon collaterals	Generates and transmits electrical impulses (action potentials) away from the cell body toward other cellular targets
Parts of Axon • Axon Hillock	• Site of origin of axon from neuron cell body • Area is unmyelinated and characteristically devoid of Nissl substance
• Initial segment	• Region distal to axon hillock • Serves as site of initiation for an action potential due to high density of voltage-gated Na + channels
• Synaptic terminal (terminal bouton)	• Dilated portion of the terminal part of an axon • Contain synaptic (endocytotic) vesicles, which store neurotransmitters (chemical mediators) • Serves as the contact point between the neuron and target cell • Loss of synaptic contact between axon and target may lead to neuronal degeneration

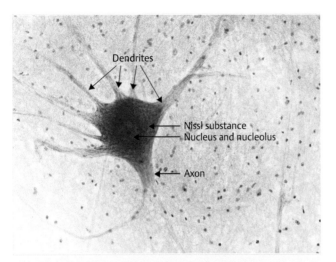

Fig. 3.3 Light microscopy of a multipolar (motor) neuron (40 × magnification; hematoxylin and eosin [H/E] stain). Note the centrally placed nucleus, prominent nucleolus, and abundant rough endoplasmic reticulum (Nissl substance). These structural features are characteristic features associated with cells undergoing active protein synthesis. Neurons exhibit polarity based on the flow of electrical signals along their membrane. Signals are received at the dendrites, passed along the cell body, and propagated along the axon toward the target.

- Microtubules in association with other motor proteins facilitate the translocation of intracellular material along the length of the axon.
- Transport occurs bidirectionally, at a fast or slow rate, depending on the product transported.
- Axonal transport away from the cell body toward the axon terminal is termed **anterograde**, while transport from the axon terminal toward the cell body is called **retrograde**.
- Types of axonal transport include the following:
  - **Fast anterograde axonal transport** typically involves the movement of endocytic vesicles containing substances that have a functional role at the axon terminus. The enzymes, proteins, and macromolecules necessary for neurotransmitter release from the synaptic terminal utilize this transport mechanism.
  - **Slow anterograde axonal transport** involves the movement of soluble cytoplasmic substances, motor proteins, and cytoskeletal proteins which are necessary for proper synaptic transmission. Slow axonal transport of cytoskeletal proteins is essential for axonal outgrowth during development and axonal regeneration following injury.
  - **Fast retrograde axonal transport** may involve the passage of exogenous soluble (trophic) growth factors from the axon terminal, or the transport of worn-out synaptic membrane vesicles to be carried toward the cell body for degradation or recycling. Viruses and neurotoxins may infect axon terminals of peripheral nerves and pass to cell bodies by retrograde transport.

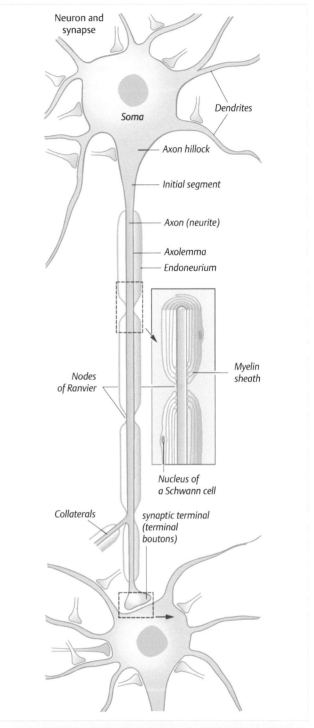

Fig. 3.4 Schematic of a neuron cell body and nerve cell processes (neurites). Neurons may contain one or more unmyelinated dendrites that function to receive, integrate, and transmit an electrical signal toward the neuron cell body. Each neuron contains only one axon which may be myelinated or unmyelinated and functions to generate and transmit action potentials away from the neuron cell body. The axon hillock represents the site of origin of the axon from the cell body. The unmyelinated initial segment of the axon lies just distal to the hillock and represents an area of high Na + channel density and the point of initiation for an action potential. The distal part of the axon exhibits branching into several collateral axons that end as specialized presynaptic terminals known as terminal boutons. (Modified with permission from Silbernagl S, Despopoulos A. Color Atlas of Physiology. Sixth Edition. © Thieme 2009.)

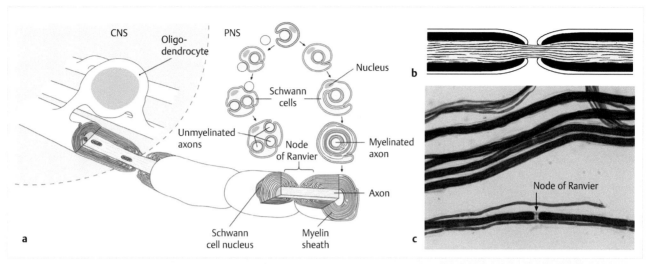

Fig. 3.5 **(a)** Schematic of cells responsible for axon myelination in the central nervous system (CNS) and peripheral nervous system (PNS). Neuroglial cells deposit a lipid sheath, known as myelin around axons. In the CNS the oligodendrocytes, a type of neuroglial cell, myelinates multiple sections known as an internodal segment on multiple axons. The ability of a single cell to myelinate more than one axon helps to conserve space within the CNS. In the PNS, the neuroglial Schwann cell myelinates one internodal segment of a single axon. **(b)** Schematic image and **(c)** light microscopy demonstrating a node of Ranvier in a myelinated axon (40 × magnification; Osmium stain). Small gaps in the myelin sheath, known as nodes of Ranvier, contain exposed Na + ion channels and serve as sites for membrane depolarization. Myelin insulates the axon, increasing the electrical resistance of the membrane, and prevents decay of the action potential. Nodes of Ranvier increase the conduction speed by permitting the action potential to "jump" rapidly from one node to the next through the process of saltatory conduction. (▶ Fig. 3.5a: Reproduced with permission from Schuenke M, Schulte E, Schumacher U. THIEME Atlas of Anatomy Third Edition, Vol 3. © Thieme 2020. Illustrations by Markus Voll and Karl Wesker. ▶ Fig. 3.5b: Reproduced with permission from Kahle W, Frotscher M. Color Atlas of Human Anatomy. Sixth Edition, Vol 3. © Thieme 2011.)

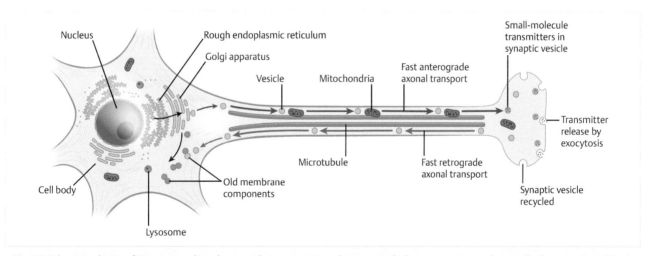

Fig. 3.6 Schematic showing fast anterograde and retrograde transport. Axonal transport which moves proteins and organelles between the cell body and axon terminal is essential for neuronal survival, synaptic transmission, and regeneration.

3.2.4 Neuronal Communication: Synapses (▶ Fig. 3.7)

- Neurons are excitable, polarized cells that receive and transmit electrochemical signals in one direction. The signal received by the dendrite passes to the cell body, and then to the terminal part to the axon where transmission of the impulse to another cell occurs.
- At the terminal end of the axon, the electrical impulse initiates **synaptic transmission**, which serves as the

mechanism of communication between a neuron and its cellular target.
- Neurotransmission, which occurs at specialized points of contact called **synapses**, may be classified as **electrical** or **chemical** based on the mechanism of signal transduction (▶ Fig. 3.7) (▶ Table 3.3).
  ○ In **electrical synapses**, two neurons are physically and electrically coupled by small intercellular channels, called **gap junctions**. Gap junctions provide low electrical resistance and allow for the rapid propagation of an action

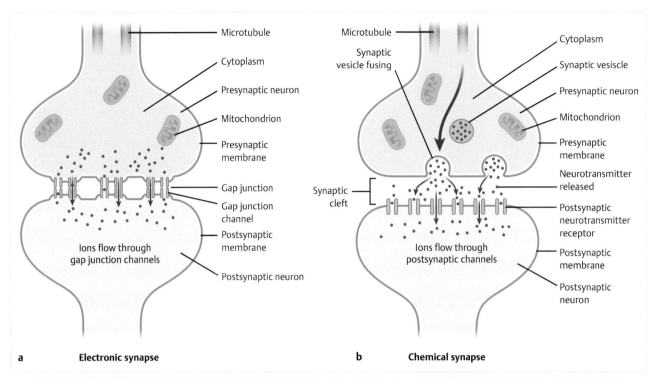

a   **Electronic synapse**   **b**   **Chemical synapse**

Fig. 3.7 (a,b) Schematic illustration of electrical (**a**) and chemical (**b**) synapses. Synapses are sites of functional contact between two neurons, a neuron and an effector cell, or a neuron and a sensory receptor. Synapses may be excitatory or inhibitory and consist of a presynaptic membrane, synaptic cleft, and a postsynaptic membrane. Electrical synapses (**a**) consist of a physical and electrical coupling of two neurons together by gap junctions. The gap junction allows ions to flow bidirectionally between cells. Chemical synapses (**b**) are unidirectional and use neurotransmitters released from the presynaptic terminal to bind to the receptors on the postsynaptic membrane and creates either an excitatory membrane depolarization (EPSP) or inhibitory (IPSP) hyperpolarization of the postsynaptic membrane. EPSP increases the potential of generating an action potential by the postsynaptic neuron, whereas an IPSP decreases the chance of the postsynaptic neuron firing.

Table 3.3 Overview of sites of synaptic neurotransmission

Points of synaptic contact	Type of contact
Between neurons in the central nervous system	Chemical or electrical
Motor neurons and skeletal muscle fiber (Neuromuscular junction)	Chemical
Preganglionic autonomic fibers and postganglionic cell body	Chemical
Postganglionic autonomic fiber and effector organ	Chemical

Note: Synapses do not occur in the dorsal root ganglia or cranial sensory ganglia.

potential to pass directly from the presynaptic neuron to a postsynaptic neuron.

○ In **chemical neurotransmission**, a small intercellular space, or **synaptic cleft** separates the presynaptic neuron and postsynaptic target. Chemical synapses involve the release of a chemical mediator, called a **neurotransmitter** from the **presynaptic terminal** of the neuron. The neurotransmitter diffuses across the synaptic cleft and

then binds to specific receptors located on the **postsynaptic membrane**.

– Points of synaptic contact vary, but **axodendritic synapses**, which occur between a presynaptic axon terminating on a postsynaptic dendrite, are most common (▶ Fig. 3.8).

– A detailed description of neurotransmission is covered in Chapter 4.

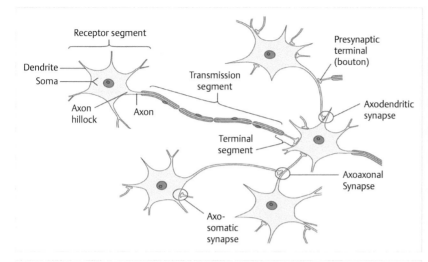

Fig. 3.8 Schematic showing points of synaptic contact. Synapses may be classified by the site of synaptic contact. Synaptic contact occurs most often between a presynaptic axon and a postsynaptic dendrite. Other points of synaptic contact may occur between two axons (axon-axonal) or between the axon and neuron cell body (axosomatic). (Reproduced with permission from Gilroy AM, MacPherson BR. Atlas of Anatomy. Third Edition. © Thieme 2016. Illustrations by Markus Voll and Karl Wesker.)

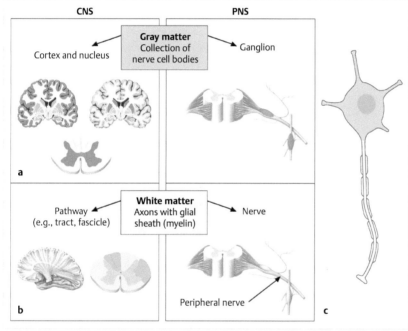

Fig. 3.9 Location of neuron cell bodies and nerve fibers in the central nervous system (CNS) and peripheral nervous system (PNS). The regions containing neuron cell bodies (*pink*) and axons (*green*) in the CNS are analogous to structures in the PNS. In the CNS, groups of functionally related neuron cell bodies form nuclei and reside in the gray matter (*pink*) of the brain and spinal cord (**a**). Clusters of myelinated axons form tracts (*green*) and reside within the white matter of the CNS (**b**). In the PNS, groups of neuron cell bodies form ganglia (*pink*) (**c**), whereas groups of axons are referred to as peripheral nerves. (Reproduced with permission from Schuenke M, Schulte E, Schumacher U. THIEME Atlas of Anatomy Second Edition, Vol 3. © Thieme 2016. Illustrations by Markus Voll and Karl Wesker.)

Clinical Correlation Box 3.2: Alzheimer Disease due to Synaptic Damage

Alzheimer disease is the most common form of senile dementia and is characterized by progressive memory loss that results from synaptic damage, degeneration of nerve processes, plaque formation within the cerebral cortex, and the accumulation of neurofibrillary tangles associated with neuronal cell death.

- Plaques represent abnormal build-up of clusters of β-amyloid proteins between synaptic terminals which may disrupt synaptic signaling and lead to degeneration of nerve processes. Plaques form as nerve processes degenerate at presynaptic terminals and become wrapped with aggregations of β-amyloid proteins. Neurofibrillary tangles develop from the improper folding of the microtubule associated protein, Tau. Defects in Tau protein synthesis lead to disruption in axonal transport, neuronal cell death, and the extracellular accumulation of Tau as neurofibrillary tangles.

3.2.5 Organization of Neurons in the CNS and PNS (▶ Fig. 3.9a–d)

- Neurons reside in both the CNS and PNS as functional groups of cells bodies; however, the arrangement between the two regions varies and is described below (▶ Table 3.4).

3.2.6 Central Nervous System (▶ Fig. 3.9a, b)

- In the CNS, the cell bodies of neurons and dendrites reside the gray matter and may be organized in **laminae (layers/sheets)** or aggregate to form functionally associated groups of cell bodies known as **nuclei** (▶ Fig. 3.9a).
- The axons extending from the cell bodies may be myelinated or unmyelinated and form functionally related bundles of fibers called **tracts** or **fasciculi** which pass through the white matter of CNS. Tracts are usually named and connect nuclei

Table 3.4 Summary of neurons and axons in CNS and PNS

Structural term	Location	
	CNS	PNS
Group of neuron cell bodies	Nuclei	Ganglia
Group of Axons	Tract (named)	Peripheral nerve (named)

Abbreviations: CNS, central nervous system; PNS, peripheral nervous system.

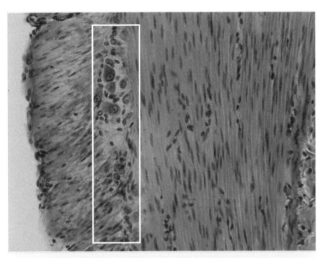

Fig. 3.10 Light microscopy demonstrating visceral motor neuron cell bodies in an autonomic ganglion. Wall of the ileum (20 × magnification; hematoxylin and eosin [H/E] stain). Autonomic ganglia associated with the peripheral nervous system (PNS) may be found near an organ or within the wall (intramural) of visceral organs. Autonomic neuron cell bodies are part of two neuron relay chain. One cell body resides in nuclei of the central nervous system (CNS) and the second cell body is found in the PNS. The autonomic nervous system, which includes the parasympathetic and sympathetic systems, consists of neuron cell bodies and axons. Neuron cell bodies shown in this image appear as large, pink cells. The nucleus and nucleolus are visible.

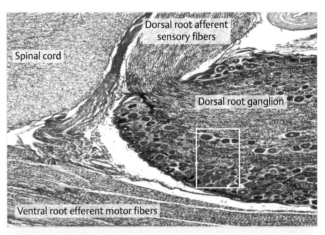

Fig. 3.11 Light microscopy demonstrating sensory neuron cell bodies in the dorsal root (spinal) ganglion. (4 × magnification; silver stain of dorsal root ganglion and spinal cord). Sensory cell bodies appear as large round cells with a centrally placed nucleus. Sensory nerve fibers are shown passing through ganglion and continue as dorsal root afferent fibers. The dorsal root ganglion and sensory (afferent) nerve fibers are in the peripheral nervous system (PNS). The afferent fibers convey sensory information toward the central nervous system (CNS). Nerve fibers carrying motor (efferent) impulses from the CNS are shown passing through the ventral root toward peripheral targets.

between different regions of the brain and spinal cord (▶ Fig. 3.9b).

3.2.7 Peripheral Nervous System (▶ Fig. 3.9c, d)

- In the PNS, aggregations of functionally related neuronal cell bodies lie outside the CNS and form encapsulated structures known as **ganglia** (▶ Fig. 3.9c). Ganglia are associated with the autonomic nervous system, the dorsal roots of the spinal nerves, and some of the sensory cranial nerves (CN V, VII, VIII, IX, and X) (▶ Fig. 3.10, ▶ Fig. 3.11).
- The axons or nerve fibers found in the PNS represent cranial and spinal nerve fibers. The axons form bundles of functionally related fibers known as **peripheral nerves** (▶ Fig. 3.9d).

- Each peripheral nerve is enveloped in three layers of connective tissue which provide structural and vascular support (▶ Fig. 3.12a, b).
- The connective tissue layers, arranged from deep to superficial, include the: **endoneurium, perineurium,** and **epineurium**.
  - **Endoneurium** is an inner layer of loose connective, which invests each axon, and serves as an important component in axonal regeneration following injury.
  - **Perineurium** forms the middle layer of connective tissue, which bundles groups of axons together as **fascicles.**
  - **Epineurium** consists of an outer layer of dense connective tissue that encircles the entire group of fascicles and forms the external covering of the peripheral nerve fiber bundle.
- Peripheral nerves are named and functionally classified as **mixed, motor (efferent),** or **sensory (afferent)** based on the type of nerve fiber carried in the peripheral nerve.
- Mixed nerves contain both motor and sensory axons, while efferent and afferent nerves carry only motor or sensory fibers, respectively.

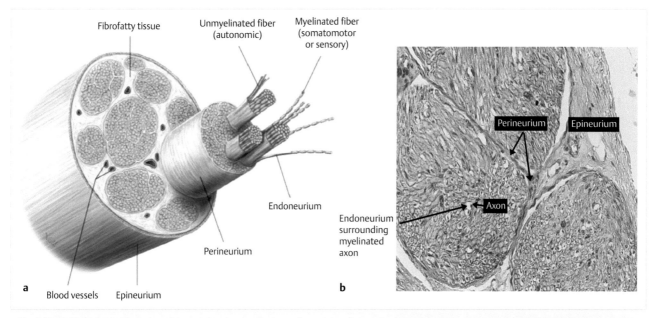

Fig. 3.12 Structural components and connective tissue coverings of a peripheral nerve in the peripheral nervous system (PNS). **(a)** Schematic of peripheral nerve in cross-section. Peripheral nerves represent cranial or spinal nerves that carry sensory, motor, or autonomic input. Nerve fibers may be classified by function, fiber diameter, the extent of myelination, and conduction speed. Spinal nerves are functionally classified as mixed nerves that carry both motor (efferent) and sensory (afferent) fibers. In comparison, some cranial nerves may be classified as mixed nerves, or only as sensory, or only motor. **(b)** Light microscopy demonstrating the connective tissue layers surrounding a peripheral nerve (20 × magnification; hematoxylin and eosin [H/E] stain). Peripheral nerves consist of bundles of myelinated or unmyelinated axons enveloped with three layers of connective tissue (CT). The CT layers arranged from superficial to deep, include an endoneurium, perineurium, and epineurium. The individual axons in the section shown appear as small *pink* circles surrounded by the myelin sheath (*white*). The endoneurium surrounds each axon, and is important in axonal regeneration following nerve damage. The middle layer of CT, known as the perineurium, bundles groups of individual axons together to form fascicles. The outer CT layer is the epineurium which bundles nerve fascicles together. (▶ Fig. 3.12a: Reproduced with permission from Schuenke M, Schulte E, Schumacher U. THIEME Atlas of Anatomy Second Edition, Vol 1. © Thieme 2014. Illustrations by Markus Voll and Karl Wesker.)

- All spinal nerves as they emerge from the vertebral column are classified as **mixed nerves** and carry both motor (efferent) and sensory (afferent) fibers. In comparison, some cranial nerves may be mixed nerves, while others may carry only afferent (sensory) fibers or only efferent (motor) fibers.
  - **Afferent fibers** of spinal or cranial nerves convey sensory information from peripheral receptors *toward* the CNS. The neuronal cell bodies for these afferent (sensory) fibers are in sensory ganglia located in the PNS.
  - **Efferent fibers** transmit motor impulses *away* from the CNS to peripheral effectors such as muscle or glands. The cell bodies of efferent (motor) fibers reside in either the spinal cord or as cranial motor nuclei within the brainstem of the CNS. Additionally, some efferent (motor) cell bodies associated with the autonomic nervous system lie in autonomic ganglia.

3.2.8 Classification of Nerve Fibers (▶ Table 3.5 and ▶ Table 3.6)

- Individual peripheral afferent and efferent nerve fibers vary in axonal diameter and the extent of myelination. These morphological differences correlate with the speed of transmission (**conduction velocity**) and serve as the basis for nerve fiber classification.

- In general, an increase in the cross-sectional diameter of the axon, which is proportional to conduction velocity will increase the speed of impulse transmission.
- Peripheral nerve fibers classified by **conduction velocity** are designated as **Type A, B,** and **C**. Type A and B are both myelinated, while C fibers are unmyelinated. Type A and C groups may contain motor or sensory fibers. The type A group, which exhibits the fastest conduction speed, is further subdivided as **Aα, Aβ, Aγ,** and **Aδ**, based on the type of information transmitted (▶ Table 3.5).
  - Aα and Aγ fibers carry somatic efferent (GSE) information, while B fibers and some C-fibers convey visceral efferent (GVE) information associated with the autonomic system.
  - Aβ, Aδ, and some C-fibers transmit somatic (GSA) and visceral (GVA) afferent input from the peripheral receptors.
- An alternative classification scheme based on **axonal diameter** categorizes afferent nerve fibers numerically, in descending order, **as groups I, II, III,** or **IV**. In this system group I, II, and III fibers are myelinated. Unmyelinated fibers which exhibit the smallest axonal diameter are group IV (▶ Table 3.6).
- Given the correlation between conduction velocity and axonal diameter, there is considerable overlap in the nomenclature of nerve classification. (Nerve fibers, as indicated in ▶ Table 3.5 and ▶ Table 3.6, may also be functionally classified.)

Table 3.5 Classification of peripheral motor (efferent) axons

Fiber classification Motor axon	Conduction velocity (m/s)	Diameter (µm)	Nerve type Motor axon	Terminal location	Function
Aα (alpha) fiber	Fast 15–120	Large 12–20	Myelinated Somatic efferents	Extrafusal fibers of skeletal muscle *Fibers of α motor neurons	Skeletal muscle contraction
Aγ (gamma) fiber	Medium 10–50	Medium 2–10	Lightly myelinated somatic efferent	Muscle spindle of intrafusal fiber *Fibers of γ motor neurons	Contraction of muscle stimulates intrafusal muscle spindles
B fiber	Slow 3–15	Small <3	Lightly myelinated Visceral efferents	Preganglionic autonomic fibers	Synapse on ganglia
C fiber	Slowest 0.5–2	Small <1	Unmyelinated Visceral efferents	Postganglionic autonomic fibers	• Smooth muscle contraction • glandular secretion Modulate cardiac contraction

Table 3.6 Classification of peripheral sensory (afferent) axons

Fiber classification Sensory axon	Conduction velocity (m/s)	Diameter (µm)	Nerve type Sensory axon	Terminal location (receptor)	Sensory function
Type I (Ia) (Aα) (alpha)	Fast 70–120	Large 12–20	Myelinated Somatic afferent fiber	Muscle spindle Intrafusal fibers skeletal muscle	Proprioceptive (Position and movement) Muscle stretch
Type I (Ib) (Aα) (alpha)	Fast 70–120	Large 12–20	Myelinated Somatic afferent fiber	Golgi tendon organ Myotendinous junction	Proprioceptive (Position and movement) Muscle tension
Type II (Aβ) (beta)	Medium 10–50	Medium 2–10	Myelinated Somatic afferent fiber	Skin Mucosa Ligaments Muscle Joints Viscera	Tactile Discriminative (2pt) Vibration Stretch Pressure Stereognosis
Type III (Aδ) (delta)	Slow 3–15	Small <3	Lightly myelinated • Somatic afferent fibers • Visceral afferents fibers	Free nerve ending Ubiquitous	Fast, sharp pain Temperature (cold) Pressure (mechanical) Crude touch
Type IV C-fiber	Slowest 0.5–2	Small <1	Unmyelinated • Somatic afferent fibers • Visceral afferents	Free nerve ending Ubiquitous	Slow, dull pain Temperature (warm) Pressure/pinch

Clinical Correlation Box 3.3: Neuronal Injury, Axonal Degeneration, and Regeneration

- Nerve injuries can occur in both the PNS and CNS with variable outcomes and lead to damage to the neuronal cell body and nerve fibers. Damage can occur from **ischemia** (decrease blood supply) or trauma, such as compressions injuries, nerve entrapment, avulsion, stretching, cutting of the nerve fibers, or by degenerative nerve diseases (neuropathies).
- The severity of the injury to the nerve fiber and the proximity of the damage to the cell body impact neuronal cell survival and axonal regeneration. In response to nerve injuries, several characteristic changes may occur in the cell body and axon in the regions proximal and distal to the site of injury.
  - **Changes proximal to the injury** may include degeneration of the proximal portion of the axon, in a process known as **retrograde axonal degeneration**. At the point of injury, degeneration begins to spread retrograde, toward the cell body. If the damage occurs close to the cell body, the process of chromatolysis occurs and may lead to neuronal cell death. **Chromatolysis** histologically appears as swelling of the cell body, peripheral displacement of the nucleus, and the disappearance of Nissl substance. Neuronal cell death may occur in the CNS and PNS and is irreparable.
  - **Changes distal to the site of injury** involve axonal fragmentation, degenerations, and phagocytosis axonal debris by microglial cells or macrophages. The process of axonal degeneration occurring distal to nerve injury is known as **anterograde axonal degeneration** or **Wallerian degeneration**. Wallerian degeneration may occur in the CNS and PNS.

- Axonal regeneration (recovery) varies between the CNS and PNS.
- Typically, axonal damage within the CNS leads to loss of function without the possibility of regeneration.
- In the PNS, the extent of damage to the nerve fiber and the connective tissue coverings serves as the basis for describing peripheral nerve injuries.
  - **Neuropraxia** is a mild form of injury in which there is a focal block of nerve impulses, often caused by transient ischemia or mild compression. The nerve fibers and connective tissue remain intact without Wallerian degeneration.
  - More significant compression injuries leading to partial damage to the connective tissue coverings cause **axonotmesis** and **neurotmesis**. Axonotmesis may lead to Wallerian degeneration; however, the axon may be able to distally regenerate if the endoneurial connective tissue sheath surrounding individual nerve fibers is still intact. Schwann cells, a type of neuroglial cells in the PNS, will aid in axonal guidance. If the connective sheath is disrupted, which may be associated with more severe cases of axonotmesis and with neurotmesis, surgical intervention may be necessary.
- Associated outcomes due to axonal injury include sensory loss, paresthesia, motor dysfunction, and muscle atrophy due to the loss of synaptic contact. In turn, this may lead to neuronal degeneration of the pre- and postsynaptic neurons, or target cells.

▶ Fig. 3.13

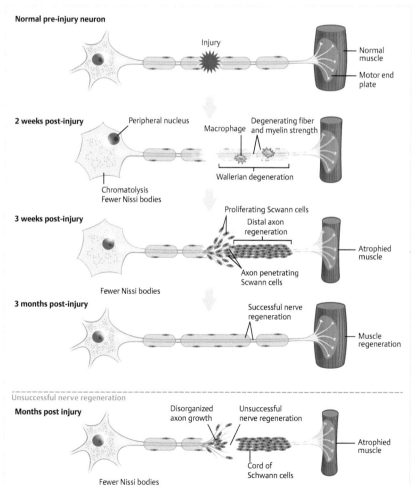

Fig. 3.13 Schematic diagram showing morphological changes to the neuron cell body and the proximal and distal regions of a myelinated axon following nerve injury. Potential outcomes depend on the extent and location of the nerve injury; however, they may include chromatolysis of the cell body, degeneration of the distal axon (Wallerian; anterograde axonal degeneration), and loss of synaptic contact with the target. This may cause a loss of sensation, muscle atrophy, or motor dysfunction. Typically, the proximal part of the axon remains attached to the cell body and continues to live, while the section distal to the injury degenerates. The proximal axon may potentially regenerate distally and reform synaptic connections with targets if the endoneurium and Schwann cells surrounding the axon remain viable. If the proximal axon is unable to penetrate the existing Schwann cell sheath, the axon exhibits disorganized growth and forms a traumatic neuroma.

Normal pre-injury neuron

Injury

Normal muscle

Motor end plate

2 weeks post-injury

Peripheral nucleus

Macrophage

Degenerating fiber and myelin strength

Wallerian degeneration

Chromatolysis
Fewer Nissl bodies

3 weeks post-injury

Proliferating Scwann cells

Distal axon regeneration

Atrophied muscle

Axon penetrating Scwann cells

Fewer Nissl bodies

3 months post-injury

Successful nerve regeneration

Muscle regeneration

Unsuccessful nerve regeneration

Months post injury

Disorganized axon growth

Unsuccessful nerve regeneration

Atrophied muscle

Cord of Schwann cells

Fewer Nissl bodies

3.3 Classification of Neurons in the Nervous System

- Neurons and supportive glial cells may be classified based on their morphology, function, and location within the CNS and PNS.

3.3.1 Morphological Neuronal Classification

- Neurons exhibit considerable diversity in shape and size but can be morphologically classified into three broad groups: **pseudounipolar, bipolar,** and **multipolar.** The structural classification depends on the morphological appearance and the number of cell processes extending from the cell body (▶ Fig. 3.14, ▶ Table 3.7).

- **Pseudounipolar (Unipolar) neurons** possess a single process that emerges from the cell body and branches into a peripheral and a central cell process. The peripheral branch transmits input from sensory receptors in peripheral tissue toward the neuronal cell body and the central process carries information from the cell body to the spinal cord or brainstem.
  - Pseudounipolar cell bodies reside within the **dorsal root (spinal) ganglia** or **cranial sensory ganglia** in the PNS.
- **Bipolar neurons** possess a single axon and a single dendrite that emerge from opposite poles of the cell body.

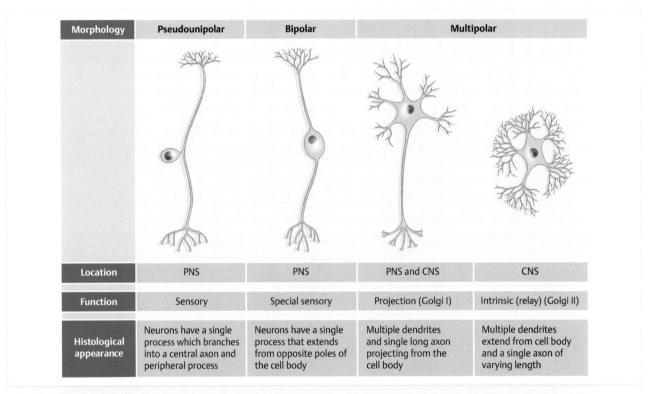

Morphology	Pseudounipolar	Bipolar	Multipolar	
Location	PNS	PNS	PNS and CNS	CNS
Function	Sensory	Special sensory	Projection (Golgi I)	Intrinsic (relay) (Golgi II)
Histological appearance	Neurons have a single process which branches into a central axon and peripheral process	Neurons have a single process that extends from opposite poles of the cell body	Multiple dendrites and single long axon projecting from the cell body	Multiple dendrites extend from cell body and a single axon of varying length

Fig. 3.14 Diagram and table depicting the morphological and functional classification of neurons. Neuron classification depends on the morphological appearance and the number of dendritic cell processes extending from the neuron cell body. The morphological appearance correlates with function. Neurons may be morphologically described as pseudounipolar, bipolar, and multipolar.

Table 3.7 Classification scheme of neurons

Location	PNS	PNS	PNS and CNS	CNS
Morphology	Pseudounipolar	Bipolar	Multipolar	Multipolar
Functional	Sensory	Special sensory	Projection (Golgi I)	Intrinsic (Golgi II)
Histology	Neurons have a single process which branches into a central axon and peripheral process	Neurons have a single process that extends from opposite poles of the cell body	Multiple dendrites and single long axon projecting from the cell body Axon may extend into periphery or project between different regions of the CNS	Multiple dendrites extend from cell body and a single axon of varying length Cell body and process remain in the CNS

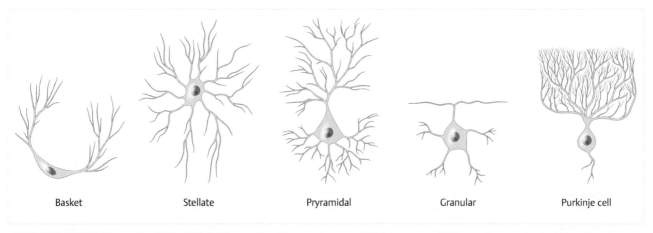

Basket   Stellate   Pryramidal   Granular   Purkinje cell

Fig. 3.15 Schematic diagram illustrating different types of multipolar neurons. Multipolar neurons exhibit a single axon of variable length and more than one dendrite extending from the cell body. Multipolar neurons function in the execution of motor responses or the integration of sensory and motor impulses.

○ Bipolar neuronal cell bodies are found in the PNS within the olfactory epithelium, the retina of the eye, and the **special sensory ganglia** of the vestibulocochlear nerve (CN VIII).

• **Multipolar neurons** are structurally and functionally diverse, comprising the largest morphological group of neurons.

○ Multipolar neurons may be found in the gray matter of the CNS or associated with the autonomic ganglia in the PNS.

○ Depending on their function and location, multipolar neurons may appear basket-shaped, stellate, pyramidal, granular, or have a special shape such as the Purkinje cell (▶ Fig. 3.15).

○ Histologically, multipolar neurons exhibit a single axon and more than one dendrite extending from the soma. The length of the axon varies and serves as criteria for further subdividing multipolar neurons into two groups: **Type I Golgi neurons** and **Type II Golgi neurons**.

– **Type I Golgi neurons,** also known as **projection neurons** or **principal neurons**, possess long axons that extend from the soma in the gray matter of the CNS to terminate at distant sites. The axons of projection neurons form long fiber tracts that may project between different regions within the CNS. Alternatively, the axons of multipolar projection neurons may extend from the CNS into the PNS.

– In contrast, **Type II Golgi neurons**, also known as **local circuit neurons**, represent a type of **integrative interneuron** with short axons that remain near their cell body in the (same region of the) CNS and terminate on local neuronal targets. Local circuit interneurons serve to functionally link different neurons together, modulate neuronal activity in local regions of the brain and spinal cord, and form reflex arcs.

3.3.2 Functional Neuronal Classification

• Neurons can be functionally classified, into three main groups; **afferent, efferent,** and **integrative,** based upon the type of information transmitted and the direction of the impulse. Each of these functional groups correlates to the type of information transmitted, the location of the cell body, and the neuronal morphology discussed in the previous section (▶ Table 3.8).

• **Afferent Neurons,** also known as **sensory afferent neurons,** receive information from peripheral sensory organs and transmit this input from the PNS to the CNS. Afferent neurons reside in the sensory ganglia of the PNS and send nerve fibers toward the CNS (▶ Fig. 3.16).

• Types of sensory input include somatic sensory information from the body, visceral input from organs and glands, and special sensory input from sensory receptors of the eyes, ears, nose, and mouth.

○ **Afferent sensory neurons,** which function to transmit somatic sensory and visceral input from receptors in the skin joints, muscle, and visceral organs to the CNS are known as **primary sensory neurons** or **first-order neurons**.

○ Afferent sensory neurons may also be designated as **general somatic afferent (GSA) neurons** if they convey sensations from the body or **general visceral afferent (GVA) neurons** if they transmit visceral sensations from organs or blood vessels.

– Primary sensory neurons are morphologically classified as pseudounipolar neurons and reside in the **dorsal root (spinal) ganglia** and **cranial sensory ganglia** within the PNS.

– The spinal and cranial nerve fibers that project from primary sensory neurons are known as **primary sensory afferent fibers.**

– Primary sensory afferent nerve fibers carry somatic (GSA) and visceral (GVA) input associated with pain, temperature, proprioception, and visceral sensations from peripheral sensory receptors, toward the neuronal cell bodies in the ganglia, and then enter the dorsal horn of the spinal cord or the brainstem.

○ **Special sensory afferent neurons** are found in the PNS and transmit special sensations such as smell, light, taste,

Table 3.8 Summary of neurons based on function, morphology, and location

Morphological classification	Functional classification and examples	Examples of location of cell body
Pseudounipolar	PNS (Afferent) Somatic sensory (GSA) (body) (Afferent) Visceral sensory (GVA) (organs)	PNS • Dorsal root spinal ganglia (GSA; GVA) • Some cranial ganglia (GSA; GVA)
Bipolar	PNS Afferent special sensory	PNS • Olfactory epithelium • Vestibulocochlear ganglia of CN VIII • Retina of eye
Multipolar	Efferent of PNS • Postganglionic visceral (motor) efferent (GVE) Efferent CNS • Preganglionic visceral (motor) efferent (GVE) • Somatic efferent (GSE) (lower motor) Integrative CNS • Purkinje, Granular, basket, etc. • Pyramidal (upper motor neurons), granular, fusiform, horizontal cells of Cajal, etc. • Dorsal horn of spinal cord	PNS Autonomic ganglia: postganglionic neurons CNS • Lateral horn spinal cord (GVE) • Ventral horn spinal cord (GSE) • Cranial motor nuclei (SVE) • Cerebellar cortex and deep cerebellar nuclei • Cerebral cortex and basal ganglia • Spinal cord

Abbreviations: CNS, central nervous system; GSA, general somatic afferent; GSE, general somatic efferent; GVA, general visceral afferent; GVE, general visceral efferent; PNS, peripheral nervous system; SVE, special visceral efferent.

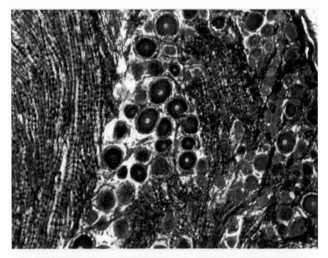

Fig. 3.16 Light microscopy demonstrating the dorsal root ganglion containing primary afferent neurons and associated nerve processes (40× magnification; hematoxylin and eosin [H/E] stain). The primary afferent neurons in the ganglion morphologically correspond to pseudounipolar neurons, which appear as large round cells, a centrally placed nucleus, and surrounded by smaller neuroglial cells called satellite cells.

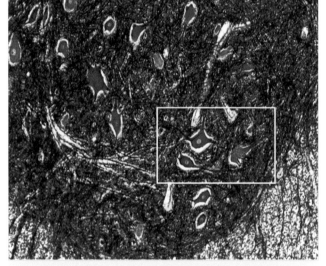

Fig. 3.17 Light microscopy demonstrating somatic motor (efferent) neurons in the ventral horn of the spinal cord (40× magnification; hematoxylin and eosin [H/E] stain). The motor neurons shown in the image are large cells with multiple cellular processes that represent multipolar neurons associated with the execution of voluntary motor functions.

and sound. The detection of special sensations occurs through special sensory receptors found within the olfactory epithelium, the retina of the eye, the taste buds of the oral cavity, and the vestibulocochlear apparatus.

- Special sensory afferent neurons that reside in the olfactory epithelium, the retina of the eye, and vestibulocochlear ganglia are morphologically characterized as bipolar neurons.
- A notable exception is the neuron cell bodies of special sensory afferent fibers that convey taste. Taste neurons are morphologically classified as pseudounipolar neurons and reside in peripheral cranial sensory ganglia.

- **Efferent neurons** that conduct impulses from the central nervous system to muscles, glands, and organs in the periphery are functionally classified as **motor neurons** and morphologically correspond to multipolar neurons. The cell bodies of efferent motor neurons reside in the gray matter of CNS or peripheral ganglia depending on their function.
- Types of efferent motor neurons include **somatic motor**, **special visceral motor**, and **autonomic (visceral motor) neurons** (▶ Fig. 3.17).
  ○ The cell bodies of **somatic** (GSE) and **special visceral efferent neurons** (SVE) lie in the ventral horn of the spinal

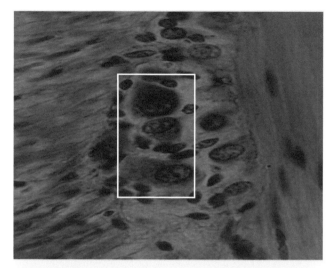

Fig. 3.18 Light microscopy demonstrating visceral motor neurons in an autonomic ganglion found in the wall of a visceral organ (40× magnification; hematoxylin and eosin [H/E] stain). Visceral motor neurons are part of a two-neuron relay chain consisting of preganglionic motor neurons and postganglionic motor neurons. The visceral motor neurons shown in the boxed region represent postganglionic motor neurons found in an autonomic ganglion. Visceral motor neurons are multipolar neurons that elicit involuntary motor responses.

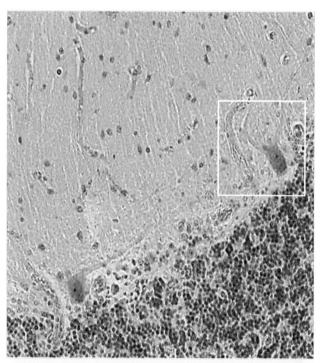

Fig. 3.19 Light microscopy demonstrating integrative neurons in the cerebellum (40× magnification; hematoxylin and eosin [H/E] stain). Purkinje neurons shown in the boxed area are the largest neurons found in the central nervous system (CNS) and are morphologically classified as multipolar neurons, characterized by the extensive branching (arborization) of dendrites extending from the cell body. The axons of Purkinje neurons provide the only output of the cerebellar cortex.

cord, and some cranial nerve nuclei of the brainstem. These neurons are also known as lower motor neurons (LMN). The axons of lower motor neurons extend into the PNS to terminate on skeletal muscle of the head, neck, trunk, or limbs.

○ **Visceral motor neurons** of the autonomic nervous system form a two-neuron chain consisting of **preganglionic motor neurons** and **postganglionic motor neurons**. Preganglionic neurons represent the first group of neurons and have cell bodies located in the brainstem or lateral horn of the spinal cord (T1–L2; S2–S4). The second group of neurons, known as **postganglionic neurons**, have cell bodies located in the **autonomic ganglia** of the PNS (▶ Fig. 3.18).

– The nerve fibers, known as **visceral efferent nerve fibers (preganglionic fibers)**, extend from the CNS to synapse with postganglionic neurons in peripheral autonomic ganglia.

– **Postganglionic nerve fibers** project from the ganglia and travel with mixed peripheral nerves to innervate smooth muscle, glands, and cardiac muscle.

• **Integrative neurons,** also known as **interneurons, projection,** or **relay neurons**, represent a diverse group and comprise the largest class of neurons found in the CNS (▶ Fig. 3.19).

• Integrative neurons are morphologically classified as multipolar and function to form neuronal circuits, process information, integrate afferent and efferent inputs, and coordinate reflex activity.

• In comparison to afferent and efferent neurons that contain cell processes in the periphery, the cell body and nerve processes of the integrative neuron reside only in the CNS.

Integrative neurons may be further classified based on the length of axons as **local circuit interneurons** and **relay (projection) neurons**.

○ **Interneurons** that form local circuits possess short axons that remain near their cell body in the CNS to terminate on local neuronal targets. These neurons are equivalent to type II Golgi multipolar neurons and modulate afferent input and motor responses.

○ **Relay neurons** typically possess long axons which project between different regions of the CNS and serve to functionally connect circuits of neurons. Many of the long axons of integrative relay neurons comprise functionally related ascending and descending axonal tracts that transmit motor and sensory information.

3.4 Neuroglial Cells

3.4.1 General Characteristics of Neuroglial Cells

• Neuroglial cells represent a diverse group of specialized non-neural support cells found in high abundance throughout the PNS and CNS. Glial cells outnumber neurons, but are typically smaller in size than neurons, lack axons, and dendrites, and possess only one type of cell process extending from the cell body.

- In comparison to neurons, neuroglial cells do not transmit electrical signals or form chemical synaptic contacts.
- Neuroglial cells perform numerous functions which include the following:
  - Maintain the ionic environment.
  - Modulate synaptic activity through the uptake of neurotransmitters.
  - Aid in recovery following neuronal injury.
  - Provide scaffolding for neuronal migration and axonal guidance during development.
  - Provide electrical insulation by myelinating axons.
  - Protect neurons within the CNS by maintaining the blood–brain barrier, glial limitans, and blood–CSF barrier.

3.4.2 Neuroglial Cells in the Central Nervous System (▶ Table 3.9)

- Histologically, neuroglial display variation in morphology, such as shape, size, and cell process density which serve as criteria for glial classification in the CNS and PNS (▶ Fig. 3.20).

- Two principal groups of glial cells found in the central nervous system include **microglial** and **macroglial** cells.
  - **Microglial cells**, the smallest of the neuroglial cells and play an important role in immune defense and phagocytosis in regions of the CNS following neuronal injury and disease.
  - **Macroglial cells** arise from neuroectoderm and are further subdivided into **astrocytes (astroglial)**, **oligodendrocytes**, and **ependymal cells** (▶ Fig. 3.21).

3.4.3 Neuroglial Cells in the Peripheral Nervous System

- In the PNS, glial cells arise from neural crest cells and include **Schwann cells** and **Satellite cells** (▶ Table 3.10).
  - **Schwann cells** are responsible for the myelination of peripheral nerve fibers and represent the functional equivalent to oligodendrocytes.
  - **Satellite cells** appear as small-cells surrounding neuronal cell bodies found in sensory and visceral motor ganglia. Satellite cells function to maintain ionic and metabolic homeostasis (▶ Fig. 3.22).

Table 3.9 Neuroglial cells of CNS

Cell types	Structural appearance	Location CNS	Function	Germ layer
Microglial	Smallest glial cells, short process	White matter and gray matter	Phagocytosis during inflammation and disease following CNS injury	Hematopoietic-derived precursors (mesoderm)
		Macroglial cells:		
Astrocytes[a] • Fibrous	Small cell bodies, long process, vascular feet	White matter	Maintain [K + ion] and metabolic environment Modulate neurotransmission Remove excess excitatory neurotransmitters Maintain blood–brain barrier	Neuroectoderm
• Protoplasmic	Small cell body, short processes	Gray matter	Maintain ionic environment Contribute to glial limitans barrier	Neuroectoderm

• Specialized astrocytes
  ○ Radial (developmental)
  ○ Bergmann
  ○ Pituicytes
  ○ Müller
	Variety of shapes	Exhibit differential and restricted distribution in CNS	Function based on location: provides structural and metabolic support	Neuroectoderm

Oligodendrocytes	Small cell body, short delicate process	White matter Gray matter Interspersed between nerves	Myelination of axons in CNS A single oligodendrocyte myelinates multiple axonal (internodal) segments of several different axons	Neuroectoderm
Ependymal • Ependymocytes	Cuboidal epithelium with microvilli	Line ventricles and central canal	CSF circulation and absorption	Neuroectoderm
• Choroidal	Cuboidal epithelium with tight junction	Cover choroid vascular plexus	Produce CSF; contribute to blood–CSF barrier	Neuroectoderm
• Tanycytes	Epithelial cells	Line third ventricle	Transport of substances from CSF to hypophyseal portal system	Neuroectoderm

Abbreviations: CNS, central nervous system; CSF, cerebrospinal fluid.
[a]Represent largest group of glial cells.

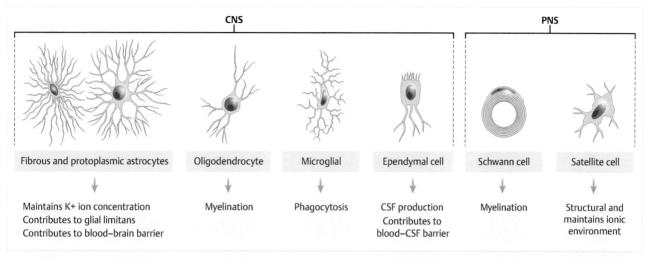

Fig. 3.20 Schematic diagram of neuroglial (glial) cells distributed in the central nervous system (CNS) and peripheral nervous system (PNS). Glial cells represent non-neural cells that provide numerous supportive functions essential for the maintenance of neuronal function. Glial cells found in the CNS include astrocytes, oligodendrocytes, ependymal, and small microglial cells. Glial cells in the PNS include Schwann cells and satellite cells.

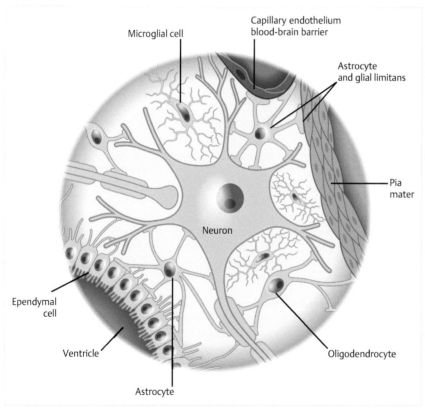

Fig. 3.21 Distribution and functional interactions of glial cells in the brain: astrocytes, oligodendrocytes, ependymal cells, and microglial cells. Astrocytes that provide metabolic and ionic support to neurons also contact the basement membrane of the pia mater, forming the glial limitans, and maintain the blood–brain barrier. Oligodendrocytes function to myelinate axons in the central nervous system (CNS). Ependymal cells play a role in the production and circulation of cerebrospinal fluid (CSF).

Table 3.10 Neuroglial cells PNS

Neuroglial cell PNS	Structural appearance	Location PNS	Function	Germ layer
Schwann cell	Small elongated cells	Surround segments of peripheral axons in PNS	• Myelinates one (internodal) segment of a single axon • Plasma membrane of cell forms a single layer around unmyelinated axons • Aid in axonal regrowth and remyelination following injury to peripheral axon	Neural crest
Satellite cells	Small cuboidal to squamous-shaped cells	Surrounds cell bodies sensory and autonomic ganglion	Structural support; maintain ionic environment	Neural crest

Abbreviation: PNS, peripheral nervous system.

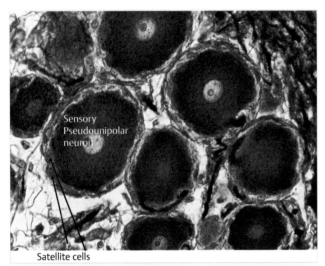

Fig. 3.22 Light microscopy of satellite cells surrounding the sensory cell body (40× magnification; silver stain). Satellite cells appear as small gold-stained cells surrounding the sensory pseudounipolar neuron in the dorsal root ganglion. Satellite cells are functionally analogous to astrocytes found in the central nervous system (CNS) and function to maintain the ionic environment.

3.5 Histological Appearance of CNS

- The gray matter in the spinal cord and brainstem is centrally located and surrounded by white matter. In the cerebellum and cerebrum, the pattern is reversed, and the white matter lies internal to the gray matter.

3.5.1 Spinal Cord Histology (▶ Fig. 3.23a, b)

- The spinal cord functions to conduct impulses between the brain and the body.
- The histological appearance of the spinal cord cut in a transverse section demonstrates the white matter is peripherally located and surrounds the centrally placed gray matter which is shaped like a butterfly or the letter "H."

- Each side of the gray matter consists of a **dorsal** and **ventral horn** and is connected by a band of gray matter called the **gray commissure**. The **central canal,** which is located within the gray commissure, is lined by ependymal cells.
- In the thoracolumbar (T1–L2) and sacral regions (S2–S4) of the spinal cord an **intermediate (lateral) horn** is also present in the gray matter.
- The cell bodies of interneurons, projection (integrative) neurons, and somatic (ventral) motor neurons form nuclei in the gray matter that exhibit differential distribution within the dorsal, lateral, and ventral horns.
  - The nuclei within each horn are longitudinally organized as **columns** of cells extending from one vertebral level to another.
  - The cell columns histologically appear as ten layers (laminae), known as the **Rexed laminae** (▶ Fig. 3.24).
- The **dorsal (posterior) horn** or **posterior column** consists mainly of relay interneurons and projection neurons associated with the **Rexed laminae (I, II, III, IV, V, IV).** These regions of the Rexed laminae receive sensory information from the body (somatic) and organs (visceral). Interneurons may form local circuit connections and reflex arcs, while projection neurons may transmit the information along axonal tracts to higher regions of the brain for conscious and unconscious processing.
- The Rexed lamina (VII) of the **lateral horn** is also known as the **intermediolateral cell column (IMLC).** The IMLC contains the cell bodies of preganglionic autonomic neurons, along with interneurons, and projections neurons, that provide visceral motor innervation to smooth muscle, glands, and the heart.
- The Rexed laminae (VIII, IX) of the **ventral (anterior) horn** receives input from descending cortical motor tracts and contains α (alpha) and γ (gamma) lower motor (somatic motor) neurons that innervate and modulate skeletal muscle contractions (▶ Fig. 3.25a).
- In the white matter the axonal tracts are organized into **three funiculi (columns).** The term funiculus refers to cordlike and is a descriptive term for the axonal tracts comprising the **dorsal, lateral,** and **ventral columns of white matter.** Each column (funiculus) consists of several functionally related groups of **axonal tracts (fasciculi)** that

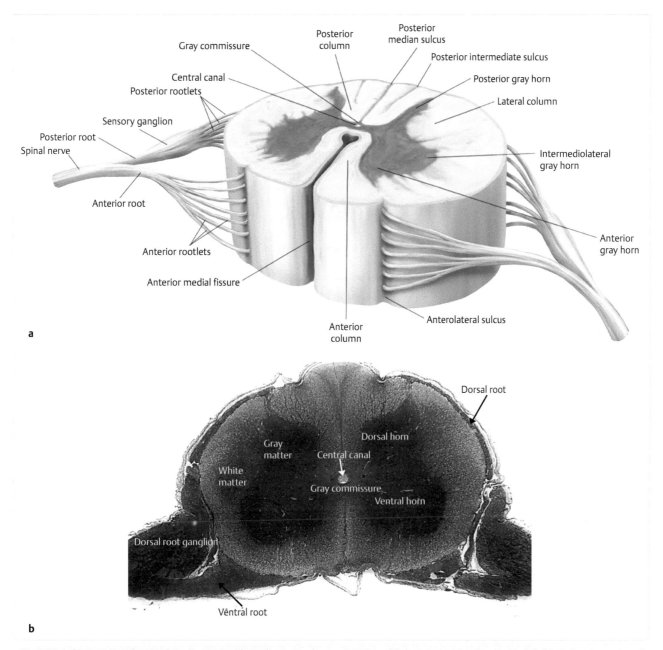

Fig. 3.23 (a,b) Anatomy of a spinal cord segment. Three-dimensional representation, oblique anterior view from upper left **(a)**. Light microscopy of spinal cord cut in cross-section (2.5 × magnification; silver stain) **(b)**. The white matter of the spinal cord and brainstem is peripherally located and surrounds the internally placed gray matter. The arrangement of white and gray matter found in the spinal cord is reversed in the cerebellum and cerebral cortex, and the white matter lies internal to the gray matter. In the spinal cord, the gray matter appears butterfly-shaped or as the letter "H" and surrounds the fluid-filled central canal, which is part of the ventricular system. Each side of the gray matter consists of the dorsal (posterior) horn and a ventral (anterior) horn. A lateral horn is present in the thoracolumbar (T1–L2) and sacral (S2–S4) regions of the spinal cord. A narrow band of gray matter known as the gray commissure connects each side. The location of the ventral (motor) root, the dorsal (sensory) root, and the dorsal root ganglion which contains pseudounipolar sensory neurons are also shown in the field of view. (Reproduced with permission from Schuenke M, Schulte E, Schumacher U. THIEME Atlas of Anatomy Third Edition, Vol 3. © Thieme 2020. Illustrations by Markus Voll and Karl Wesker.)

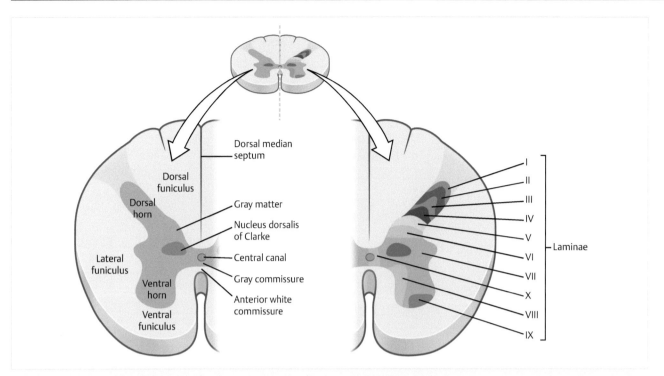

Fig. 3.24 The location of the Rexed laminae in the spinal cord. Clusters of functionally similar neurons (nuclei) are arranged in the dorsal, lateral, and ventral horns of the spinal cord in 10 zones. The zones, referred to as Rexed laminae, represent a layered configuration of integrative and motor neurons that receive and transmit sensory and motor input. The dorsal horn, which receives primary afferent (sensory) fibers, contains nuclei associated with Rexed lamina I, II, III, V, and IV. The lateral horn, found in the thoracolumbar and sacral regions, contains preganglionic autonomic nuclei associated with Rexed lamina VII. The ventral horn contains somatic motor nuclei found in Rexed lamina VIII and IX.

transmit information to different levels of the spinal cord and brain (▶ Fig. 3.25b).

3.5.2 Brainstem Histology

- The brainstem represents the most caudal region of the brain, sitting just above the spinal cord and next to the cerebellum. The brainstem, which consists of the medulla, pons, and the mesencephalon (midbrain), functions to regulate autonomic activities and relay information between the body, spinal cord, cerebral cortex, and cerebellum.
- The brainstem is structurally similar in organization to that of the spinal cord; consisting of nuclei in the gray matter, and ascending and descending tracts in the white matter. However, the histological appearance of the gray and white matter in the brainstem is not as distinct. The modified appearance is due to the presence of the fourth ventricle, the emergence of the cranial nerves, and the physical connection to the cerebellum.
- Neurons of the gray matter are arranged into three functionally related groups of nuclei: the cranial nerve nuclei associated with **CN III-CN XII**, the nuclei of the **reticular formation**, and the **pontine nuclei**.

3.5.3 Cerebellum Histology

- The cerebellum functions to maintain postural stability, balance, muscle tone, and serves to coordinate, correct, and

modulate voluntary motor activity based on sensory input from the spinal cord, brainstem, cerebrum, and the vestibular system of the inner ear.
- Macroscopically, the cerebellum consists of two lateral **hemispheres** which flank a narrow midline region, called the **vermis** (▶ Fig. 3.26a, b).
- Three deep fissures divide the cerebellar hemispheres and vermis along the transverse axis into three main lobes: an **anterior lobe**, a **posterior (middle) lobe**, and the **flocculonodular lobe**.
- The cerebellar surface of each lobe appears deeply grooved with intervening fissures and numerous transverse folds, known as **folia**, which separate the lobes into **lobules.**
- The gray matter follows the convoluted surface of the cerebellar folia, forming an outer cortical region, called the **cerebellar cortex.**
- The cortical gray matter surrounds a large, centrally located area of **subcortical white matter.** Embedded deep within the subcortical white matter are several masses of gray matter, arranged as four paired clusters of neurons, which comprise the **deep cerebellar nuclei.**
- The white matter contains several excitatory axonal fibers, known as **mossy** and **climbing fibers**. The excitatory afferent fibers that enter the cerebellum pass from the spinal cord, brainstem, and cerebral cortex, project to the deep cerebellar nuclei and specific neurons in the cerebellar cortex. The axons arising from the deep nuclei form the sole cerebellar efferent (outflow) pathways from

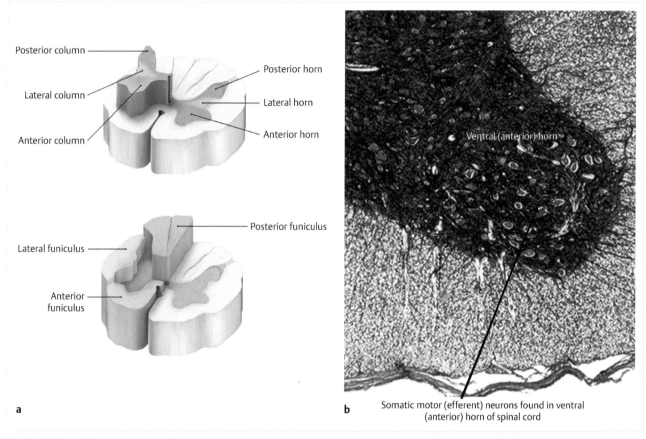

Posterior column

Lateral column

Anterior column

Posterior horn

Lateral horn

Anterior horn

Posterior funiculus

Lateral funiculus

Anterior funiculus

Ventral (anterior) horn

a

b Somatic motor (efferent) neurons found in ventral (anterior) horn of spinal cord

Fig. 3.25 Three-dimensional schematic representation of a spinal cord segment with gray matter and white matter highlighted (Left anterior oblique and superior view). **(a)** The gray matter consists of neurons, dendrites, and myelinated and unmyelinated axons which project in and out of the gray matter. The neurons form nuclei within each horn that are longitudinally organized as columns of cells extending from one vertebral column to the next. The white matter contains axonal tracts organized into three funiculi (columns). Note the location of the posterior (dorsal), lateral, and anterior (ventral) columns which contain neurons, and the corresponding locations of the posterior (dorsal), lateral, and anterior (ventral) funiculi containing the axonal tracts. **(b)** Light microscopy of the ventral horn of the spinal cord (20 × magnification; cross-section, silver stain). The ventral (anterior) horn contains alpha and gamma lower motor (somatic motor) neurons. Based on the location of the lower motor neurons in the ventral horn, these cells are sometimes referred to as ventral (anterior) horn cells. Lower motor neurons are multipolar. (▶ Fig. 3.25a: Reproduced with permission from Schuenke M, Schulte E, Schumacher U. THIEME Atlas of Anatomy Second Edition, Vol 3. © Thieme 2016. Illustrations by Markus Voll and Karl Wesker.)

the cerebellum. The efferent cerebellar pathways contribute primarily the indirect motor paths of the extrapyramidal system.

○ The cerebellum attaches to the brainstem through three axonal tracts, the **inferior, middle,** and **superior peduncles**, through which the efferent and afferent fiber tracts pass to connect the cerebellum to the spinal cord, brainstem, cerebrum, and vestibular system.

○ The afferent fiber tracts that arise from the spinal cord, brainstem, cerebrum, and vestibular system enter primarily through the inferior and middle peduncles, whereas efferent output passes mainly through the superior peduncles.

• Microscopically, the cortical gray matter of the cerebellum contains five different types of neurons, which along with their nerve fibers and associated neuroglial cells, are differential distributed between three **laminae** (layers).

• The layers of **cerebellar cortex** include: an external **molecular layer,** the middle **Purkinje cell layer,** and the internal **granular layer** (▶ Fig. 3.27a, b).

○ The superficial layer of cerebellar cortex, known as the **molecular layer**, lies just below the meninges and consists of two types of **inhibitory interneurons**: the **outer stellate cells** and **inner basket cells**. The interneurons are interspersed among the dendrites of the Purkinje cells.

○ The **Purkinje layer** is the thinnest layer of the cortex, containing a single, parallel layer of large, multipolar projection (**type I Golgi**) neurons, known as **Purkinje cells**. Purkinje cells function as inhibitory neurons and represent the characteristic cell type associated with the cerebellum. Each cell appears flask-shaped with extensive dendritic fans extending toward the external molecular layer and an axon projecting through the inner granular layer to enter the white matter.

– The axons of Purkinje cells serve as the sole efferent output from the cerebellar cortex, and project through the white matter to synapse on neurons in the deep cerebellar nuclei. Some Purkinje axons also pass directly to the vestibular nuclei.

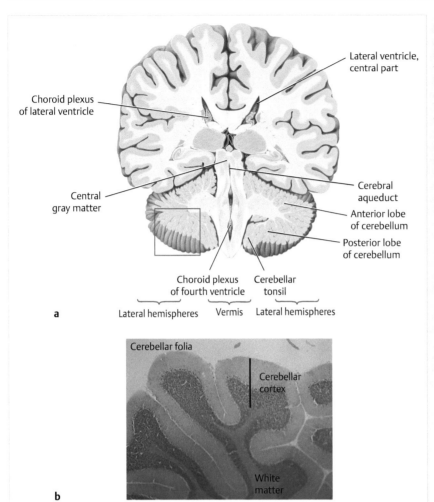

Choroid plexus
of lateral ventricle

Central
gray matter

Lateral ventricle,
central part

Cerebral
aqueduct

Anterior lobe
of cerebellum

Posterior lobe
of cerebellum

Choroid plexus
of fourth ventricle

Cerebellar
tonsil

a

Lateral hemispheres   Vermis   Lateral hemispheres

Cerebellar folia

Cerebellar
cortex

White
matter

b

Fig. 3.26 (a) Coronal section through cerebrum and cerebellum. The cerebellum consists of two lateral hemispheres joined in the midline by the vermis. Three horizontal fissures subdivide the hemispheres and vermis into three lobes: anterior, posterior, and flocculonodular lobes. The cerebellum is connected to other regions of the brain by three pairs of (cerebellar) peduncles (not shown). Afferent and efferent axonal tracts pass ipsilaterally through the peduncle to the ipsilateral cerebellar cortex. **(b)** Light microscopy of the cerebellum depicting extensive folds (folia) and fissures of the cerebellar cortex (20 × magnification; hematoxylin and eosin [H/E] stain). The cerebellar cortex consists of an outer cortical layer of gray matter that surrounds a central medullary region of white matter containing myelinated axons. Note the white matter extending into the folia. Embedded within the white matter are four clusters of paired nuclei, known as the deep cerebellar nuclei (not shown) that receive input from specific regions of the cerebellar hemispheres. (Fig. 3.26a: Reproduced with permission from Schuenke M, Schulte E, Schumacher U. THIEME Atlas of Anatomy Third Edition, Vol 3. © Thieme 2020. Illustrations by Markus Voll and Karl Wesker.)

- The axonal tracts passing from the Purkinje cells to the vestibular nuclei represent the only axonal path to originate directly from the cerebellar cortex and leave the cerebellum.
- All other output signals arise from the deep cerebellar nuclei and project to other regions in the CNS to modify or correct motor output of movements.

  ○ The layer closest to the white matter, the **granular layer**, is composed of small, tightly packed relay interneurons (**type Golgi II**), known as **granule cells**. Granule cells represent the most numerous neurons in the cerebellum and are the main **excitatory** neurons in the cerebellar cortex. **Golgi (inner stellate) cells** are inhibitory interneurons scattered among the granule cells.

3.5.4 Cerebrum Histology

- The cerebrum is the largest part of the brain, located superiorly and anteriorly to the brainstem and cerebellum. It is functionally important for mediating all higher mental functions, including conscious sensory processing, planning and generating voluntary movements, and providing awareness of emotions. It is also necessary for cognition, memory formation, storage, and retrieval, language, and speech production.
- The cerebrum consists of two hemispheres, each containing a region of gray and white matter. The gross macroscopic appearance of the cerebrum shows that the **gray matter** follows the convoluted perimeter of the cerebral hemispheres, forming an outer mantle, known as the **cerebral cortex** (▶ Fig. 3.28a, b).

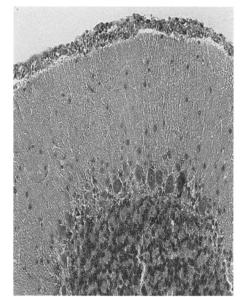

a

Fig. 3.27 (a,b) Functional histology of the cerebellar cortex. **(a)** Light microscopy of the cerebellar cortex taken through a cerebellar fold (folium) (20× magnification, transverse section, hematoxylin and eosin [H/E] stain). The gray matter of the cerebellar cortex contains three cell layers: an outer molecular, a middle Purkinje layer, and an inner granular layer. **(b)** Schematic diagram of the three layers of the cerebellar cortex, showing the five neuronal cell types that are differentially distributed between the three layers. The white matter forms the central medullary region and contains several axonal nerve tracts comprised of excitatory afferent fibers that terminate on neurons in the deep cerebellar nuclei and the cerebellar cortex. The afferent fiber tracts originate from the spinal cord, brainstem, cerebrum, and vestibular system and comprise many of the ascending unconscious somatosensory pathways of the head and body. Efferent fibers originating from Purkinje cells of the cortex and neurons in the deep cerebellar nuclei project to the vestibular system to maintain balance and coordinate eye movement. Efferent fibers also project to the spinal cord, brainstem, and cerebral cortex to maintain posture control and muscle tone, and serves to modulate, coordinate, and correct voluntary motor activity. The efferent cerebellar pathways contribute primarily to the indirect motor paths. (▶ Fig. 3.27b: Reproduced with permission from Greenstein B, Greenstein A. Neuroanatomy and Neurophysiology. © Thieme 2000.)

Basket cell   Stellate cell

Molecular layer / Purkinje cell layer / Granular layer — cerebellar cortex

Granule cell / Golgi cell / Mossy fiber cell rosette / Purkinje cell / Climbing fiber

Molecular layer

Purkinje layer

Granular layer

Cellular organization

Cerzebellar nuclei — Efferent cerebellar fiber

b

- The white matter, containing myelinated axons and neuroglial cells, lies deep to cortex and functions to connect the cerebrum to the opposing hemisphere and other regions of the brain and spinal cord.
- Distinct masses of gray matter containing various nuclei associated with basal ganglia are visible deep within the white matter and in regions surrounding the ventricles.
• Histologically the neurons, nerve fibers, and neuroglial cells of the cortical gray matter exhibit a laminar or layered arrangement that is reflective of development (Table 3.11).

- The largest cortical region, designated as the **neocortex**, contains six stratified layers (I–VI) of cells that lie parallel to the surface. The neurons within the various layers interact with one another through vertical connections and form functional cortical columns (▶ Fig. 3.29).
- Each layer, which is delineated based on the morphological appearance of the predominant cell type, differs in its functional properties and types of connections. Variations in the laminar arrangement reflect functional differences between the motor, sensory, and association regions of the cortex.

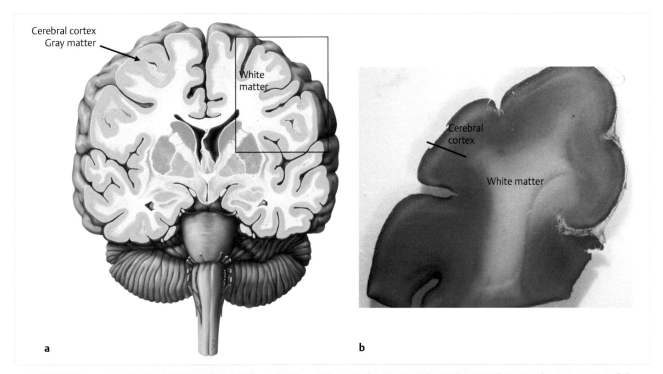

Fig. 3.28 (a) Coronal section through the right and left cerebral hemispheres in the telencephalon. Schematic illustrates the organization of the outer cortical gray matter, centrally located white matter, the basal (deep cortical gray) nuclei, and the position of the right and left lateral ventricles near the midline. The two cerebral hemispheres are separated by the medial longitudinal fissure and exhibit extensive folding to form gyri and sulci. The superficial gray matter contains cortical neurons and follows the convoluted surface to form the outer mantle region. Gray matter is also present subcortical, in the base of the hemispheres, and comprise the basal (deep cortical gray) nuclei. Additional subcortical structures are not visible. The white matter lies internal to the gray matter and contains several axon fiber groups including projection fibers of the ascending and descending fiber tracts, association fibers that connect different cortical areas within one hemisphere, and commissural fibers which connect the cortical regions of both hemispheres. The commissural fibers of the corpus callosum are visible and lie just inferior to the median longitudinal fissure. The projection fibers of the internal capsule, which are shown separating the basal nuclei, convey ascending and descending tracts that pass to and from the cortex. **(b)** Light microscopy of the cerebral cortex demonstrating the appearance of the outer cortical gray matter and subcortical white matter (10 × magnification, silver stain). (▶ Fig. 3.28a: Reproduced with permission from Schuenke M, Schulte E, Schumacher U. THIEME Atlas of Anatomy Second Edition, Vol 3. © Thieme 2016. Illustrations by Markus Voll and Karl Wesker.)

- Cortical neurons which are morphologically characterized as multipolar neurons comprise two broad groups: **Pyramidal cells** and **nonpyramidal cells** or local (association) interneurons.
- The **pyramidal cell** is a type of multipolar cortical projection (type I Golgi) neuron, functionally classified as an **upper motor neuron,** and represents the predominant neuron of the cortex. Pyramidal cells, which are found in layers II–VI, establish efferent connections between the cerebral cortex and other areas of the brain and spinal cord. The **pyramidal cell of Betz** is an extremely large pyramidal cell (UMN) and a histological characteristic of the cerebral cortex (▶ Fig. 3.30).
- **Interneurons** establish local connections and function to modulate pyramidal cell activity. Interneurons exhibit differential distribution within the cortical layers and include **granule (stellate) cells, fusiform cells, Martinotti cells**, and **horizontal cells of Cajal.**

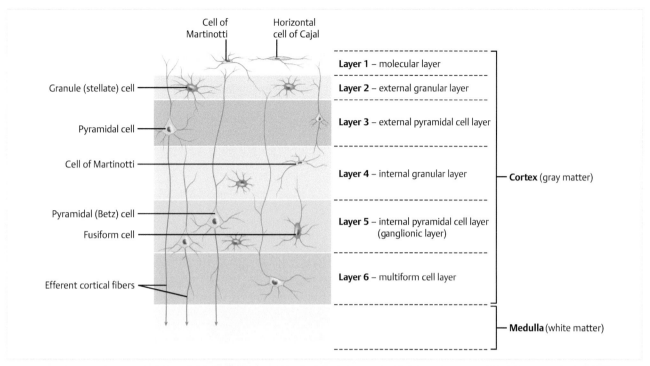

Fig. 3.29 Schematic diagram depicting the six layers of the cerebral cortex (neocortex) and the arrangement of the two principal types of cortical neurons, the pyramidal and granule cells, within these layers. Each layer is named according to the predominant cell type. The neurons within the six layers interact with one another through vertical connections that form functional columns (not shown). Variations in the composition and arrangement within the six layers exist and reflect functional differences associated with different regions of the cerebrum. The sensory regions of the cortex exhibit a granular appearance due to the expansion of granular layers (layers II and IV), which represent the point of termination for ascending sensory fibers. Conversely, the motor cortex shows thinning of the granular layers but shows an expansion of pyramidal layers (III and V). Large pyramidal cells of layer V represent a distinctive histological feature of the cerebral cortex. Pyramidal cells are multipolar neurons that serve as the main cortical efferent (output) neuron.

Table 3.11 Histological laminar organization of cerebral cortex

Layer I	The **molecular layer** lies adjacent to pial surface and contains mainly dendrites, axons, a few neuroglial cells, and interneurons, known as the horizontal cells of Cajal
Layer II	The **external (outer) granular layer** contains small pyramidal cells and a dense population of inhibitory interneurons called granule cells. Small pyramidal cells project to different cortical areas. This layer serves mainly to establish intracortical connections
Layer III	The **external (outer) pyramidal layer** contains medium-sized pyramidal neurons that gives rise to association fibers and commissural fibers and some granule cells
Layer IV	The **internal granular layer** contains numerous small granule cells that receive primarily afferent input from the thalamus. The size of this layer varies based on the functional region of the cortex. Sensory cortical areas exhibit a larger region IV than the motor cortex. Layer IV is either small or absent in the motor cortex
Layer V	The **internal pyramidal layer** is typically the largest layer within the cortex, containing pyramidal cells which vary in size depending on the functional region of the cortex. Connects with subcortical regions, including basal ganglia, brainstem, spinal cord Large pyramidal cells, known as Betz cells, are classified as upper motor neurons and are characteristic of the cortical regions associated with motor function. Upper motor neurons (UMN) of Betz cells send efferent projection to the lower motor neurons (LMN) in the spinal cord and cranial nerve motor nuclei
Layer VI	The **polymorphic or fusiform layer** contains numerous fusiform-shaped interneurons, granule cells, Martinotti cells, and some pyramidal cells that form association and projections fibers that connect with primarily the thalamus

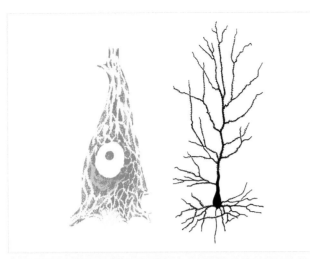

Fig. 3.30 Schematic illustrating large pyramidal cells of cortical layer V (pyramidal cell of Betz) in the cerebral motor cortex. Pyramidal neurons are a distinctive histological feature of the cerebral cortex and correspond to upper motor neurons of the primary motor cortex. The axons of the large pyramidal neurons contribute to the corticobulbar and corticospinal voluntary motor tracts that project to the brainstem and spinal cord, respectively. (Reproduced with permission from Kahle W, Frotscher M. Color Atlas of Human Anatomy. Sixth Edition, Vol 3. © Thieme 2011.)

Questions and Answers

1. Each of the following types of neurons is found in ganglia throughout the body **EXCEPT** one. Which one is the exception?
   a) Visceral motor
   b) Somatic sensory
   c) Somatic motor
   d) Special sensory

Level 2: Moderate

Answer C: Somatic motor neurons are the exception. Somatic neurons are found in the ventral (anterior) horn of the spinal cord and in the brainstem, so they are situated within the CNS. Visceral motor (**A**) are found in CNS (lateral horn) but are also found in the PNS. Visceral motor neurons are part of the autonomic nervous system and the postganglionic neurons reside in ganglia. Somatic sensory neurons (**B**) are pseudounipolar neurons found in the dorsal root ganglia and some cranial sensory ganglia. Special sensory neurons (**D**) of the vestibulocochlear nerve (CN VIII) are found in ganglia.

2. The neurons found in the ventral horn of the spinal cord are morphologically classified as _____.
   a) Visceral motor
   b) Interneurons
   c) Bipolar
   d) Multipolar
   e) Pseudounipolar

Level 1: Easy

Answer D: Multipolar. Neurons may be classified based on function or morphology. Choices (**A**) and (**B**) represent functional classifications. Choices (**C**), (**D**), and (**E**) are morphological classifications. Ventral horn neurons are morphologically multipolar neurons (**E**); functionally they are a type of projection neuron and may also be classified as lower motor neurons or somatic motor neurons.

3. Completely severing the ulnar nerve in the wrist will damage each of the following **EXCEPT** one. Which is the exception?
   a) Satellite cells
   b) Cutaneous sensation to the skin covering digiti minimi
   c) Epineurium
   d) Motor innervation to hypothenar eminence
   e) Myelin sheath

Level 3: Difficult

Answer A: Satellite cells are the exception. They are confined primarily to region around the cell body of sensory and autonomic neurons and are found in the ganglia. When cutting the ulnar nerve at the wrist the satellite cells will not be affected since the anatomical location of the dorsal root ganglia is located just outside the vertebral column and therefore distant from the site of injury. The ulnar nerve is a peripheral nerve carrying both motor and sensory fibers (**B** and **D**), so both fiber types are damaged, and the muscle and skin innervated by these areas reflects the damage. Peripheral nerves are surrounded by three layers of the epineurium (**C**), perineurium, and endoneurium (not listed). The myelin sheath (**E**) surrounds the axons of somatic motor fibers and most sensory fibers so it would also be severed.

4. A multipolar neuron that synapses on a sweat gland and elicits secretion is functionally classified as a(an)

   _____.
   a) Special sensory neuron
   b) Somatic motor neuron
   c) Interneuron
   d) Visceral motor neuron
   e) Somatic sensory neuron

Level 1: Easy

Answer D: Visceral motor. The visceral motor neurons represent a functional classification and are examples of a type of multipolar neuron. They carry autonomic nerve fibers which innervate smooth muscle and glands. The remaining choices provide innervation to other areas. Somatic motor neurons (**B**) are multipolar but carry somatic efferent fibers and provide innervation to skeletal muscle. Interneurons (**C**) are integrative or perform relay functions. Interneurons are also classified as multipolar. Special sensory (**A**) and somatic sensory (**E**) provide sensory innervation and do not elicit secretory motor function from glands.

5. Complete the following statement correctly. Primary sensory neurons that carry general somatic sensory afferent fibers _____.

a) Are located in the dorsal horn of the spinal cord
b) Transmit pain, temperature and touch from the skin
c) Are derived from neuroectoderm
d) Have receptors in the olfactory mucosa
e) Are classified as multipolar neurons

Level 2: Moderate

Answer B: Transmit pain, temperature, and touch from skin. Primary sensory neurons are pseudounipolar neurons that carry somatic sensory afferent fibers or general visceral afferent fibers.

Somatic sensory afferent fibers carry sensations from peripheral receptors in the body and are associated with skin, muscles, and joints. These neurons are located in dorsal root ganglia and are derived from neural crest cells, not neuroectoderm (**C**). Neurons found in the dorsal horn (**A**) are interneurons that receive sensory input from primary afferent neurons. Receptors found in the olfactory mucosa (**D**) are special sensory afferent bipolar neurons. Receptors found in the visceral wall are classified as general visceral afferents neurons. Somatic sensory neurons are pseudounipolar, not multipolar (**E**).

4 Neurophysiology

Gilbert M. Willett

Learning Objectives

1. Describe the molecular composition of a neuron membrane.
2. Describe the process of neuron depolarization.
3. Compare the two main types of neuron synapses.
4. Explain how neurotransmitters assist in neuronal function.
5. Given a specific neurotransmitter, describe its basic function.

4.1 Neurophysiology Overview

Consistent with other systems of the human body, the nervous system structure (anatomy) and function (physiology) are intricately linked. Thus, a thorough knowledge of nervous system anatomy and histology is essential for understanding neurophysiology.

4.2 Cell Membrane

- Neuron membranes are complex molecular structures mostly made up of lipids and proteins. They exhibit unique adaptations for cellular information-processing functions.
  - The membrane maintains the intracellular environment and separates the neuron from surrounding cells and the aqueous extracellular environment. Signaling must pass through the membrane.
  - Two opposing rows of phospholipid molecules comprise the neuron membrane:
    - The "head" end of each molecule is a polar (charged) phosphate group that is hydrophilic (attracted to aqueous environment).
    - The "tail" end of each molecule consists of two nonpolar (neutral) lipid extensions from the "head" that are hydrophobic (repelled by fluids) (▶ Fig. 4.1).
      - Cholesterol molecules insert between the tails, preventing permeability of small water molecules and enhancing membrane flexibility.
    - Large proteins are interspersed between the phospholipid molecules of the neuron membrane (the number of different types of proteins in a cell membrane vary from approximately 100 to only a few). There are two primary classifications (see ▶ Fig. 4.1):
      - **Integral** (transmembrane) proteins span the entire thickness of the cell membrane, enabling transport between extra- and intracellular environments. They are tightly embedded within and bound to the surrounding phospholipid molecules of the membrane.
        - **Channel** proteins allow small ions to **passively** move through the cell membrane (i.e., potassium [K^+] leak channels) (▶ Fig. 4.2).
        - **Carrier** proteins have ion-specific bonding sites which may transport ions passively (with gradient) or actively (against a gradient) across the membrane, depending on whether an energy source is available (i.e., sodium/potassium pump—ATP needed).

- **Peripheral** proteins are loosely adherent to other membrane proteins or to the inner or outer membrane surface through hydrogen bonds.
- This enables disconnection without affecting the structure of the membrane.
- Functions include acting as:
  - Receptors.
  - Enzymes.
  - Reaction catalysts.
  - Structural support.
  - Movement facilitation (e.g., microfilament, intermediate filament, and microtubule components).

4.3 Action Potentials

When a neuron is resting (not firing), its axon membrane is polarized at −70 mV. This polarization results from intracellular fluid being relatively negative in comparison to the extracellular fluid. The polarized state is achieved by integral channel and carrier proteins in the cell membrane distributing ions across the membrane (e.g., sodium [Na^+] potassium [K^+] pump carrier proteins and K^+ channel proteins). Ion movement creates electrical signals.

- **Resting potential** is the difference in electrical charge between the extra- and intracellular sides of the neuron cell membrane (−70 mV).
  - Resting potential is created by:
    - Extra-/intracellular K^+ concentration gradient.

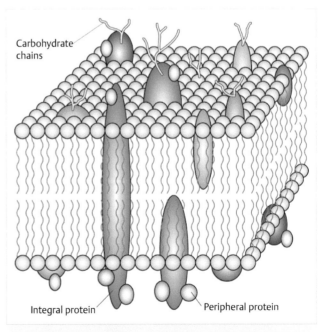

Fig. 4.1 Neuron membrane molecular structure. (Reproduced with permission from Michael J, Sircar S. Fundamentals of Medical Physiology. © Thieme 2011.)

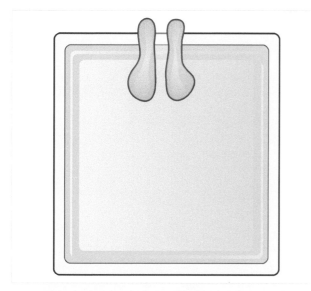

Fig. 4.2 Neuron membrane channel protein.

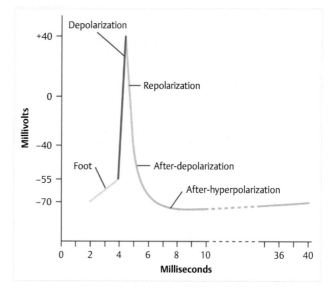

Fig. 4.3 Neuron action potential steps. (Reproduced with permission from Michael J, Sircar S. Fundamentals of Medical Physiology. © Thieme 2011.)

- Cell membrane permeability to K^+, Na^+, and chloride ions (Cl^-).
- Osmotic pressure (selective membrane permeability to water but not all solute particles).
- Example: Na^+–K^+ pump carrier "transport" proteins move large numbers of Na^+ out of the cell, creating a positive extracellular charge. Simultaneously, these proteins move some K^+ into the cell's cytoplasm. The cell becomes positive on the outside and negative on the inside because more Na^+ ions are moved outside the cell than K^+ ions are moved inside.
- If a resting neuron is adequately stimulated, the neuron will transmit an impulse or signal known as an **action potential**.
  - An **action potential** is the movement of ions across the neuron's membrane resulting in (1) rapid depolarization (charge moves toward 0 mV; i.e., no difference in charge) followed by (2) repolarization, (3) brief hyperpolarization (overshoot, meaning greater than −70 mV), and return to (4) normal resting potential of −70 mV. Nerve impulses are transmitted via action potentials.
  - Steps of an action potential (▶ Fig. 4.3, also see example below):
    - Step #1: **Depolarization**—resultant from a "sufficient" stimulus
      - If the signal is strong enough for the membrane to reach the threshold level of −55 mV (threshold potential), an action potential will be triggered.
      - Depolarization is opening of neuron membrane Na^+ channels, allowing extracellular Na^+ to rush into the cell.
      - These Na^+ channels are called **voltage-gated ion channels** because they can open and close in response to an electrical signal.
      - Threshold level stimulation activates opening of numerous voltage-gated ion channels. The amount of

Na^+ inside the cell increases and the cell membrane charge reverses (i.e., the inside of the cell becomes positively charged and the outside becomes negatively charged).
      - A stimulus may be generated by activation of sensory receptor organs (e.g., mechanically gated channels) or
      - By neurotransmitter release at a synapse (ligand gated channels).
    - Step #2: **Repolarization**—when the intracellular membrane potential reaches approximately + 30 mV ("peak action potential"), the voltage-gated Na^+ channels close and voltage-gated K^+ channels open.
      - Potassium ions move outside the cell membrane and Na^+ stays inside. This rapidly repolarizes the cell. However, the resulting polarization is now due to a greater amount of intracellular Na^+ versus K^+ (the Na^+–K^+ ion ratio is different compared to the initial "resting potential" polarization).
      - **Absolute refractory** period:
        - The cell membranes are unable to depolarize while the membrane potential is above −55 mV (occurs during depolarization and the initial part of repolarization).
      - **Relative refractory** period:
        - Occurs near the latter aspect of the repolarization phase as the membrane potential moves toward −55 mV.
        - The K^+ channels close.
    - Step #3: **Hyperpolarization** (i.e., the membrane potential moves lower than normal resting potential of > −70 mV; i.e., it "overshoots"). This is due to a brief increase in intracellular Na^+ ions relative to the normal resting potential ratio of Na^+–K^+ ions.

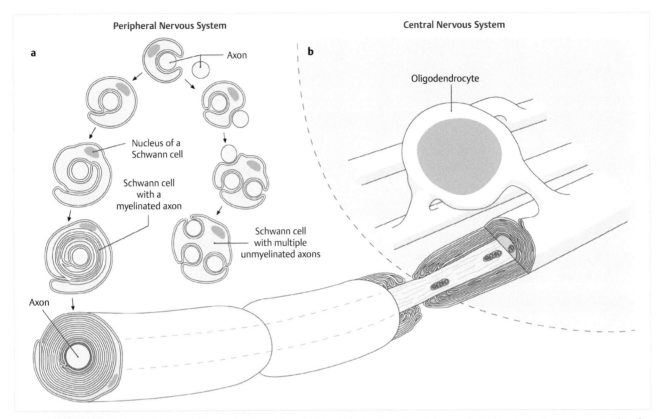

Peripheral Nervous System

Central Nervous System

a

Axon

Nucleus of a
Schwann cell

Schwann cell
with a
myelinated axon

Schwann cell
with multiple
unmyelinated axons

Axon

b

Oligodendrocyte

Fig. 4.4 (a,b) Myelinated axon with nodes of Ranvier. (Reproduced with permission from Schuenke M, Schulte E, Schumacher U. THIEME Atlas of Anatomy Third Edition, Vol 3. © Thieme 2020. Illustrations by Markus Voll and Karl Wesker.)

- The Na$^+$–K$^+$ pump moves intracellular Na$^+$ ions out to the extracellular environment in exchange for K$^+$ ions. This returns the neuron membrane to its normal intracellular Na$^+$–K$^+$ ion ratio and polarized resting state.
- The Na$^+$–K$^+$ ion exchange helps to re-establish diffusion gradients and resting potential.
  □ The Na$^+$–K$^+$ pump is not directly involved in the firing of an action potential.
- The relative refractory period continues during this step.
– Step #4: **Resting potential**—the membrane potential returns to –70 mV. Resting potential is restored and the relative refractory period ends.
○ Important concepts of neuron signaling:
– The **refractory period** ensures that an **action potential** will only travel forward. As an action potential moves forward along an axon, a new action potential is incapable of occurring until the membrane resting potential is re-established behind it. This limits the number of signals/impulses a neuron can generate over a period of time.
  - During the **absolute refractory** period, an action potential **cannot be produced** regardless of the stimulus strength. Voltage-gated Na$^+$ channels are either already open or inactivated, thus making them incapable of producing an action potential.
  - During the **relative refractory** period, voltage-gated Na + channels are recovering from inactivation. If the

neuron receives a sufficiently strong stimulus (greater than normal), it may generate another action potential.
– **Saltatory conduction** (from Latin *saltare*, meaning "to leap"): Myelinated axons conduct signals faster than unmyelinated due to a phenomenon known as saltatory conduction.
  - In unmyelinated axons, Na$^+$ channels must open sequentially along the axon for the signal to propagate.
  - Myelinated axons enable the signal to continue along the axon through myelin insulated segments without the need for channel opening. Sodium channel opening only occurs periodically at uninsulated spots along the axon known as "**nodes of Ranvier**" (▶ Fig. 4.4).
- **Oligodendrocytes** are cells in the central nervous system that myelinate multiple neurons.
- **Schwan cells** are in peripheral nervous system; they myelinate individual neurons.

4.4 Synapses

- Neurons communicate by conducting signals from one to another using connections known as **synapses**. The number of synapses between neurons in the brain are believed to be in the "trillions."
- Connections occur in several different ways:
  ○ Between axons (axoaxonic synapse),
  ○ Between an axon and a cell body (axosomatic), or
  ○ Between an axon and a dendrite (axodendritic).

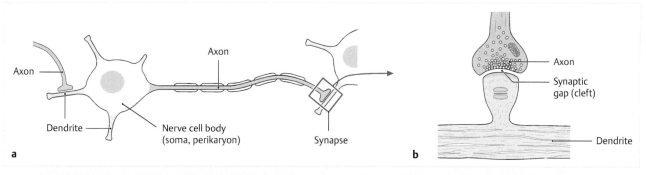

Fig. 4.5 (a,b) Neuron chemical synapse. (Reproduced with permission from Schuenke M, Schulte E, Schumacher U. THIEME Atlas of Anatomy Second Edition, Vol 3. © Thieme 2016. Illustrations by Markus Voll and Karl Wesker.)

- Synapses are either electrical (signal is transmitted from one cell to the other via polarization change) or chemical (signal is transmitted using neurotransmitters/chemicals). The majority of synapses are chemical.
  - **Electrical synapses** consist of a direct physical connection (**gap junction**) between the two neurons which allows ions to flow directly from one cell to the next.
    - Electrical synapses enable the fastest form of communication between neurons.
    - These synapses allow bidirectional signaling (current can flow either way).
    - Groups of neurons connected by electrical synapses are capable of firing together in a synchronized fashion.
    - Electrical synapses lack the ability to modulate signaling (they are unable to vary signal intensity or alter signal type—excitatory versus inhibitory).
  - **Chemical synapses** consist of (Fig. 4.5):
    - A neuron with a **presynaptic ending** that contains neurotransmitter filled vesicles,
    - A neuron with a **postsynaptic ending** that contains neurotransmitter **receptors** located in the cell membrane, and
    - A **synaptic cleft** between these two specialized "endings."
- A neuron action potential (electrical signal) triggers the presynaptic neuron to release **neurotransmitters** (chemical signal). These molecules bind to receptors on the postsynaptic cell which facilitates action potential firing or inhibition in the postsynaptic neuron (▶ Fig. 4.5).
  - Chemical synapses are slower to transmit impulses than electrical synapses due to the time it takes for the process of neurotransmitter release and reception to occur.
  - Neurotransmitter signaling may make the postsynaptic neuron either more *or* less likely to reach an action potential (excitatory postsynaptic potential neurotransmitter [EPSP] or inhibitory postsynaptic potential neurotransmitter [IPSP]) (▶ Fig. 4.6).
  - Neuron signaling intensity can vary. It may be influenced by the amount of neurotransmitter released and number of receptors available. Changes in these two factors also are important for **neuroplasticity.**
    - Neuroplasticity is associated with physiologic changes in the neuron, such as:

- Changes in production of amount of neurotransmitter chemicals in presynaptic endings.
- Changes in number of receptors available on postsynaptic endings.
- Changes in numbers of axons or dendrites on a neuron.
- Changes in number of neurons (growth).

4.5 Neurotransmitters and Receptors

Neurotransmitters are the essential molecules used by neurons for converting electrical signals (action potentials) into chemical-based communication signals at synapses. Neurotransmitters are sometimes referred to as **neurocrines** (neuron secretions).

- Release of a neurotransmitter at a chemical synapse occurs when an action potential reaches the terminal end of an axon.
  - The action potential opens voltage-gated Ca^{2+} channels in the axon membrane adjacent to the synaptic vesicles.
    - The Ca^{2+} influx facilitates vesicle fusion to the membrane and subsequent neurotransmitter release.
      - These synaptic vesicles are recycled by the cell.
  - There are at least 50 known neurotransmitters and even greater numbers and variability in postsynaptic receptors for these chemicals.
    - The study of neurotransmission is an area where knowledge is rapidly expanding and changing.
  - The important basic concepts that need to be understood about neurotransmitters include:
    - Most prevalent types of presynaptic chemicals (neurotransmitters) released,
    - Categories of postsynaptic receptors, and
    - The general effects these substances have on nerve cell Ionotropic receptors change shape activity.
    (See ▶ Table 4.1 for a summary of the most common, well-known neurotransmitters.)
- **Neurotransmitter receptors** are located in the postsynaptic cell membrane. These receptors have specific neurotransmitter bonding sites which facilitate signal transmission between cells. There are two broad receptor classifications:

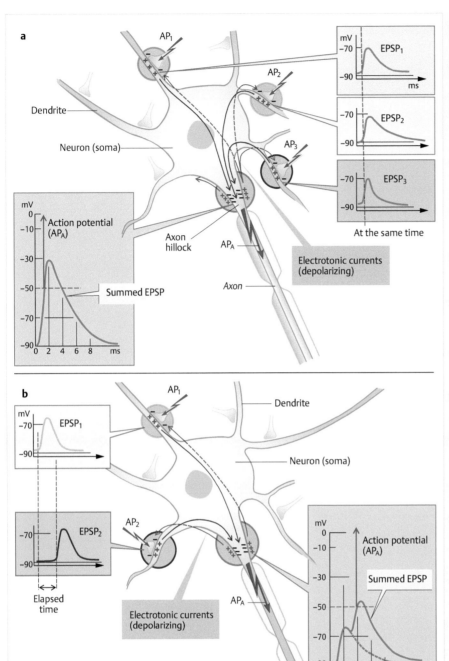

Fig. 4.6 (a,b) Examples of an action potential created by summation of excitatory neurotransmitter signaling. (Reproduced with permission from TannerThies R. Physiology: An Illustrated Review. © Thieme 2012.)

○ **Ionotropic receptors** (ligand-activated ion channels, see ▶ Fig. 4.7):
 – These **integral carrier proteins** span the postsynaptic cell membrane and respond to the binding of a specific neurotransmitter (also known as a ligand or molecule/ion).
  ▪ Ionotropic receptors change shape when a neurotransmitter binds to them. The change in shape creates a small channel opening that only allows a specific ion to flow through.

 ▪ Typically, K+, Na+, Cl−, and Ca2+ ions travel through ionotropic receptors.
 ▪ Ionotropic receptors are quick to open and close. The ion flow stops as soon as the neurotransmitter is no longer bound to its receptors.
  □ In most cases, the neurotransmitter is rapidly removed from the synapse by enzyme breakdown or neighboring cell reuptake.

Table 4.1 Common neurotransmitters

Neurotransmitter	Receptor Type	Nervous System	Functional Role
Unique chemical class			
Acetylcholine (ACh) secreted by cholinergic neurons	Ionotropic (nicotinic) GCPR (muscarinic)	PNS (neuromuscular junction), CNS, ANS	Enables muscle contraction, learning, and memory; both excitatory and inhibitory functions
Amines (basic nitrogenous compounds formed mainly by decarboxylation of amino acids)			
Norepinephrine (secreted by adrenergic /noradrenergic neurons)	GCPR	ANS, CNS	Alertness and arousal; both excitatory and inhibitory functions
Dopamine	GPCR	CNS	Reward activity/motivation; influences movement, learning, attention, and emotion; primarily inhibitory
Serotonin (5-hydroxytryptamine or 5-HT)	Ionotropic GPCR	CNS	Regulates mood, anxiety, appetite, sleep cycle, and body temperature; inhibits pain pathways in the spinal cord; involved in circadian rhythmicity and neuroendocrine function; primarily inhibitory
Histamine	GPCR	CNS	Increases wakefulness, stomach acid production, and itchiness, decreases hunger; primarily excitatory
Amino acids			
GABA (gamma-aminobutyric acid)	Ionotropic GPCR	CNS	Decreases anxiety and muscle tone, increases relaxation and sedation; helps improve focus; major inhibitory function
Glutamate	Ionotropic GPCR	CNS	Involved with learning and memory; involved with synapse development; major excitatory function
Purines (water-soluble nitrogen base molecules)			
Adenosine (atypical—not stored in vesicles, not released by exocytosis)	GPCR	CNS	Promotes sleep and suppresses arousal; inhibitory function
Gases			
Nitric oxide (atypical—not stored in vesicles and not released by exocytosis)	Unique "gasotransmitter" (diffuses through cell membrane)	CNS	Modulates release of other neurotransmitters; involved in learning and memory through the maintenance of long-term potentiation; primarily excitatory

Abbreviations: ANS, autonomic nervous system; CNS, central nervous system; GCPR, G-protein coupled receptors (also known as metabotropic receptors); PNS, peripheral nervous system.

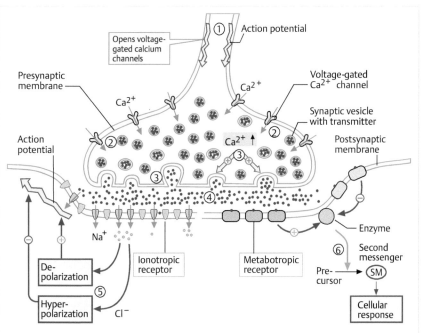

Fig. 4.7 Ionotropic (ligand-activated ion channel pathway, left side) and metabotropic (G-protein coupled receptor/second messenger pathway, right side). (Reproduced with permission from TannerThies R. Physiology: An Illustrated Review. © Thieme 2012.)

□ Receptors may have multiple subtypes which allow one neurotransmitter to have different effects on different cells.

○ **G-protein coupled receptors** (also known as metabotropic receptors, see ▶ Fig. 4.7):

– These are secondary signaling receptors, not ion channels.

▪ Neurotransmitter binding to the receptor triggers a G-protein signaling pathway.

▪ The G-protein activates one or more other molecules known as "secondary messengers."

▪ Ion channels may be opened *or* closed (or some other effect such as shape change) because of this secondary signaling.

– Once activated, the secondary messengers can travel throughout the cell and create a wider range of responses than ionotropic receptors.

□ The multistep pathway (the steps vary per receptor) results in a slower response time.

□ G-protein coupled receptors may be longer acting in some cases.

– G-protein coupled receptors may have multiple subtypes which allow the same neurotransmitter to have different effects on different cells (similar to ionotropic receptors).

○ There are several known "unique" neurotransmitters that do not require a cell membrane receptor. They simply diffuse through the cell membrane and act directly on molecules inside the cell.

– In addition, these molecules are not stored in synaptic vesicles. They include:

▪ Endocannabinoids and

▪ Gasotransmitters (soluble gases such as nitric oxide and carbon monoxide).

4.6 Clinical Correlations

Lidocaine is an injectable local anesthetic agent. It blocks fast voltage-gated sodium channels in the cell membrane of postsynaptic neurons. This prevents neuron depolarization through inhibition of action potential generation and propagation. Neurons are unable to transmit any signal, including nociceptive.

Oromandibular dystonia is a condition characterized by uncontrollable, forceful contractions/spasms of mastication muscles and/or tongue muscles. Difficulty in opening and closing the mouth creates mastication and speech related problems. Most individuals with this diagnosis experience decreased spasms and improved chewing and speech after **botulinum toxin** injection into the affected mandibular muscles. Botulinum toxin prevents neurotransmitter filled vesicles from attaching and fusing to the presynaptic cell membrane. This prevents neuron signals from reaching the muscles.

Guillain-Barré syndrome (also known as acute inflammatory demyelinating polyneuropathy) is an autoimmune disease characterized by progressive demyelination of peripheral nerves. Demyelination of a neuron will severely limit or prevent signal conduction through disruption of Na^+, K^+, and Ca^{2+} ion channel function. This creates a metabolic crisis in the cell. Guillain-Barré syndrome is believed to be triggered by an improper immune response to a prior illness, most commonly associated with a respiratory infection or a bacterial infection related episode of diarrhea (*Campylobacter jejuni*). Numbness, paresthesia, weakness, pain in the limbs, or some combination of these symptoms is frequently reported by individuals with this diagnosis. The primary sign of Guillain-Barré syndrome is progressive bilateral and relatively symmetric limb weakness progressing (sometimes to complete paralysis) over a period of 12 hours to 4 weeks. Individuals typically recover slowly over a 6- to 12-month period.

Questions and Answers

1. Which of the following central nervous system neurotransmitters is primarily excitatory in function?
   a) Norepinephrine
   b) Adenosine
   c) Dopamine
   d) Glutamate

Level 1: Easy

Answer D: Most commonly known as "monosodium glutamate" or "MSG," a flavor or taste enhancer used in food. It is the primary mediator of excitatory signals in the mammalian central nervous system and is involved in most aspects of normal brain function including cognition, memory and learning. Glutamate also regulates brain development and information related to cell survival, differentiation and elimination as well as neuron synapse formation and pruning. Amount and timing of glutamate available directly affects these functions. Either too much and too little glutamate can be deleterious for normal nervous system development and function. Thus, glutamate is essential yet potentially harmful. **(A)** Norepinephrine has both excitatory and inhibitory functions. **(B)** Adenosine has primarily inhibitory functions. **(C)** Dopamine has primarily inhibitory functions.

2. An electrical synapse exhibits this unique characteristic:
   a) Allows bidirectional signaling
   b) Ability to alter signal intensity
   c) Slower signaling process relative to a chemical synapse
   d) Inability to propagate a signal unless the neuron is myelinated

Level 1: Easy

Answer A: Although much less common than chemical synapses, electrical synapses are found in all nervous systems, including the human brain. Electrical synapses are characterized by gap junctions between pre- and postsynaptic membranes which permit current to flow passively through intercellular channels. The current flow enables postsynaptic membrane potential change which initiates (or in some instances inhibits) a postsynaptic action potential. **(B)** Electrical synapses do not have the ability alter signal intensity. **(C)** Fewer steps are involved with electrical synapses relative to chemical, therefore, electrical synapses transmit signals fastest. **(D)** Myelination does not influence the ability of the gap junctions to transmit the signal between neurons, it does affect speed of signal transmission along an axon.

3. A neuron cell membrane is best described as being comprised of:
   a) Monosaccharides and nucleic acids

b) Proteins, amino acids, and monosaccharides
c) Lipids, proteins, and cholesterol
d) Amino acids, lipids, and proteins

Level 2: Moderate

Answer C: Neuron membrane contains lipid bilayers, cholesterol (affects permeability and flexibility), and proteins (function as channels, receptors, support, etc.). **(A)** Monosaccharides are the simplest form of a carbohydrate. Nucleic acids are components of RNA and DNA. **(B)** Amino acids are the building blocks of protein, but are not found in isolation in the cell membrane. **(D)** See "b" for explanation.

4. G-protein coupled receptors only are *specifically* known for which of the following?
   a) A multi-step signaling pathway
   b) Quick to open and close
   c) A change in shape when a neurotransmitter binds to them
   d) Multiple subtypes which allow one neurotransmitter to have different effects

Level 2: Moderate

Answer A: These are secondary signaling receptors, not ion channels. When a neurotransmitter binds to a G-protein coupled receptor, a multi-step pathway is triggered. The G-protein activates one or more other molecules known as "secondary messengers." Once activated, the secondary messengers can travel throughout the cell and create a wider range of responses than ionotropic receptors. The multi-step pathway (the steps vary per receptor) results in a slower response time and may be longer acting in some cases. **(B)** Slower to open and/or close due to the multi-step pathway. **(C)** This occurs with ionotropic receptors (ligand-activated ion channels). **(D)** Occurs with both ionotropic and G-protein receptors.

5. If a patient receives a medication that prevents neuron depolarization by blocking fast voltage-gated sodium channels in the cell membrane, what sign or symptom will they be most likely to experience?
   a) Spasm of the muscles innervated by the affected nerve
   b) Paralysis of the muscles innervated by the affected nerve
   c) Profuse sweating in the area innervated by the affected nerve
   d) Hypersensitivity to touch in the area innervated by the affected nerve

Level 2: Moderate

Answer B: Blockage of fast voltage-gated sodium channels in the cell membrane of a neuron will prevent depolarization through inhibition of action potential generation and propagation. As a result, the neuron will be unable to transmit any signal (motor, sensory, or autonomic). **(A)** The muscle must be receiving motor input signaling to spasm. **(C)** Autonomic signals (sympathetic) must be propagated through the nerve to produce sweating. **(D)** Sensory (afferent) signals must be able to be propagated through the nerve to allow sensation. In this case, the individual would experience anesthesia (numbness).

Unit II

Gross Anatomy of Brain and Spinal Cord

5 Gross Topography of the Brain

5.1 Overview

The brain is composed of two cerebral hemispheres, the brainstem, and the cerebellum. These structures develop from the embryonic neural tube, which ultimately differentiates into five vesicles: **telencephalon**, **diencephalon**, **mesencephalon**, **metencephalon,** and the **myelencephalon** (▶ Fig. 5.1). The telencephalon is made up of the cerebral cortex and related subcortical structures. The diencephalon is made up of the **thalamus**, **hypothalamus**, **epithalamus,** and **subthalamus**. The mesencephalon (**midbrain**) is composed of several structures located in close proximity to the cerebral aqueduct such as the **mesencephalic reticular area**, **red nucleus**, **substantia nigra**, and motor and sensory pathways among others. The metencephalon includes the **pons** and **cerebellum**. The myelencephalon is made up of the **medulla** along with associated nuclei and pathways. The mesencephalon, metencephalon, and myelencephalon collectively make up what is known as the **brainstem**.

5.2 Neuroanatomical Terms

- Planes (▶ Fig. 5.2)
  - **Sagittal plane**: Divides the body into two symmetrical halves.
  - **Parasagittal plane**: Parallel to the sagittal plane.
  - **Frontal/coronal plane**: Perpendicular to the sagittal plane. Separates the body into anterior and posterior equal halves.
- Axes (▶ Fig. 5.3)
  - **Rostrocaudal:** Early in development, the human embryo has a linear axis. In this model, **rostral** means the front of the brain and **caudal** indicates the back of the brain. However, due to flexures that are produced in the developing central nervous system (CNS), the axes change. In humans, a prominent flexure develops at the level of the midbrain that changes the axis from linear to a more curved orientation. This means that at or below the level of the midbrain, rostral is toward the cortex and caudal is toward the sacrum.
  - **Dorsoventral:** Rostral to the midbrain, dorsal indicates the top of the brain and ventral refers to the bottom of the brain. At the level of the flexure/midbrain or inferiorly, the term **superior** is often used rather than **dorsal,** and **inferior** rather than **ventral**. At the level of the lower medulla/spinal cord, the **neuroaxis** is once again linear so ventral (**anterior**) and dorsal (**posterior**) are appropriate.

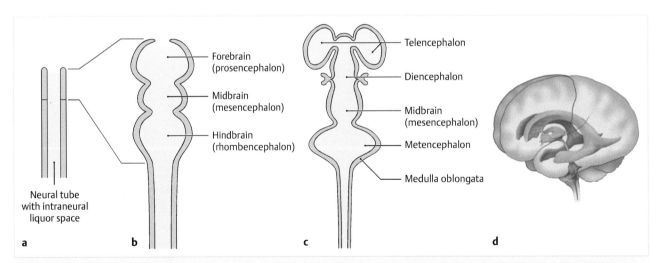

Fig. 5.1 **(a)** Undifferentiated neural tube. **(b)** Three primary vesicles develop from the undifferentiated neural tube. **(c)** Five secondary vesicles develop from the primary vesicles. **(d)** The secondary vesicles eventually differentiate into adult structures. Note: The cavity of the neural tube also differentiates at the same time resulting in the formation of the four ventricles (I–IV) and the connecting as well as the aqueduct which leads to the central canal of the spinal cord. (Reproduced with permission from Schuenke M, Schulte E, Schumacher U. THIEME Atlas of Anatomy. Second Edition, Vol 3. © Thieme 2016. Illustrations by Markus Voll and Karl Wesker.)

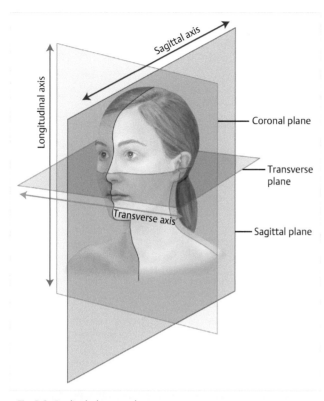

Fig. 5.2 Cardinal planes and axes.

○ **Flexures**: Differential growth of the neural tube produces flexures in the developing embryo during weeks 4 to 5 (▶ Fig. 5.4). The cephalic flexure is the only one that persists later in development.
  – **Cephalic:** Between midbrain and hindbrain.
  – **Pontine:** Between metencephalon and myelencephalon.
  – **Cervical:** Between the brain and spinal cord.

5.3 Telencephalon

• The cerebral hemispheres are the largest component of the human brain. The outer layer is called the **cortex**, which is made up of neurons and supporting cells. It is commonly referred to as the **gray matter** due to its gray color. Deep to the gray matter is the **white matter** which is composed of myelinated tracts. It is the myelinated fibers that give it the white-ish color.
• The cerebral hemispheres are separated by a long, deep midline groove known as the **longitudinal (sagittal) fissure** (▶ Fig. 5.5).
• The convoluted appearance of the cerebral hemispheres is due to ridges called **sulci** and the grooves between them known as **fissures**.
  ○ The presence of the sulci and gyri serves to increase the surface area of the cortex.
  ○ Approximately two-thirds of the cortex is hidden by the convoluted surface.

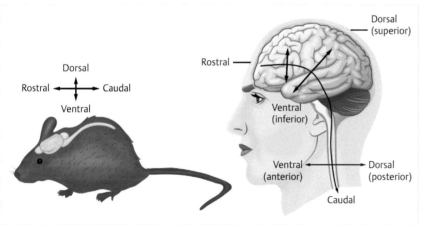

Fig. 5.3 Axes of the CNS in a rat (linear orientation) and a human whose CNS has a flexure in the midbrain, changing the axis in that area. CNS, central nervous system.

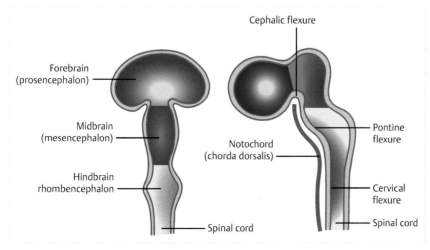

Fig. 5.4 Flexures arise in the neural tube changing the orientation of the developing embryo.

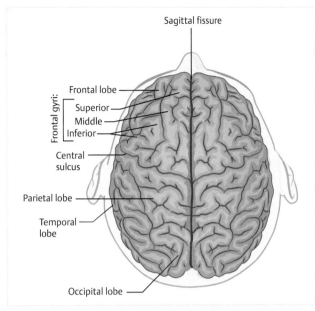

Fig. 5.5 A deep midline groove (sagittal fissure) separates the cerebral hemispheres.

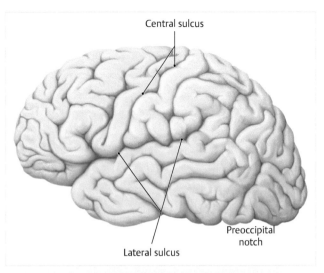

Fig. 5.6 Cerebrum. Left lateral view. The surface anatomy of the cerebrum can be divided macroscopically into four lobes: frontal, parietal, temporal, and occipital. The surface contours of the cerebrum are defined by convolutions (gyri) and depressions (sulci). (Reproduced with permission from Schuenke M, Schulte E, Schumacher U. THIEME Atlas of Anatomy Third Edition, Vol 3. © Thieme 2020. Illustrations by Markus Voll and Karl Wesker.)

Table 5.1 Functions of the cerebrum

Brain Structure	Lobe	Function
Cerebrum (telencephalon)	Frontal	Motor movement; motor aspect of speech (Broca's area); reasoning; personality; problem solving
	Parietal	Sensory perceptions related to pain, temperature, touch, and pressure; spatial orientation and perception; sensory aspect of language (Wernicke's area)
	Temporal	Auditory perceptions; learning; memory
	Occipital	Vision
	Insula	Associated with visceral functions, e.g., taste

(Reproduced with permission from Baker EW. Anatomy for Dental Medicine. Second Edition. © Thieme 2017)

- Gyri and sulci are somewhat variable between individuals; however, there are several that are fairly consistent and will be discussed in this chapter, particularly those that define the lobes of the cortex.
  - The **central**, **parieto-occipital**, and **lateral sulci** as well as the **preoccipital notch** are used as boundaries to demarcate the **frontal**, **parietal**, **temporal**, and **occipital lobes** of the cerebral hemispheres (▶ Fig. 5.6) (▶ Table 5.1).
- Main sulci
  - Central sulcus
    - Separates the motor (**precentral gyrus**) and the sensory strip (**postcentral gyrus**).
    - Separates the frontal from the parietal lobe.
    - Runs from the superior margin of the hemisphere, approximately at the midpoint, and continues inferiorly at a slightly oblique angle (inferiorly and anteriorly), until it meets the lateral fissure.

- Parieto-occipital sulcus
  - Lies on the medial aspect of the brain.
  - Begins on superior margin of cortex and passes inferiorly and anteriorly to meet the **calcarine sulcus**.
  - Separates the parietal lobe from the occipital lobe.
- Lateral sulcus
  - Separates the frontal and parietal lobes from the temporal lobe.
  - Mainly visible on the inferior and lateral surface of the brain.
  - The **insula** lies deep to the lateral sulcus. This structure cannot be viewed unless the lateral sulcus is separated.
- Preoccipital notch
  - Formed by the petrous ridge of the temporal bone, it can be seen as an indentation in the inferior temporal gyrus.
  - Located on the lateral surface of the temporal lobe.
  - Contributes to the delineation of the occipital lobe by drawing an arbitrary line from the superior aspect of the parieto-occipital sulcus to the preoccipital notch (parietotemporal lateral line).
- Lobes and main gyri
  - Frontal lobe (▶ Fig. 5.7)
    - Largest of the cerebral lobes.
    - Lies anterior to the central sulcus and superior to the lateral sulcus.
    - Composed of four gyri:
      - **Precentral gyrus** that parallels the central sulcus.
      - Three horizontal gyri: **superior**, **middle**, and **inferior frontal gyri.**
    - The gyri of the frontal lobe create functional areas (▶ Fig. 5.8):
      - Primary motor cortex (M1)
        - Origin of the corticospinal tract as well as part of the corticobulbar tract. Sends projections to the basal ganglia and the thalamus.

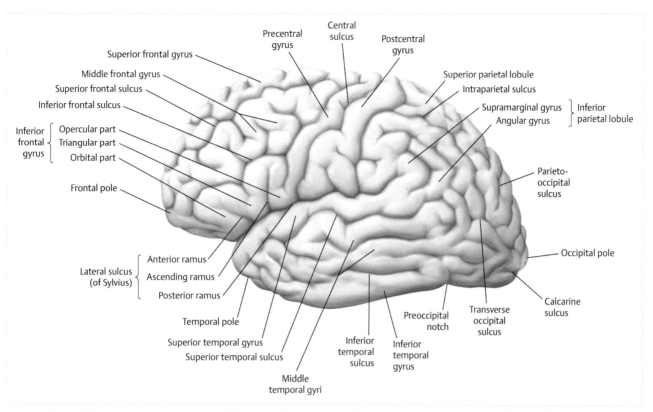

Fig. 5.7 Frontal lobe lies anterior to the central sulcus and superior to the lateral sulcus. Gyri includes: superior, middle, and inferior frontal gyrus. (Reproduced with permission from Gilroy AM, MacPherson BR. Atlas of Anatomy. Third Edition. © Thieme 2016. Illustrations by Markus Voll and Karl Wesker.)

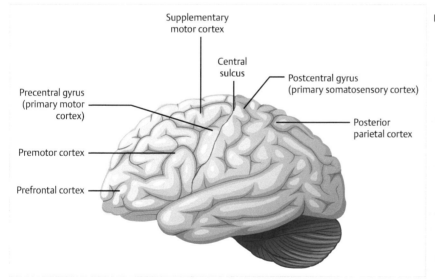

Fig. 5.8 Functional areas of the frontal lobe.

- ▫ The precentral gyrus is **somatotopically** arranged creating a **motor homunculus**. Somatotopy refers to specific areas of the motor strip that are functionally associated with specific and distinct areas of the body (▶ Fig. 5.9).
- ▪ **Premotor cortex (PMC)**
- ▫ Lies immediately anterior to the precentral gyrus and has many of the same connections as the motor strip.

Most of the output from the premotor cortex is to the precentral gyrus with some projections to the brainstem and spinal cord. It receives input from the sensory cortex as well as the basal ganglia by way of the thalamus. The premotor cortex is critical for the planning of movement and selection of appropriate responses based on learned associations.

- ▪ **Supplemental motor area (SMA)**

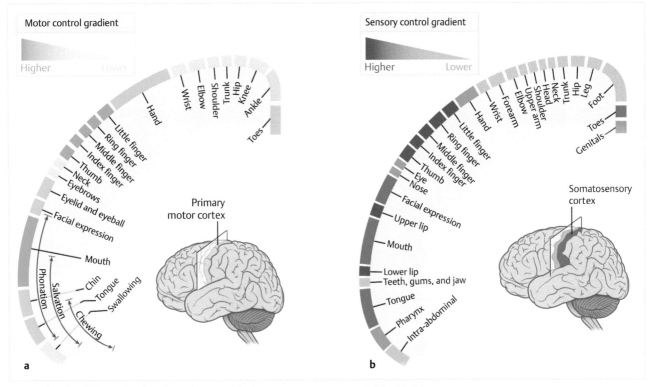

Fig. 5.9 (a,b) The precentral gyrus is somatotopically arranged creating a motor homunculus.

□ Extension of the premotor cortex that reaches to the medial aspect of the hemisphere. Outputs from the SMA project to the precentral gyrus, basal ganglia, and thalamus. It also has connections to the contralateral SMA. Function includes complex motor tasks and coordinating movements of both hands. Studies have shown that this area becomes active prior to movement and is thought to be involved in the initiation of movement.

- **Frontal eye fields**
  □ Located in the middle frontal gyrus and part of the inferior frontal gyrus rostral to the premotor area.
  □ Involved in voluntary eye movement. Initiates gaze response to stimuli.
- **Broca's area**
  □ Part of the inferior frontal gyrus on the dominant side (usually the left). It is involved in the motor aspects of speech (▶ Fig. 5.10) (Clinical Correlation Box 5.1).

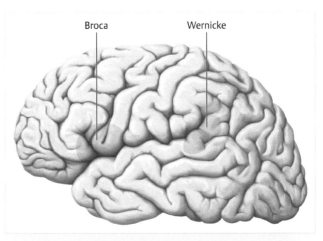

Fig. 5.10 Broca's area is located (partially) in the inferior frontal gyrus. It is involved in the motor aspects of speech. (Reproduced with permission from Schuenke M, Schulte E, Schumacher U. THIEME Atlas of Anatomy Third Edition, Vol 3. © Thieme 2020. Illustrations by Markus Voll and Karl Wesker.)

Clinical Correlation Box 5.1: Broca's Aphasia

People with Broca's aphasia have difficulty speaking while their comprehension remains intact. These individuals have problems with grammar and their spoken sentences are very short. They may understand speech fairly well, especially if it is grammatically simple. More complex sentence structure is challenging for them. Patients may be able to read but writing is usually limited. This type of aphasia is the result of damage to the dominant inferior frontal gyrus (usually the left).

- **Prefrontal cortex (PFC)**
  □ The remainder of the frontal lobe is called the **prefrontal cortex**.
  □ It is very well developed in humans and continues to develop postnatally. It deals with activities such as decision-making, planning complex cognitive behavior, personality expression, and social behavior (**executive function**).

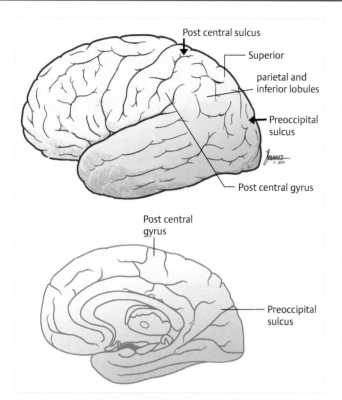

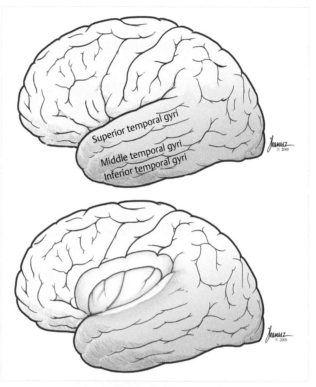

Fig. 5.11 The parietal lobe lies posterior to the central sulcus and extends to the parietal-occipital sulcus. The inferolateral boundary is the lateral sulcus. (Modified with permission from Alberstone CD, Benzel EC, Najm IM, et al. Anatomic Basis of Neurologic Diagnosis. © Thieme 2009.)

Fig. 5.12 The temporal lobe lies inferior to the lateral sulcus. It contains the superior, middle, and inferior temporal gyri. (Modified with permission from Alberstone CD, Benzel EC, Najm IM, et al. Anatomic Basis of Neurologic Diagnosis. © Thieme 2009.)

- □ It can also be subdivided functionally, although less consistent, and lesions in these areas produce mixed symptoms.
  - ✓ **Lateral PFC:** Cognitive support for behavior, speech, and reasoning.
  - ✓ **Medial PFC:** Motility, attention, and emotion.
  - ✓ **Inferior PFC:** Personality
- ○ **Parietal lobe**
  - – The parietal lobe lies posterior to the central sulcus and continues posteriorly to the parietal-occipital sulcus located on the medial surface. From the lateral surface, the posterior border is an "imaginary line that is drawn from the parieto-occipital sulcus on the superior margin to the **preoccipital notch** on the inferior margin of the hemisphere." The inferolateral boundary is the lateral sulcus, which separates it from the temporal lobe (▶ Fig. 5.11).
  - – The lateral surface is divided into the **postcentral gyrus** and **superior and inferior lobules**.
    - ▪ The postcentral gyrus (S1) is posterior to the central sulcus and parallels it. It extends posteriorly to the **postcentral sulcus**. It is the primary somatosensory cortex and receives sensory information from the body and viscera. It also receives proprioceptive information.
    - ▪ The inferior parietal lobule contains **Wernicke's area**, which is important in comprehension of language and reading (language input) (Clinical Correlation Box 5.2).
    - ▪ The superior parietal lobule is involved in spatial orientation and body image.
- ○ **Temporal lobe** (▶ Fig. 5.12)

- – It occupies the cortex inferior to the lateral sulcus.
- – It contains the **superior**, **middle**, and **inferior temporal gyri**.
- – A portion of the superior aspect of the temporal lobe (superior temporal gyrus) is known as the **primary auditory cortex**.
- – Wernicke's area also encompasses the posterior part of the superior temporal gyrus of one hemisphere (usually the left). Thus, Wernicke's area is made up of part of the inferior parietal gyrus and portions of the superior temporal gyrus.
- – A significant amount of the temporal lobe (especially the inferior aspect) is involved in higher order processing of visual information.
- – The medial aspect of the temporal lobe is involved in learning and memory.

Clinical Correlation Box 5.2: Wernicke's Aphasia

Individuals with this disorder have difficulty grasping the meaning of spoken word. Their ability to produce speech is not impaired although much of what they say does not make sense. Reading and writing may be affected. Intellectual and cognitive abilities are intact. This condition is the result of damage to specific parts of the temporal and parietal lobes known as Wernicke's area.

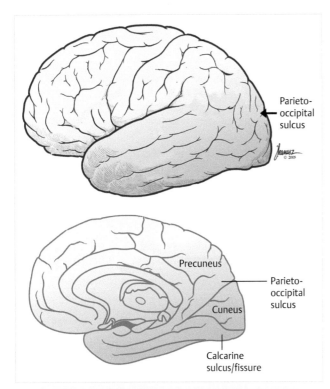

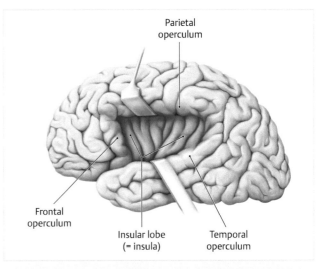

Fig. 5.14 Insular cortex. Lateral view of the retracted left cerebral hemisphere. Part of the cerebral cortex sinks below the surface during development forming the insula (or insular lobe). (Reproduced with permission from Schuenke M, Schulte E, Schumacher U. THIEME Atlas of Anatomy Third Edition, Vol 3. © Thieme 2020. Illustrations by Markus Voll and Karl Wesker.)

Fig. 5.13 The occipital lobe lies posterior to the parieto-occipital sulcus. (Modified with permission from Alberstone CD, Benzel EC, Najm IM, et al. Anatomic Basis of Neurologic Diagnosis. © Thieme 2009.)

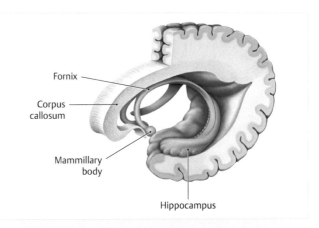

Fig. 5.15 The limbic system, which exchanges and integrates information between the telencephalon, diencephalon, and mesencephalon, regulates drive and affective behavior and plays a crucial role in memory. (Reproduced with permission from Schuenke M, Schulte E, Schumacher U. THIEME Atlas of Anatomy Third Edition, Vol 3. © Thieme 2020. Illustrations by Markus Voll and Karl Wesker.)

○ **Occipital lobe** (▶ Fig. 5.13)
  – Located posterior to the parieto-occipital sulcus and lies on the **tentorium cerebelli**.
  – Prominent fissures present on the medial aspect define the **cuneus**. The cuneus receives visual information from the opposite visual field.
    ▪ **Calcarine fissure/sulcus**
      □ Location of the primary visual cortex (within walls).
    ▪ **Parieto-occipital sulcus**
      □ Separates occipital from parietal lobe.
      □ Divides cuneus from precuneas.
  – Remainder of the lobe is referred to as the **visual association cortex**.
    ▪ Visual association cortex also extends into the temporal lobe.
    ▪ Interprets signals and recognizes forms.
○ **Insular cortex** (▶ Fig. 5.14)
  – Lies deep to the lateral sulcus. Can only be seen if lateral sulcus is retracted.
  – Represents fusion of the telencephalon and diencephalon during embryonic development.
  – Thought to be involved in nociception, regulation of the autonomic nervous system (ANS), homeostasis, speech production, and emotions.
○ **Limbic lobe**
  – Located on the inferomedial aspect of the cerebral hemispheres.
  – Not a "true" lobe but made up of several cortical regions and subcortical structures including the **hippocampus**,

amygdala, **septal nuclei**, **cingulate cortex,** and **parahippocampal cortex** (▶ Fig. 5.15).
  – The **hippocampus** is a forebrain structure located within the medial temporal lobe.
  – The **amygdala** is located within the anterior temporal lobe within the **uncus**. It lies anterior to the hippocampus.
  – **Septal nuclei** are subcortical nuclei that have connections to emotion generating areas.
  – The **cingulate cortex** is located on the medial aspect of the cerebral cortex and is a subset of the limbic cortex.

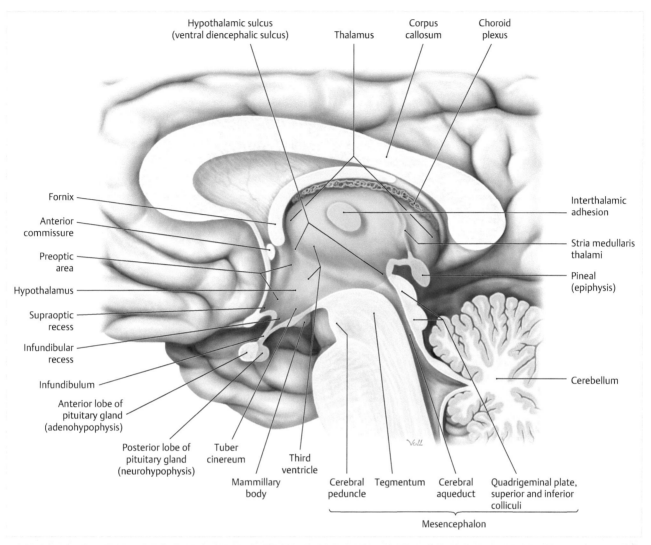

Fig. 5.16 The diencephalon is located below the corpus callosum, part of the telencephalon, and above the mesencephalon (midbrain). The thalamus makes up four-fifths of the entire diencephalon, but the only parts of the diencephalon that can be seen externally are the hypothalamus (visible from the basal aspect) and portions of the epithalamus (pineal gland, visible from the occipital aspect). The diencephalon is involved in endocrine functioning and autonomic coordination of the pineal gland, the posterior lobe of the pituitary gland (neurohypophysis), and the hypothalamus. It also acts as a relay station for sensory information and somatic motor control (via the thalamus). (Reproduced with permission from Schuenke M, Schulte E, Schumacher U. THIEME Atlas of Anatomy Third Edition, Vol 3. © Thieme 2020. Illustrations by Markus Voll and Karl Wesker.)

– The **parahippocampal cortex** surrounds the hippocampus. It is important in memory encoding and retrieval.
– The **limbic system** is involved in memory and learning, drive-related behavior, and emotions.

5.4 Diencephalon

The diencephalon consists of the **thalamus, hypothalamus, subthalamus,** and **epithalamus** (▶ Fig. 5.16). These structures have wide-ranging and diverse activity (see Chapter 18) (▶ Table 5.2).

- The **thalamus** is a major part of the diencephalon (▶ Fig. 5.17).

○ Consists of groups of nuclei that lie on either side of the third ventricle.
○ Receives sensory input and relays information to the cortex.
○ Plays a role in motor loops involving cerebellum, cortex, and basal ganglia.
○ Receives limbic projections.

- The **hypothalamus** is located inferior to the thalamus and separated from it by the **hypothalamic sulcus** within the wall of the third ventricle. It also forms the floor of the ventricle (▶ Fig. 5.18) (▶ Table 5.3).

○ The inferior surface includes the **infundibulum**, which is the connection between the pituitary and the hypothalamus.
○ **Mammillary bodies** are present on the inferior surface.

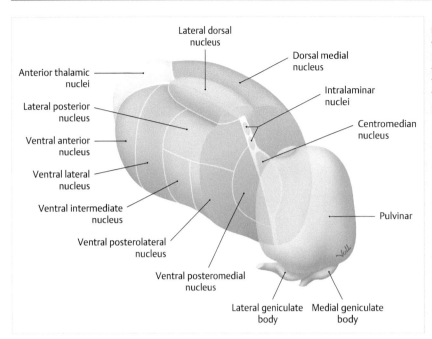

Anterior thalamic nuclei

Lateral posterior nucleus

Ventral anterior nucleus

Ventral lateral nucleus

Ventral intermediate nucleus

Ventral posterolateral nucleus

Ventral posteromedial nucleus

Lateral dorsal nucleus

Dorsal medial nucleus

Intralaminar nuclei

Centromedian nucleus

Pulvinar

Lateral geniculate body   Medial geniculate body

Fig. 5.17 The thalamus is a major component of the diencephalon and is made up of several nuclear groups. (Reproduced with permission from Schuenke M, Schulte E, Schumacher U. THIEME Atlas of Anatomy Third Edition, Vol 3. © Thieme 2020. Illustrations by Markus Voll and Karl Wesker.)

Table 5.2 Function of the diencephalon

Part	Structures	Function
Epithalamus	• Pineal gland • Habenula	Regulation of circadian rhythms; linking of olfactory system to brain
Thalamus	• Thalamus	Relay center for the somatosensory system and parts of the motor system
Subthalamus	• Subthalamic nucleus • Zona incerta • Globus pallidus	Relay of sensory information (somatomotor zone of diencephalon)
Hypothalamus	• Optic chiasm, optic tract • Tuber cinereum • Posterior lobe of pituitary gland (neurohypophysis) • Mammillary bodies	Coordination of autonomic nervous system with endocrine system; participation in the visual pathway

(Reproduced with permission from Baker EW. Anatomy for Dental Medicine. Second Edition. © Thieme 2017)

Table 5.3 Function of the hypothalamus

Region or Nucleus	Function	Lesion
Anterior preoptic region	Maintains constant body temperature	Central hypothermia
Posterior region	Responds to temperature changes, e.g., sweating	Hypothermia
Midanterior and posterior regions	Activate sympathetic nervous system	Autonomic dysfunction
Paraventricular and anterior regions	Activate parasympathetic nervous system	Autonomic dysfunction
Supraoptic and paraventricular nuclei	Regulate water balance	• Diabetes insipidus • Hyponatremia (low Na^+)
Anterior nuclei	Regulate appetite and food intake	• Lesion of medial part causes obesity • Lesion of lateral part causes anorexia and emaciation

(Reproduced with permission from Baker EW. Anatomy for Dental Medicine. Second Edition. © Thieme 2017)

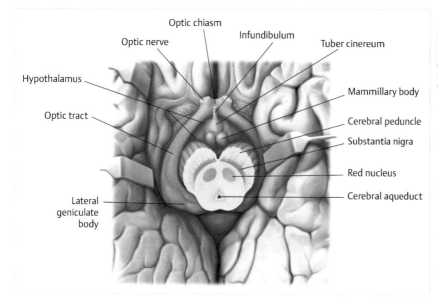

Fig. 5.18 The hypothalamus is located inferior to the thalamus. (Reproduced with permission from Schuenke M, Schulte E, Schumacher U. THIEME Atlas of Anatomy Third Edition, Vol 3. © Thieme 2020. Illustrations by Markus Voll and Karl Wesker.)

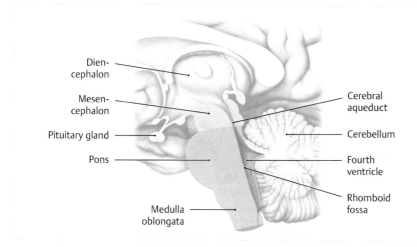

Fig. 5.19 The mesencephalon is the smallest and most rostral part component of the midbrain. (Reproduced with permission from Schuenke M, Schulte E, Schumacher U. THIEME Atlas of Anatomy Third Edition, Vol 3. © Thieme 2020. Illustrations by Markus Voll and Karl Wesker.)

- Controls the ANS, and along with the pituitary, the endocrine system.
- Plays a role in the limbic system.
- The **epithalamus** is composed of the pineal gland and other neural structures whose function is somewhat less defined in humans compared to other species.
  - Regulates circadian rhythms.
  - Involved in the limbic system.
- The **subthalamus** lies between the thalamus and the midbrain.
  - A significant amount of the subthalamus is made up by subthalamic nuclei. Functionally, they are considered part of the basal ganglia.

5.5 Mesencephalon

Also known as the **midbrain**, the **mesencephalon** is the smallest and most rostral part of the brainstem (▶ Fig. 5.19). The major components are the **tectum**, **tegmentum,** and the **cerebral peduncles** (▶ Fig. 5.20). The midbrain contains several cranial nerve nuclei.

- In mammals, the tectum contains two pairs of **colliculi** (▶ Fig. 5.21).
  - The **inferior colliculus** has an auditory function. It is the largest nuclei in the human auditory system.
  - The **superior colliculus** is involved in vision.
- The tegmentum lies ventral to the tectum.
  - Contains the reticular formation, tracts, periaqueductal gray, red nucleus, and substantia nigra.
- The cerebral peduncles contain ascending and descending tracts that run to and from the cerebrum.

5.6 Metencephalon

The **metencephalon** is made up of the **pons** and **cerebellum**. This structure houses many of the ascending and descending tracts of the CNS as well as part of the reticular formation.

- Pons (▶ Fig. 5.22)
  - It creates a large "bulge" or prominence on the ventral surface of the brain. It is often referred to as the "bridge" to the cerebellum. There are three **cerebellar peduncles** that attach the cerebellum to the brainstem. The middle

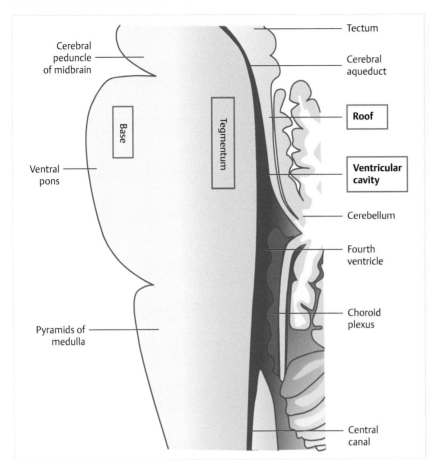

Cerebral peduncle of midbrain

Base

Ventral pons

Tegmentum

Pyramids of medulla

Tectum

Cerebral aqueduct

Roof

Ventricular cavity

Cerebellum

Fourth ventricle

Choroid plexus

Central canal

Fig. 5.20 The major parts of the mesencephalon are: tectum, tegmentum, and cerebral peduncles. (Reproduced with permission from Alberstone CD, Benzel EC, Najm IM, et al. Anatomic Basis of Neurologic Diagnosis. © Thieme 2009.)

cerebellar peduncle primarily contains afferents from pontine nuclei.

○ The pons is the middle component of the brainstem, lying inferior to the midbrain.

○ The **fourth ventricle** lies within the pons and/or upper part of medulla.

○ **CN V** emerges from the lateral aspect of the pons.

○ CNs VI, VII, and VIII exit at the pontomedullary junction.

• Cerebellum (▶ Fig. 5.23)

○ Known as "little brain," the cerebellum lies at the posterior-inferior aspect of the brain (see Chapter 18).

○ Typically considered a motor structure; however, it does not initiate motor commands. Rather, the cerebellum modifies motor activity so that it is more fluid and accurate.

○ Functions include:

– Maintenance of posture.

– Coordination of voluntary movements.

– Motor learning.

– Cognitive function.

5.7 Myelencephalon

The myelencephalon is the most caudal of the embryonic vesicles. It is derived from the embryonic hindbrain and ultimately develops into the **medulla oblongata** (▶ Fig. 5.24a, b).

• The medulla oblongata lies superior to the spinal cord. It is the most caudal of the brainstem structures.

• It provides a conduit for ascending and descending tracts running between the brain and the rest of the body.

• The **medullary pyramids** and the **decussation of the pyramids** are characteristic structures on the ventral surface of the medulla.

• A portion of the **fourth ventricle** lies within the medulla.

• The **nucleus cuneatus** and **nucleus gracilis** are found in the medulla. These structures transmit sensory information to the thalamus.

• Part of the **reticular formation** runs within the medulla.

• It contains several **cranial nerve nuclei** (CNs IX, X, XI, and XII).

• The **respiratory** and **cardiovascular centers** are located within the medulla. These centers are a collection of nuclei located in the medullary reticular formation. Their function is to regulate breathing, heart rate, and blood pressure.

• The **olivary nucleus**, which transmits information from the cortex, diencephalon, and brainstem to the cerebellum, is present in the medulla. It is also involved in motor control and sensory processing as well as cognition.

5.8 Medial Surface of the Cerebral Hemispheres

There are many components of the brain that are only visible from the medial aspect. These include gyri, sulci, and white matter structures (▶ Fig. 5.25).

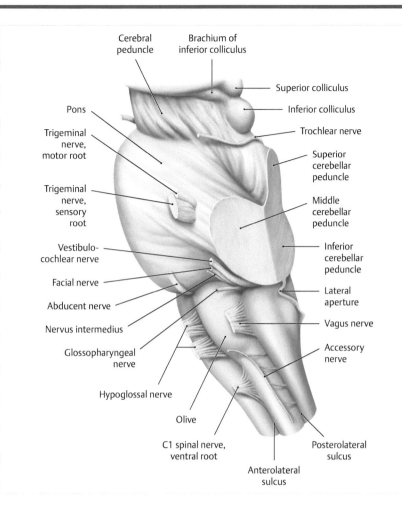

Cerebral peduncle

Brachium of inferior colliculus

Superior colliculus

Inferior colliculus

Pons

Trigeminal nerve, motor root

Trochlear nerve

Superior cerebellar peduncle

Trigeminal nerve, sensory root

Middle cerebellar peduncle

Vestibulo-cochlear nerve

Inferior cerebellar peduncle

Facial nerve

Lateral aperture

Abducent nerve

Vagus nerve

Nervus intermedius

Glossopharyngeal nerve

Accessory nerve

Hypoglossal nerve

Olive

C1 spinal nerve, ventral root

Posterolateral sulcus

Anterolateral sulcus

Fig. 5.21 The tectum contains colliculi. The inferior colliculus has auditory functions while the superior colliculus is involved in vision. (Reproduced with permission from Schuenke M, Schulte E, Schumacher U. THIEME Atlas of Anatomy Third Edition, Vol 3. © Thieme 2020. Illustrations by Markus Voll and Karl Wesker.)

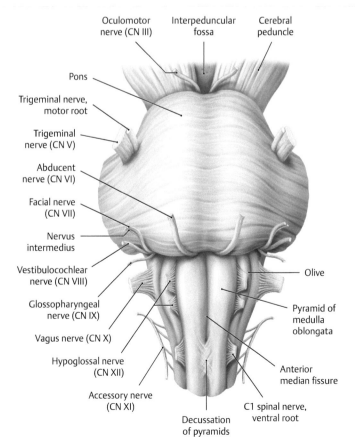

Oculomotor nerve (CN III)

Interpeduncular fossa

Cerebral peduncle

Pons

Trigeminal nerve, motor root

Trigeminal nerve (CN V)

Abducent nerve (CN VI)

Facial nerve (CN VII)

Nervus intermedius

Vestibulocochlear nerve (CN VIII)

Glossopharyngeal nerve (CN IX)

Vagus nerve (CN X)

Hypoglossal nerve (CN XII)

Accessory nerve (CN XI)

Decussation of pyramids

C1 spinal nerve, ventral root

Anterior median fissure

Pyramid of medulla oblongata

Olive

Fig. 5.22 The pons is a large structure on the ventral surface of the brainstem that lies inferior to the midbrain. It is often referred to as the "bridge" to the cerebellum. (Reproduced with permission from Schuenke M, Schulte E, Schumacher U. THIEME Atlas of Anatomy Third Edition, Vol 3. © Thieme 2020. Illustrations by Markus Voll and Karl Wesker.)

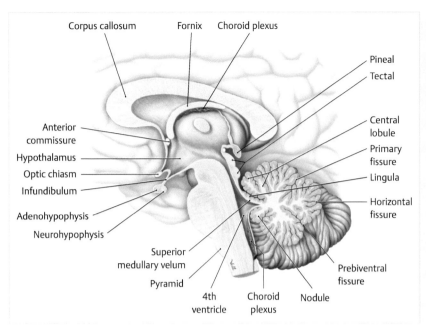

Corpus callosum   Fornix   Choroid plexus

Pineal

Tectal

Anterior commissure

Central lobule

Hypothalamus

Primary fissure

Optic chiasm

Lingula

Infundibulum

Horizontal fissure

Adenohypophysis

Neurohypophysis

Superior medullary velum

Prebiventral fissure

Pyramid

4th ventricle   Choroid plexus   Nodule

Fig. 5.23 The cerebellum is part of the metencephalon. It lies at the posterior-inferior aspect of the brain. It is involved in motor activity. (Reproduced with permission from Schuenke M, Schulte E, Schumacher U. THIEME Atlas of Anatomy Third Edition, Vol 3. © Thieme 2020. Illustrations by Markus Voll and Karl Wesker.)

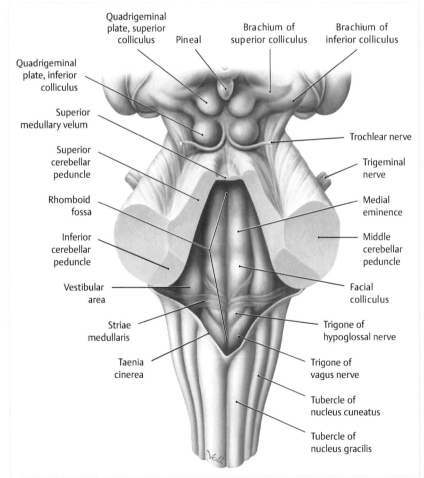

Quadrigeminal plate, superior colliculus

Pineal

Brachium of superior colliculus

Brachium of inferior colliculus

Quadrigeminal plate, inferior colliculus

Trochlear nerve

Superior medullary velum

Trigeminal nerve

Superior cerebellar peduncle

Medial eminence

Rhomboid fossa

Middle cerebellar peduncle

Inferior cerebellar peduncle

Vestibular area

Facial colliculus

Striae medullaris

Trigone of hypoglossal nerve

Taenia cinerea

Trigone of vagus nerve

Tubercle of nucleus cuneatus

Tubercle of nucleus gracilis

Fig. 5.24 The medulla oblongata is derived from the myelencephalon. It is the most caudal of the brainstem structures and lies superior to the spinal cord. It provides a conduit for tracts running between the brain and the body. (Reproduced with permission from Schuenke M, Schulte E, Schumacher U. THIEME Atlas of Anatomy Third Edition, Vol 3. © Thieme 2020. Illustrations by Markus Voll and Karl Wesker.)

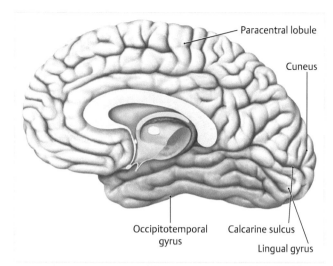

Fig. 5.25 Many of the brain's components, such as the corpus collosum, are only visible from the medial aspect. Occipitotemporal gyrus is made up of the lower two gyri (medial and lateral). It is also known as the fusiform gyrus. (Reproduced with permission from Schuenke M, Schulte E, Schumacher U. THIEME Atlas of Anatomy Third Edition, Vol 3. © Thieme 2020. Illustrations by Markus Voll and Karl Wesker.)

- Corpus callosum (Clinical Correlation Box 5.3)
  - The corpus callosum is a large band of myelinated fibers that connect the two cerebral hemispheres. It lies at the bottom of the longitudinal fissure.
  - The function of the structure is to integrate motor, sensory, and cognitive information between the two hemispheres.
  - It is a C-shaped structure and can be divided into specific components.
    - **Rostrum**: Thin part of the anterior end. Downward and posterior projection from the genu.
    - **Genu**: Curved anterior end.
    - **Body**: Area between the genu and splenium.
    - **Splenium**: Posterior aspect.

- Cingulate gyrus
  - Lies on the medial aspect of the hemispheres and adjacent to the corpus callosum.
  - Considered a major component of the limbic system. It is involved in emotions and behavior. Recently, cognitive functions have also been attributed to the cingulate gyrus.
- Paracentral lobule
  - Surrounds the indentation of the central sulcus on the medial aspect of the hemispheres.
  - The anterior part is a continuation of the precentral gyrus (motor) and the posterior part is a continuation of the postcentral gyrus (sensory).
- Cuneus
  - Small lobule in the occipital lobe.
  - Bounded by calcarine sulcus and parieto-occipital sulcus.
  - Part of the visual association cortex, which is responsible for higher order processing of visual information.
- Calcarine sulcus
  - Located on the medial aspect of the occipital lobe and divides the visual cortex.
  - Contains the primary visual cortex.
- Lingual gyrus
  - Lies inferior to the calcarine sulcus.
  - Continues anteriorly as the **parahippocampal gyrus.** This gyrus surrounds the hippocampus and is part of the limbic system.
  - Attributed with visual activity.
- Occipitotemporal gyrus
  - Composed of temporal portion (anterior) and occipital portion (posterior).
  - Considered to be involved in higher order visual processing.

5.9 Inferior Aspect of the Cerebral Hemispheres

The inferior surface of the hemisphere contains the following structures (▶ Fig. 5.26):
- **Olfactory bulb** and **tract** are located on the inferior surface of the frontal lobe and are involved in **olfaction**.
- Several **orbital gyri** are found on the inferior surface of the frontal lobe. These gyri play a role in olfaction.
- **Optic chiasm** is a midline structure where fibers from both optic nerves decussate.
- **Optic tracts** are a continuation of the optic nerve extending from the optic chiasm to the lateral geniculate body of the thalamus.
- **Mammillary bodies** are part of the diencephalon that lie on either side of the tuber cinereum. They are part of the limbic system and are involved in memory.
- **Tuber cinereum** is a mass of gray matter that is continuous with the infundibulum of the pituitary.
- **Hypothalamus** is the most ventral part of the diencephalon. It extends from the optic chiasm to the mammillary bodies.
- **Lateral** and **medial occipitotemporal gyri** have both temporal and occipital components and lie on the basal surface of the temporal and occipital lobes.

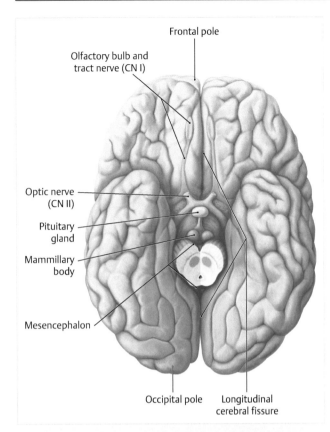

Frontal pole

Olfactory bulb and
tract nerve (CN I)

Optic nerve
(CN II)

Pituitary
gland

Mammillary
body

Mesencephalon

Occipital pole   Longitudinal
cerebral fissure

Fig. 5.26 Basal (inferior) view with the brainstem removed. Structures on the inferior surface of the brain includes: olfactory bulb and tract, optic chiasm and tracts, hypothalamus, and mammillary bodies. (Reproduced with permission from Schuenke M, Schulte E, Schumacher U. THIEME Atlas of Anatomy Third Edition, Vol 3. © Thieme 2020. Illustrations by Markus Voll and Karl Wesker.)

Questions and Answers

1. A 27-year-old male was involved in a motorcycle accident. MRI results show damage to the left superior margin of the brain, anterior to the central sulcus and adjacent to the longitudinal fissure. Which of the following symptoms would you expect to see in this patient?
   a) Sensory deficits on the face
   b) Motor deficits in the extremities
   c) Motor deficits in the face
   d) Loss of language comprehension

Level 3: Difficult

Answer C: Based on the motor homunculus, the area described in the question reflects the part of the cortex that is responsible for generating motor command for the face. (A) Sensory deficit's would require damage to the cortex in the postcentral gyrus which is posterior to the central sulcus. (B) Motor loss in the extremities would mean the trauma occurred

to the inferolateral aspect of the parietal lobe based on the motor homunculus. (D) Wernicke's area is responsible for language comprehension and it is located in the inferior parietal gyri and the superior temporal gyri.

2. The primary visual cortex is located in which of the following areas?
   a) Calcarine sulcus
   b) Parieto-occipital sulcus
   c) Lateral occipitotemporal gyrus
   d) Cuneus

Level 2: Medium

Answer A: The primary visual cortex is located within the walls of the calcarine sulcus. (B) The parieto-occipital sulcus is a fissure located on the medial aspect of the hemispheres that is the anterior boundary of the occipital lobe. (C) The lateral occipitotemporal gyri is part of the visual association area. (D) The cuneus is also part of the visual association cortex.

3. Which of the following structures of the mesencephalon is involved in hearing.
   a) Superior colliculus
   b) Inferior colliculus
   c) Tegmentum
   d) Cerebral peduncles

Level 1: Easy

Answer B: Inferior colliculus that is part of the tectum (midbrain) is involved in the auditory system. (A) Superior colliculus is also part of the tectum however, it is involved in vision. (C) The tegmentum lies ventral to the tectum and is not involved in hearing. (D) Cerebral peduncles are located in the midbrain and contains motor and sensory tracts running to and from the cerebellum.

4. An unconscious 50-year-old female is admitted to the ER. Preliminary observations indicate increased intracranial pressure. Imaging studies document a subdural hematoma with herniation of the medulla oblongata. The patient ultimately died from cardiac arrest. Damage to which of the following structures was most likely the cause of death?
   a) Nucleus cuneatus
   b) Reticular formation
   c) Fourth ventricle
   d) Olivary nucleus

Level 3: Difficult

Answer B: The cardiovascular center nuclei, which are responsible for regulation of the cardiovascular system, are located in the reticular formation of the medulla. (A) Nucleus cuneatus carries sensory information from T6 and above. (C) Damage/blockage of the fourth ventricle may have been the cause of the increased intracranial pressure but not the direct cause of the cardiac arrest. (D) The olivary nucleus is involved in motor control and sensory processing. Its major output is to the cerebellum.

5. Which of the following structures on the medial aspect of the cerebrum is responsible for coordination of sensory and motor information between the two hemispheres.
   a) Cingulate gyrus
   b) Paracentral lobule
   c) Lingual gyrus
   d) Corpus callosum

Level 1: Easy

   Answer D: The function of the corpus callosum is to coordinate information between the two hemispheres. **(A)** Cingulate gyrus is part of the limbic system. **(B)** Paracentral lobule is a continuation of the pre and postcentral gyrus. **(C)** Lingual gyrus is involved in visual activity.

6 Blood Supply of the Brain

6.1 Overview of the Blood Supply to the Brain

Most of the blood supply to the brain comes from paired vessels, the **internal carotid** and the **vertebral arteries** (▶ Fig. 6.1). The internal carotid supplies the majority of the brain while the vertebral arteries provide blood to the posterior aspect of the **cerebrum**, the **brain stem,** and the **cerebellum**. A large anastomosis on the inferior surface of the brain, the **circle of Willis**, connects the anterior and posterior circulation. The **blood–brain barrier** is a physiological and anatomical system present in the circulatory system of the brain that controls the bidirectional movement of molecules. **Superficial** and **deep cerebral veins** drain the brain tissue and empty into **dural venous sinuses**, which in turn drain into the **internal jugular vein** and **venous plexi**.

6.2 Anterior Circulation of the Brain

The anterior circulation of the brain is derived from the internal carotid artery (**ICA**) (▶ Fig. 6.2a). The internal carotid

originates from the common carotid, which is a branch of the **subclavian artery**. After ascending through the neck, the ICA enters the **carotid canal** and begins its **intracranial course** (▶ Fig. 6.2b). The pathway of the ICA is commonly divided into four segments:

- The **cervical portion** begins at the bifurcation of the **common carotid** (at the level of C4) in the neck and continues until it reaches the carotid canal.
- The **petrous portion** begins in the carotid canal, which is located in the petrous part of the temporal bone. After entering the canal, it curves forward and medially. As it exits, it travels superior to **foramen lacerum**, which in life is filled with cartilage, and then enters the **cavernous sinus**.
- The **cavernous portion** lies between layers of dura forming the cavernous sinus. It initially ascends toward the **posterior clinoid process**, then curves forward along the side of the body of the **sphenoid bone,** and finally turns upward and ascends alongside the **anterior clinoid process**. The resulting S-shaped configuration of the ICA, which is made up of the cavernous and, to a smaller extent, the cerebral portion, is referred to as the **carotid siphon** and is often used as a radiographic landmark.
  - The **ophthalmic artery** is given off just as the ICA emerges from the cavernous sinus (▶ Fig. 6.2c).
  - It enters the orbit through the optic foramen, inferior and lateral to the **optic nerve**.
  - Once in the orbit, it passes superior to the optic nerve along with the **nasociliary nerve**.
- The **cerebral portion** begins after the vessel perforates the dura medial to the anterior clinoid process. Here, the ICA passes between the optic and occulomotor nerves and travels toward the lateral cerebral fissure where it gives off its terminal branches, the **anterior** and **middle cerebral arteries**.

6.2.1 The Anterior Cerebral Artery (ACA)

The ICA supplies the majority of the cerebrum. After giving off the ophthalmic artery, the ICA continues in a superior direction alongside the optic chiasm. Eventually, it will bifurcate into the anterior and middle cerebral arteries but before it does so, the **anterior choroidal** and **posterior communicating arteries** are given off (▶ Fig. 6.2d).

- The anterior choroidal artery supplies the optic tract, the choroid plexus, portions of the internal capsule, the thalamus, and the hippocampus.
  - The anterior choroidal artery is frequently involved in **cerebrovascular** incidents.
- The posterior communicating artery passes posteriorly and joins the posterior cerebral artery.
- The anterior cerebral artery enters the longitudinal fissure of the brain that separates the cerebral hemispheres where it branches and arches posteriorly.
  - The ACA closely follows the **corpus collosum** and supplies the medial aspect of the **frontal** and **parietal lobes** of the brain (▶ Fig. 6.2e).

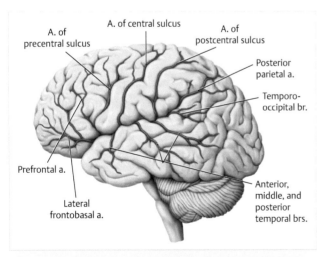

A. of precentral sulcus
A. of central sulcus
A. of postcentral sulcus
Posterior parietal a.
Temporo-occipital br.
Prefrontal a.
Lateral frontobasal a.
Anterior, middle, and posterior temporal brs.

Fig. 6.1 Lateral view of arteries in the left hemisphere. (Reproduced with permission from Schuenke M, Schulte E, Schumacher U. THIEME Atlas of Anatomy Third Edition, Vol 3. © Thieme 2020. Illustrations by Markus Voll and Karl Wesker.)

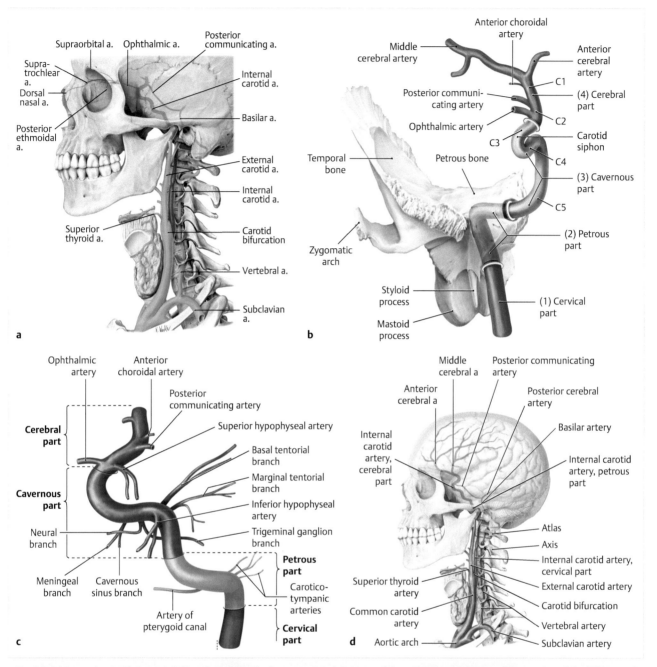

Fig. 6.2 (a) Internal carotid artery. Left lateral view. **(b)** The four anatomical divisions of the internal carotid artery. Anterior view of the left internal carotid artery. The internal carotid artery consists of four topographically distinct parts between the carotid bifurcation and the point where it divides into the anterior and middle cerebral arteries. The parts are as follows: (1) Cervical part located in the lateral pharyngeal space; (2) petrous part located in the carotid canal of the petrous bone; (3) cavernous part which follows an S-shaped curve in the cavernous sinus; (4) cerebral part located in the chiasmatic cistern of the subarachnoid space. **(c)** The petrous part of the internal carotid artery (traversing the carotid canal) and the cavernous part (traversing the cavernous sinus) have a role in supplying extracerebral structures of the head. They give off additional small branches that supply local structures and are usually named for the areas they supply. Of the branches not supplying the brain, of special importance is the ophthalmic artery, which arises from the cerebral part of the internal carotid artery. Note: The ophthalmic artery forms an anastomosis with the artery of the pterygoid canal derived from the maxillary artery. **(d)** The ICA supplies most of the cerebrum. After giving off the ophthalmic artery, it bifurcates into the anterior and middle cerebral arteries. (Reproduced with permission from Schuenke M, Schulte E, Schumacher U. THIEME Atlas of Anatomy Third Edition, Vol 3. © Thieme 2020. Illustrations by Markus Voll and Karl Wesker.)

(Continued)

○ Some of the branches supply the dorsolateral surface of each hemisphere.
○ The **anterior communicating artery** joins the anterior cerebral arteries from both sides.

○ Distal to the anterior communicating artery, the anterior cerebral artery continues as the **pericallosal** artery, which runs alongside the corpus callosum.

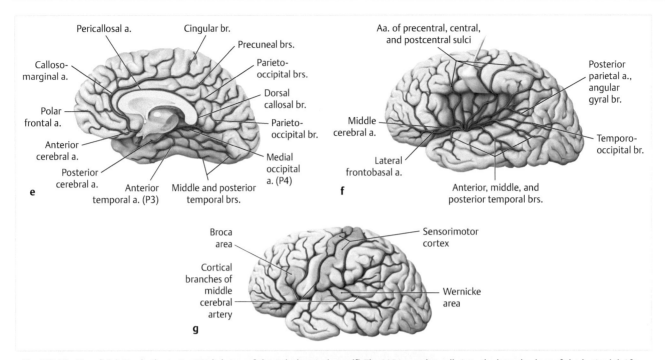

Fig. 6.2 (*Continued*) **(e)** Cerebral arteries. Medial view of the right hemisphere. **(f)** The MCA runs laterally into the lateral sulcus of the brain. **(g)** After entering the lateral sulcus, the MCA sends branches to the insula. ICA, internal carotid artery; MCA, middle cerebral artery. (Reproduced with permission from Schuenke M, Schulte E, Schumacher U. THIEME Atlas of Anatomy Third Edition, Vol 3. © Thieme 2020. Illustrations by Markus Voll and Karl Wesker.)

6.2.2 The Middle Cerebral Artery (MCA)

The **middle cerebral artery** (**MCA**) is the larger of the two terminal branches of the ICA. It runs laterally into the **lateral sulcus** of the brain (▶ Fig. 6.2f).
- After entering the lateral sulcus, the MCA sends branches to the **insula** (▶ Fig. 6.2g).
- It then emerges from the lateral sulcus to supply a large part of the lateral surface of the cerebral hemispheres.
  - The MCA supplies a significant portion of the pre- and postcentral gyri.
    - Occlusion of the MCA results in both motor and sensory deficits.
    - The area supplied by the MCA is involved in language; thus, occlusion can also result in language problems.

6.3 Posterior Circulation of the Brain

The posterior circulation of the brain is provided by paired vertebral arteries that join to form a single basilar artery. For that reason, it is often referred to as the **vertebrobasilar circulation**.
- The vertebral artery is a branch of the subclavian artery (▶ Fig. 6.3a).
- The **cervical** part of the vertebral arteries enters the **transverse foramina** of C6 vertebrae and continues to ascend through the foramina of C1 vertebrae.

- After exiting the C1 foramen, the vertebral artery perforates the dura and the arachnoid meninges and ascends through the **foramen magnum**.
- The vertebral arteries join to form the **basilar artery** at the caudal border of the **pons** (▶ Fig. 6.3b).
- The basilar artery traverses the **clivus** (**occipital bone**), and then divides into two **posterior cerebral arteries** (**PCAs**) at the level of the **midbrain** (▶ Fig. 6.3c).
  - Before bifurcating, the PCA gives off numerous branches including the **anterior inferior cerebellar artery** (**AICA**) the **superior cerebellar artery** and **pontine arteries**.
  - The AICA supplies the inferior surface of the **cerebellum** and parts of the pons.
- The posterior cerebral arteries supply the medial and inferior surfaces of the **occipital** and **temporal lobes** of the brain (▶ Fig. 6.2e).
  - The PCA also sends smaller branches to the structures of the diencephalon.

6.4 Circle of Willis

The **circle of Willis** connects the anterior and posterior circulation of the brain (▶ Fig. 6.4a). It is an anastomosis located on the inferior surface of the brain (▶ Fig. 6.3b). This arterial ring (▶ Fig. 6.4b) is formed by the following arteries:
- Anterior communicating artery.
- Anterior cerebral arteries.
- Internal carotid arteries.

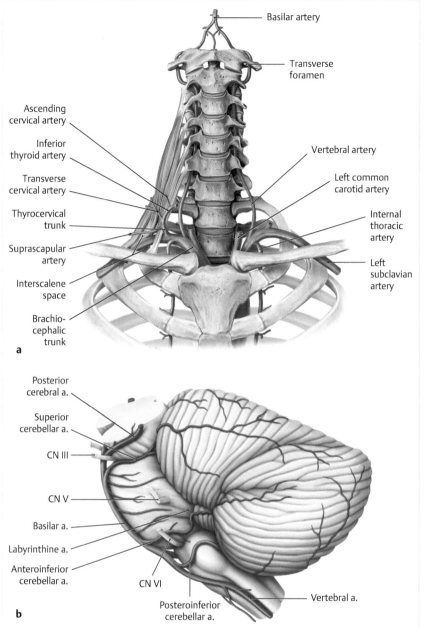

Basilar artery

Transverse foramen

Ascending cervical artery

Inferior thyroid artery

Transverse cervical artery

Thyrocervical trunk

Suprascapular artery

Interscalene space

Brachio-cephalic trunk

Vertebral artery

Left common carotid artery

Internal thoracic artery

Left subclavian artery

a

Posterior cerebral a.

Superior cerebellar a.

CN III

CN V

Basilar a.

Labyrinthine a.

Anteroinferior cerebellar a.

CN VI

Posteroinferior cerebellar a.

Vertebral a.

b

Fig. 6.3 (a) Each vertebral artery arises from the posterior aspect of the subclavian artery on each side and ascends through the foramina in the transverse processes of the cervical vertebrae (C6–C1). **(b)** After entering the skull through the foramen magnum, the vertebral arteries unite to form the basilar artery. (Reproduced with permission from Schuenke M, Schulte E, Schumacher U. THIEME Atlas of Anatomy Third Edition, Vol 3. © Thieme 2020. Illustrations by Markus Voll and Karl Wesker.)

(*Continued*)

- Posterior communicating arteries.
- Posterior cerebral arteries
  - Under normal circumstances, little blood actually flows through the circle due to pressure differentials.
    - In the case of occlusion of one of the major vessels, the anastomoses can maintain blood flow to the brain tissue and prevent neurological damage resulting from ischemia.
    - Anatomic variants are common, some of which can have a negative effect on patency.

6.5 Blood–Brain Barrier

The **blood–brain barrier** (**BBB**) (▶ Fig. 6.5) is a highly selective membrane diffusion barrier that prevents potentially noxious molecules from leaving the blood and entering the extracellular fluid (**ECF**) compartment of the central nervous system (CNS). By regulating the transport of molecules across a barrier, the CNS is able to maintain a stable environment.

- The BBB **endothelial cells** are unique compared to those of the rest of the body because they lack **fenestrations**.
- The endothelial cells of the BBB have more extensive **tight junctions**.
- The BBB has limited **pinocytic vesicular transport**.
- Most of the CNS is protected by the BBB; however, there are areas in the brain that lack this specialized barrier. The structures that lack a BBB are collectively called **circumventricular organs** because they are situated in the midline of the **ventricular system**.
  - Some of the areas of the brain lacking a BBB are:

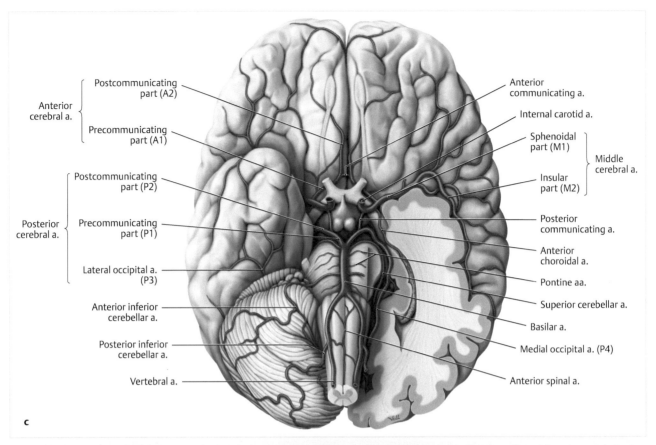

Fig. 6.3 (*Continued*) (**c**) The basilar artery divides into two posterior cerebral arteries. (Reproduced with permission from Schuenke M, Schulte E, Schumacher U. THIEME Atlas of Anatomy Third Edition, Vol 3. © Thieme 2020. Illustrations by Markus Voll and Karl Wesker.)

– Pituitary gland.
– Area postrema.
– Pineal gland.
– Endothelium of the choroid plexus.

6.6 Venous Drainage in the Brain

The **cerebral venous system** (▶ Fig. 6.6a) is unique in that it does not follow the cerebral arterial system. In general, cerebral veins are fairly superficial, lying on the deep surface of the arachnoid layer (subarachnoid space) (see Chapter 8).

- Cerebral veins are thin, lacking a muscular layer, and valveless.
- Most cortical veins pierce the arachnoid and meningeal dural layer to empty into the dural venous sinuses (see Chapter 8).
- **Cerebral veins** can be divided into a **superficial** and **deep system** (▶ Fig. 6.6b).
  ○ The superficial system is composed of sagittal sinuses and cortical veins that drain the superficial surfaces of both hemispheres. This venus system is highly variable.
  – The superficial veins can be divided into a **superior** and **inferior group**.
    ▪ The superior group empties into the **superior** and **inferior sagittal sinus**.
    ▪ The inferior group empties into the **transverse** and **cavernous sinus**.

- The most consistent of the superficial veins include:
  ▪ **Superficial middle cerebral vein:** Drains a significant part of the temporal lobe into the cavernous or **sphenoparietal sinus**.
  ▪ **Superior anastomotic vein:** Runs across the parietal lobe and connects the superior middle cerebral vein to the **superior sagittal sinus**.
  ▪ **Inferior anastomotic vein:** Travels across the temporal lobe and connects the superficial middle cerebral vein to the **transverse sinus**.
  ○ The deep system is made up of the lateral and straight sinuses and the deeper cortical veins.
  – Typically, more constant than the superficial veins and are often used as radiological landmarks.
  – Major deep veins include:
    ▪ Internal cerebral vein
      □ Formed by the union of three smaller veins posterior to the foramen of Monroe.
        ✓ Drains the choroid plexus, septum pellucidum, and thalamus.
      □ Travels posteriorly in the roof of the third ventricle and unites to form the great cerebral vein.
    ▪ Great cerebral vein (of Galen)
      □ Passes posteriorly behind the splenium of the corpus collosum.
      □ Receives basal veins and posterior fossa veins.
      □ Drains into the transverse sinus.

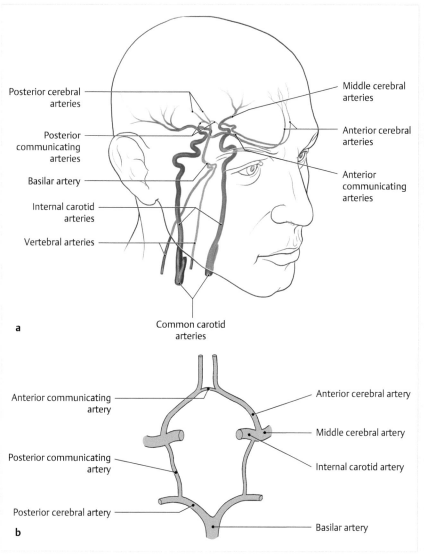

Fig. 6.4 **(a)** Blood supply to the brain. Schematic of circle of Willis in situ. **(b)** Schematic of isolated circle of Willis. The brain is supplied by four arteries that leave the root of the neck separately, the left and right internal carotid arteries and the left and right vertebral arteries. The circle of Willis is a means by which the brain can receive blood when one or more of its major arterial contributors becomes narrowed or blocked. (Fig. 6.4a: Reproduced with permission from Baker EW. Anatomy for Dental Medicine. Second Edition. © Thieme 2015. Illustrations by Markus Voll and Karl Wesker. Fig. 6.4b: Reproduced with permission from Schuenke M, Schulte E, Schumacher U. THIEME Atlas of Anatomy Third Edition, Vol 3. © Thieme 2020. Illustrations by Markus Voll and Karl Wesker.)

- Deep middle cerebral vein
  - Formed near the optic chiasm.
  - Drains the insula, basal ganglia, and orbital surface of the frontal lobe.

Clinical Correlation Box 6.1: Transient Ischemic Attacks

Transient ischemic attacks (TIAs) are sometimes referred to as "mini-strokes" but clinically are considered to be a warning signal. This cerebral event begins like a **stroke** but, on average, only lasts for minutes and leaves no noticeable symptoms or deficits. Individuals that have experienced TIAs are at risk for more serious strokes. Blood clots are the most common cause of a TIA.

Clinical Correlation Box 6.2: Brain Aneurysm (▶ Fig. 6.7)

A **cerebral aneurysm** is a weakened area in the wall of an artery that results in a ballooning or bulging at the weakened spot which is at risk of rupture. Most cerebral aneurysms are of the **saccular** or "berry" type and 85% of these occur in the circle of Willis. There is a familial tendency to develop aneurysms or they can develop due to atherosclerosis and aging. Most cerebral aneurysms do not produce symptoms and are fairly small which generally have a lower risk of rupture. When a brain aneurysm does rupture, it results in a subarachnoid hemorrhage.

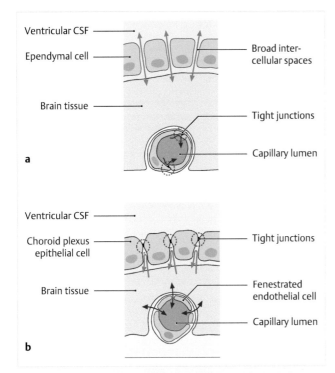

Ventricular CSF

Ependymal cell

Broad inter-
cellular spaces

Brain tissue

Tight junctions

Capillary lumen

a

Ventricular CSF

Choroid plexus
epithelial cell

Tight junctions

Brain tissue

Fenestrated
endothelial cell

Capillary lumen

b

Fig. 6.5 Blood–brain barrier and blood–CSF barrier. **(a)** The blood–brain barrier in normal brain tissue consists mainly of the tight junctions between capillary endothelial cells. It prevents the paracellular diffusion of hydrophilic substances from CNS capillaries into surrounding tissues and in the opposite direction as well. Essential hydrophilic substances that are needed by CNS must be channeled through the barrier with the aid of transport mechanisms. **(b)** The blood–brain barrier is absent in fenestrated capillary endothelial cells in the choroid plexus and other circumventricular organs which allow substances to pass freely from the bloodstream into the brain tissue and vice versa. Tight junctions in the overlying ependyma (choroid plexus epithelium) create a two-way barrier between the brain tissue and ventricular CSF in these regions. The diffusion barrier shifts from the vascular endothelium to the cells of the ependyma and choroid plexus. CNS, central nervous system; CSF, cerebrospinal fluid. (Reproduced with permission from Schuenke M, Schulte E, Schumacher U. THIEME Atlas of Anatomy Second Edition, Vol 3. © Thieme 2016. Illustrations by Markus Voll and Karl Wesker.)

Clinical Correlation Box 6.3: Hemorrhages

The cause of intracranial bleeding or hemorrhages is usually the result of trauma. These injuries can occur without obvious damage to the superficial structures such as the scalp or the cranium itself. Hematomas can develop as a result of the blood collecting in areas outside the vessels which can eventually cause compression on the brain tissue.

- **Epidural hematomas** (▶ Fig. 6.8) occur between the skull and the dural layer of meninges. This commonly occurs as a result of tearing the **middle meningeal artery** from a skull fracture. The extravasated blood pools between the periosteal layer of dura and the cranium resulting in increased pressure on the brain. Symptoms vary but may include: confusion, loss of consciousness, headache, vomiting, slurred speech, and weakness in areas of the body.
- **Subdural hematomas** (▶ Fig. 6.9) are a collection of blood below the inner layer of dura but superior to the arachnoid layer and the brain. There is no naturally occurring space at this level and it is caused by extravasated blood creating the space. This type of hematoma is the most common type of traumatic intracranial lesion and is usually the result of trauma that can be severe or less significant and even spontaneous. Subdural hematomas are often venous in origin. Patients may appear normal for days or may lose consciousness immediately. Symptoms depend on the rate of bleeding and may include: headache, confusion, change in behavior, dizziness, and vomiting.
- **Subarachnoid hematoma** (▶ Fig. 6.10) is an extravasation of blood into the subarachnoid space between the pial and arachnoid meninges. It most often occurs as a result of trauma resulting in an arterial bleed but can be due to the rupture of a saccular aneurysm. Symptoms may include: headache, dizziness, visual changes, and seizures.

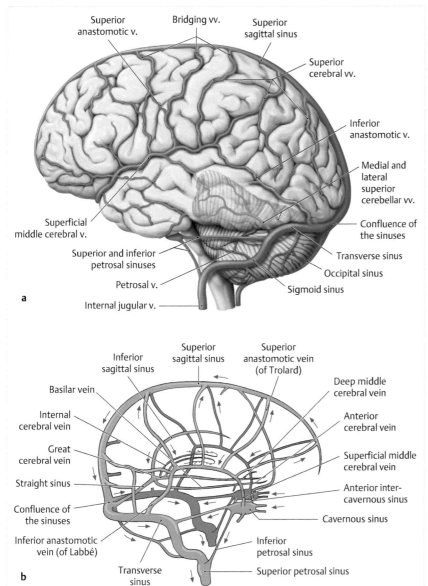

a

Superior anastomotic v.

Bridging vv.

Superior sagittal sinus

Superior cerebral vv.

Inferior anastomotic v.

Medial and lateral superior cerebellar vv.

Confluence of the sinuses

Superficial middle cerebral v.

Superior and inferior petrosal sinuses

Petrosal v.

Internal jugular v.

Transverse sinus

Occipital sinus

Sigmoid sinus

b

Inferior sagittal sinus

Superior sagittal sinus

Superior anastomotic vein (of Trolard)

Deep middle cerebral vein

Basilar vein

Internal cerebral vein

Anterior cerebral vein

Great cerebral vein

Superficial middle cerebral vein

Straight sinus

Anterior inter-cavernous sinus

Confluence of the sinuses

Cavernous sinus

Inferior anastomotic vein (of Labbé)

Inferior petrosal sinus

Transverse sinus

Superior petrosal sinus

Fig. 6.6 **(a)** Superficial cerebral veins. Lateral view of the left hemisphere. **(b)** Dural sinus tributaries from the cerebral veins. Right lateral view. Venous blood collected deep within the brain drains to the dural sinuses through superficial and deep cerebral veins. The red arrows in the diagram show the principal directions of venous blood flow in the major sinuses. (▶ Fig. 6.6a: Reproduced with permission from Gilroy AM, MacPherson BR. Atlas of Anatomy. Third Edition. © Thieme 2016. Illustrations by Markus Voll and Karl Wesker. ▶ Fig. 6.6b: Reproduced with permission from Schuenke M, Schulte E, Schumacher U. THIEME Atlas of Anatomy Second Edition, Vol 3. © Thieme 2016. Illustrations by Markus Voll and Karl Wesker.)

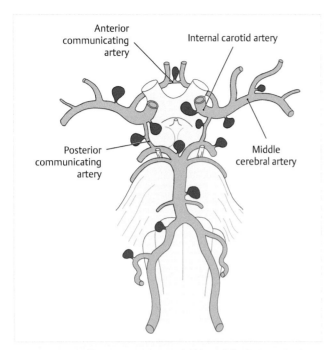

Fig. 6.7 Sites of berry aneurysms at the base of the brain. (Reproduced with permission from Schuenke M, Schulte E, Schumacher U. THIEME Atlas of Anatomy Second Edition, Vol 3. © Thieme 2016. Illustrations by Markus Voll and Karl Wesker.)

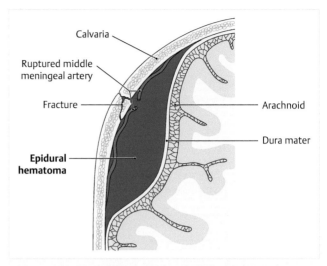

Fig. 6.8 Epidural hematoma. Extracerebral hemorrhages are defined as bleeding between the calvaria and brain. Because the bony calvaria is immobile, the developing hematoma exerts pressure on the soft brain. Depending on the source of the hemorrhage (arterial or venous), this may produce a rapidly or slowly developing incompressible mass with a rise of intracranial pressure that may damage not only the brain tissue at the bleeding site but also in more remote brain areas. (Reproduced with permission from Schuenke M, Schulte E, Schumacher U. THIEME Atlas of Anatomy Second Edition, Vol 3. © Thieme 2016. Illustrations by Markus Voll and Karl Wesker.)

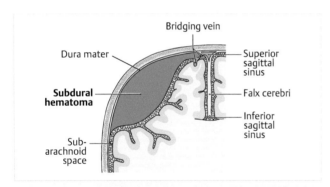

Fig. 6.9 Subdual hematoma. Collection of blood between the lower layer of dura and the arachnoid layer. Subdural hematomas are often venous in origin. (Reproduced with permission from Schuenke M, Schulte E, Schumacher U. THIEME Atlas of Anatomy Second Edition, Vol 3. © Thieme 2016. Illustrations by Markus Voll and Karl Wesker.)

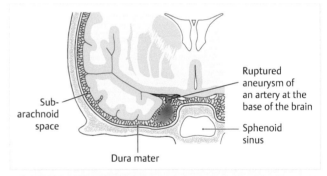

Fig. 6.10 Subarachnoid hematoma. An extravasation of blood into the subarachnoid space (between the pial and arachnoid layers). (Reproduced with permission from Schuenke M, Schulte E, Schumacher U. THIEME Atlas of Anatomy Second Edition, Vol 3. © Thieme 2016. Illustrations by Markus Voll and Karl Wesker.)

Questions and Answers

1. The anterior circulation of the brain is derived from which of the following arteries?
   a) External carotid
   b) Vertebral
   c) Internal carotid
   d) Maxillary

Level 1: Easy
   Answer C is correct. **(A)**. The external carotid supplies the face and neck. **(B)** Vertebral artery supplies the posterior circulation to the brain. **(D)** Maxillary artery supplies the head.

2. Which portion of the internal carotid is referred to as the carotid siphon?
   a) Cervical
   b) Petrous
   c) Cavernous
   d) Cerebral

Level 1: Easy
   Answer C is correct. **(A)** Cervical portion is in the neck. **(B)** Petrous portion is in carotid canal. **(D)** Cerebral portion is after the ICA exits the cavernous sinus and terminates as the ACA and MCA.

3. Occlusion of the MCA would result in which of the following clinical presentations?
   a) Sensory deficits
   b) Motor deficits
   c) Language difficulties
   d) All of the above

Level 2: Moderate
   Answer D is correct. An individual with occlusion of the MCA may experience sensory, motor and language issues.

4. The anterior communicating artery connects which of the following arteries forming the circle of Willis?
   a) Anterior cerebral
   b) Posterior cerebral
   c) Middle cerebral
   d) Internal carotid

Level 1: Easy
   Answer A is correct. **(A)** The posterior communicating artery originates from the IC and joins the ipsilateral posterior cerebral artery to form part of the circle of Willis. **(C)** Middle cerebral artery is a branch of the internal carotid **(D)** and communicates with the posterior communicating artery and the anterior cerebral artery.

5. The posterior cerebral artery is a branch of which of the following arteries?
   a) Internal carotid
   b) Basilar
   c) Vertebral
   d) Circle of Willis

Level 1: Easy
   Answer B is correct. **(A)** The internal carotid artery is a branch of the common carotid. **(C)** The vertebral artery is a branch off the subclavian artery. **(D)** The circle of Willis is an anastomotic structure joining the anterior and posterior circulation of the brain.

7 Ventricles and Cerebrospinal Fluid (CSF)

Learning Objectives

1. Identify the ventricles of the brain and their embryonic origin.
2. Describe the flow of CSF through the adult brain and spinal cord.
3. Describe the choroid plexus.
4. Differentiate between CSF and plasma in terms of chemical composition.
5. Explain how CSF returns to the venous system.

7.1 Overview of the Ventricles and CSF

The **ventricles** of the brain are a series of interconnected, fluid-filled spaces (▶ Fig. 7.1). The ventricular system is composed of paired **lateral ventricles**, the **third ventricle**, and the **fourth ventricle**. These four cavities develop from the lumen of the embryonic neural tube. The **choroid plexus** found within the ventricles produces cerebrospinal fluid (CSF) which fills the ventricular spaces and the subarachnoid space. The CSF moves through the ventricular system and the subarachnoid space via small foramen that connects all four ventricles. It is eventually returned to the venous circulation through arachnoid villi found in the subarachnoid layer of the meninges.

7.2 Ventricles

The paired lateral ventricles develop in the lumen of the prosencephalon and are the largest of the cavities making up the ventricular system. The single third ventricle develops in the diencephalon and the unpaired fourth ventricle originates in developing rhombencephalon. The fourth ventricle narrows at the caudal end to form the **central canal** of the spinal cord. The four ventricles communicate with one another through foramina. The fourth ventricle also connects to the subarachnoid space of the brain and spinal cord via **apertures**. The cerebral ventricular network facilitates the movement and resorption of CSF.

- The **lateral ventricles** are large C-shaped structures that reside in each of the cerebral hemispheres. Each lateral ventricle has five distinctive parts, **anterior horn**, **body**, **posterior horn**, **inferior horn**, and **atrium** (▶ Fig. 7.2a).
  - The lateral ventricles communicate with the third ventricle by way of the **interventricular foramen** (**foramina of Monro**) (▶ Fig. 7.2b, c).
- The third ventricle is a narrow, single structure in the midline of the brain.
  - A circular-shaped structure in the center of the ventricle when viewed from the lateral aspect represents the **interthalamic adhesion.** The interthalamic adhesion is a **commissure** connecting the two **thalamic lobes**.
  - The third ventricle communicates with the fourth ventricle through the **cerebral aqueduct** (**aqueduct of Sylvius**) (▶ Fig. 7.2b, c).

- The fourth ventricle lies between the cerebellum posteriorly and the pons and medulla anteriorly. Rostrally, it connects to the cerebral aqueduct and caudally, it narrows into the **central canal** of the spinal cord (▶ Fig. 7.2b, c).
  - There are three apertures connecting the fourth ventricle, and thus the entire ventricular system, with the subarachnoid space. The apertures are the unpaired **median aperture** (**foramen of Magendie**) and the paired **lateral apertures** (**foramina of Luschka**).
    - The apertures of the fourth ventricle allow communication with large subarachnoid cisterns.
    - The median aperture connects the fourth ventricle with the **cisterna magna**.
    - The lateral apertures connect the fourth ventricle with the **pontine cistern**.
- The **central canal** is derived from the primitive neural tube.
  - The central canal extends from the fourth ventricle to the conus medullaris of the spinal cord.
  - It is lined with ependymal cells and contains CSF.
  - Its function is not clearly understood in humans.
  - By the second decade, it fills with cellular debris and is no longer patent.

7.3 Flow of CSF through the Ventricular System

New CSF is produced at a rate of approximately 500 mL/day. However, at any given time there is only around 200 mL present within the ventricles and subarachnoid space. This means that the CSF must be turned over several times a day. To achieve this, it must be able to move to the sites of resorption. The foramina that connect the ventricular system facilitate this movement (▶ Fig. 7.3a).

- Starting superiorly, the CSF formed in the lateral ventricles passes through the interventricular foramen to reach the third ventricle.
- From the third ventricle, the CSF moves to the fourth ventricle through the cerebral aqueduct.
- From the fourth ventricle, the CSF proceeds through the median and lateral apertures into the subarachnoid cisterns, the cisterna magna and pontine cistern, respectively.
  - From these cisterns, the CSF flows around the cerebral hemispheres and up toward the superior sagittal sinus where resorption occurs through arachnoid villi and granulations.
    - The movement of CSF into the venous system is dependent on a pressure gradient. Pressure in the venous system is lower than that of the subarachnoid space facilitating the movement of CSF from the subarachnoid space (high pressure) into the venous sinuses (low pressure) (▶ Fig. 7.3b).
  - Some CSF will travel from the cranial cisterns into the subarachnoid space surrounding the spinal cord. Here, it will move caudally toward the lumbar cistern and then rostrally, back toward the cranial cisterns.
    - Some CSF will be returned to the venous system via arachnoid villi associated with spinal nerve roots.

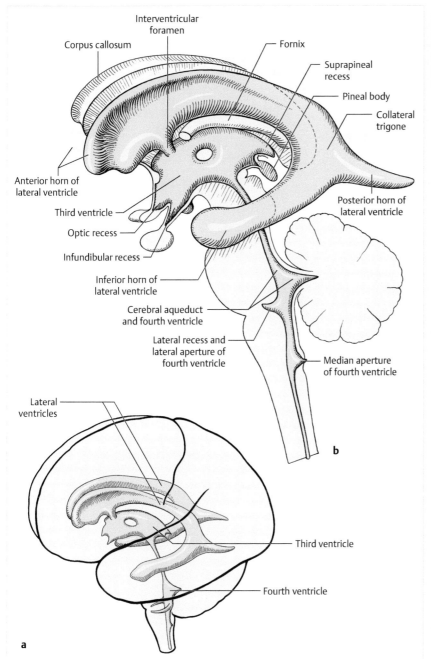

Fig. 7.1 (a,b) The ventricular system is a series of interconnected spaces filled with CSF. CSF, cerebrospinal fluid. (Reproduced with permission from Baehr M, Frotscher M. Duus' Topical Diagnosis in Neurology. Fourth Edition. © Thieme 2005.)

7.4 Choroid Plexus and CSF

7.4.1 Choroid Plexus

The choroid plexus (CP) is a specialized tissue that is highly vascularized and located in the ventricles of the brain. Developmentally, it appears first on the dorsal aspect of the neural tube and eventually will be present in all ventricles (▶ Fig. 7.4a).

- The CP consists of an outer layer of cuboidal epithelial cells that surround fenestrated capillaries and connective tissue. Adjacent epithelial cells are held together by tight junctions forming the blood–CSF barrier (▶ Fig. 7.4b, c).

- The CP can receive blood from the anterior or posterior circulation.
- Although CSF is considered a filtrate of blood, its precise composition is altered from that of plasma by active transport.
  ○ CSF has lower concentrations of glucose, protein, potassium, calcium, and magnesium when compared to plasma. It also has a lower pH and very few cells.

7.4.2 Cerebral Spinal Fluid

CSF is considered a filtrate of plasma that is clear and colorless. However, its chemistry is somewhat different than that of

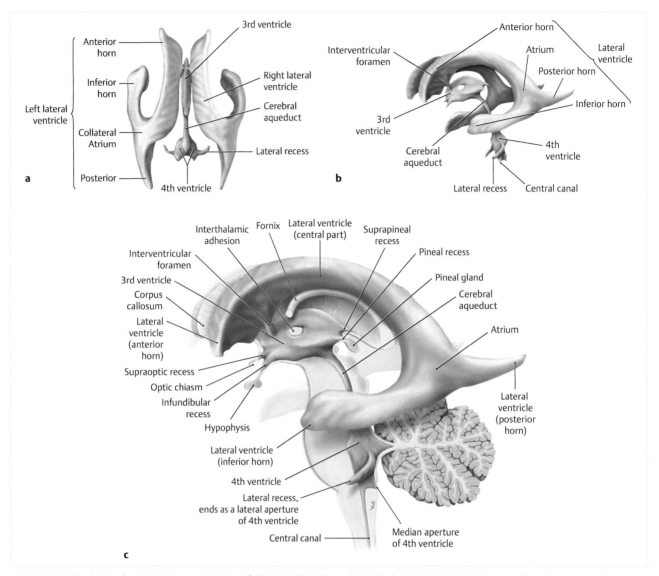

Fig. 7.2 (a) The ventricular system is a continuation of the central spinal canal into the brain. Cast specimens are used to demonstrate the connections between the four ventricular cavities. Superior view. **(b)** The lateral ventricles communicate with the third ventricle via the interventricular foramen. The third ventricle communicates with the fourth ventricle through the cerebral aqueduct. **(c)** The fourth ventricle narrows into the central canal of the spinal cord. (Reproduced with permission from Schuenke M, Schulte E, Schumacher U. THIEME Atlas of Anatomy Third Edition, Vol 3. © Thieme 2020. Illustrations by Markus Voll and Karl Wesker.)

plasma. There is evidence that in addition to blood filtration, active transport of certain molecules does occur. In general, there are few cells, little protein, lower K^+, and fewer amino acids compared to plasma. The pCO_2 in CSF is higher than plasma; thus, the pH is lower. In addition, glucose concentrations are lower in CSF. Most of the CSF is produced in the ventricles by specialized tissue known as the **choroid plexus**.

- Functions of CSF:
  - Helps maintain homeostasis:
    - Provides a constant controlled environment for neural and glial cells.
  - Provides signals for development via growth factors and other growth promoting molecules.
  - Potentially plays a role in signal transduction by providing a route for hormones to move within the brain and between the brain and the rest of the body.
  - Provides a mechanical cushion to protect the brain from trauma.
  - Acts as a lymphatic system for the brain.

Clinical Correlation Box 7.1: Dandy-Walker Syndrome

Dandy-Walker syndrome is a genetic abnormality that results in the malformation of the cerebellum. The **vermis** (medial zone) of the cerebellum is abnormally small or absent and as a result the fourth ventricle is pathologically large. Dandy-Walker syndrome is also associated with abnormalities in other parts of the brain that can lead to **aqueductal stenosis** resulting in **hydrocephalus**. Affected individuals have problems with movement, coordination, intellect, and other neurological functions.

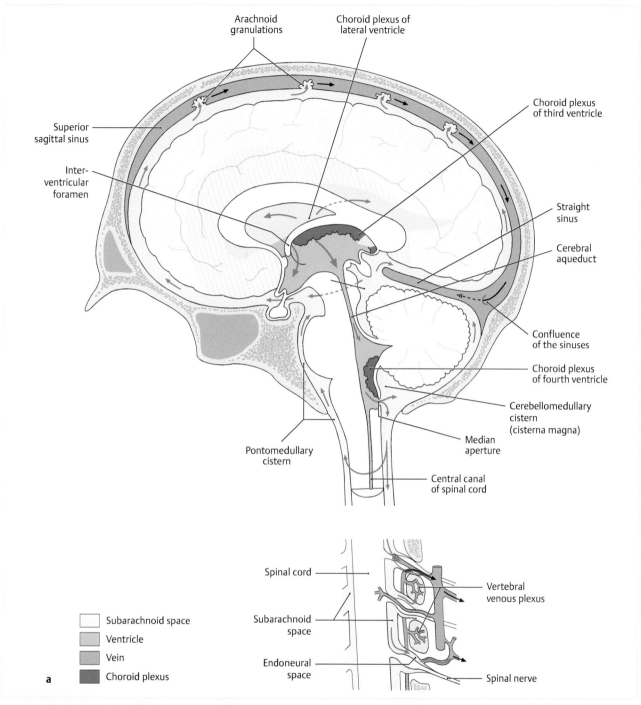

Fig. 7.3 (a) Flow of CSF through the ventricular system.

(Continued)

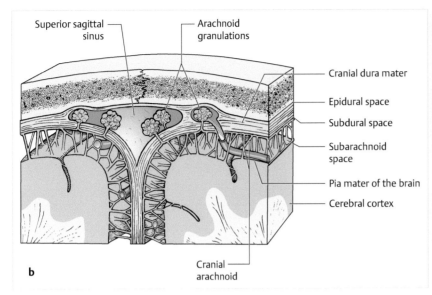

Superior sagittal sinus
Arachnoid granulations
Cranial dura mater
Epidural space
Subdural space
Subarachnoid space
Pia mater of the brain
Cerebral cortex
Cranial arachnoid

b

Fig. 7.3 (*Continued*) **(b)** CSF moves from the ventricular system into the venous system via a pressure gradient. CSF, cerebrospinal fluid. (Fig. 7.3a: Reproduced with permission from Schuenke M, Schulte E, Schumacher U. THIEME Atlas of Anatomy Second Edition, Vol 3. © Thieme 2016. Illustrations by Markus Voll and Karl Wesker. Fig. 7.3b: Reproduced with permission from Baehr M, Frotscher M. Duus' Topical Diagnosis in Neurology. Fourth Edition. © Thieme 2005.)

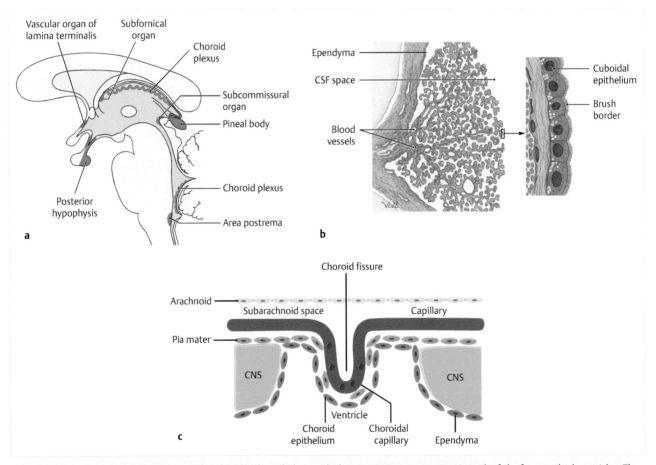

Fig. 7.4 **(a)** Cerebrospinal fluid (CSF) is produced in the choroid plexus, which is present to some extent in each of the four cerebral ventricles. The cerebral ventricles and subarachnoid space have a combined capacity of approximately 150 mL of CSF (20% in the ventricles and 80% in the subarachnoid space). This volume is completely replaced two to four times daily, so that approximately 500 mL of CSF is produced each day. Obstruction of CSF drainage will therefore cause a rise in intracranial pressure. **(b)** The choroid plexus (CP) contains epithelial cells that surround fenestrated capillaries. **(c)** The cuboidal epithelial cells of the CP surround the capillaries. Adjacent epithelial cells are held together by tight junctions forming the blood–CSF barrier. (▶ Fig. 7.4a,b: Reproduced with permission from Schuenke M, Schulte E, Schumacher U. THIEME Atlas of Anatomy Second Edition, Vol 3. © Thieme 2016. Illustrations by Markus Voll and Karl Wesker.)

Hydrocephalus of the brain is the result of an imbalance between the amount of CSF that is produced and the rate at which it is absorbed back into the venous system. Hydrocephalus can be classified as **obstructive** and **nonobstructive**. **Nonobstructive hydrocephaly** occurs when CSF is not absorbed normally resulting in increased volume in the brain. **Obstructive hydrocephaly** occurs when the CSF does not flow normally due to an obstruction. In the case of **overproduction hydrocephalus**, the CSF is overproduced and cannot be resorbed properly.

- The different types of hydrocephaly include:
  - **Congenital hydrocephalus**
    - Aqueductal stenosis
      - Narrowing of the cerebral aqueduct.
    - Neural tube defects
  - **Acquired hydrocephalus**
    - Caused by trauma, brain tumors, cysts, hemorrhage, or infection.

Questions and Answers

1. The fourth ventricle develops in which of the embryonic structures?
   a) Prosencephalon
   b) Diencephalon
   c) Mesencephalon
   d) Rhombincephalon

Level 1: Easy

   Answer D: The fourth ventricle develops on the Prosencephalon; the lateral ventricles develop in **(A)** the Prosencephhalon; the third ventricle develops in **(B)** the Diencephalon. There is no ventricle in the Mesencephalon **(C)**.

2. The lateral ventricles communicate with the third ventricle via which of the following structures?
   a) Interventricular foramen
   b) Cerebral aqueduct
   c) Central canal
   d) Median aperture

Level 2: Moderate

   Answer A: The lateral ventricles communicate to the third ventricle via the interventricular foramen. **(B)** The third

ventricle communicates with the fourth ventricle through the cerebral aqueduct. **(C)** Central canal is formed from the narrowing of the fourth ventricle and continues down the spinal cord. **(D)** The median aperture connects the fourth ventricle to the cisterna magna.

3. CSF is located in which of the following spaces?
   a) Epidural
   b) Subarachnoid
   c) Subdural
   d) Subpial

Level 1: Easy

   Answer B: CSF is located and travels in the subarachnoid space. **(A)** The epidural space is a potential space located between the dura and the skull. **(C)** The subdural space is a potential space located between the dura and the arachnoid layer. **(D)** There is no such potential or real space at the pial level. The pia is tightly adherent to the brain tissue.

4. Which of the following structures does not facilitate communication between the fourth ventricle with the subarachnoid space?
   a) Median aperture
   b) Lateral aperture
   c) Cisterna Magna
   d) Cerebral aqueduct

Level 2: Moderate

   Answer D: The cerebral aqueduct connects the third and the fourth ventricles. **(A)** The median aperture connects the fourth ventricle with the cisterna magna. **(B)** The lateral aperture connects the fourth ventricle with the pontine cistern. **(C)** The cisterna magna is a subarachnoid cistern.

5. The choroid plexus is located in which of the following ventricles?
   a) Lateral
   b) Third
   c) Fourth
   d) A and C
   e) All of the above

Level 1: Easy

   Answer E: Choroid plexus can be found to some degree in *ALL* of the ventricles.

8 The Meninges

Learning Objectives

1. Name the three meningeal layers.
2. Describe the function of the meninges.
3. List and describe the location of the dural septa.
4. List and describe the dural sinuses.
5. Explain the blood supply to the meninges.
6. Describe the innervation of the dura mater.

8.1 Overview of the Meninges

The brain and spinal cord reside in bony structures (skull and vertebral column), which provide protection from external forces. Additionally, the central nervous system (CNS) is encased in membranous coverings called the **meninges**, which help to stabilize the structures particularly during body movements (▶ Fig. 8.1). The three meningeal layers, from the outermost to the innermost are: the **dura mater**, the **arachnoid mater**, and the **pia mater**. The space between the arachnoid and pial layer is called the **subarachnoid space**. The subarachnoid space is filled with **cerebrospinal fluid** (**CSF**), which is a colorless liquid that is somewhat similar to **plasma**. All three meningeal layers are continuous around the spinal cord. The dura mater consists of two parts referred to as **periosteal** and

meningeal layers. The meningeal dural layer creates **septi** that protrude into cranial cavities and separate different aspects of the brain. At several points along the dural reflections, the two layers separate to form venous channels called **sinuses** that drain the **cerebral veins**. The dura mater has its own blood supply from meningeal arteries, the largest of which is the **middle meningeal artery**. Unlike the brain and other meninges, the dura mater is sensitive to pain. It is largely innervated by the **trigeminal nerve** (**CN V**) with contributions from the **vagus** and upper **cervical nerves**.

8.2 Meningeal Layers

There are three distinct meningeal layers that make up the coverings of the brain and spinal cord. From superficial to deep direction, the layers are called the dura mater, the arachnoid mater, and the pia mater (▶ Fig. 8.2a–c).

- All three **connective tissue** layers are derived from the **menix-primitiva**, a meningeal mesenchyme originating from embryonic **mesoderm** and **neural crest**.
- The tough, fibrous dura is the most appreciable of the layers and is often called the **pachymenix**, referring to its "thickness." The word pachy is derived from the Greek word *pachy*, meaning "tough or thick." *Mater* is the Latin word for "mother."

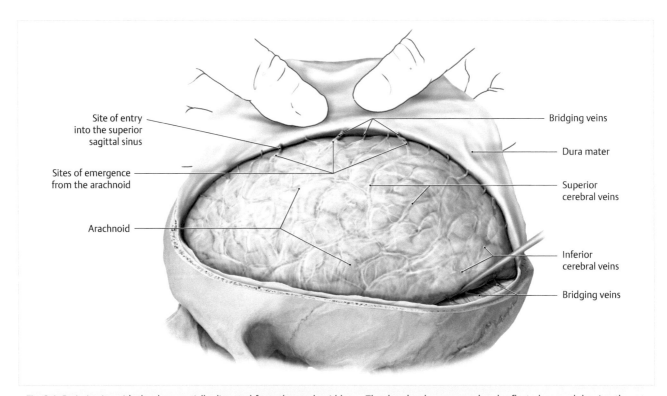

Fig. 8.1 Brain in situ with the dura partially dissected from the arachnoid layer. The dura has been opened and reflected upward, leaving the underlying arachnoid and pia mater on the brain. Because the arachnoid is so thin, the underlying subarachnoid space and the vessels that lie within it can be seen. (Reproduced with permission from Schuenke M, Schulte E, Schumacher U. THIEME Atlas of Anatomy Second Edition, Vol 3. © Thieme 2016. Illustrations by Markus Voll and Karl Wesker.)

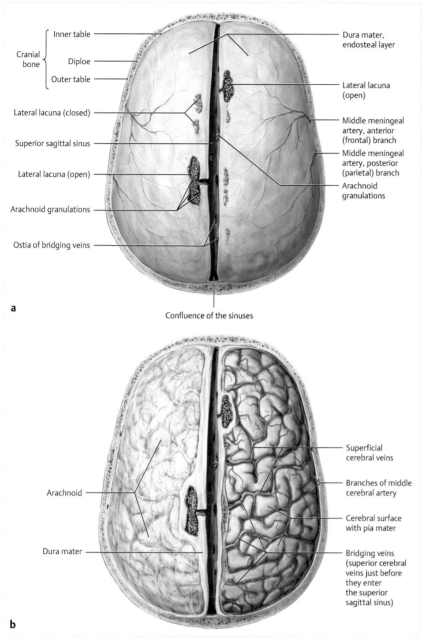

Fig. 8.2 **(a)** Brain and meninges in situ. Superior view of the cranial cavity with the calvarium removed. **(b)** The calvarium has been removed, and the superior sagittal sinus and its lateral lacunae have been opened.

(Continued)

- The arachnoid and pial layers are significantly thinner and more delicate than the dura. These inner layers are continuous with each other and are often called the **leptomeninges**. *Lepto* is the Greek word meaning "fine." *Arachnoid* is the Greek word for "spider" and *pia* is the Latin term for "tender or loving."
- The dural mater has two components: a **periosteal** layer that is attached to the inner aspect of the skull and a meningeal layer that covers the brain.
- The arachnoid layer is attached to the inner surface of the meningeal dura. It is separated from the pial layer by the **subarachnoid space**, which contains **CSF** and blood vessels (▶ Fig. 8.2d).

- The arachnoid layer characteristically has small projections called **arachnoid villi** that are important for the recirculation of CSF.
- Aggregates of villi that project into dural sinuses and facilitate the transfer of CSF are called **arachnoid granulations**. They are most commonly associated with the transverse and superior sagittal sinuses.
- The pial layer is intimately associated with the surface of the brain and extends down into the **sulci**, which are grooves that cover the surface of the brain.
- The meningeal dura, arachnoid, and pia layers surrounding the brain are continuous on the spinal cord.

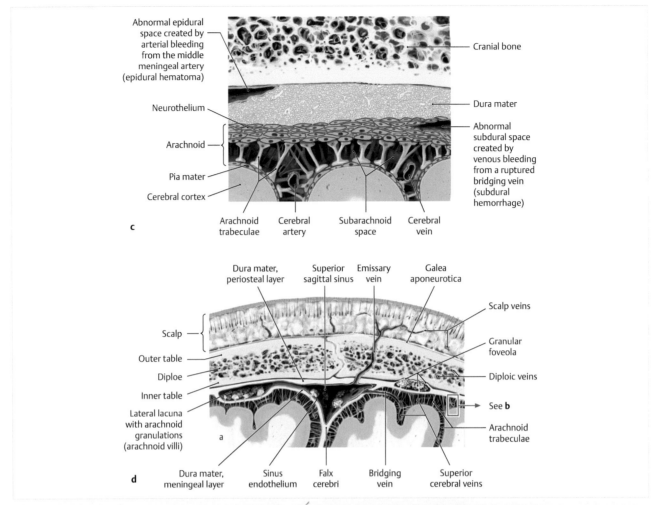

Fig. 8.2 (*Continued*) **(c)** From superficial to deep, the layers are: dura, arachnoid, and pia mater. **(d)** The dura has two components, a periosteal layer and a meningeal layer. The arachnoid layer is attached to the inner aspect of the meningeal dura. It is separated from the pia by the subarachnoid space. (Reproduced with permission from Schuenke M, Schulte E, Schumacher U. THIEME Atlas of Anatomy Second Edition, Vol 3. © Thieme 2016. Illustrations by Markus Voll and Karl Wesker.)

8.3 Function of the Meninges

The meninges, in particular the dura, provide protection from mechanical damage due to trauma and also serve as a framework for the venous drainage of the brain.

- Under normal conditions, there is no *actual* space on the superior or inferior surface of the dura. That is because the dura is tightly adherent to the inner surface of the skull and the arachnoid layer is adherent to the inner surface of the dura.
  - In pathological conditions, such as hemorrhages, the epidural and subdural *potential* spaces can be involved (▶ Fig. 8.3a, b).

8.4 Dural Septa

The meningeal layer of dura creates folds or reflections that are called **dural septa**. These reflections create compartments in the brain (▶ Fig. 8.4).

- The **falx cerebri** runs between the two **cerebral hemispheres**. The term falx is derived from the Greek word *falx*, which means sickle.
  - The falx cerebri occupies the **longitudinal fissure.** It is attached to the **crista galli** (a bony projection above the **cribiform plate** in the **anterior cranial fossa**) anteriorly and the **tentorium cerebelli** posteriorly.
- The falx cerebelli separates the cerebellar hemispheres.

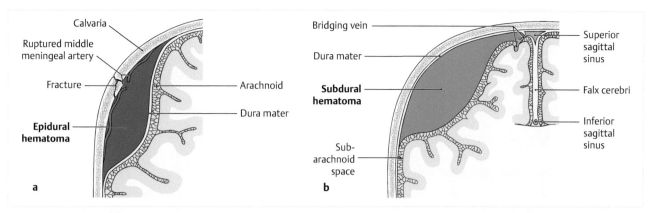

Fig. 8.3 (a, b) After trauma, hemorrhages can develop in the potential spaces. (Reproduced with permission from Schuenke M, Schulte E, Schumacher U. THIEME Atlas of Anatomy Second Edition, Vol 3. © Thieme 2016. Illustrations by Markus Voll and Karl Wesker.)

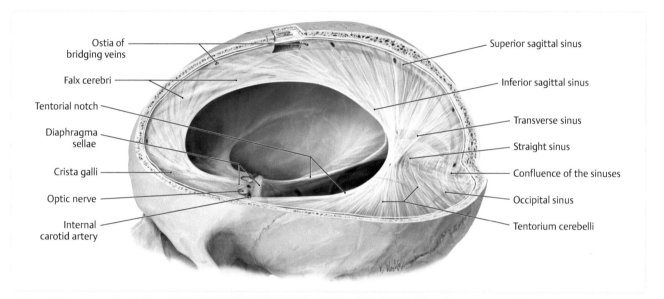

Fig. 8.4 The dural septa, which are folds of the meningeal dural layer, create compartments. (Reproduced with permission from Schuenke M, Schulte E, Schumacher U. THIEME Atlas of Anatomy Second Edition, Vol 3. © Thieme 2016. Illustrations by Markus Voll and Karl Wesker.)

- The tentorium cerebelli separates the cerebrum from the cerebellum.
  - The horizontal orientation of the tentorium cerebelli divides the cranial cavity into a **supratentorial** and an **infratentorial** compartment.
- The **diaphragm sellae**, which is also a dural reflection, forms the roof of the **hypophyseal fossa**. The **infundibulum** of the **pituitary** passes through a small opening in the diaphragm sellae.

8.5 Dural Sinuses

Although the periosteal and meningeal layers of dura are continuous both physically and histologically, there are several points along the edges where the connective tissue forms venous channels that are called **dural venous sinuses** into which the cerebral veins drain. The venous sinuses are valveless and permit blood to return to the systemic circulation in a low-pressure system (▶ Fig. 8.5).

- The **superior sagittal sinus** runs in the superior aspect of the falx cerebri in an anterior-posterior orientation.
- The **inferior sagittal sinus** runs in the inferior edge of the falx cerebri and returns blood, along with the **great cerebral vein**, into the **straight sinus**.
- The **straight sinus** is found at the junction of the falx cerebri and the tentorium cerebelli. It runs posteriorly toward the **confluence of sinuses**.
- The confluence of sinuses is the dilated terminal end of the superior sagittal sinus. It is located near the internal **occipital protuberance**.

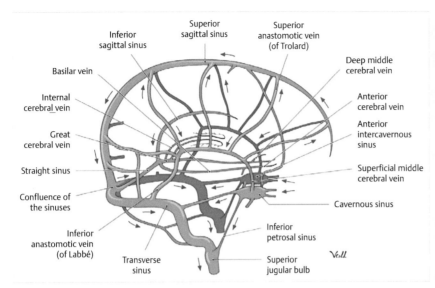

Fig. 8.5 Venous channels (dural venous sinuses) develop between the periosteal and meningeal layers of dura. (Reproduced with permission from Schuenke M, Schulte E, Schumacher U. THIEME Atlas of Anatomy Third Edition, Vol 3. © Thieme 2020. Illustrations by Markus Voll and Karl Wesker.)

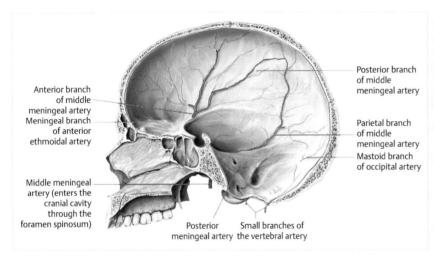

Fig. 8.6 The primary arterial sources of the dura are: middle meningeal, accessory meningeal, and posterior meningeal arteries. (Reproduced with permission from Schuenke M, Schulte E, Schumacher U. THIEME Atlas of Anatomy Second Edition, Vol 3. © Thieme 2016. Illustrations by Markus Voll and Karl Wesker.)

- ○ It receives blood from the superior sagittal, straight, and **occipital** sinuses.
- ○ It is the origin of the **transverse sinuses**.
- The paired transverse sinuses are formed from the superior sagittal sinus and the straight sinus (confluence of sinuses).
  - ○ The sinuses are typically asymmetrical with one larger than the other. One, usually the larger of the two, is the direct continuation of the superior sagittal sinus while the other is an extension of the straight sinus.
  - ○ The transverse sinus emerges from the tentorium as the **sigmoid sinus**.
- The sigmoid sinus forms an "S" shape as it proceeds toward the internal jugular vein where it empties.
- The occipital sinus is the smallest of the dural sinuses. Some of its tributaries join the transverse sinus. It terminates at the confluence of sinuses.
- The **superior petrosal sinus** runs within the tentorium along the **petrous temporal bone**.
  - ○ The superior petrosal sinus carries blood from the **cavernous sinus** to the transverse sinus.

- The **inferior petrosal sinus** is located in a depression between the temporal and occipital bones.
  - ○ The inferior petrosal sinus carries blood from the cavernous sinus and empties directly into the internal jugular vein.

8.6 Blood Supply to the Meninges

The arterial blood supply to the pia and arachnoid layers is primarily from branches of **cerebral vessels** located within the **subarachnoid space**. Numerous vessels, located between the periosteal dura and the skull, supply the dura. **Diploic, emissary,** and **cerebral veins** transport blood to the dural venous sinuses. The arteries to the dura supply the **calvaria** as well. The arterial supply to the dura is primarily the **middle meningeal, accessory meningeal,** and **posterior meningeal arteries** and their branches (▶ Fig. 8.6). The middle meningeal artery is a branch of the **maxillary artery,** a derivative of the internal carotid (IC). It enters the cranium through **foramen spinosum**

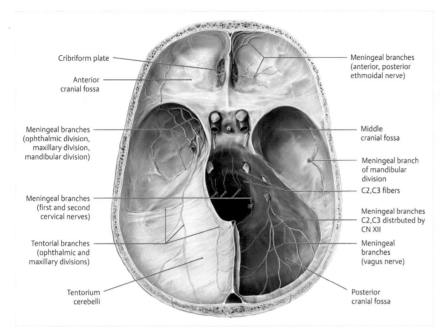

Cribriform plate

Anterior
cranial fossa

Meningeal branches
(ophthalmic division,
maxillary division,
mandibular division)

Meningeal branches
(first and second
cervical nerves)

Tentorial branches
(ophthalmic and
maxillary divisions)

Tentorium
cerebelli

Meningeal branches
(anterior, posterior
ethmoidal nerve)

Middle
cranial fossa

Meningeal branch
of mandibular
division

C2,C3 fibers

Meningeal branches
C2,C3 distrbuted by
CN XII

Meningeal
branches
(vagus nerve)

Posterior
cranial fossa

Fig. 8.7 Sensory afferent fibers innervate the dura. (Reproduced with permission from Schuenke M, Schulte E, Schumacher U. THIEME Atlas of Anatomy Second Edition, Vol 3. © Thieme 2016. Illustrations by Markus Voll and Karl Wesker.)

and ultimately splits into an anterior and posterior branch. The accessory meningeal, a branch of the maxillary artery if present, enters the cranium through the **foramen ovale** and supplies the temporal region. The majority of the posterior fossa is supplied by the posterior meningeal artery which typically is a branch of the **vertebral artery** although this can be somewhat variable. Small areas of the dura are also supplied by branches of the **occipital, ophthalmic,** and **vertebral arteries**.

8.7 Innervation of the Meninges

Innervation of the meninges is limited to **sensory afferent fibers** from the dura mater although there are **sympathetic fibers** that accompany blood vessels of the pia and dural layers (▶ Fig. 8.7). The sensory innervation of the dura is largely provided by the **trigeminal nerve (CN V)** with fewer contributions from the **vagus nerve (CN X)**, the upper three **cervical nerves (C1–C3),** and **meningeal branches** of C2 and C3 carried on the **hyoglossal nerve (CN XII)**. The **ophthalmic division (V1)** of the **trigeminal nerve** primarily supplies the supratentorial aspect of the dura while the infratentorial compartment is supplied by C1–C3 and the vagus nerve (CN X). Both the vagus (CN X) and the hypoglossal nerves (CN XII) carry meningeal nerve branches from C2 and C3 to the dura of the posterior cranial fossa.

- The **anterior cranial fossa** is supplied by:
  - **Ophthalmic division** of the trigeminal nerve (CN V)
    - Nasociliary branch
      - Anterior and posterior ethmoidal nerves
- The **middle cranial fossa** is supplied by:
  - Meningeal branches of the **ophthalmic (V1)**, **maxillary (V2)**, and **mandibular (V3)** branches of the trigeminal nerve.

- The posterior cranial fossa is supplied by:
  - The upper three **cervical nerves** (C1–C3).
  - Meningeal branches of the C2 and C3 cervical nerves carried on the hypoglossal (CN XII) and vagus (CN X) nerves.
  - Meningeal branches of the vagus nerve (CN X).

Clinical Correlation Box 8.1: Meningiomas

A **meningioma** is a tumor that originates in the arachnoid layer of the meninges.[1] The majority of meningiomas are benign, although in rare cases, they can be malignant. This type of tumor is most common in older women but can be found in men and children. Due to their slow growth pattern, meningiomas often go undetected for years and do not always require immediate treatment. However, these benign tumors can grow quite large and depending on location, may be disabling or life threatening.

Clinical Correlation Box 8.2: Headaches

In general, damage to the brain does not produce pain. However, irritation of structures within the cranium, e.g., arteries, venous sinuses, and dura, can produce head pain such as headaches. Distortion or traction of the dura produced by intracranial masses or increased cranial pressure is thought to be the source of many headaches. Headaches can also be induced following a lumbar puncture where CSF is removed for laboratory analysis. The removal of CSF results in a decrease of intracranial volume and pressure. The change in pressure can result in traction of the dura and subsequent stimulation of pain receptors located in the dura causing headache which can be exacerbated or relieved by postural movements.

Clinical Correlation Box 8.3: Meningitis

Meningitis is the inflammation of the meninges of the brain and spinal cord. Studies have shown that typically infectious meningitis involves the leptomeninges (arachnoid and pia) while other causes, such as carcinomatous and chemical, affect the pachymeninges (Kioumehr et al., 1995). The two main causes of meningitis are viruses and bacteria with viral being the more common of the two. Both viral and bacterial meningitis are spread from person to person. Fungi, parasites, drugs, or trauma can also cause meningitis. The classic triad of symptoms includes stiff neck, fever, and headache. Other symptoms include, but are not limited to, vomiting, seizures, photophobia, and delirium. There are vaccines available for some of the more common types of vaccines seen in the United States.

Reference

1. American Association of Neurological Surgeons, 2012. https://www.aans.org/Patients/Neurosurgical-Conditions-and-Treatments/Meningiomas

Questions and Answers

1. The meningeal layer that extends down into the sulci is?
   a) Periosteal dura
   b) Meningeal dura
   c) Arachnoid
   d) Pia
   e) All of the above

Level 2: Moderate

Answer D is correct. The pial layer dives down into the sulci. **(A)** The periosteal dura is tightly adherent to the calvaria. **(B)** The meningeal dura creates reflections that divides the cranial cavity if four distinct locations. **(C)** The arachnoid layer is adherent to the inner layer of dura and follows its contours.

2. The falx cerebri is located in which of the following structures?
   a) Superior sagittal fissure
   b) Lateral sulcus
   c) Transverse cerebral fissure
   d) Diaphragma sellae
   e) None of the above

Level 1: Easy

Answer A is correct. **(B)** Lateral sulcus does not contain a dural septum. **(C)** The tentorium cerebelli is found within the transverse cerebral fissure. **(D)** The diaphragm sellae forms the roof of the hypophyseal fossa.

3. Which of the following sinuses does not drain into the confluence of sinuses?
   a) Superior sagittal sinus
   b) Inferior sagittal sinus
   c) Right transverse sinus
   d) Occipital sinus

Level 2: Moderate

Answer C is correct. The transvers sinus drains away from the confluence of sinuses. **(A)** The superior sagittal sinus and **(B)** The inferior sagittal sinus.

4. The blood supply to the anterior cranial fossa is supplied by which of the following arteries?
   a) Ascending pharyngeal
   b) Vertebral
   c) Accessory branch of the middle meningeal
   d) Ophthalmic

Level 2: Moderate

Answer D is correct. **(A)** The ascending pharyngeal supplies the middle *AND* posterior cranial fossa. **(B)** The vertebral artery supplies the posterior cranial fossa. **(C)** Accessory branch of the middle meningeal supplies the middle cranial fossa.

5. Which of the following nerves provide the majority of the sensory afferents to the dura mater?
   a) CN V
   b) C3
   c) CN X
   d) CN XII

Level 2: Moderate

Answer A. is correct. **(B)** C3; **(C)** CN X; and **(D)** CN XII all provide minor contributions to the innervation of the dura.

9 Cranial Nerves

9.1 Overview of Cranial Nerves

- Cranial nerves are a set of 12 paired peripheral nerves that arise directly from the brain and innervate the structures of the head and neck. Each cranial nerve is named according to its structure or function and sequentially numbered with Roman numerals (CNs I–XII). The numerical classification reflects the rostral to caudal position of the cranial nerves as each nerve enters or exits the cerebrum and brainstem (▶ Fig. 9.1).
- Cranial nerves carry motor, sensory, and autonomic fibers, along with several unique nerve fibers, which reflect the special functional attributes of the head. The types of fibers carried by the nerves serve as the basis for classifying the neurons of the cranial nerves into functional components/modalities (▶ Table 9.1).
- In comparison to spinal nerves that pass through the intervertebral foramina in an orderly arrangement, the cranial nerves arise from various levels of the brain and travel through numerous fissures and foramina in the cranium (skull) (▶ Fig. 9.2). Among the 12 cranial nerves, the CN I (olfactory) and CN II (optic) nerves develop as outgrowths of the forebrain directly and are considered extensions of the central nervous system (CNS). The remaining cranial nerves, CNs III to XII, develop in association with the brainstem and enter and exit from distinct regions of the midbrain, pons, and medulla.
- The following sections discuss the functional components of the cranial nerves, the location of the motor and sensory nuclei, and the general distribution path of each cranial nerve. The specific ascending pathways of the special senses are covered in Chapter 15, while more detailed descriptions for the trigeminal (CN V), facial (CN VII), glossopharyngeal (CN IX), vagus (CN X), and hypoglossal (CN XII) nerves are provided in Chapters 20 and 21.

9.2 Functional Modalities of Cranial Nerves

9.2.1 Classification of Functional Fiber Types

- Cranial nerves transmit motor, sensory, or autonomic input and function in a manner analogous to spinal nerves. However, cranial nerves exhibit a more complex innervation pattern due to the functional and structural diversity of the head and neck region.
- Cranial nerves that convey special sensory input for taste, sight, sound, and smell carry ancillary types of nerve fibers to accommodate the functional complexity of the head.
- Collectively, seven types of nerve fibers may emanate from cranial nerve motor and sensory neurons and convey the functional modalities associated with the cranial nerves.
- Each cranial nerve carries one to five of the functional fiber types.
- The seven fiber types include four types of **motor (efferent)** fibers and three **sensory (afferent)** fiber types. Motor and sensory fibers are classified as **general** or **special** and further designated as **somatic (body-related)** or **visceral** components.
- A short-hand designation for the types of neurons and associated fibers uses a three-letter classification scheme.
  - The **first letter** is either **G = general** or **S = special**. General refers to neurons common to both the head and body. Special refers to types of neurons found only in the head.
  - The **second letter** is **S = somatic** or **V = visceral**. Somatic refers to the types of neurons that innervate somite-derived structures, such as skeletal muscle, connective tissue, and skin of the body. Visceral refers to neurons that supply the internal organs, mucosa, glands, blood vessels, and structures derived from the pharyngeal arches.
  - The **third letter** is either **A = afferent** or **E = efferent**. Afferent refers to sensory neurons and associated fibers that convey somatic and visceral sensations. Efferent refers to motor neurons that supply skeletal and smooth muscle, along with providing glandular secretion.
- Based on this classification scheme, the seven modalities are designated as follows.
  - General functional modalities found in the cranial nerves are analogous to those carried by the spinal nerves and include general somatic efferent (GSE), general somatic afferent (GSA), general visceral efferent (GVE), and general visceral afferent (GVA).
  - Special functional components that are unique to the head and found *only* in the cranial nerves include special visceral

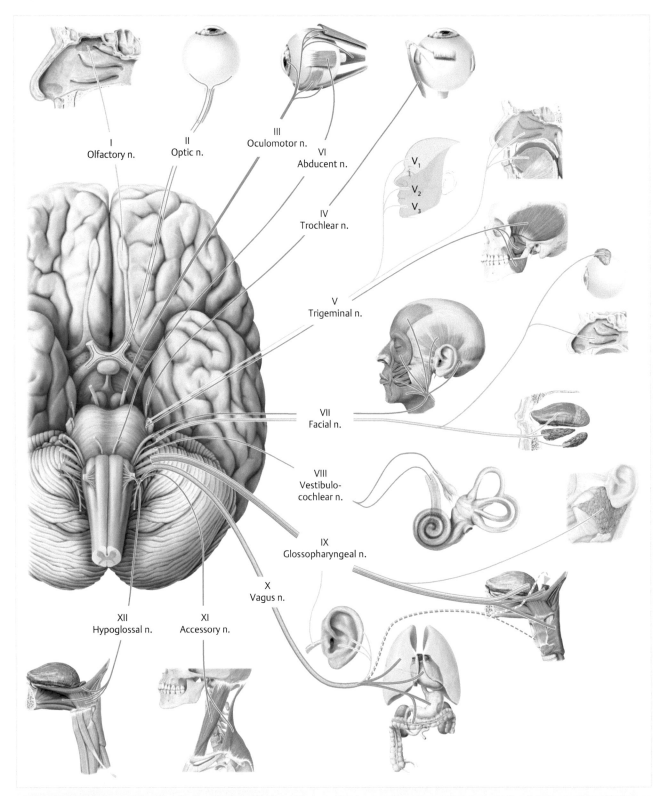

Fig. 9.1 Cranial nerves. Inferior (basal) view. The 12 pairs of cranial nerves (CNs) are numbered according to the order of their emergence from the brainstem. Note: The sensory and motor fibers of the cranial nerves enter and exit the brainstem at the same sites. In comparison, the sensory and motor fibers of spinal nerves enter and leave through posterior and anterior roots, respectively. (Reproduced with permission from Schuenke M, Schulte E, Schumacher U. THIEME Atlas of Anatomy Third Edition, Vol 3. © Thieme 2020. Illustrations by Markus Voll and Karl Wesker.)

I
Olfactory n.

II
Optic n.

III
Oculomotor n.

VI
Abducent n.

IV
Trochlear n.

V_1
V_2
V_3

V
Trigeminal n.

VII
Facial n.

VIII
Vestibulo-
cochlear n.

IX
Glossopharyngeal n.

X
Vagus n.

XII
Hypoglossal n.

XI
Accessory n.

Table 9.1 General overview of cranial nerves

Cranial Nerve Name	Roman Numeral	Location	Fissure/ Foramina	General Function	Functional Modality
Olfactory	CN I	Telencephalon	Cribriform plate	Olfaction	SVA
Optic	CN II	Diencephalon	Optic canal	Vision	SSA
Oculomotor	CN III	Midbrain	Superior orbital fissure	Eye movement; Oculomotor nerve: Superior branch • Levator palpebrae • Superior rectus Inferior branch • Medial rectus • Inferior rectus • Inferior oblique Pupillary constriction; visual accommodation	GSE GVE
Trochlear	CN IV	Midbrain	Superior orbital fissure	Eye movement Motor to superior oblique	GSE
Trigeminal	CN V	Pons	• Superior orbital fissure (V1) • Foramen rotundum (V2) • Foramen ovale (V3)	General sensation of pain, temperature, proprioception from orofacial region Motor to muscles of mastication	SVE GSA
Abducens	CN VI	Pons	Superior orbital fissure	Eye movements Motor to lateral rectus	GSE
Facial	CN VII	Pons	Internal auditory meatus → stylomastoid foramen	Motor to muscles of facial expression; taste, lacrimation, salivation; general sensation around ear	SVE GVE GSA GVA SVA
Vestibulocochlear	CN VIII	Pons Medulla	Internal auditory meatus	Hearing and balance	SSA
Glossopharyngeal	CN IX	Medulla	Jugular foramen	Sensation to oropharynx; carotid reflex, taste; parotid salivation, motor to stylopharyngeus muscle	SVE GVE GSA GVA SVA
Vagus	CN X	Medulla	Jugular foramen	Sensation to larynx, motor to most palatal, pharyngeal, and all laryngeal muscles; aortic reflex; taste; parasympathetic to heart, lungs, and gut	SVE GVE GSA GVA SVA
Accessory **	CN XI	Spinal component: C1–C6 of spinal cord	Jugular foramen	Motor to: Sternocleidomastoid Trapezius	GSE/SVE **controversy in origin
Hypoglossal	CN XII	Medulla	Hypoglossal canal	Motor to tongue muscles (extrinsic and intrinsic tongue muscles except palatoglossus)	GSE

Abbreviations: GSA, general somatic afferent; GSE, general somatic efferent; GVA, general visceral afferent; GVE, general visceral efferent; SSA, special somatic afferent; SVA, special visceral afferent; SVE, special visceral efferent.

Notes: * Motor and sensory fibers of cranial nerves exit and enter the skull through the same foramina.

** There is controversy in the literature regarding the existence of a cranial component of the spinal accessory nerve. Recent evidence suggests that the accessory nerve has no connection to the vagus and lacks a cranial component. There is additional controversy whether accessory motor nucleus is GSE or SVE.

Openings between internal surface of cranial base and other spaces

Anterior cranial fossa

Anterior ethmoidal foramen

- Anterior ethmoidal nerve, artery and vein

→ *Orbit*

Cribriform plate

- Olfactory nerves (I)
- Anterior ethmoidal nerve, artery and vein

→ *Nasal cavity*

Middle cranial fossa

Optic canal

- Optic nerve (II)
- Ophthalmic artery

→ *Orbit*

Superior orbital fissure

① Superior ophthalmic vein
② Ophthalmic nerve (V₁)
   2a Lacrimal nerve
   2b Frontal nerve
   2c Nasociliary nerve
③ Abducens nerve (VI)
④ Oculomotor nerve (III)
⑤ Trochlear nerve (IV)

→ *Orbit*

Hiatus for lesser petrosal nerve

- Greater petrosal nerve (parasympathetic, from IX)
- Superior tympanic artery

→ *Tympanic cavity*

Hiatus for greater petrosal nerve

- Greater petrosal nerve (parasympathetic, from VII)
- Stylomastoid vein and artery

→ *Facial canal*

Posterior cranial fossa

Porus and internal acoustic meatus

- Labyrinthine artery and veins
① Facial nerve (with intermediate nerve) (VII)
② Vestibulocochlear nerve (V₃)

→ *Facial canal, inner ear*

Openings between internal and external surface of cranial base

Middle cranial fossa

Foramen rotundum

- Maxillary nerve (V₂)

Foramen ovale

- Mandibular nerve (V₃)
- Pterygoid meningeal artery
- Venous plexus of foramen ovale

Carotid canal

- Internal carotid artery
- Internal carotid plexus (sympathetic)
- Internal carotid venous plexus

Foramen lacerum

(covered by internal carotid artery)

- Deep petrosal nerve
- Greater petrosal nerve (parasympathetic, from VII)

Foramen spinosum

- Middle meningeal artery
- Meningeal branch of mandibular nerve (V₃)

Petrosphenoidal fissure

- Lesser petrosal nerve (parasympathetic, from IX)

Posterior cranial fossa

Jugular foramen

① Glossopharyngeal nerve (IX)
② Vagus nerve (X)
③ Inferior petrosal sinus
④ Accessory nerve (XI)
⑤ Posterior meningeal artery
⑥ Internal jugular vein

Foramen magnum

See right-hand side

Hypoglossal canal

- Hypoglossal nerve (XII)
- Venous plexus of hypoglossal canal

Condylar canal

- Condylar emissary vein (inconstant)

Mastoid foramen

- Mastoid emissary vein
- Mastoid branch of occipital artery

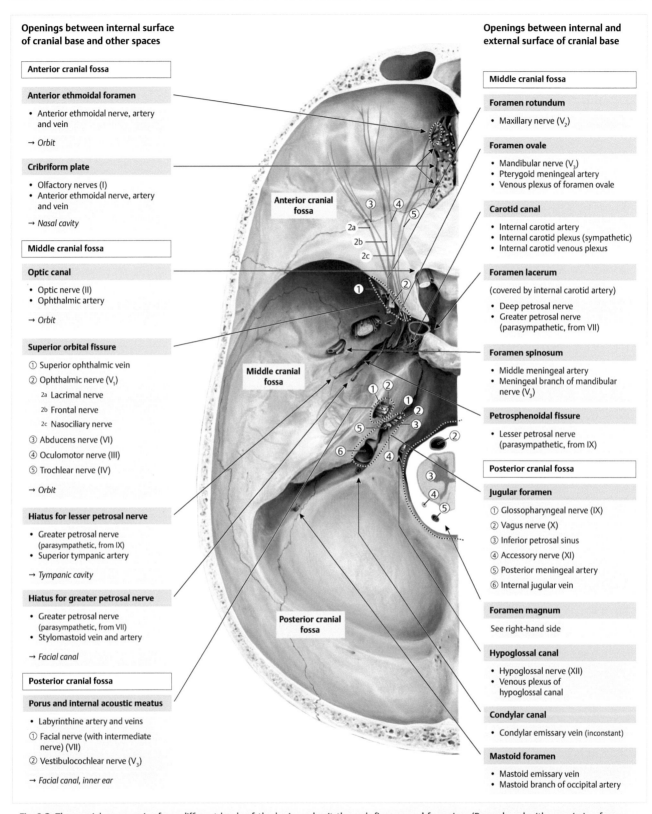

Fig. 9.2 The cranial nerves arise from different levels of the brain and exit through fissures and foramina. (Reproduced with permission from Schuenke M, Schulte E, Schumacher U. THIEME Atlas of Anatomy Second Edition, Vol 3. © Thieme 2016. Illustrations by Markus Voll and Karl Wesker.)

Table 9.2 Categories of cranial nerve functional components

Motor (Efferent)		
Nerve Fiber Modality	**Function**	**Cranial Nerve**
General somatic efferent (GSE)	• Voluntary motor to skeletal muscle of eye and tongue; muscles derived from somites	**CN III** (oculomotor nerve) **CN IV** (trochlear) **CN VI** (abducens) **CN XII** (hypoglossal)
General visceral efferent (GVE)	• Autonomic (involuntary motor) innervation to glands, smooth muscle, and cardiac muscle • In the head, GVE neurons are from the cranial portion of the parasympathetic system	**CN III** (oculomotor nerve) **CNVII** (facial nerve) **CN IX** (glossopharyngeal) **CN X** (vagus)
Special visceral efferent (SVE)	• Voluntary motor to skeletal muscles derived from pharyngeal (branchiomeric) arch mesoderm • Pharyngeal arch muscles perform specialized functions of mastication, facial expression, phonation, and deglutition	**CN V** (trigeminal) **CN VII** (facial) **CN IX** (glossopharyngeal) **CN X** (vagus) **CN XI*** (accessory)

*There is a discrepancy in the literature on whether the accessory nerve is considered GSE or SVE.

Sensory (Afferent)		
Nerve Fiber Modality	**Function**	**Cranial Nerve**
General visceral afferent (GVA)	• Transmit visceral sensations such as distention, stretch, or pain from interoceptors in visceral organs and from baroreceptors and chemoreceptors that help regulate blood pressure and heart rate • Contribute to autonomic visceral reflex arcs with GVE fibers	**CN VII** (facial) **CN IX** (glossopharyngeal) **CN X** (vagus)
Special visceral afferent (SVA)	• Transmit taste sensation and smell from chemoreceptors associated with taste buds and the olfactory mucosa	**CN I** (olfactory nerve) (taste) **CN VII** (facial) **CN IX** (glossopharyngeal) **CN X** (vagus)
General somatic afferent (GSA)	• Transmit pain, temperature, touch, and positional information from exteroceptors and proprioceptors found in the skin, mucosa, muscles, and joints	**CN V** (trigeminal) **CN VII** (facial) **CN IX** (glossopharyngeal) **CN X** (vagus)
Special somatic afferent (SSA)	• Transmit the special sense of sight, hearing, and balance from exteroceptive input	**CN II** (optic nerve) (sight) **CN VIII** (vestibulocochlear (hearing, balance)

afferent (SVA), special somatic afferent (SSA), and special visceral efferent (SVE).

• The different functional modalities carried by the cranial nerves can serve as a basis for classifying the cranial nerves (► Table 9.2).
  ○ **CNs III, IV, VI,** and **XII** carry **GSE fibers** and provide voluntary motor function to the extrinsic skeletal musculature of the eye and tongue. GSE fibers found in the head are homologous to fibers carried by spinal nerves.
    – CNs III, IV, VI, and XII possess a small sensory component that transmits proprioceptive input from extraocular and tongue muscles.
  ○ **CNs I, II,** and **VIII** carry only **special sensory** fibers. Special sensory modalities include vision, auditory, balance (vestibular), and taste. These special sensory sensations are unique attributes of cranial nerves and include **SSA** and **SVA**, based on the type of receptor stimulation. SSA receptors respond to light and mechanical stimulation, while SVA fibers utilize chemoreceptors and respond to chemical stimuli.

– The **optic (CN II)** and **vestibulocochlear (CN VIII)** carry **SSA fibers**. For the eye, specialized neuroepithelial cells, known as **rods** and **cones**, reside within the retinal epithelium and serve as sensory receptors or **photoreceptors**. The sensory receptors for the vestibulocochlear apparatus are neuroepithelial cells known as **hair cells**, which are specific to the organ of Corti, the semicircular canals, the utricle, and the saccule of the inner ear. The sensory neurons of the vestibulocochlear apparatus convey information about hearing and balance.

– The **olfactory nerve (CN I)** carries **SVA fibers** associated with the sense of smell. Olfactory receptors are bipolar neurons found within the olfactory epithelium lining the roof of the nasal cavity and act as chemoreceptors to mediate the sense of smell (olfaction).

– It is important to note that **SVA fibers** are also associated with chemoreceptors that detect the special sensation of **taste**. Specialized neuroepithelial cells found within **taste buds** synapse with the SVA fibers of **CNs VII, IX,** and **X** to mediate the sensation of taste (**gustation**).

○ **CNs V, VII, IX,** and **X** are mixed nerves that carry both **motor (SVE)** and **sensory (GSA)** fibers.

– The motor fibers carried by **CNs V, VII, IX,** and **X** are classified as SVE fibers because the SVE neurons provide motor innervation to a unique group of skeletal muscles that develop from pharyngeal arch (branchiomeric) mesoderm. These voluntary skeletal muscles function in visceral tasks such as eating, swallowing, phonation, and speaking, which are distinct functions to the head. Pharyngeal arch derived muscles are morphologically identical to skeletal muscles in the body; however, the neurons of these efferent fibers have a distinct location in the brainstem. The accessory nerve, CN XI, also carries motor fibers to skeletal muscle; however, there is controversy in the literature concerning the classification of the fibers as GSE or SVE. The basis for the controversy of the accessory nerve stems from the location of the neuron cell bodies in the spinal cord and the origin of the neck skeletal muscles. The motor fibers of the accessory nerve innervate the trapezius and sternocleidomastoid muscles.

– The **GSA** fibers transmit pain, temperature, crude and discriminative touch, as well as stereognostic, proprioceptive (positional), and kinesthetic (movement) inputs from the skin, temporomandibular joint (TMJ), muscles, and mucous membranes of the orofacial and pharyngeal regions.

▪ **CN V** transmits the majority of GSA input from the head, face, and oral cavity, with minor contributions provided from the region of the ear by **CNs VII, IX,** and **X**. CNs IX and X also convey GSA information from the mucosa of the ear, auditory tube, oropharynx, and laryngeal region.

– GSA fibers in the head are functionally identical to fibers in spinal nerves.

○ **CNs III, VII, IX**, and **X** carry autonomic **(GVE) fibers** from the cranial portion of the **parasympathetic** nervous system. The parasympathetic fibers are analogous to those carried by the sacral spinal nerves.

– GVE fibers provide motor innervation to smooth muscle and secretomotor innervation for glandular secretion.

▪ The cell bodies of the GVE neurons are part of a two-neuron relay chain, with the first cell body located in the gray matter of the CNS and the second cell body located in peripheral autonomic ganglia.

9.2.2 Cranial Nuclei

• The olfactory and optic cranial nerves develop as outgrowths of the developing forebrain and do not possess cranial nerve nuclei in the brainstem.

• During development, motor and sensory neurons of CNs III to XII become organized within the alar and basal plates of the brainstem into seven functionally similar groups of neuronal cell bodies known as **nuclei**.

• In the adult, the groups of functionally related neurons are arranged in the gray matter throughout the long axis of the brainstem as six discontinuous **columns of nuclei**.

○ The motor and sensory functional columns exhibit a medial to lateral arrangement, with the motor nuclei lying medial to the nuclei of the sensory columns (▶ Fig. 9.3).

○ Each column of nuclei serves a different **motor (efferent)** or **sensory (afferent)** function and corresponds to the functional modalities carried by the cranial nerve fiber types.

○ In the adult brainstem, there are **three columns of sensory nuclei** on which primary afferent fibers terminate and **three columns of motor nuclei** from which efferent fibers originate.

9.2.3 General Overview of Motor and Sensory Pathways

• In a manner analogous to spinal nerves, the transmission of motor and sensory input from cranial nerves occurs through distinct multisynaptic nerve pathways in which the signal passes between a chain of several sequentially arranged neurons.

• In general, the first neuron in the relay chain is the first to propagate information and synapses on the second neuron in the chain. The location of the first neuron varies between the sensory and motor pathways. Sensory, first-order neurons are found in the peripheral nervous system (PNS), while motor neurons are in the CNS. The second-order neuron usually resides in cranial nerve nuclei.

○ **Sensory pathways,** also known as **ascending pathways,** are groups of axons that form **ascending tracts** and function to transmit information from peripheral receptors to cranial sensory nuclei and then to higher regions of the brain for conscious and unconscious processing.

○ **Motor pathways,** also known as **descending pathways,** consist of groups of axons **(tracts)** that descend from neurons in the cortex, hypothalamus, and brainstem and function to modulate efferent neurons situated within cranial nerve motor nuclei of the brainstem or within the spinal cord.

• Afferent sensory pathways consist of three major neurons: the primary, secondary, and tertiary neurons (▶ Fig. 9.4).

○ For afferent sensory paths, the **primary afferent (first-order)** neuron typically resides in the PNS within **cranial sensory ganglia.** Cranial sensory ganglia are homologous structures to the dorsal root (spinal) ganglia.

○ The peripheral axons of first-order neurons receive input from various types of sensory receptors, while the central axonal processes transmit the information to the integrative **second-order neurons** found within **cranial sensory nuclei** of the gray matter of the brainstem. A synapse does not occur in the sensory ganglion.

○ Axons of second-order sensory neurons, which may decussate (cross the midline), form ascending tracts that synapse on **third-order integrative (relay) neurons** in the **thalamus.** Relay fibers from the thalamus project to the **primary somatosensory cortex** for conscious processing.

• Alternatively, axons of ascending tract may terminate in the cerebellum or on integrative neurons in visceral autonomic reflex centers of the hypothalamus and the reticular formation of the brainstem to modulate autonomic functions.

• The **efferent motor pathways** involved in mediating voluntary motor activity consist of two principal neurons: the **upper motor neurons (UMNs)**, also known as

Classification of cranial nerve fibers and nuclei				
This color coding is used to indicate fiber and nuclei classifications.				
	Fiber type	Example	Fiber type	Example
	General somatic efferent (somatomotor function)	Innervate skeletal muscles	General somatic afferent (somatic sensation)	Conduct impulses from skin, skeletal muscle spindles
	General visceral efferent (visceromotor function)	Innervate smooth muscle of the viscera, intraocular muscles, heart, salivary glands, etc.	Special somatic afferent	Conduct impulses from retina, auditory and vestibular apparatuses
	Special visceral efferent	Innervate skeletal muscles derived from branchial arches	General visceral afferent (visceral sensation)	
			Special visceral afferent	Conduct impulses from taste buds, olfactory mucosa

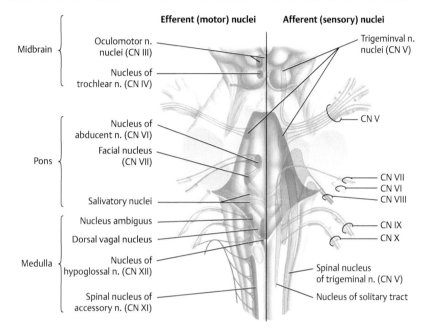

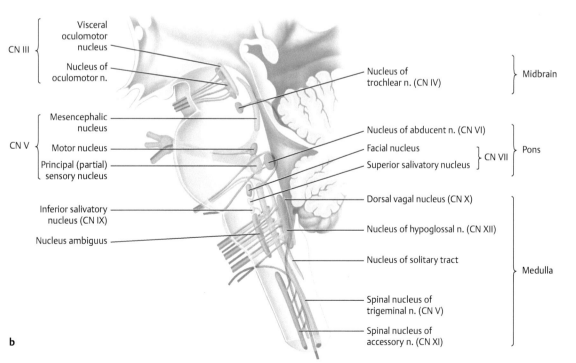

Fig. 9.3 (a,b) In the adult, groups of functionally related neurons are arranged into six columns within the gray matter. (Reproduced with permission from Schuenke M, Schulte E, Schumacher U. THIEME Atlas of Anatomy Third Edition, Vol 3. © Thieme 2020. Illustrations by Markus Voll and Karl Wesker.)

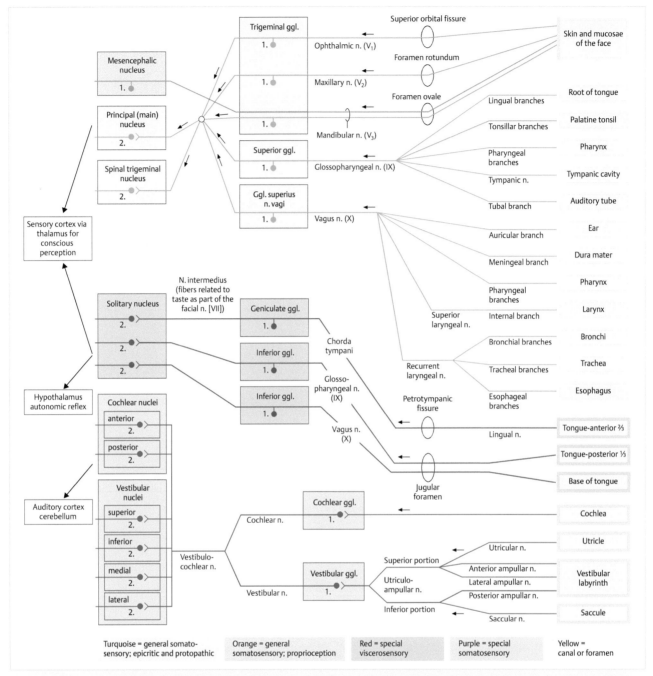

Fig. 9.4 Afferent sensory pathways include primary, secondary, and tertiary neurons. (Reproduced with permission from Schuenke M, Schulte E, Schumacher U. THIEME Atlas of Anatomy Second Edition, Vol 3. © Thieme 2016. Illustrations by Markus Voll and Karl Wesker.)

supranuclear neurons, and the **lower motor neurons (LMNs),** which comprise cranial motor nuclei (▶ Fig. 9.5a).
- For voluntary motor activity, UMNs reside in the **primary motor cortex,** the **premotor motor cortex (PMC),** and **supplementary motor areas (SMAs). Supranuclear (UMN)** neurons represent **first-order motor neurons** and function in the execution and planning of voluntary movements as well as maintaining posture and balance.
- Axons originating from UMNs form **descending fiber tracts** that synapse on the **LMNs** found within the **cranial nerve motor nuclei** or spinal cord.

- Fibers projecting from LMNs in cranial motor nuclei terminate on skeletal muscle to elicit contraction and movement.
- The **efferent paths** that mediate **autonomic** functions utilize a three-neuron circuit:
  - For involuntary visceromotor activity associated with the autonomic nervous system, **supranuclear (preautonomic)** neurons reside within **hypothalamic nuclei** and integrative nuclei of the **brainstem** and **reticular formation.**
  - Axonal tracts descend from preautonomic neurons to synapse on preganglionic parasympathetic neurons in

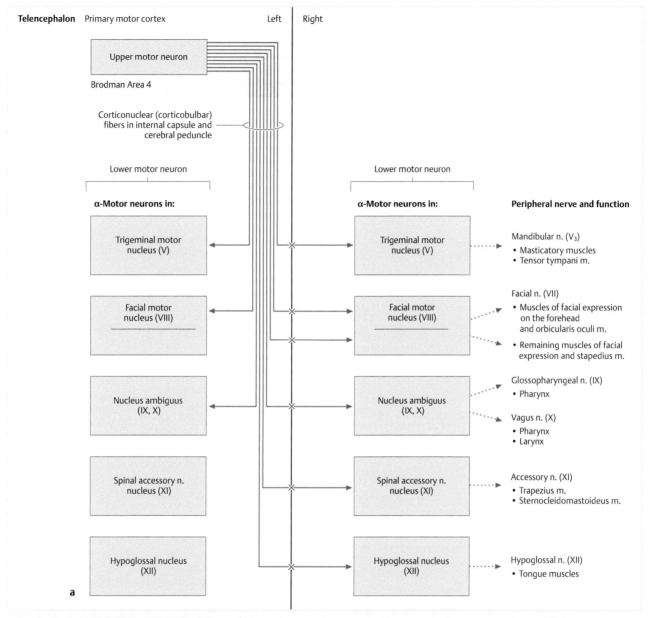

Fig. 9.5 (a) The GSE and SVE neurons of the efferent motor pathway mediate voluntary motor activity. (Fig. 9.5a: Reproduced with permission from Schuenke M, Schulte E, Schumacher U. THIEME Atlas of Anatomy Second Edition, Vol 3. © Thieme 2016. Illustrations by Markus Voll and Karl Wesker.)

(Continued)

cranial visceral motor (GVE) nuclei or synapse on preganglionic sympathetic neurons of the **intermediolateral column (IMLC)** of the spinal cord at T1–L2 vertebral level.

  ○ Preganglionic fibers project to the PNS to synapse on postganglionic cell bodies in **autonomic ganglia**.

• Postganglionic fibers originate from autonomic ganglia and terminate on smooth muscle, cardiac muscle, and glands to modulate effector output.

  ○ In the head and neck, postganglionic parasympathetic and sympathetic fibers accompany or "hitch-hike" with cranial nerves or blood vessels found within the local vicinity for distribution to their target organ (▶ Fig. 9.5b).

9.2.4 Cranial Nerve Sensory Pathways: Ganglia and Nuclei

• Among the four sensory modalities carried by the cranial nerves, there are three corresponding columns of sensory nuclei found in the brainstem. Each column of sensory nuclei contains second-order interneurons and receives input from central afferent fibers of the first-order neurons which lie within cranial sensory ganglia in the PNS (▶ Table 9.3).

• The eight cranial sensory ganglia include the **trigeminal (semilunar) ganglion** (**CN V**), **geniculate ganglion** (**CN VII**), **vestibular** and **spiral ganglion** (**CN VIII**),

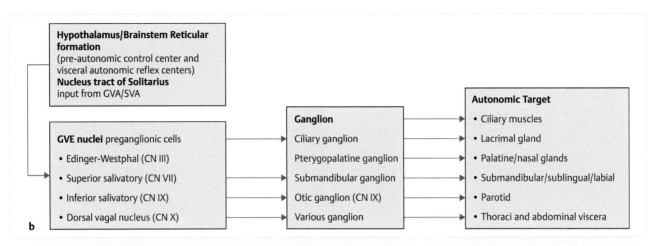

Fig. 9.5 (*Continued*) **(b)** GVE neurons of visceral efferent motor pathway mediate autonomic function. Postganglionic autonomic fibers originate in autonomic ganglia and terminate on their target structures. In the head and neck, theses fibers travel with cranial nerves or blood vessels. GSE, general somatic efferent; GVE, general visceral efferent; SVE, special visceral efferent. (Reproduced with permission from Schuenke M, Schulte E, Schumacher U. THIEME Atlas of Anatomy Third Edition, Vol 3. © Thieme 2020. Illustrations by Markus Voll and Karl Wesker.)

Table 9.3 Cranial sensory ganglia and nuclei of the brainstem

Cranial Nerve	Type of Afferent Neuron	Name of Sensory Ganglia (location of first-order neurons)	Name of Cranial Nerve Nuclei (location of second-order neurons)
Trigeminal (CN V)	GSA	Trigeminal (semilunar) • Pseudounipolar neurons	Trigeminal nuclear complex: • Mesencephalic nucleus of V** • Main (principal/chief) sensory nucleus of V • Spinal trigeminal nucleus
Facial (CN VII)	GSA	Geniculate • Pseudounipolar neurons	Spinal trigeminal nucleus
	SVA GVA	Geniculate • Pseudounipolar neurons	Rostral Nucleus solitarius Caudal nucleus solitarius
Vestibulocochlear (CN VIII)	SSA	Vestibular (Scarpa) ganglion • Bipolar neurons	Vestibular nuclei
		Cochlear (spiral) ganglion • Bipolar neurons	Cochlear nuclei
Glossopharyngeal (CN IX)	GSA	Superior ganglion of CN IX • Pseudounipolar neurons	Spinal trigeminal nucleus
	SVA GVA	Inferior ganglion (petrous) of CN IX • Pseudounipolar neurons	Nucleus solitarius
Vagus (CN X)	GSA	Superior (jugular) ganglion of CN X • Pseudounipolar neurons	Spinal trigeminal nucleus
	SVA GVA	Inferior (nodose) ganglion of CN X • Pseudounipolar neurons	Nucleus solitarius

Abbreviations: GSA, general somatic afferent; GVA, general visceral afferent; SSA, special somatic afferent; SVA, special visceral afferent.
Notes: *Terms in parentheses indicate alternative nomenclature.
** Mesencephalic nucleus of V is unique and contains first-order neurons.

superior and **inferior (petrous) ganglion of CN IX**, and the **superior (jugular)** and **inferior (nodose) ganglion of CN X**.
○ The first-order (primary afferent) neurons found within the ganglia are primarily **pseudounipolar neurons.** A notable exception to this pattern is that of the **vestibular** and **cochlear** (**spiral**) **ganglia,** which contain **bipolar sensory neurons.**

○ CNs I (olfactory) and II (optic) deviate from this pattern and do not have sensory ganglia. The primary afferent neurons are specialized neuroepithelial cells found in the olfactory mucosa and retinal epithelium, respectively.
• **Cranial sensory nuclei** contain second-order interneurons and serve as terminal, integrative, or relay stations for sensory input. The three columns of cranial sensory nuclei include the following:

Table 9.4 General overview of sensory pathways

Overview of Sensory Pathways						
Modality	Cranial Nerve	Origin of Peripheral Afferent Input	Sensory Ganglia (first-order neuron) Synapse Doesn't Occur	Cranial Sensory Nuclei (second-order neurons; axons form ascending tracts)	Target of Nuclei	Termination
GSA	CN V CN VII CN IX CN X	Peripheral receptors detect pain, temperature, discriminative touch, crude touch, and proprioception from face, ear, oral cavity, and oropharyngeal region	Trigeminal ganglion (CN V) Geniculate ganglion (CN VII) Superior ganglion (CN IX) Superior ganglion (CN X)	Trigeminal nuclear complex: Receives input from all three divisions of CN V Spinal trigeminal nucleus receives afferent input from CNs V, VII, IX, and X	Thalamus (VPM) (third-order integrative/relay neurons)	• Somatosensory cortex for conscious processing (parietal lobe) • Somatosensory association cortex for interpreting size, texture, weight of object (stereognostic)
GVA	CN VII CN IX CN X	• Peripheral receptors detect stretch, distention, pain, and thermal sensations from pharyngeal and laryngeal mucosa, and thoracic and abdominal viscera • Special mechanoreceptors (baroreceptors) detect pressure changes • Chemoreceptors detect changes in pressure and O_2 and CO_2 levels	Geniculate ganglion (CN VII) Inferior (petrous) ganglion (CN IX) Inferior (nodose) ganglion (CN X)	Nucleus solitarius (caudal)	• Hypothalamic nuclei containing preautonomic /integrative neurons • Autonomic visceral reflex centers in brainstem reticular formation • NTS fibers project to cranial GVE nuclei for vasomotor control	• Depends on path; most involve autonomic preganglionic nuclei controlling autonomic functions (salivary, respiratory, gastrointestinal cardiac)
SVA**	CN VII CN IX CN X	Specialized neuroepithelial cells found in taste buds contain chemoreceptors (taste receptors) to detect taste	Geniculate ganglion (CN VII) Inferior (petrous) ganglion (CN IX) Inferior (nodose) ganglion (CN X)	Nucleus solitarius (rostral)	Thalamus VPM (third-order integrative/relay neurons)	• Primary gustatory area of cortex for conscious processing and taste perception • Autonomic visceral reflex centers in brainstem (salivary centers)

SSA**	CN VIII
	Two nerves that run together
		• Specialized mechanoreceptors (hair cells) detect movement and sound
		• Vestibular system: Hair cells in maculae of utricle, saccule, and cristae ampullaris
			Vestibular ganglion (of Scarpa) (bipolar neurons)	Vestibular nuclei	• Vestibular path balance and reflexes
					  ○ Cerebellum
					  ○ Brainstem motor nuclei
					  ○ Spinal cord motor nuclei
						• Cerebellum and lower motor neurons in nuclei of CNs III, IV, and VI and spinal cord coordinate eye and head movement

		• Auditory system: Hairs cells in organ of Corti of cochlea	Cochlear (spiral) ganglion (bipolar neurons)	Cochlear nuclei	• Auditory path: Inferior colliculus (nucleus in midbrain)	• Primary auditory cortex (temporal lobe)

Abbreviations: GSA, general somatic afferent; GVA, general visceral afferent; GVE, general visceral efferent; NTS, nucleus tractus solitarius; SSA, special somatic afferent; SVA, special visceral afferent; VPM, ventral posteromedial medial.

Note: ** SVA and SSA inputs from olfactory (CN I) and optic (CN II) are excluded; a detailed path is included in Chapter 15.

- **GSA nuclei** receive primary afferent fibers carrying pain, temperature, touch, and proprioceptive input from receptors in the skin, muscle, and joints. The **trigeminal (CN V)** nerve transmits most of the GSA information from the head, along with smaller contributions from **facial (CN VII), glossopharyngeal (CN IX)**, and **vagus (CN X) nerves**.
  - The GSA nuclei comprise the **trigeminal nuclear complex** which consists of three groups of sensory nuclei:
    - **Mesencephalic trigeminal nucleus (mesencephalic nucleus of V)**—contains first-order afferent neurons and receives proprioceptive input from jaw-closing muscles and the periodontal ligament (PDL).
    - **Main (chief/principal) sensory nucleus of V**—receives fine discriminative touch and some proprioceptive input.
    - **Spinal trigeminal nucleus (spinal nucleus of V)**—receives pain, temperature, and crude touch from CNs V, VII, IX, and X.
  - **GVA** and **SVA** fibers terminate on the same nuclei, the **nucleus solitarius**. The nucleus, also known as the **nucleus tractus solitarius (NTS)** or the **solitary nucleus**, consists of a rostral and causal division. The **rostral** part of the nucleus solitarius receives **taste** fibers carried by **CNs VII, IX**, and **X**, while the **caudal** portion of the nucleus receives **visceral afferent** input from blood vessels, internal organs, and the mucous membranes lining the oropharynx, and larynx via **CNs IX** and **X**.
    - The nucleus solitarius, which lies in the medulla, serves as the principal relay station for first-order visceral and gustatory neurons. The nucleus solitarius functions in the integration of visceral and autonomic responses.
  - **SSA** fibers arise from the vestibular and cochlear (spiral) ganglion and terminate on four vestibular and two cochlear nuclei, respectively.
- Fibers originating from second-order neurons within the cranial sensory nuclei of the brainstem typically decussate and then ascend to specific nuclei of the thalamus.
  - Alternatively, some cranial nuclei may project to the cerebellum, hypothalamus, or autonomic reflex centers in the reticular formation.
- Fibers project from thalamic relay neurons to specific regions of the cortex including the gustatory cortex, somatosensory cortex, and auditory cortex (▶ Table 9.4).
- The olfactory (CN I) and optic nerve (CN II), which develop as outgrowths of the forebrain, deviate from the sensory path configuration described above.
  - The cell bodies of first-order neurons for the **olfactory (CN I)** and **optic (CN II)** nerves reside in the olfactory mucosa of the nose and retinal sensory epithelium of the eye, respectively. The primary afferent fibers then synapse on second-order neurons located within the olfactory bulb and retinal epithelium.

9.2.5 Cranial Motor Pathways: Nuclei and Ganglia

- There are **three columns** of **motor nuclei** within the brainstem: **GSE, SVE**, and **GVE** columns (▶ Table 9.5, ▶ Fig. 9.5a).
- **Somatic motor nuclei** are the most medially positioned column in the brainstem and contain alpha and gamma multipolar LMNs. **GSE fibers** project from **LMNs** to skeletal muscles derived from somites. **CNs III, IV, IX**, and **XII** each have a separate motor nucleus that is named for the cranial nerve. GSE nuclei include the **oculomotor (CN III), trochlear (CN IV), abducens (CN VI)**, and **hypoglossal (CN XII)** motor nuclei.
- **Special visceral efferent nuclei** associated with **CNs V, VII, IX**, and **X** contain **LMNs** that innervate skeletal muscles derived from pharyngeal arch mesoderm. These muscles mediate chewing, swallowing, phonation, and articulation. The pharyngeal arch muscles include the muscles of mastication, facial expression, as well as the palatal, pharyngeal, and laryngeal musculature.
- The SVE motor nuclei include the **trigeminal motor nucleus (CN V), facial motor nucleus (CN VII)**, and **nucleus ambiguus (CNs IX and X)**.
  - It should be noted that the **accessory nerve (CN XI)** originates in the **accessory nucleus** that lies outside the brainstem and is situated in the ventral horn of the upper cervical levels (C1–C6) of the spinal cord. The nucleus contains LMNs which innervate the trapezius and sternocleidomastoid muscles. There is controversy in the literature on whether the nucleus is GSE or SVE in origin.
- The GSE and SVE cranial nerve motor nuclei receive bilateral or contralateral central efferent input from cortical UMNs.
- Cortical UMNs reside in the primary motor, the premotor, and supplementary motor cortices of the frontal lobe, and function to control the planning and execution of movement through the modulation of LMNs found within cranial GSE and SVE motor nuclei.
  - Cranial motor nerve nuclei may receive additional efferent input from the cerebellar and subcortical nuclei.
  - Many of the cranial motor nuclei involved in oropharyngeal functions also receive direct input from the reticular formation. These neurons act as central pattern generators (CPGs) and mediate rhythmic orofacial movements.
- The GVE column consists of four nuclei: the Edinger-Westphal nucleus of CN III, the superior salivatory of CN VII, the inferior salivatory nuclei of CN IX, and the dorsal motor nucleus (CN X) (▶ Fig. 9.6).
  - The nuclei which comprise the **GVE** column lie between the GSE and SVE columns in the brainstem and correspond to multipolar **preganglionic neurons** from the cranial portion of the **parasympathetic** nervous system.

Table 9.5 Overview of motor path

Overview of Motor Pathways					
Modality	Cranial Nerve	Central Efferent Input	Cranial Motor Nuclei	Target of Efferent Fibers	Termination

GSE	CN III
	CN IV
	CN VI
	CN XII
		• Extraocular muscles receive input from cortical areas, reticular formation, vestibular nuclei, and cerebellum; provide central input for ocular and vestibulo-ocular reflexes
		• Cortical neurons (UMN) provide contralateral input to hypoglossal nerve
		• UMN axons form descending corticobulbar tracts
			GSE nuclei
			• Each nucleus consists of cell bodies of GSE neurons also known as lower motor neurons (LMNs)
			  ○ Oculomotor nucleus (CN III)
			  ○ Trochlear nucleus (CN IV)
			  ○ Abducens (CN VI)
			  ○ Hypoglossal nucleus (CN XII)
			• Nuclei serve as point of origin for GSE fiber
				Skeletal muscle derived from somites	Extraocular eye muscles Oculomotor nerve (CN III)
					Superior branch
					• Levator palpebrae
					• Superior rectus
					Inferior branch
					• Medial rectus
					• Inferior rectus
					• Inferior oblique
					Trochlear nerve (CN IV)
					• Superior oblique
					Abducens nerve (CN VI)
					• Lateral rectus
					Tongue muscles (CN XII)
					Intrinsic and all extrinsic muscles except palato-glossus muscle

SVE	CN V CN VII CN IX CN X *CN XI	• Cortical neurons (upper motor neurons) provide primarily bilateral input to SVE motor nuclei • UMN axons form descending corticobulbar tracts *UMN project contralaterally to LMN neurons in lower facial nuclei of CN VII	SVE nuclei • Each nucleus consists of cell bodies of SVE neurons also known as lower motor neurons (LMNs) • Trigeminal motor nucleus (CN V) • Facial motor nucleus (CN VII) • Nucleus ambiguus (CNs IX and X) • Nuclei serve as point of origin for SVE fiber	Skeletal muscle derived from pharyngeal arches	• Muscles of mastication, tensor muscles, anterior digastric (CN V) • Facial expression muscles, posterior digastric, stylohyoid, stapedius (CN VII) • Pharyngeal and palatal muscles (CNs IX and X) • Extrinsic and intrinsic laryngeal muscles (CN X)
GVE	CN III CN VII CN IX CN X	• Direct GVA input from nucleus solitarius as part of autonomic visceral reflex arcs • Input from hypothalamus via preautonomic (integrative) neurons found in hypothalamic nuclei • Receive input from visceral autonomic reflex control centers of brainstem	GVE nuclei • Origin of preganglionic parasympathetic neurons and preganglionic fibers • Edinger-Westphal (CN III) • Superior salivatory (CN VII) • Inferior salivatory (CN IX) • Dorsal vagal (CN X)	**Parasympathetic ganglia** • Origin of postganglionic neurons and postganglionic fibers • Ciliary (CN III) • Pterygopalatine (CN VII) • Submandibular (CN VII) • Otic (CN IX) • Intramural (CN X)	• Smooth muscle of eye, respiratory, GI tract above splenic flexure • Cardiac muscle • Secretomotor to parotid, submandibular, sublingual, nasal, palatal, laryngeal, and minor salivary glands

Abbreviations: GI, gastrointestinal; GSE, general somatic efferent; GVA, general visceral afferent; GVE, general visceral efferent; LMN, lower motor neuron; SVE, special visceral efferent; UMN, upper motor neuron.

○ Preganglionic parasympathetic neurons of GVE motor nuclei receive central input, primarily from **integrative (preautonomic) neurons** found in the hypothalamic nuclei and visceral reflex control centers of the brainstem.

  – Preganglionic neurons may also receive direct input from GVA and SVA second-order interneurons in the nucleus solitarius which are associated with CNs VII, IX, and X. These fibers mediate salivatory, vasomotor, and respiratory reflex arcs.

• The preganglionic parasympathetic nerve fibers synapse on a second group of visceral motor neurons known as **postganglionic neurons**.

• Cell bodies of postganglionic parasympathetic neurons are found in the PNS within **parasympathetic ganglia** of the head and include:
  ○ Ciliary ganglia (CN III).
  ○ Pterygopalatine and submandibular ganglion (CN VII).
  ○ Otic ganglion (CN IX).

• The parasympathetic postganglionic cell bodies associated with the **vagus (CN X)** lie outside the head, near or in the wall (intramural ganglion) of their target organ as indistinct, unnamed groups of neurons.

• Axons of cranial postganglionic parasympathetic neurons synapse on target organs such as salivary, nasal, and lacrimal

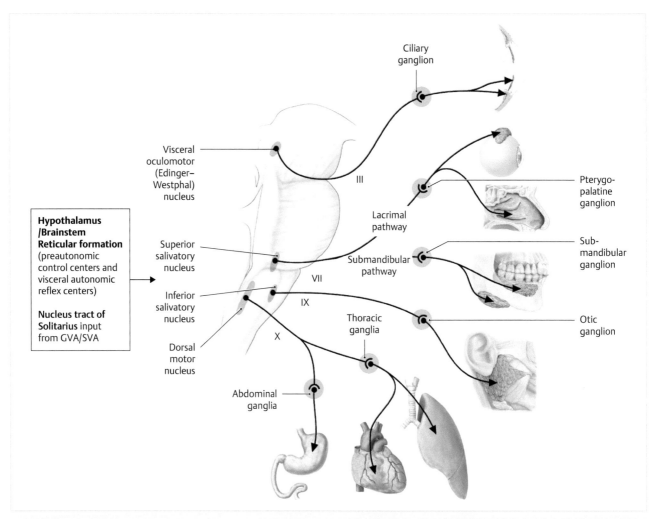

Fig. 9.6 The GVE column consists of four nuclei. These nuclei lie between the GSE and SVE columns in the brainstem. Each of the nuclei have an associated ganglion and cranial nerve. GSE, general somatic efferent; GVE, general visceral efferent; SVE, special visceral efferent. (Reproduced with permission from Schuenke M, Schulte E, Schumacher U. THIEME Atlas of Anatomy Third Edition, Vol 3. © Thieme 2020. Illustrations by Markus Voll and Karl Wesker.)

glands, and the smooth muscle associated with the eye. The postganglionic fibers that terminate on structures within the head accompany branches of the trigeminal division (V1–V3) to reach their target organs. Postganglionic parasympathetic nerve fibers from the vagus target muscles of the heart, respiratory, and gastrointestinal tract.

9.3 Summary of Cranial Nerves

- The following section provides summary tables outlining the general path of the cranial nerves (▶ Fig. 9.7, ▶ Fig. 9.8, ▶ Fig. 9.9, ▶ Fig. 9.10, ▶ Fig. 9.11, ▶ Fig. 9.12, ▶ Fig. 9.13, ▶ Fig. 9.14, ▶ Fig. 9.15, ▶ Fig. 9.16, ▶ Fig. 9.17, ▶ Fig. 9.18, ▶ Fig. 9.19, ▶ Table 9.8, ▶ Table 9.9, ▶ Table 9.10,

▶ Table 9.11, ▶ Table 9.12, ▶ Table 9.13, ▶ Table 9.14, ▶ Table 9.15, ▶ Table 9.16, ▶ Table 9.17). A summary of important cranial nerve reflexes is shown in ▶ Table 9.18. A detailed description of the special sensory pathways involving CNs I, II, VII, VIII, IX, and X can be found in Chapter 15. A comprehensive description of CNs V, VII, IX, X, and XII and their functional role in the orofacial region are covered in Chapters 20 to 22.

9.4 Summary of Cranial Nerve Testing

- See ▶ Table 9.19.

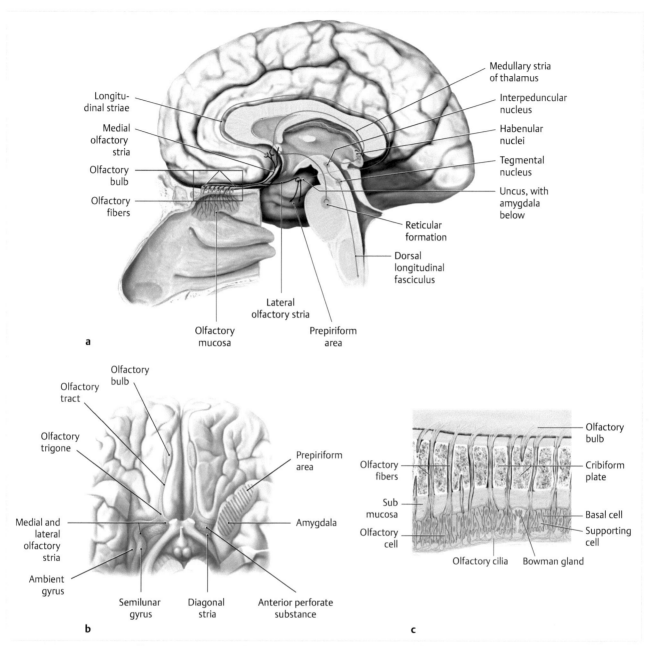

Fig. 9.7 (a–c) Olfactory Nerve (CN I) (SVA) Olfactory tract viewed in a midsagittal plane (a) and inferiorly (b). The olfactory mucosa located in the roof of the nasal cavity contains numerous olfactory receptor cells (boxed region (a). Each olfactory receptor cell represents a primary bipolar afferent neuron comprised of a short peripheral axon containing cilia with chemoreceptors embedded within olfactory epithelium (c). Olfactory stimulation of chemoreceptors is conveyed by the central axons of the bipolar neurons as SVA input. The SVA fibers of olfactory neurons pass through the cribriform plate of the ethmoid bone and synapse on second-order neurons, known as mitral cells, in the olfactory bulb. The axons of secondary neurons form the olfactory tract and project directly, without pre-cortical thalamic relays, to olfactory areas of the frontal lobe. (Reproduced with permission from Schuenke M, Schulte E, Schumacher U. THIEME Atlas of Anatomy Third Edition, Vol 3. © Thieme 2020. Illustrations by Markus Voll and Karl Wesker.)

Table 9.6 Olfactory nerve (CN I)

Cranial Nerve	Origin	General Course	Termination	Functional Role
CN I Olfactory nerve SVA (special visceral afferent) Special sense (smell)	Primary afferent bipolar neurons in the olfactory epithelium of the nasal mucosa	• Second-order neurons (mitral cell) in the olfactory bulb	• Olfactory tract projects directly without thalamic relays to primary olfactory cortical areas	Function to detect odorant molecules (olfactory stimuli)

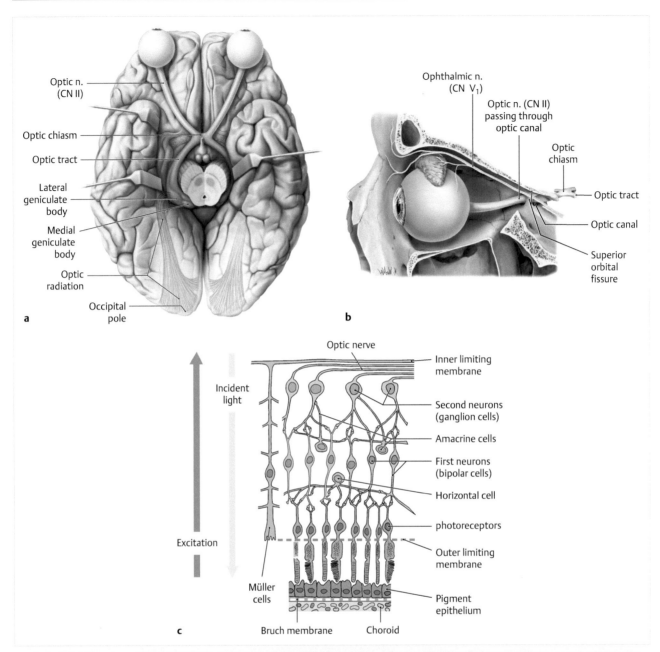

Fig. 9.8 (a–c) Optic Nerve (CN II)(SSA) **(a)** Inferior view of the brain illustrating optic nerve, optic chiasm, and optic tract. **(b)** Lateral view of left orbit with optic nerve shown passing through the optic canal. The optic nerve transmits visual input via a four-neuron pathway from the retina to the visual cortex. **(c)** Retinal photoreceptors known as rods and cones are first-order neurons that convert photons into electrical impulses and then transmit the impulses to bipolar cells (second-order neurons) and ganglion cells (third-order) found in the retinal epithelium. Ganglion cells form the optic nerve which pass through optic chiasm to form the right and left optic tracts. Most of the special somatic afferent (SSA) fibers are carried by optic tract synapse in the lateral geniculate ganglion and then projected to the visual cortex of the occipital lobe. (Reproduced with permission from Schuenke M, Schulte E, Schumacher U. THIEME Atlas of Anatomy Third Edition, Vol 3. © Thieme 2020. Illustrations by Markus Voll and Karl Wesker.)

Table 9.7 Optic nerve (CN II)

Cranial Nerve	Origin	General Course	Termination	Functional Role
CN II **Optic nerve** **SSA** (special somatic afferent) **Special sense** (vision)	• Rod/cone photoreceptors represent primary afferent neurons that convert light stimuli into electrical impulses	• Second-order bipolar cells in retinal epithelium receive signals and transmit to ganglion cells of the retinal epithelium • Axons of retinal ganglion cells form the **optic nerve** • The optic nerves pass through the **optic chiasm** • Fibers emerge from chiasm as right and left **optic tracts** • Nasal fibers cross at optic chiasm; temporal fibers pass ipsilaterally at chiasm • Each optic tract contains nasal retina fibers of one eye and temporal retina fibers of the opposite eye • Optic tracts pass to lateral geniculate nuclei to visual cortex in occipital lobe	• **Optic tract** synapse in **lateral geniculate nucleus of the thalamus** • Fibers from lateral geniculate nucleus projecting to the **visual cortex** of the **occipital lobe**	SSA fibers of the optic nerve mediate vision Serves as afferent limb of pupillary light reflexes Decussation of fibers at optic chiasm provide binocular vision and depth perception

Table 9.8 Oculomotor nerve (CN III)

Cranial Nerve	Origin	General Course	Termination	Functional Role
CN III **Oculomotor** **GSE** (general somatic efferent) **Motor (somatic)**	• GSE neurons **Oculomotor nuclei** in the **rostral midbrain**	• GSE fibers exit the midbrain, pass through the cavernous sinus, enter orbit via superior orbital fissure • GSE motor fibers divide into a superior and inferior branch	• Superior division: Levator palpebrae and superior rectus muscles • The inferior division: Medial rectus, inferior rectus, inferior oblique muscles	Innervates all extraocular muscle except lateral rectus and superior oblique
GVE (general visceral efferent) **Parasympathetic (visceral motor)**	GVE neurons lie in the **Edinger-Westphal** nucleus in midbrain	• Preganglionic fibers synapse on **ciliary ganglion** located in the orbit • Postganglionic fibers travel with the **short ciliary nerves** of **V1** division	• Postganglionic fibers terminate on smooth muscle comprising the **ciliary body** and **sphincter pupillae muscle** of the iris	Mediates pupillary constriction and accommodation (focus on close objects)

Table 9.9 Trochlear nerve (CN IV)

Cranial Nerve	Origin	General Course	Termination	Functional Role
CN IV **Trochlear nerve** **GSE** (general visceral efferent) **Motor (somatic)**	GSE neurons **Trochlear motor nucleus** in the caudal midbrain	• GSE fibers from each nucleus **cross** over each other in the **midline** of midbrain • Fibers exit from the **dorsal surface** of midbrain • Pass through cavernous sinus; enters orbit via the superior orbital fissure	• GSE fibers terminate on the **superior oblique muscle**	Functions to direct the pupil inward (intorsion), downward (depression), and abduct

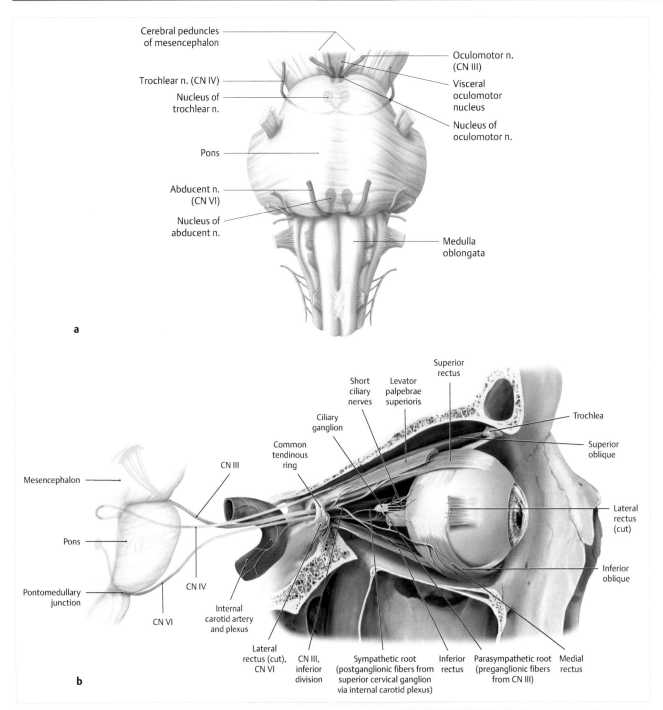

Cerebral peduncles
of mesencephalon

Oculomotor n.
(CN III)

Trochlear n. (CN IV)

Visceral
oculomotor
nucleus

Nucleus of
trochlear n.

Nucleus of
oculomotor n.

Pons

Abducent n.
(CN VI)

Nucleus of
abducent n.

Medulla
oblongata

a

Superior
rectus

Short
ciliary
nerves

Levator
palpebrae
superioris

Ciliary
ganglion

Trochlea

Superior
oblique

CN III

Common
tendinous
ring

Mesencephalon

Lateral
rectus
(cut)

Pons

Inferior
oblique

Pontomedullary
junction

CN IV

Internal
carotid artery
and plexus

CN VI

Lateral
rectus (cut),
CN VI

CN III,
inferior
division

Sympathetic root
(postganglionic fibers from
superior cervical ganglion
via internal carotid plexus)

Inferior
rectus

Parasympathetic root
(preganglionic fibers
from CN III)

Medial
rectus

b

Fig. 9.9 (a,b) The oculomotor (CN III), trochlear (CN IV), and abducent (CN VI) nerves provide general somatic efferent (GSE) innervation to the extraocular muscles. (a) Anterior view of brainstem demonstrating the location of the general somatic motor (GSE) nuclei of the cranial nerves innervating the extraocular muscles. The trochlear nerve is the only cranial nerve in which all the fibers decussate (cross) to the opposite side. It is also the only cranial nerve to emerge from the dorsal surface of the brainstem. (b) Right orbit, lateral view with the temporal wall removed. The path of oculomotor, trochlear, and abducent cranial nerves. Cranial nerves III, IV, and VI enter the orbit through the superior orbital fissure, lateral of the optic canal. CN III and VI pass through the tendinous ring while CN IV passes lateral to the ring. The ciliary ganglion, which contains postganglionic (GVE) parasympathetic neurons, transmits parasympathetic, sympathetic, and sensory fiber to and from the intraocular muscles via short ciliary nerves. Only preganglionic parasympathetic fibers traveling with oculomotor nerve (CN III) synapse in the ganglion. Postganglionic sympathetic (GVE) fibers traveling from the superior cervical ganglion pass through the ganglion. General somatic afferent (GSA) fibers from the eyeball travel via the short ciliary nerves to the nasociliary branch of CN V1. (Reproduced with permission from Schuenke M, Schulte E, Schumacher U. THIEME Atlas of Anatomy Third Edition, Vol 3. © Thieme 2020. Illustrations by Markus Voll and Karl Wesker.)

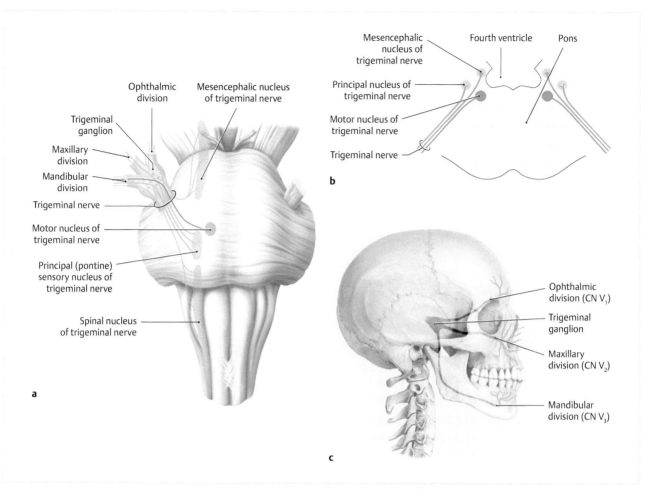

Fig. 9.10 (a–c) Trigeminal nerve nuclei and distribution pattern. **(a)** Anterior view of the brainstem at the level of the trigeminal sensory ganglion and pons. The trigeminal nerve carries most of the general somatic sensation (GSA) from the face, nasal, and oral mucosa. Primary afferent neurons reside in the trigeminal ganglion and first synapse in the large trigeminal sensory nuclear complex that extends along the brainstem and into the spinal cord. The three sensory nuclei shown are named for their location and include the mesencephalic nucleus, principal (pontine, chief) sensory nucleus, and the spinal nucleus of CN V. The mesencephalic nucleus is the only trigeminal sensory to contain primary afferent proprioceptive neurons for muscles of mastication. The remaining trigeminal nuclei contain second-order afferent neurons for epicritic and protopathic sensations. A small motor component provides special visceromotor (SVE) innervation to the muscles of mastication. The efferent fibers arise from the lower motor neurons in the trigeminal motor nucleus. **(b)** cross-section through the pons at the level of the trigeminal nerve (the three sensory nuclei are located at different levels). **(c)** Lateral view of trigeminal nerve divisions and distribution pattern. Three trigeminal nerve divisions include the ophthalmic (CN V1), maxillary (CN V2), and mandibular (CN V3). (Reproduced with permission from Schuenke M, Schulte E, Schumacher U. THIEME Atlas of Anatomy Third Edition, Vol 3. © Thieme 2020. Illustrations by Markus Voll and Karl Wesker.)

Table 9.10 Trigeminal nerve (CN V)

Cranial Nerve	Origin	General Course	Termination	Functional Role
CN V **Trigeminal nerve** **GSA** (general somatic afferent) **Sensory**	• GSA primary afferent neurons **Trigeminal (semilunar) ganglion** ○ Cell bodies for primary afferent proprioceptive neurons reside in **mesencephalic nucleus of V** Three divisions: • **Ophthalmic division (V1)** • **Maxillary division (V2)** • **Mandibular division (V3)**	• Sensory fibers from sensory root enters brainstem level mid-pons • Sensory root synapses on second-order neurons found within **trigeminal sensory nuclear complex**	• Ascending path via trigeminothalamic tract • Project to ventral posterior medial (VPM) thalamic • Thalamic fibers project to the orofacial region of postcentral gyrus in **somatosensory cortex in the parietal lobe**	Somatosensory input (pain, temperature, discriminative tactile proprioceptive) from anterior face, oral cavity, nasal cavity, conjunctiva eye, teeth; meninges (dura); proprioceptive PDL, TMJ, jaw closing muscles, extraocular muscles Mediates afferent limb of several sensorimotor reflexes
SVE (special visceral efferent—pharyngeal arch muscle) **Motor** (voluntary motor)	**SVE neurons**, the **motor nucleus of V** in the **mid-pons**	SVE fibers travel with **mandibular division (V3)**	Efferent fibers innervate the muscles derived from **first** pharyngeal arch (masseter, temporalis, medial, and lateral pterygoids), along with the mylohyoid, anterior digastric, tensor tympani, tensor veli palatini muscles	• Mediates mastication; facilitates jaw movements necessary for swallowing and articulation Mediates efferent limb of jaw reflex

Abbreviations: PDL, periodontal ligament; TMJ, temporomandibular joint.

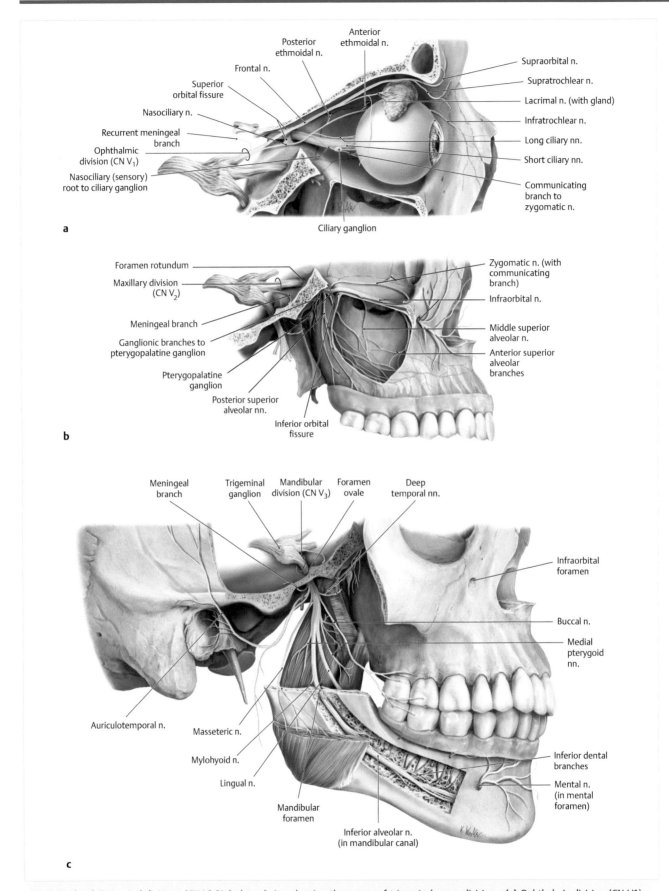

Fig. 9.11 (a–c) Trigeminal divisions (CN V) Right lateral view showing the course of trigeminal nerve divisions. **(a)** Ophthalmic division (CN V1), partially opened right orbit. **(b)** Maxillary division (CN V2), partially opened right maxillary sinus with zygomatic arch removed. **(c)** Mandibular division (CN V3), partially opened mandible with zygomatic arch removed. (Reproduced with permission from Schuenke M, Schulte E, Schumacher U. THIEME Atlas of Anatomy Third Edition, Vol 3. © Thieme 2020. Illustrations by Markus Voll and Karl Wesker.)

Table 9.11 Abducens nerve (CN VI)

Cranial Nerve	Origin	General Course	Termination	Functional Role
CN VI **Abducens nerve** **GSE** (general somatic efferent) **Motor (somatic)**	GSE neurons **Abducens motor nucleus** in the **caudal pons**	• GSE fibers exit the caudal pons • Fibers pass through the cavernous sinus, enter orbit	• GSE fibers innervate the lateral rectus muscle	Functions to abduct the eye

Table 9.12 Facial nerve (CN VII)

Cranial Nerve	Origin	General Course	Termination	Functional Role
CN VII **Facial nerve** **GSA** (general somatic afferent) **Sensory**	• GSA fibers arise from peripheral receptors, travel via **intermediate nerve** GSA primary afferent neurons reside in the **geniculate ganglion**	• Primary afferent fibers synapse on **spinal trigeminal nucleus** and **chief sensory nucleus of V** • Ascending path via trigeminothalamic tract to VPM of thalamus	Thalamic fibers terminate in somatosensory cortex for conscious processing	Transmits pain, temperature, crude touch, and general sensation from small area of external ear
GVA (general visceral afferent) **Sensory**	• **GVA** primary afferent fibers travel via **intermediate nerve,** first-order neurons of **geniculate ganglion**	• Primary afferent fibers synapse on **caudal** portion of **nucleus tract of solitarius (NTS)**	• Fibers of NTS project to reticular formation and hypothalamus for autonomic and reflexive input	GVA fibers transmit visceral input from sensory receptors found in the mucous membranes of nasopharynx and soft palate (minor contribution)
SVA (special visceral afferent) **Special sense** (taste)	• Primary afferents travel via **intermediate nerve** SVA primary afferent neurons reside in the **geniculate ganglion**	Primary afferent fibers synapse on second-order neurons in **rostral** part of **nucleus tract of solitarius (NTS)** in the medulla	• NTS fibers project to VPM thalamus Tertiary fibers terminate in **gustatory (taste) area** of the **cortex**	Mediates taste from anterior two-thirds of tongue; hard and soft palates
SVE (special visceral efferent—pharyngeal arch muscle) **Motor** (voluntary motor)	• SVE neurons located in the facial motor nucleus of CN VII within the caudal pons • The SVE fibers travel in facial nerve proper SVE fibers and afferent fibers of CN VII from intermediate nerve (nervus intermedius) travel the same path	• Motor root loops around abducens (CN VI) • The SVE fibers of motor and sensory fibers pass through the **internal acoustic meatus** and **facial canal**	• SVE innervate the muscles of second pharyngeal arch (PA 2) • (facial expression muscle stylohyoid, stapedius posterior digastric muscles)	• Voluntary motor innervation to ipsilateral muscles of second pharyngeal arch • Mediates facial movements necessary for chewing, speech, swallowing, and facial expression Mediates efferent limb of corneal reflex
GVE (general visceral efferent) **Parasympathetic** (visceral motor—secretion)	• GVE neurons Superior salivatory nucleus in the caudal pons GVE travels with the intermediate nerve to follow either lacrimal or submandibular pathway	• Lacrimal path: GVE preganglionic synapse on **pterygopalatine ganglion** • **Submandibular pathway:** GVE synapse on the **submandibular ganglion** Postganglionic fibers of lacrimal path accompany V2 to glands Postganglionic fibers from sublingual follow V3 to glands	• **Lacrimal pathway:** Postganglionic fibers terminate on lacrimal glands associated with nasal, pharyngeal, and palatal mucosa **Submandibular pathway:** Postganglionic fibers terminate on the submandibular sublingual glands; minor labial and lingual salivary glands	Mediates secretomotor activity of all orofacial glands except parotid, circumvallate salivary glands, and buccal glands

Abbreviation: VPM, ventral posterior medial.

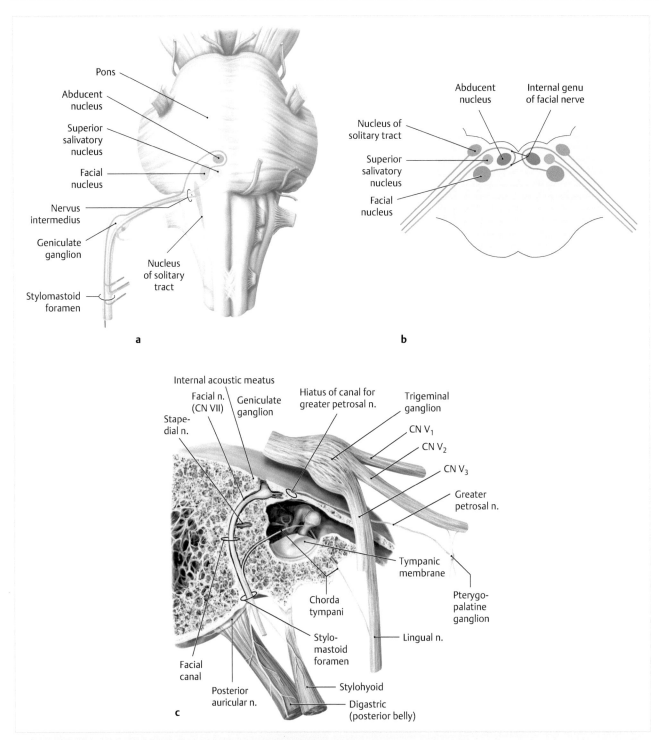

Fig. 9.12 (a–c) Facial nerve nuclei and principal branches. **(a)** Anterior view of the brainstem demonstrating the level of the facial motor and sensory nerve nuclei and the emergence of the facial nerve proper and nervus intermedius from the lower pons. Different sensory and motor nuclei are associated with different fiber modalities carried by the facial nerve and nervus intermedius. The nervus intermedius transmits taste (SVA), general somatic sensations (GSA), and preganglionic parasympathetic visceral motor fibers (GVE). The facial nerve is the principal motor nerve to the muscles of facial expression that develop from the second pharyngeal arch. The special visceral (SVE) fibers are voluntary motor fibers that arise from lower motor neurons in the facial motor nucleus. **(b)** Cross-section through the lower pons, showing the path of the special visceral efferent (SVE) fibers looping around the abducent nucleus to form the internal genu (bend). **(c)** Right lateral view of right temporal bone demonstrating the course of the facial nerve. Both the motor and sensory roots of the facial nerve travel together from the lower pons and then pass through the internal auditory meatus. facial canal. (Reproduced with permission from Schuenke M, Schulte E, Schumacher U. THIEME Atlas of Anatomy Third Edition, Vol 3. © Thieme 2020. Illustrations by Markus Voll and Karl Wesker.)

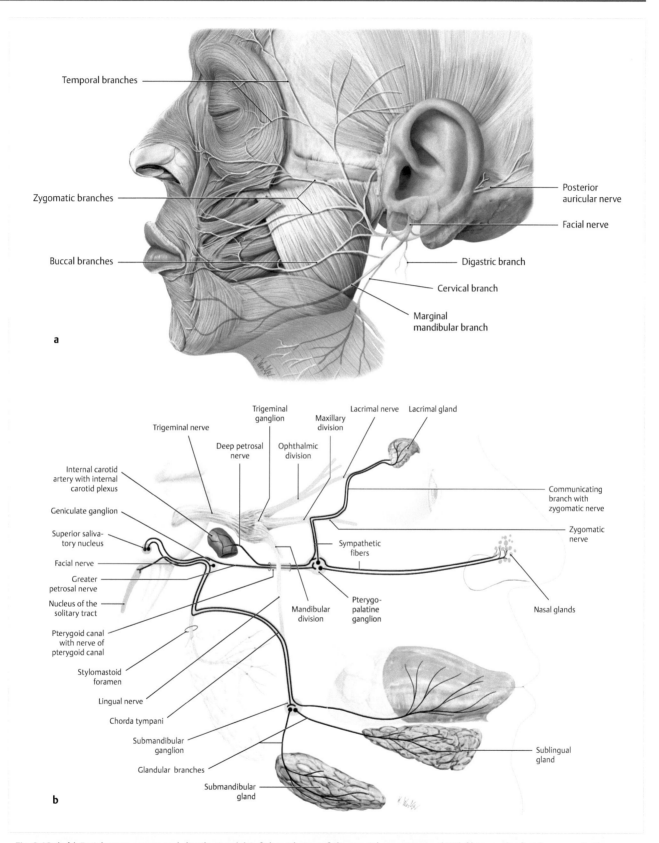

Fig. 9.13 (a,b) Facial nerve course and distribution **(a)** Left lateral view of the special visceromotor (SVE) fibers as the facial nerve exits the stylomastoid foramen. (Reproduced with permission from Schuenke M, Schulte E, Schumacher U. THIEME Atlas of Anatomy Third Edition, Vol 3. © Thieme 2020. Illustrations by Markus Voll and Karl Wesker.) **(b)** Facial nerve ganglia are associated with parasympathetic (GVE) and taste fibers (SVA) of the facial nerve. Autonomic and taste fibers travel with the greater petrosal and chorda tympani nerves, respectively before accompanying branches of trigeminal nerve. (Reproduced with permission from Schuenke M, Schulte E, Schumacher U. THIEME Atlas of Anatomy Third Edition, Vol 3. © Thieme 2020. Illustrations by Markus Voll and Karl Wesker.)

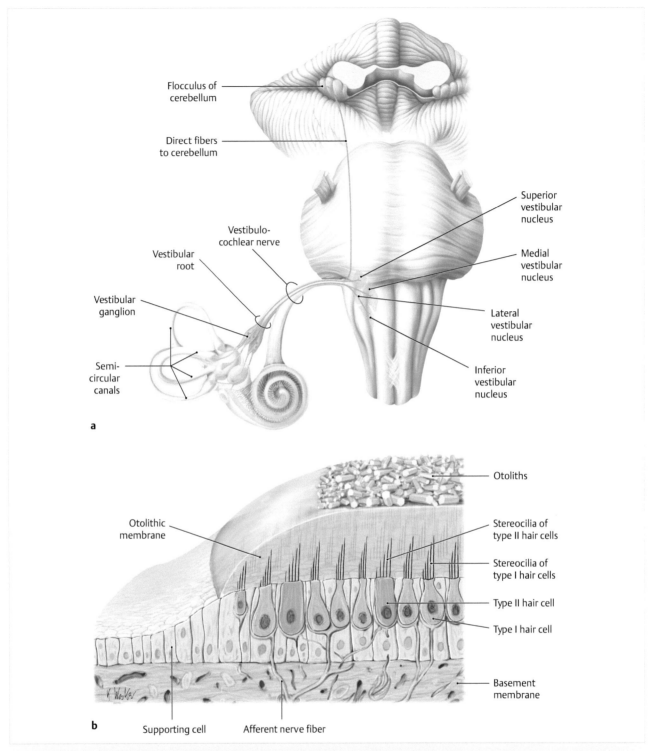

Flocculus of cerebellum

Direct fibers to cerebellum

Vestibulo-cochlear nerve

Vestibular root

Vestibular ganglion

Semi-circular canals

Superior vestibular nucleus

Medial vestibular nucleus

Lateral vestibular nucleus

Inferior vestibular nucleus

a

Otolithic membrane

Otoliths

Stereocilia of type II hair cells

Stereocilia of type I hair cells

Type II hair cell

Type I hair cell

Basement membrane

b Supporting cell   Afferent nerve fiber

Fig. 9.14 (a–d) Vestibulocochlear nerve (CN VIII) and nuclei in the brainstem. The vestibulocochlear nerve carries special somatic afferent (SSA) fibers to their respective cranial nuclei in pons and medulla. The vestibulocochlear nerve consists of two functional divisions; a vestibular division that maintains balance and equilibrium, and a cochlear division that mediates hearing. **(a)** Anterior view of the medulla oblongata and pons shows the location of the vestibular nuclei, vestibulocochlear nerve root, and vestibular ganglion. The vestibular ganglion contains primary afferent bipolar neurons that transmit sensory information about positional changes and rotational movements from the utricle, saccule, and semicircular canals to vestibular nuclei. **(b)** schematic view of maculae of the utricle. The macule of the sensory epithelium contains sensory hair cells with apical stereocilia projecting into the otolith membrane.

(*Continued*)

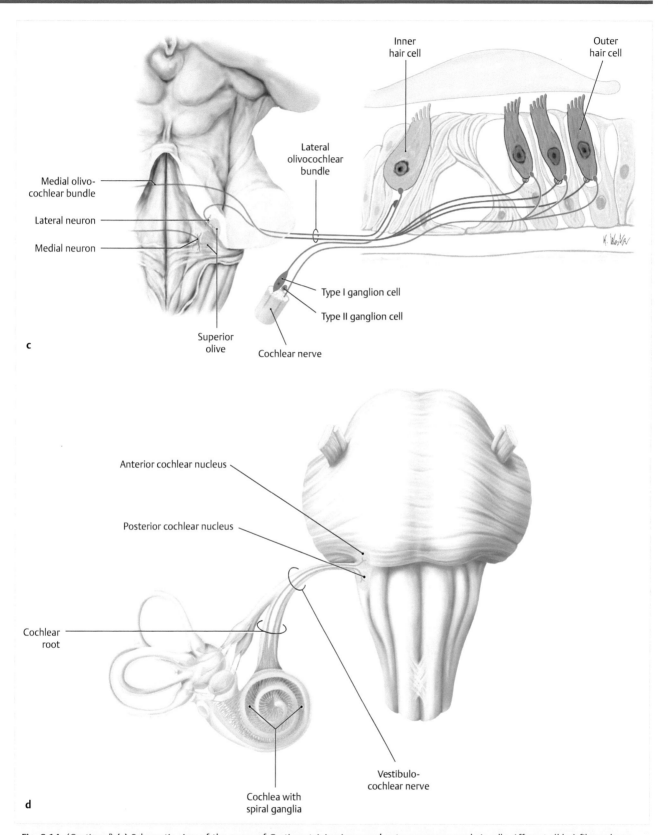

c

Medial olivo-cochlear bundle
Lateral neuron
Medial neuron
Superior olive
Cochlear nerve
Type I ganglion cell
Type II ganglion cell
Lateral olivocochlear bundle
Inner hair cell
Outer hair cell

d

Anterior cochlear nucleus
Posterior cochlear nucleus
Cochlear root
Cochlea with spiral ganglia
Vestibulo-cochlear nerve

Fig. 9.14 (*Continued*) **(c)** Schematic view of the organ of Corti containing inner and outer neurosensory hair cells. Afferent (*blue*) fibers shown traveling from the hair cells in the organ of Corti via the cochlear nerve root to the spiral ganglia in the cochlea. The cell bodies for the bipolar afferent neurons reside in the spiral ganglion. Primary afferent fibers pass through each ganglion without synapsing and project to cerebellum, vestibular and cochlear nuclei. (Reproduced with permission from Schuenke M, Schulte E, Schumacher U. THIEME Atlas of Anatomy Third Edition, Vol 3. © Thieme 2020. Illustrations by Markus Voll and Karl Wesker.)

Table 9.13 Vestibulocochlear nerve (CN VIII)

Cranial Nerve	Origin	General Course	Termination	Functional Role
Vestibulocochlear nerve (CN VIII) SSA (special somatic afferent fibers) Special sense (hearing/balance)	• **Primary afferent cell bodies** of SSA fibers are bipolar neurons found in: **Vestibular ganglion** in the internal auditory meatus	• Central fibers project directly to: ○ **Four vestibular nuclei** in the lower pons and upper medulla ○ **Cerebellum**	• Terminate in: ○ Cerebellum ○ LMN in spinal cord brainstem, including motor nuclei of extraocular muscles Thalamus for cortical processing	Vestibular nerve provides input about positional changes and rotational movements of the head; serves to maintain balance and equilibrium
	Auditory system: • Primary afferent cell bodies of SSA fibers are **bipolar neurons** found in: **Cochlear ganglion**, the modiolus of the cochlea, within the temporal bone	Central fibers project directly to the **dorsal** and **ventral cochlear nuclei** in the upper medulla	Ascending auditory pathway pass through thalamus and terminates in **auditory cortex** of superior temporal gyrus	Cochlear nerve mediates hearing Cochlear nerve mediates the **stapedial reflex**—a protective acoustic reflex induced in response to loud noises at certain thresholds

Abbreviation: LMN, lower motor neuron.

Table 9.14 Glossopharyngeal nerve (CN IX)

Cranial Nerve	Origin	General Course	Termination	Functional Role
Glossopharyngeal nerve CN IX GSA (general somatic afferent) Sensory	• GSA primary afferent neurons reside in the **superior glossopharyngeal ganglion**	• Primary afferent fibers synapse on **spinal trigeminal nucleus and chief sensory nucleus of V** • Ascending path via trigeminothalamic tract to VPM of thalamus	Thalamic fibers terminate in somatosensory cortex for conscious processing	• Transmits pain, temperature, and touch from the posterior one-third of tongue, internal aspect of the tympanic membrane, the tympanic cavity of the middle ear, and the auditory tube GSA fibers innervate the external auditory meatus and pinnae of the ear through the small, **auricular (CN X) branch** of the vagus
GVA (general visceral afferent) Sensory	• **GVA** primary afferent neurons reside in the **inferior (petrous) ganglion**	• GVA fibers synapse on **caudal** portion of **nucleus tract of solitarius (NTS)**	• Fibers terminate in reticular formation and hypothalamus for autonomic and reflexive input • NTS project to GVE neurons in dorsal motor nucleus of CN X carotid sinus baroreflex	• GVA fibers of CN IX form sensory component of pharyngeal nerve plexus • Visceral input from mucous membranes of oropharynx, tonsils, soft palate, and pharyngeal wall; monitor arterial blood pressure, blood pH, and O_2/CO_2 saturation levels • Mediates the afferent limb of the **gag reflex** Mediates vasomotor reflex (**carotid sinus baroreflex**)
SVA (special visceral afferent) Special sense (taste)	SVA **primary** afferent neurons reside in the **inferior (petrous) ganglion**	SVA synapse in **rostral** part of **nucleus tract of solitarius (NTS)** in the upper medulla	• Afferent pathways project to VPM thalamus Tertiary fibers terminate in gustatory (taste) area of the cortex	Mediates taste from posterior one-third of tongue (circumvallate and foliate papillae) and oropharynx
SVE (special visceral efferent—pharyngeal arch muscle) Motor (voluntary motor)	• SVE neurons **nucleus ambiguus** in the medulla	SVE fibers exit the medulla and skull	• SVE innervate **stylopharyngeus muscle** derived from the **third pharyngeal arch mesoderm**	Voluntary motor innervation to ipsilateral muscles Mediates voluntary muscle elevation of stylopharyngeus, a muscle of the pharynx, during swallowing and speech
GVE (general visceral efferent) Parasympathetic (visceral motor—secretion)	**GVE neurons inferior salivatory nucleus** in the **medulla**	GVE preganglionic fibers synapse on the **otic ganglion**	• Postganglionic fibers follow a branch of V3 and terminate on parotid gland	Mediates salivary secretions of parotid, minor salivary glands of circumvallate and foliate papillae of tongue, and buccal glands

Abbreviation: VPM, ventral posterior medial.

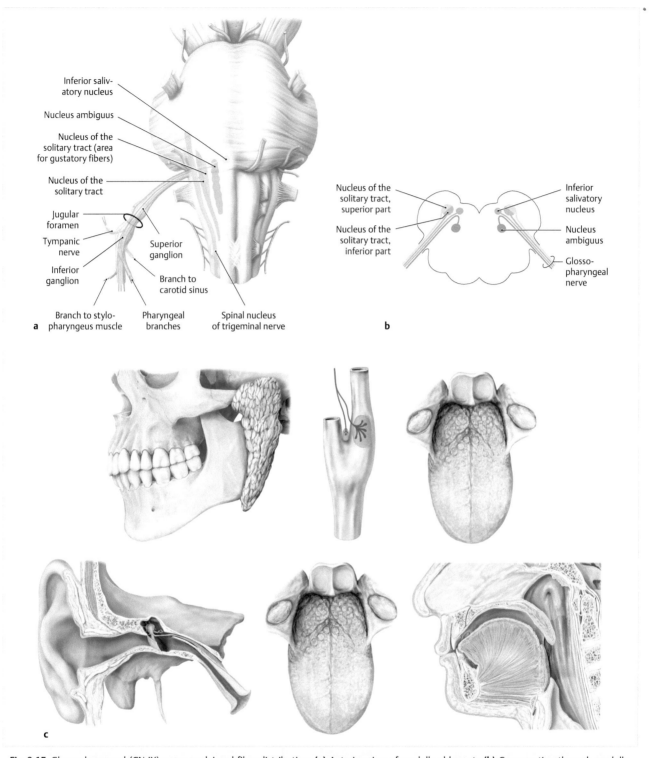

Inferior saliv-atory nucleus

Nucleus ambiguus

Nucleus of the solitary tract (area for gustatory fibers)

Nucleus of the solitary tract

Jugular foramen

Tympanic nerve

Inferior ganglion

Superior ganglion

Branch to carotid sinus

Branch to stylo-pharyngeus muscle

Pharyngeal branches

Spinal nucleus of trigeminal nerve

a

Nucleus of the solitary tract, superior part

Nucleus of the solitary tract, inferior part

Inferior salivatory nucleus

Nucleus ambiguus

Glosso-pharyngeal nerve

b

c

Fig. 9.15 Glossopharyngeal (CN IX) nerve nuclei and fiber distribution. **(a)** Anterior view of medulla oblongata **(b)** Cross-section through medulla oblongata at the level of emergence of the glossopharyngeal nerve. The spinal trigeminal nucleus is not shown. The glossopharyngeal nerve is a mixed nerve carrying both motor (SVE, GVE) and sensory (GVA, SVA, and GSA) fibers. Each fiber modality is associated with a specific motor or sensory nuclei and designated as either purple (SVE), blue (GVE), green (GVA, SVA), or yellow (GSA). The glossopharyngeal provides motor innervation via special visceral efferent (SVE) fiber to the stylopharyngeus muscle derived from the third pharyngeal arch. The special visceral (SVE) fibers are voluntary motor fibers that arise from lower motor neurons in the nucleus ambiguus (purple). (Reproduced with permission from Schuenke M, Schulte E, Schumacher U. THIEME Atlas of Anatomy Third Edition, Vol 3. © Thieme 2020. Illustrations by Markus Voll and Karl Wesker.) **(c)** Schematic depicting CN IX fiber distribution. The Inferior salivatory nucleus contains preganglionic parasympathetic visceromotor (GVE) neurons. GVE fibers synapse in the otic ganglion, and then continue as postganglionic fibers to innervate the parotid gland (*blue*). General visceral afferent (GVA) fibers convey changes in blood pressure from baroreceptors in the carotid sinus and blood oxygen saturation levels from chemoreceptors in the carotid body (*green*). The primary afferent neurons of GVA fibers reside in the inferior petrosal ganglion and project to the inferior (caudal) part of the nucleus of the solitary tract. Special visceral afferent (SVA) fibers transmit taste from the posterior 1/3 of tongue. The primary afferent SVA neurons are in the inferior ganglion of IX and project to the superior (rostral) part of the nucleus of the solitary tract (*green*). General somatic afferent (GSA) fiber carry sensations from the posterior one-third of the tongue, eustachian tube, and oropharynx (*yellow*). Primary afferent GSA neurons reside in the superior ganglion of IX and synapse in the spinal trigeminal nucleus.

Table 9.15 Vagus nerve (CN X)

Cranial Nerve	Origin	General Course	Termination	Functional Role
Vagus nerve **CN X** **GSA** (general somatic afferent) **Sensory**	• GSA primary afferent neurons reside in the **superior vagal (jugular) ganglion**	• Primary afferent fibers synapse on **spinal trigeminal nucleus** Secondary afferents follow ascending trigeminal paths to **VPM of thalamus**	Thalamic fibers terminate in somatosensory cortex for conscious processing	Transmits pain, temperature, and touch from the external auditory meatus and pinnae of the ear through the small, **auricular** (CN X) branch of the vagus
GVA (general visceral afferent) **Sensory**	**GVA primary afferent neurons reside in the inferior (petrous) ganglion**	• GVA primary fibers synapse in **caudal** portion of **nucleus tract of solitarius (NTS)** in the upper medulla	• NTS fibers project to reticular formation and hypothalamus • NTS projects to GVE neurons in the dorsal motor nucleus of CN X and nucleus ambiguus; for modulation of the heart rate	• GVA input from mucous membranes of larynx, including the epiglottis root of tongue, supraglottic and infraglottic regions • Monitor arterial blood pressure, blood pH, and O_2/CO_2 • GVA innervation of CN X mediates: ○ **Swallowing reflex** ○ **Cough reflex** to clear airway **Adductor laryngeal reflex** (glottic closure reflex) to prevent aspiration
SVA (special visceral afferent) **Special sense** (taste)	SVA primary afferent neurons reside in the **inferior (nodose) ganglion**	SVA fibers synapse on **rostral** part of **nucleus tract of solitarius (NTS)** in the medulla	• Ascending path to VPM of the thalamus Terminate in **gustatory (taste) area** of the **cortex**	Mediates taste from taste buds in epiglottic mucosa
SVE (special visceral efferent— pharyngeal arch muscle) **Motor** (voluntary motor)	**SVE motor neurons** found in the **nucleus ambiguus** in the medulla	**SVE fibers** descend in the neck; some fibers continue to thorax and abdomen	• SVE fibers terminate on **muscles** derived from the **fourth and sixth pharyngeal arch mesoderm** • Innervate the **intrinsic** and **extrinsic laryngeal muscles** • **Palatoglossus** muscle of the tongue • **All pharyngeal** and **palatal muscles** except: Stylopharyngeus (CN IX) and tensor veli palatini muscle (CN V3)	• Vagal SVE fibers form principal efferent (motor) component of **pharyngeal plexus of nerves** • SVE mediates airway protection, controls respiration and phonation • Vagal SVE fibers facilitate **articulation** (speech) and **deglutition** (swallowing) • SVE mediates the efferent limb of several protective reflexes including: ○ **Cough reflex** ○ **Gag reflex** ○ **Laryngeal adductor reflex**
GVE (general visceral efferent) **Parasympathetic** (visceral motor—smooth muscle, heart, secretion)	• **GVE neurons** lie in **dorsal nucleus of the vagus** in the medulla	GVE Preganglionic fibers synapse on **intramural ganglia** (within the or near organ wall)	Postganglionic fibers terminate in glands and **smooth and cardiac muscles** associated with cardiovascular, respiratory, and gastrointestinal (GI) systems	• Modulates peristalsis of GI tract and bronchoconstriction • Glandular secretions in the larynx, trachea, and bronchi and abdominal organs Decrease heart rate and cardiac output * vasomotor reflex responses

Abbreviation: VPM, ventral posterior medial.

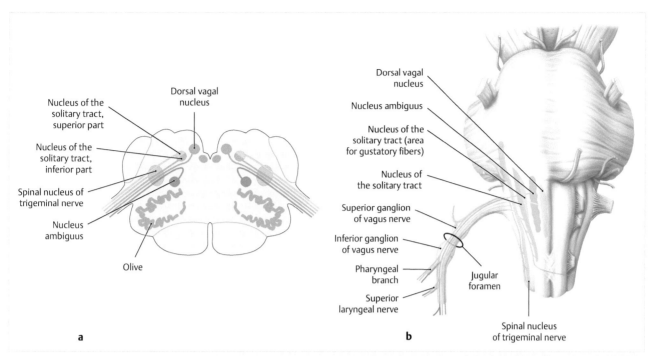

Fig. 9.16 Nuclei of the vagus (CN X) **(a)** anterior view of medulla oblongata demonstrating the location of Vagus nerve nuclei, site of vagus nerve emergence, and superior and inferior sensory ganglia of CN X. **(b)** cross-section through medulla at the level of vagus nerve nuclei. The vagus nerve is a mixed nerve carrying both motor (SVE, GVE) and sensory (GVA, SVA, and GSA) fibers. Each fiber modality is associated with a specific motor or sensory nuclei and designated as either purple (SVE), *blue* (GVE), *green* (GVA, SVA), or *yellow* (GSA). Special visceral efferent (SVE) fibers of the vagus provide voluntary motor innervation to all pharyngeal and palatal muscles except the stylopharyngeus, tensor veli palatini, and the laryngeal muscles, and palatoglossus. Lower motor neurons of SVE fibers reside in the nucleus ambiguus and contribute to the pharyngeal plexus. Visceral motor (GVE) fibers arise from the dorsal motor nucleus and provide parasympathetic innervation to glands and smooth muscle of the respiratory and GI tract. Cervical cardiac branches contribute to the cardiac plexus to modify cardiac muscle contraction. General visceral afferent (GVA) fibers carry sensory innervation from chemoreceptors of the aortic body and baroreceptors of the aortic arch to the inferior (caudal) part of the nucleus tract of solitarius. GVA innervation from the mucosa of the larynx, trachea, bronchi, and abdomen mediate several visceral reflexes. Special visceral afferent (SVA) fibers convey taste sensations from the root of the tongue and epiglottic regions to the rostral part of the nucleus tract of solitarius. General somatic afferent (GSA) fibers carry information from the external ear and auditory canal to the spinal trigeminal nucleus. (Reproduced with permission from Schuenke M, Schulte E, Schumacher U. THIEME Atlas of Anatomy Third Edition, Vol 3. © Thieme 2020. Illustrations by Markus Voll and Karl Wesker.)

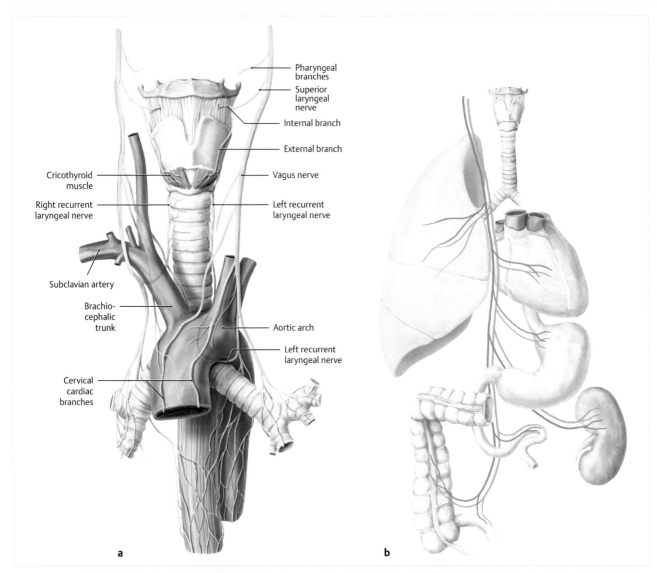

Cricothyroid muscle

Right recurrent laryngeal nerve

Subclavian artery

Brachio-cephalic trunk

Cervical cardiac branches

Pharyngeal branches

Superior laryngeal nerve

Internal branch

External branch

Vagus nerve

Left recurrent laryngeal nerve

Aortic arch

Left recurrent laryngeal nerve

a

b

Fig. 9.17 (a,b) Distribution of the vagus (CN X) nerve in the region of neck, thoracic and abdominal regions. **(a)** Anterior view of the neck showing bilateral distribution of the four branches of vagus nerve: (1) Pharyngeal branches, (2) superior laryngeal divides into the internal laryngeal and external laryngeal nerve (3) recurrent laryngeal and (4) cervical cardiac branches. **(b)** In the thorax and abdomen, right and left vagal trunks to convey general viscera sensory (GVA) and parasympathetic (GVE) fibers to glands and smooth muscle found wall of the foregut and midgut as part of several autonomic plexuses. (Reproduced with permission from Schuenke M, Schulte E, Schumacher U. THIEME Atlas of Anatomy Third Edition, Vol 3. © Thieme 2020. Illustrations by Markus Voll and Karl Wesker.)

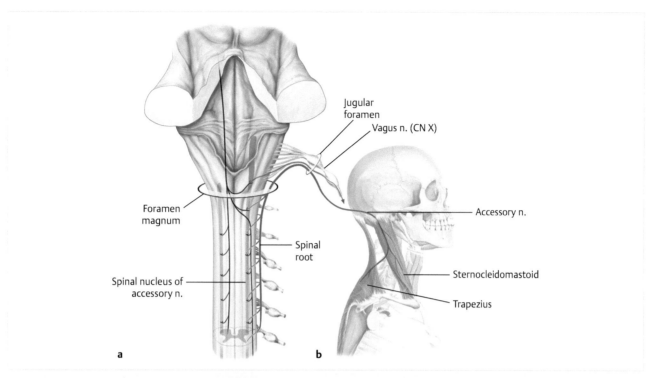

Fig. 9.18 (a,b) Accessory nerve (CN XI) **(a)** Posterior view of brainstem with cerebellum removed and cervical spinal cord showing the path of the spinal accessory nerve from lower motor neurons in the ventral horn of C1-C6 and passage through the foramen magnum. Motor fibers travel with special visceral efferent fibers of the vagus nerve that originate from lower motor neurons in the nucleus ambiguus. Spinal accessory nerve (CN XI), Vagus (CN (X), and Glossopharyngeal (CN IX) exit the skull via jugular foramen **(b)** right lateral view of sternocleidomastoid and trapezius receive innervation from spinal accessory nerve (CN XI). (Reproduced with permission from Schuenke M, Schulte E, Schumacher U. THIEME Atlas of Anatomy Third Edition, Vol 3. © Thieme 2020. Illustrations by Markus Voll and Karl Wesker.)

Table 9.16 Accessory nerve (CN XI)

Cranial Nerve	Origin	General Course	Termination	Functional Role
CN XI Accessory nerve GSE/SVE** (general somatic efferent/special visceral efferent) Motor (voluntary motor)	• **Spinal component:** Motor neurons in the **accessory nucleus** situated in the ventral horn of **spinal cord** at the level of C1–C6 • **Cranial component** **Begins in nucleus ambiguus	• Fibers ascend rostrally within the vertebral column • Enter skull via foramen magnum • Accompany vagus and glossopharyngeal nerves to exit skull via jugular foramen Fibers pass in neck to reach target muscles	• Motor fibers of the spinal component innervate the **trapezius** and **sternocleidomas**toid muscles	Sternocleidomastoid turns head to opposite side, bilaterally

Note: **Controversy in literature on whether accessory nerve is GSE or SVE and the presence or absence of a cranial nuclei component.

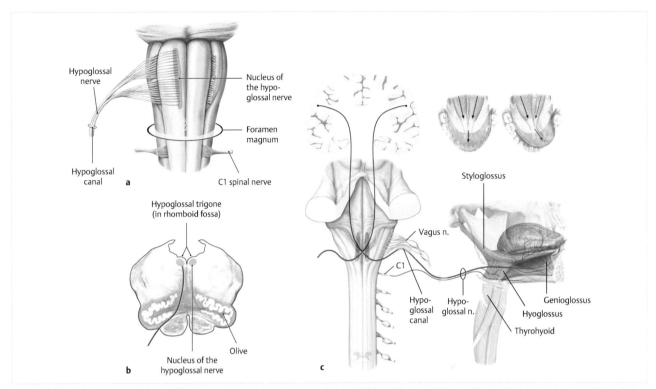

Fig. 9.19 (a–c) Hypoglossal nerve (CN XII) nuclei and fiber distribution. **(a)** Anterior view of medulla oblongata demonstrating the location of the lower motor neurons of the hypoglossal motor nuclei and the emergence of general somatic efferent (GSE) fibers. **(b)** cross-section through medulla oblongata at the level of hypoglossal motor nuclei. The hypoglossal nuclei lie close to the midline and raise the floor of the rhomboid fossa to form the hypoglossal trigone. **(c)** Path of the hypoglossal nerve, posterior view of brainstem with cerebellum removed. The upper motor neurons synapse on contralateral lower motor neurons located in the hypoglossal nucleus. The hypoglossal nerve which carries only GSE fibers exits the hypoglossal canal and pass forward to enter the oral cavity. The hypoglossal nerve innervates all intrinsic and extrinsic tongue muscles except the palatoglossus. C1 motor fibers which innervate the thyrohyoid and geniohyoid muscles run with the hypoglossal nerve. (Reproduced with permission from Schuenke M, Schulte E, Schumacher U. THIEME Atlas of Anatomy Third Edition, Vol 3. © Thieme 2020. Illustrations by Markus Voll and Karl Wesker.)

Table 9.17 Hypoglossal nerve (CN XII)

CN XII **Hypoglossal nerve** **GSE** (general somatic efferent) **Motor (somatic)**	GSE neurons found in the **hypoglossal nucleus** in the lower medulla	• GSE fibers emerge as rootlets from preolivary sulcus and exit the hypoglossal canal in the occipital bone GSE fibers descend through the neck to enter the oral cavity	• GSE fibers terminate on skeletal muscle from **occipital somites** • Innervate all intrinsic and extrinsic muscles of the tongue except for the palatoglossus (CN X) • **Intrinsic tongue muscles** include: superior and inferior longitudinal, transverse, and vertical muscles **Extrinsic tongue muscles** include: styloglossus, hyoglossus genioglossus	Hypoglossal mediates tongue movement by controlling the shape and position of the tongue Works cooperatively with trigeminal, facial, glossopharyngeal, and vagus to facilitate chewing, swallowing, phonation, and speech
CN XII **Hypoglossal nerve** **GSE** (general somatic efferent) **Motor (somatic)**	GSE neurons found in the **hypoglossal nucleus** in the lower medulla	• GSE fibers emerge as rootlets from preolivary sulcus and exit the hypoglossal canal in the occipital bone GSE fibers descend through the neck to enter the oral cavity	• GSE fibers terminate on skeletal muscle from **occipital somites** • Innervate all intrinsic and extrinsic muscles of the tongue except for the palatoglossus (CN X) • **Intrinsic tongue muscles** include: superior and inferior longitudinal, transverse, and vertical muscles **Extrinsic tongue muscles** include: **styloglossus, hyoglossus, and genioglossus**	Hypoglossal mediates tongue movement by controlling the shape and position of the tongue Works cooperatively with trigeminal, facial, glossopharyngeal, and vagus to facilitate chewing, swallowing, phonation, and speech

Table 9.18 Important reflexes mediated by cranial nerves

Reflex	Afferent Limb	Efferent Limb
Pupillary light reflex	Optic nerve (CN II) SSA	Oculomotor (CN III) GSE
Corneal reflex	Ophthalmic (CN V1) GSA	Facial nerve proper (CN VII) SVE
Lacrimation reflex	Ophthalmic (CN V1) GSA	Facial nerve proper (CN VII) SVE
Sneeze reflex	Ophthalmic (CN V2) and maxillary (CN V3) GSA	Vagus (CN X) SVE
Jaw jerk (stretch) reflex*	Mandibular (CN V3) GSA	Mandibular (CN V3) SVE
Stapedial reflex	Cochlear division of (CN VIII) SSA	Facial nerve (CN VII) SVE
Gag reflex	Glossopharyngeal (CN IX) GVA	Vagus (CN X) SVE
Carotid sinus baroreflex	Glossopharyngeal (CN IX) GVA	Vagus (CN X) GVE
Aortic sinus reflex (vasomotor)	Vagus (CN X) GVA	Vagus (CN X) GVE
Cough reflex	Vagus (CN X) GVA	Vagus (CN X) GVE and SVE Spinal GSE (C3–C5)
Laryngeal adductor reflex	Vagus (CN X) GVA	Vagus (CN X) SVE

Abbreviations: GSA, general somatic afferent; GSE, general somatic efferent; GVE, general visceral efferent; SSA, special somatic afferent; SVE, special visceral efferent.

Note: *Reflexes mediated by cranial nerves are polysynaptic except for jaw jerk reflex which is a monosynaptic stretch reflex.

Table 9.19 Clinical correlations to cranial nerve damage and testing

Cranial Nerve and Modality	Location of Neuron Cell Bodies	Functions	Testing	Clinical Correlations
Olfactory nerve (CN I) SVA	SVA Olfactory mucosa	SVA mediates olfactory sensations detected by chemoreceptors to olfactory bulb through synapse to prefrontal olfactory cortex	Sense of smell is tested in each nostril with a non-irritating stimulus since loss due nerve lesion is usually unilateral	Trauma such as skull fracture or infections (rhinitis) can cause anosmia (loss of smell) of varying degrees Loss of smell diminishes taste
Optic nerve (CN II) SSA	SSA Retinal epithelial cells	SSA mediates visual stimuli through optic nerve and tract to lateral geniculate nucleus and visual cortex	Test for acuity using Snellen chart, color blindness using Ishihara color plate, and assess visual fields for each eye Visual reflexes More extensive testing includes imaging optic disc and optic nerve	Damage due to vascular lesions, trauma, diseases such as glaucoma or demyelination of CNS may lead to partial loss of visual field, altered visual acuity, or complete blindness
Oculomotor nerve (CN III) GSE GVE	GSE Oculomotor nucleus in midbrain GVE Edinger-Westphal nucleus midbrain	GSE fibers innervate and control all ocular muscles except superior oblique and lateral rectus Moves eyes medially, up, and down GVE Preganglionic parasympathetic synapse on ciliary ganglion; postganglionic fibers innervate ciliary muscles and papillary constrictors Controls papillary constriction, near vision, and accommodation reflex	Check for: Ptosis (fallen eyelid) Pupil size Nystagmus (uncontrolled rapid eye movement) Assess eye movements by following moving target with eyes *often assessed along with CNs IV and VI **Visual reflex for GVE** Test accommodation and convergence response Method: Move a single target toward nose; eyes should move medial and	Damage to CN III due to nerve palsies, aneurysms in cavernous sinus, or diabetic neuropathy may lead to: • Double vision (diplopia) since the eyes work together • Damage to GSE fibers causes affected eye to turn down and out due to the unopposed action of lateral rectus and superior oblique • Ptosis due to loss of levator palpebrae • Strabismus (abnormal alignment of ocular fields) • Nystagmus (rapid involuntary

(*Continued*)

Table 9.19 (*Continued*) Clinical correlations to cranial nerve damage and testing

Cranial Nerve and Modality	Location of Neuron Cell Bodies	Functions	Testing	Clinical Correlations
			pupils constrict consensually **Pupillary light reflex** is consensual response: Method: Alternate shining light into each eye; pupil should constrict	movements of eyes) Damage to GVE fibers causes mydriasis (dilated pupil)
Trochlear nerve (CN IV) GSE	GSE Trochlear motor nucleus Midbrain	GSE fibers innervate superior oblique, move the eye downward and out when the eye is positioned medially	Test ocular movements with CNs III and VI	Damage or compression weakness to trochlear nerve during its course leads to nerve palsy: • Vertical diplopia • Ipsilateral extorsion (outward rotation; adduction/elevation) Patient may tilt head with downward gaze: • If the trochlear nucleus is affected the deficit is same but contralateral due to decussation of nerve
Trigeminal nerve (CN V) • Ophthalmic • (V1) • Maxillary (V2) • Mandibular (V3) GSA SVE	GSA Trigeminal ganglion (PNS) (pain, temperature, tactile) Mesencephalic nucleus Midbrain (proprioception from muscle spindles in jaw closing muscles and PDL) SVE Motor nucleus of V Upper pons	GSA fibers carrying pain/temperature/crude touch project to *spinal trigeminal nucleus (CN V)* GSA fibers carrying tactile (fine) touch and pressure project to chief sensory nucleus **CN V1 GSA** Innervates orbit, conjunctiva eye, sinuses, nasal cavity, and skin of face forehead/scalp **CN V2 GSA** Innervates skin cheek, upper lip, nose, nasal cavity, palate, superior nasopharynx, maxillary arch **CN V3 GSA** Innervates skin lower jaw, TMJ, anterior two-thirds of tongue, floor of mouth, lower lips SVE motor innervation to muscles of mastication, mylohyoid, anterior digastric, tensor tympani, and tensor veli is carried by V3	Test cutaneous sensory for each division Method: Light touch and discriminative touch to forehead, cheek, and lower jaw/chin **Corneal reflex** evaluates CNs V1 and VII Method: Lightly touch the cornea of one eye Assess **jaw jerk reflex** for motor function and proprioceptive input Method: Place an index finger on patient's chin and strike finger with tendon hammer—outcome will be slight elevation/protrusion of mandible (CN V3) Assess (masseter and temporalis) for muscle atrophy and strength Method: Palpation; jaw movement, side-to-side against resistance	Stroke, trauma, tumors, or viral infections may damage the nerve and lead to: Sensory (GSA) damage: • Trigeminal neuralgia characterized by sharp stabbing pain in one or more branches • Diminished sensation to specific affected area (V1, V2, and V3 dermatomes) • Inhibition of corneal reflex (V1) Motor (SVE) damage: • Unilateral damage of SVE fibers (V3) or motor nucleus may cause weakness—manifest as jaw deviation to side of lesion • Hypoacusis (partial loss of low-pitch sound) due to loss of tensor tympani muscle is usually insignificant
Abducens (CN VI) GSE	GSE Motor nucleus of abducens in pons	Lateral rectus abducts eye (moves laterally)	Test ocular movements with CN III and CN IV	Susceptible to damage due to cavernous sinus thrombosis during peripheral course Damage leads to muscle paralysis causing: • Medial strabismus (medial deviation on affected side) • Horizontal diplopia
Facial nerve (CN VII) SVA GVA GSA SVE GVE	SVA Geniculate ganglion (PNS) GVA Geniculate ganglion GSA Geniculate ganglion SVE Facial motor nucleus of CN VII in lower pons	SVA conveys taste from anterior two-thirds of tongue to nucleus solitarius (rostral) GVA mediates mucosal irritation (only small contribution from CN VII) Fibers project to nucleus solitarius (caudal) GSA fibers convey sensation from behind ear; GSA fibers project to spinal trigeminal nucleus (CN V) SVE innervates muscles of facial expression GVE preganglionic parasympathetic	Test sensation to anterior two-thirds of tongue Test facial expression Method: Observe facial symmetry during facial movements—smile to show teeth, whistle, close eyes against resistance, raise eyebrows/wrinkle brow Evaluate tearing ability Hard to evaluate as is decreased salivation and nasal	Damage to motor or sensory cell bodies, or nerve damage in its course may occur due to infections, neuromas, tumors in parotid gland, anesthetic during dental treatment, and trauma causing facial palsy Motor (SVE) damage: • Unilateral paralysis of upper and lower facial muscles on affected side (Bell's palsy) • Can't wrinkle forehead or close eye • Loss of corneal reflex (efferent limb)

(*Continued*)

Table 9.19 (*Continued*) Clinical correlations to cranial nerve damage and testing

Cranial Nerve and Modality	Location of Neuron Cell Bodies	Functions	Testing	Clinical Correlations
	GVE Superior salivatory nucleus in lower pons	fibers synapse in • Pterygopalatine ganglion • Submandibular ganglion Innervates majority of glands in face except parotid and minor buccal	mucous production	• Mouth pulls to unaffected side during smiling, facial droop, food pocketing due to muscle weakness • Hyperacusis—sensitivity to loud noise; paralysis of stapedius muscle GVE loss of lacrimation Sensory (SVA, GSA) damage • Loss of taste in anterior two-thirds (dysgeusia) (ageusia)
Vestibulo-cochlear (CN VIII) SSA	**SSA** Vestibular ganglion PNS (balance) Cochlear ganglion (auditory)	SSA fibers transmit vestibular and auditory signals arising from epithelial hair cells and project to the cochlear and vestibular nuclear complex and then to the cerebellum and auditory cortex	Cochlear test Method: Rub fingers together; use a tuning fork to perform Weber test and Rinne test (air vs. bone conduction) Vestibular test: Walk a straight line Test for Romberg sign: Close eyes while standing with feet together—observe swaying and instability; access vestibulo-ocular reflex	Damage to vestibular and cochlear nerve can occur separately or concurrently, depending on point of damage Hearing loss caused by • Conduction deafness • Sensorineural (nerve) damage ○ Acoustic neuromas (Schwann cell tumor) *can compress facial nerve Vestibular nerve damage caused by vestibular neuritis (nerve inflammation) leads to: • Dizziness, vomiting • Tinnitus (ringing) • Vertigo (balance) • Nystagmus
Glossopharyngeal (CN IX) • GSA • GVA • SVA • GVE • SVE	**GSA** Superior ganglion of CN IX (PNS) **GVA** Inferior petrosal ganglion of CN IX (PNS) **SVA** Inferior petrosal ganglion of IX (PNS) **GVE** Inferior salivatory nucleus Medulla **SVE** Nucleus ambiguus (motor) Medulla	GSA fibers convey sensations from mucosa of the tympanic membrane, auditory tube, lower nasopharynx, oropharynx, and tonsillar fossa of posterior one-third of tongue Fibers project to trigeminal nucleus of V and then to cortex or reflex centers GVA responds to mucosal irritation, and changes in blood pressure detected in carotid sinus and O_2/CO_2 levels in blood Fibers synapse on nucleus tract of solitarius mediating autonomic reflex SVA fibers convey taste to posterior one-third of tongue GVE parasympathetic fibers synapse on postganglionic neurons in otic ganglion; provide secretomotor innervation to parotid and minor buccal glands SVE provides motor innervation to stylopharyngeus derived third pharyngeal arch	CNs IX and X often tested together* **Gag reflex** to assess afferent function of glossopharyngeal nerve and efferent component of CN X Test taste sensation in posterior one-third of tongue Observe salivary flow from parotid duct	Due the peripheral course of CN IX, the vagus may also be involved Stroke, tumors, damage to motor nucleus or nerve during its course Outcome: Sensory deficits and autonomic reflexes most notable due to damage Sensory loss • Loss of gag reflex (afferent limb) due to damage of CN IX • Syncope (fainting) due to hypersensitive carotid reflex • Loss of taste in posterior one-third of tongue • Glossopharyngeal neuralgia (stabbing, sharp pain in oropharynx and auditory tube)
Vagus (CN X) • GSA • GVA • SVA • GVE • SVE	**GSA** Superior jugular ganglion of CN X (PNS) **GVA** Inferior nodose ganglion of CN IX (PNS) **SVA** Inferior nodose ganglion of CN	GSA fibers convey sensations from the epiglottis, laryngopharynx, larynx, thoracic, and abdominal viscera to spinal trigeminal nucleus and then to cortex or reflex centers of reticular formation GVA fibers detect mucosal irritation of the larynx, visceral distention, and stretch of baroreceptors in aortic sinus; GVA fibers mediate autonomic reflex SVA transmits taste from epiglottis/laryngopharynx	Test swallowing and soft palate elevation and phonation levels Method: Say "Ahhh" while using a tongue depressor and observe deviation of uvulae Damage to motor nucleus causes the muscle to sag on affected side; patient will exhibit unilateral deviation of uvulae to opposite side of lesion	Damage may occur to motor or sensory neurons or peripheral branches Location of lesion depends on extent of damage: Motor (SVE) damage: (unilateral) • Problems swallowing (dysphasia) due to pharyngeal and palatal weakness; muscles sag on side of lesion • Difficulty in speaking (dysarthria) • Hoarseness (dysphonia) due to damage of recurrent laryngeal

(*Continued*)

Table 9.19 (*Continued*) Clinical correlations to cranial nerve damage and testing

Cranial Nerve and Modality	Location of Neuron Cell Bodies	Functions	Testing	Clinical Correlations
	IX (PNS) **GVE** Dorsal motor nucleus of CN X **SVE** Nucleus ambiguus (motor) Medulla	**SVE** provides motor innervation via pharyngeal plexus to all palatal and pharyngeal muscles except tensor palatini (CN V3) Stylopharyngeus (CN IX) provides motor innervation to laryngeal muscle		nerve Bilateral damage to recurrent laryngeal nerve leads to asphyxiation Damage to GVE fibers may disrupt vagal reflexes involved in vomiting, vasomotor, cardiac, and respiratory control
Accessory (CN XI) GSE	**GSE/SVE** C1–C5 ventral horn cells	GSE/SVE innervates sternocleidomastoid and trapezius	Test motor function Method: Shrug of shoulders (shoulder elevation) and turn head against resistance	Motor nerve damage due to nerve impingement, radical neck resection, or cervical spinal cord or head trauma leads to: • Weakness and atrophy of sternocleidomastoid (SCM); exhibits difficulty in turning head to opposite side • Weakness of trapezius; difficulty in elevating shoulder on affected side (shoulder appears lower)
Hypoglossal (CN XII) GSE	**GSE** Motor nucleus of hypoglossal Lower medulla	GSE innervates the tongue causing bodily movement including tongue protrusion	Visual inspection: • Observe atrophy or fasciculations (unintentional muscle tremors) Listen to for ability to articulate Test motor function: • Method: Protrude and retract tongue	Unilateral motor damage of nucleus or nerve causes tongue to deviate toward affected side upon protrusion due to unopposed action of genioglossus Exhibit: Atrophy of muscle on affected side

Abbreviations: CNS, central nervous system; GSA, general somatic afferent; GSE, general somatic efferent; GVA, general visceral afferent; GVE, general visceral efferent; PDL, periodontal ligament; PNS, peripheral nervous system; SSA, special somatic afferent; SVA, special visceral afferent; SVE, special visceral efferent; TMJ, temporomandibular joint.
Note: Some cranial nerves, including CN IX and X, exhibit overlapping distribution patterns and so the modalities are not definitively tested. Some modalities, such as GVE innervation to glands, are also difficult to assess and quantify.

Questions and Answers

1. Each of the following cranial nerves passes through superior orbital fissure to the orbit EXCEPT one. Which one is the exception?
   a) Trochlear (CN IV)
   b) Optic (CN II)
   c) Abducens (CN VI)
   d) Oculomotor (CN III)
   e) Ophthalmic (CN V1)

Level 2: Moderate
   Answer B: The optic nerve enters the skull by passing through the optic canal. The optic nerve carries SSA axons from the retina of eye. The eye is found in the orbit. All other nerves pass through the superior orbital fissure to enter the orbit. The oculomotor (CN III) (**D**), the trochlear (CN IV) (**A**), and abducens (CN VI) (**C**) supply motor (GSE) innervation to the eye muscles or transmit sensory input (GSA) from the conjunctiva, mucous

membrane covering the sclera, and cornea (ophthalmic, CN V1) (**E**).

2. Which of the functional columns of the brainstem is responsible for innervating the pharyngeal arch muscles?
   a) SVE
   b) GSE
   c) GVA
   d) SVA
   e) GVE

Level 1: Easy
   Answer A: SVE carries efferent (motor) fibers to skeletal muscles derived from branchiomeric head mesoderm of the pharyngeal arches. GSE (**B**) carries motor fibers to skeletal muscle derived from the paraxial somites and is the same functional component carried by the spinal nerves. GVA (**C**) carries visceral sensory fibers from interoceptors, chemoreceptors, and baroreceptors associated with organs, and SVA (**D**) carries taste sensations from gustatory receptors associated with taste buds. GVE (**E**) carries

fibers from preganglionic parasympathetic cell bodies that mediate glandular secretion and smooth muscle contraction.

3. A construction worker injured during fall at work reports difficulty in turning his head away from the side of injury and exhibits shoulder drop on the injured side. Which cranial nerve is injured?
   a) CN X
   b) CN XII
   c) CN IX
   d) CN VII
   e) CN XI

Level 2: Moderate

Answer E: CN XI is the spinal accessory nerve which serves to mediate these actions. (**A**) CN X (vagus), (**B**) CN XII (hypoglossal), (**C**) CN IX (glossopharyngeal), and (**D**) CN VII (facial) all provide motor innervation to skeletal muscles; however, the innervation is to skeletal muscles in the larynx, pharynx, palate (CN X), tongue musculature (CN XII), stylopharyngeus muscle (CN IX), and facial muscles (CN VII).

4. Which of the following contains the primary afferent neurons (cell bodies) for sensory fibers which transmit proprioception from the masseter muscle?
   a) Chief (main) sensory nucleus of V
   b) Spinal nucleus of V
   c) Semilunar (trigeminal) ganglion
   d) Mesencephalic nucleus

Level 1: Easy

Answer D: Mesencephalic nucleus contains the cell bodies of the primary afferent neurons that transmit proprioception. The mesencephalic nucleus is the only cranial sensory nuclei in the CNS to contain primary afferent neurons. All other cranial sensory nuclei contain second-order neurons. The spinal trigeminal nucleus (**B**) contains the cell bodies of the second-order neurons for pain and temperature stimuli while the main (chief) sensory nucleus (**A**) contains the second-order neurons for tactile input. The primary afferent cell bodies for the GSA fibers are found in the trigeminal (semilunar) ganglion (**C**). The primary afferent fibers will synapse on second-order neurons in spinal trigeminal and chief sensory nuclei.

5. The primary afferent cell bodies of the cranial nerve which detect a change in pressure from baroreceptors in the carotid sinus are located in the _____.
   a) Petrosal ganglion
   b) Nucleus solitarius
   c) Nodose ganglion
   d) Otic ganglion
   e) Nucleus ambiguus

Level 2: Moderate

Answer A: The petrosal (inferior) ganglion of CN IX contains the cell bodies of SVA and GVA neurons that transmit taste (SVA) from taste buds in the posterior one-third of the tongue and GVA fibers from baroreceptors in the carotid sinus. The superior ganglion of CN IX contains GSA. The nucleus solitarius (**B**) contains the second-order neurons for the GVA fibers. The nodose (inferior ganglion of CN X) ganglion (**C**) contains the cell bodies for SVA and GVA fibers associated with the vagus nerve. GVA fibers for the vagus transmit sensory input from baroreceptors in the aortic sinus. The otic ganglion (**D**) contains the cell bodies of GVE postganglionic parasympathetic neurons associated with the glossopharyngeal nerve. These GVE fibers carry secretomotor innervation to the parotid gland. Nucleus ambiguus (**E**) contains SVE cell bodies (second-order neurons) for the vagus nerve.

10 Gross Anatomy of the Spinal Cord

1. Identify the flexures of the developing and adult brain.
2. Describe the segmental organization of the spinal cord.
3. Discuss the components of a spinal nerve.
4. Describe the external anatomy of the spinal cord.
5. Describe the internal architecture of the spinal cord.
6. Identify the columns found in the gray matter.
7. Name the columns found in the white matter.
8. Identify the Rexed laminae and describe their location and content.
9. Describe the meninges of the spinal cord.
10. Identify the blood supply to the spinal cord.

10.1 Overview of the Spinal Cord

The spinal cord along with the brain makes up the central nervous system. The spinal cord is a continuation of the distal medulla oblongata and is housed within the vertebral column. The same three layers of meninges that are associated with the brain are continuous on the spinal cord. Both the meninges and the bony vertebrae serve as a means of protection for the spinal cord against trauma. The spinal cord is also suspended in cerebrospinal fluid (CSF), which acts as a cushion and prevents injury to the delicate tissue that makes up the spinal cord. The spinal cord consists of 31 spinal segments, each of which is associated with a pair of spinal nerves. These spinal nerves allow the spinal cord to receive sensory information from receptors located in the periphery and relay that information to the cortex where it is processed and interpreted (▶ Fig. 10.1). The spinal cord also provides motor innervation to the muscles of the body via the same 31 pairs of spinal nerves. Some of the sensory and motor tracts are involved in reflex activity. The spinal cord receives blood from the vertebral artery and larger segmental arteries supplying the cervical, thoracic, lumbar, and sacral areas.

10.2 Organization of the Spinal Cord

10.2.1 Development of the Spinal Cord

- The spinal cord develops from the embryonic **neural tube**. The **rostral** portion of the tube forms the forebrain, midbrain, and hindbrain. The **caudal** portion will develop into the primitive spinal cord.
  - During the **three-vesicle stage** of embryonic development, prominent **flexures** (▶ Fig. 10.2) appear:
    - The **cephalic flexure** is the first to appear and develop at the level of the midbrain.
    - The **cervical flexure** develops later between the hindbrain and the spinal cord.
    - The **pontine flexure** is the last to appear, developing at the junction of the metencephalon and the myelencephalon.

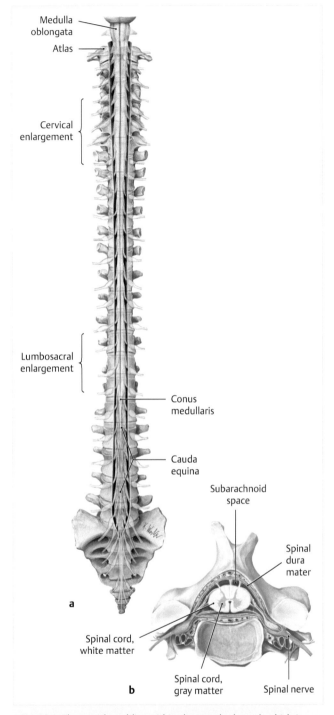

Fig. 10.1 The spinal cord lies within the vertebral canal, which is formed by the vertebral foramen of all the vertebrae stacked on top of one another and the ligaments of the vertebral column traversing the vertebrae. **(a)** The spinal cord, which is the most caudal part of the CNS, extends caudally from the first cervical vertebra, called the atlas, to the second lumbar vertebra. **(b)** Cross section through a single vertebral level demonstrating spinal cord within the vertebral canal. CNS, central nervous system. (Reproduced with permission from Schuenke M, Schulte E, Schumacher U. THIEME Atlas of Anatomy Second Edition, Vol 3. © Thieme 2016. Illustrations by Markus Voll and Karl Wesker.)

○ During the **five-vesicle stage** of development, the cephalic flexure becomes prominent while the cervical and pontine become less prominent. The persistence of the cephalic flexure results in a curved **neuroaxis** rather than the previously seen longitudinal axis present in very early embryos and lower vertebrates.

10.2.2 Segmental Organization of the Spinal Cord

- Both the developing and the adult spinal cord are composed of rostrocaudal segments derived from **mesodermal somites** (▶ Fig. 10.3).
  ○ Skeletal muscles, dermis, cartilage, tendons, and vertebrae develop from these **somites**.
- For each somite, there is a corresponding vertebra, which is described as a spinal cord segment.
  ○ In the adult, the spinal cord regions are identified as: **cervical, thoracic, lumbar, sacral,** and **coccyx**.
  ○ The 31 spinal segments are defined by the 31 spinal nerves exiting the spinal cord: 8 cervical, 12 thoracic, 5 lumbar, 5 sacral, and 1 coccygeal (▶ Fig. 10.4).
- Each spinal cord segment provides sensory and motor innervation via spinal nerves for the skin and muscle derived from the same somite (▶ Fig. 10.5).

○ Spinal nerves enter/exit the spinal cord as **dorsal** (sensory) and **ventral** (motor) **rootlets** (▶ Fig. 10.6a, b).
○ The **dorsal** and **ventral rootlets** coalesce to form the **dorsal** and **ventral roots**.
○ The dorsal root is associated with a **sensory ganglion** known as the **dorsal root ganglion** (**DRG**).
○ The dorsal and ventral roots join just distal to the DRG to form what is known as a **mixed spinal nerve**.

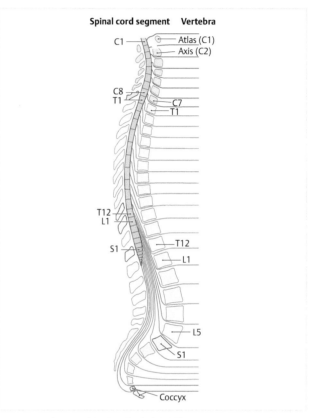

Fig. 10.4 The spinal cord is divided into four major regions: cervical, thoracic, lumbar, and sacral. There are 31 spinal nerves exiting the spinal cord. (Reproduced with permission from Schuenke M, Schulte E, Schumacher U. THIEME Atlas of Anatomy Third Edition, Vol 3. © Thieme 2020. Illustrations by Markus Voll and Karl Wesker.)

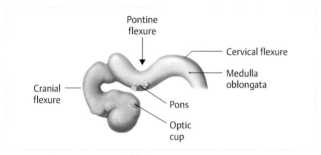

Fig. 10.2 Primary flexures develop during the three-vesicle stage of embryonic development. (Reproduced with permission from Schuenke M, Schulte E, Schumacher U. THIEME Atlas of Anatomy Third Edition, Vol 3. © Thieme 2020. Illustrations by Markus Voll and Karl Wesker.)

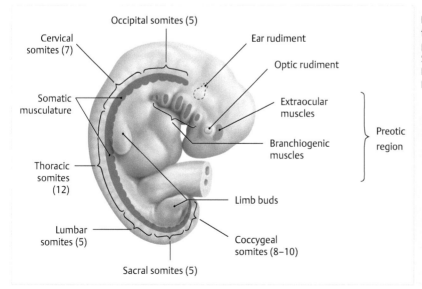

Fig. 10.3 The spinal cord develops from somites formed from paraxial mesoderm. (Reproduced with permission from Schuenke M, Schulte E, Schumacher U. THIEME Atlas of Anatomy Second Edition, Vol 1. © Thieme 2014. Illustrations by Markus Voll and Karl Wesker.)

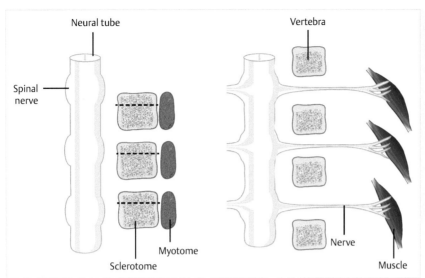

Fig. 10.5 Each spinal cord segment provides motor and sensory innervation for skin and muscle derived from the same somite.

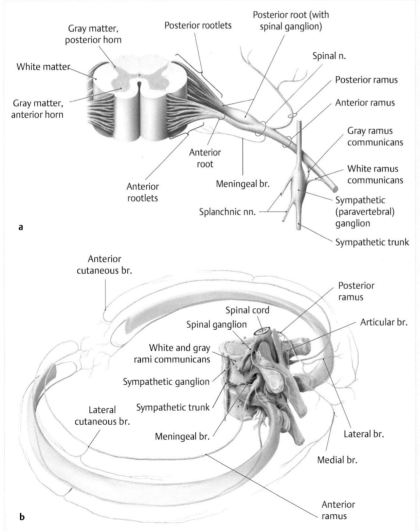

Fig. 10.6 **(a)** Afferent (sensory) posterior rootlets and efferent (motor) anterior rootlets form the posterior and anterior roots of the spinal nerve for that segment. The two roots fuse to form a mixed (motor and sensory) spinal nerve that exits the intervertebral foramen and immediately thereafter divides into an anterior and posterior ramus. **(b)** Spinal nerve branches. A superolateral view of a thoracic spinal nerve. The posterior (dorsal) rami of the spinal nerves give rise to muscular and cutaneous branches of the back. The anterior (ventral) rami of spinal nerves T1–T11 produce the intercostal nerves (T12 produces the subcostal nerve). (Reproduced with permission from Schuenke M, Schulte E, Schumacher U. THIEME Atlas of Anatomy Third Edition, Vol 3. © Thieme 2020. Illustrations by Markus Voll and Karl Wesker.)

- The mixed spinal nerve emerges from the vertebral column through the **intervertebral foramen** and then splits into **dorsal** and **ventral primary rami** that carry motor and sensory fibers to the posterior, anterior, and lateral aspect of the body. The **primary dorsal rami** innervate the deep back muscles and the skin on the back. The **primary ventral rami** innervate the limbs and the remainder of the trunk (▶ Table 10.1).
- Each mixed spinal nerve represents one of the 31 spinal segments.
  - The cervical spinal nerves/segments innervate the skin and muscle of the head, neck, and arms.
  - The thoracic spinal nerves/segments innervate the trunk.
  - The lumbar and sacral spinal nerves/segments innervate the legs and **perineal** area.
- Each spinal nerve maintains a relationship with its somite and the structures that are derived from that somite.
  - Each spinal nerve therefore (except **C1**) innervates a single **dermatome** (▶ Fig. 10.7).
  - Each dermatome represents the sensory distribution of a single spinal nerve and forms bands or contours on the body (▶ Fig. 10.8).
  - • Developmental rotation of the upper and lower extremities makes the dermatome pattern more complex than that of the chest and abdomen.
  - Dermatome patterns are clinically significant as they can aid in the diagnosis of nerve injury.

Table 10.1 Branches of a spinal nerve

Branches			Territory
Meningeal branch			Spinal meninges; ligaments of spinal column
Posterior (dorsal) ramus	Medial branches	Articular branch	Zygapophyseal joints
		Muscular branch	Intrinsic back muscles
		Cutaneous branch	Skin of posterior head, neck, back, and buttocks
	Lateral branches	Cutaneous branch	
		Muscular branch	Intrinsic back muscles
Anterior (ventral) ramus	Lateral cutaneus branches		Skin of lateral chest wall
	Anterior cutaneous branches		Skin of anterior chest wall

Note: The white and gray rami communicans carry pre- and postganglionic fibers between the sympathetic trunk and spinal nerve.
(Reproduced with permission from Gilroy AM, MacPherson BR. Atlas of Anatomy. Third Edition. © Thieme 2016. Illustrations by Markus Voll and Karl Wesker.)

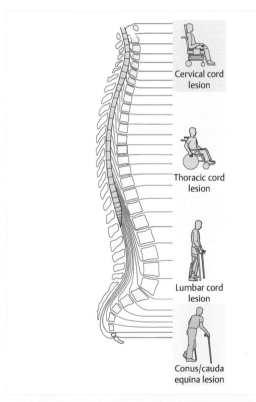

Fig. 10.7 Each spinal nerve maintains a relationship with its somite as well as the structures that are derived from that somite. Thus, each spinal nerve innervates a single dermatome. (Reproduced with permission from Schuenke M, Schulte E, Schumacher U. THIEME Atlas of Anatomy Third Edition, Vol 3. © Thieme 2020. Illustrations by Markus Voll and Karl Wesker.)

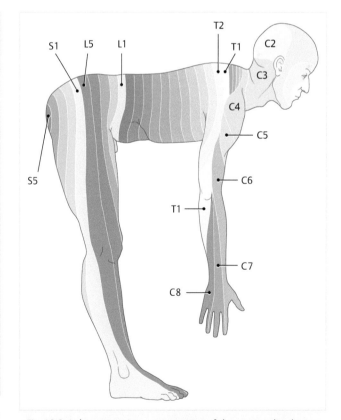

Fig. 10.8 A dermatome is a representation of the sensory distribution of a single spinal nerve. (Reproduced with permission from Schuenke M, Schulte E, Schumacher U. THIEME Atlas of Anatomy Third Edition, Vol 3. © Thieme 2020. Illustrations by Markus Voll and Karl Wesker.)

10.3 Gross Anatomy of the Spinal Cord

- The spinal cord begins at the level of the **pyramidal decussation** in the **medulla** and exits through the **foramen magnum** of the **occipital bone**. It extends inferiorly in the **vertebral canal** and terminates as the **conus medullaris**, which is at vertebral level **L2** (▶ Fig. 10.9).
- The **dural sac**, which encases the spinal cord, extends inferiorly to the level of **S2** (▶ Fig. 10.10).
- A thin filament encased in pia called the **filum terminale internum** extends from the conus medullaris. The conus medullaris becomes surrounded by dura as it passes through the caudal aspect of the dural sac. This extension of the **dural sac** is called the **filum terminale externum** or **coccygeal ligament**. The coccygeal ligament is attached to the caudal end of the coccyx, thus anchoring the spinal cord and the dural sac and preventing excessive movement (▶ Fig. 10.11) (Clinical Correlation Box 10.1).
- There are two notable enlargements of the spinal cord in the **cervical** and the **lumbar** (▶ Fig. 10.12) areas.
  - The **cervical enlargement** (**C5–T1**) corresponds to the **brachial plexus** which is a plexus of nerves innervating the upper limb.
  - The **lumbar enlargement** (**T11–S1**) represents the **lumbar** and **sacral plexi** that innervate the abdomen and lower limb.

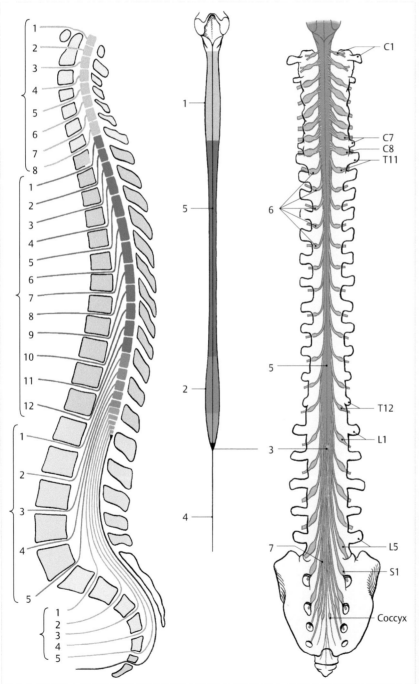

Fig. 10.9 The spinal cord begins at the pyramidal decussation and terminates as the conus medullaris which is at vertebral level L2. (Reproduced with permission from Kahle W, Frotscher M. Color Atlas of Human Anatomy. Sixth Edition, Vol 3. © Thieme 2011.)

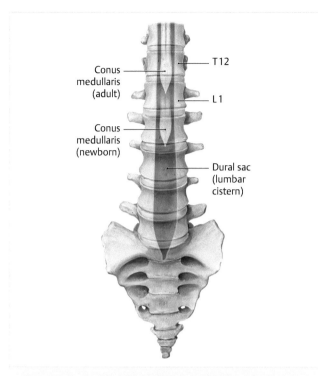

Conus medullaris (adult)

T12

L1

Conus medullaris (newborn)

Dural sac (lumbar cistern)

Fig. 10.10 The dural sac extends down to vertebral level S2 creating a space known as the lumbar cistern. (Reproduced with permission from Schuenke M, Schulte E, Schumacher U. THIEME Atlas of Anatomy Third Edition, Vol 3. © Thieme 2020. Illustrations by Markus Voll and Karl Wesker.)

Clinical Correlation Box 10.1: Tethered Cord Syndrome

Tethered cord syndrome is a neurological condition caused by tissue attachments that limits movement of the spinal cord within the spinal column. These attachments result in an abnormal stretching of the spinal cord and are highly associated (20–50%) with **spina bifida**. In this condition, the spinal cord has fat at the tip that connects to the fat that overlies the dura sac. Although the skin is closed, the spinal cord remains in the same position as the child grows (tethered) causing it to stretch and become damaged. Symptoms include lesions on lower back (dimples, tufts of hair, discoloration), back pain, leg pain, leg numbness and tingling, and deterioration in gait, among others. This condition can lead to increasing sensory and motor problems as well as loss of bladder and bowel control. If significant stretching occurs surgery may be indicated to "untether" the spinal cord.

- Early in development the growth of the spinal cord and vertebral column are fairly equal so that the spinal cord occupies the entire **vertebral canal**. After the first 3 months, the growth of the vertebral column exceeds that of the spinal cord creating a space in the caudal aspect of the vertebral canal (▶ Fig. 10.13). The space produced as a result of the differential growth is called the **lumbar cistern** (Clinical Correlation Box 10.2) (▶ Fig. 10.14).
  - The lumbar cistern is an enlargement of the **subarachnoid space** and contains the **dorsal** (sensory) and **ventral** (motor)

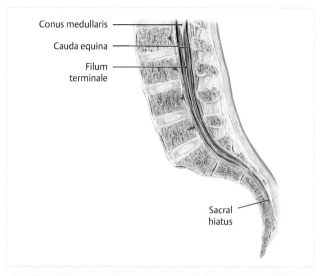

Conus medullaris

Cauda equina

Filum terminale

Sacral hiatus

Fig. 10.11 The coccygeal ligament is attached to the coccyx which anchors the spinal cord and prevents excessive movement. (Reproduced with permission from Schuenke M, Schulte E, Schumacher U. THIEME Atlas of Anatomy Third Edition, Vol 3. © Thieme 2020. Illustrations by Markus Voll and Karl Wesker.)

roots of the lumbar and sacral spinal cord segments for the legs. These floating roots in the lumbar cistern are called the **cauda equina** (Latin for horse's tail) (▶ Fig. 10.15).
- Each of the first seven cervical nerves exits the vertebral canal above the corresponding vertebrae. However, because there are only seven cervical vertebrae, the eighth cervical nerve exits between the seventh cervical vertebrae and the first thoracic vertebrae. All subsequent spinal nerves exit the vertebral column *below* their corresponding vertebrae.
- The spinal cord has several **fissures** visible from the surface (anterior and posterior) and upon cross section (▶ Fig. 10.16a–c).
  - The **anterior median fissure** divides the spinal cord into two symmetrical halves and contains the **anterior spinal artery**.
  - The **anterior lateral sulcus** is the site where the ventral rootlets exit the spinal cord.
  - The **anterior funiculus** is the area between the anterior median fissure and the anterolateral sulcus. It contains ascending and descending tracts.
  - The **posterior median sulcus** divides the spinal cord into two halves from the posterior aspect.
  - The **posterior lateral sulcus** is the site where the dorsal rootlets enter the spinal cord. It also contains the **posterior spinal artery**.
  - The **posterior funiculus** is the area between the posterior medial sulcus and the **posterolateral** sulcus. It is made up of the **fasciculus cuneatus** and **fasciculus gracilis**.
  - The **fasciculus cuneatus** is present in the upper thoracic and cervical part of the spinal cord and is separated from the fasciculus gracilis by a **septum** (**posterior intermediate sulcus**). It contains the ascending nerve fibers from the upper six thoracic and all the cervical spinal nerves.
  - The **fasciculus gracilis** is present throughout the length of the spinal cord and contains ascending fibers from the sacral, lumbar, and lower six thoracic spinal nerves.

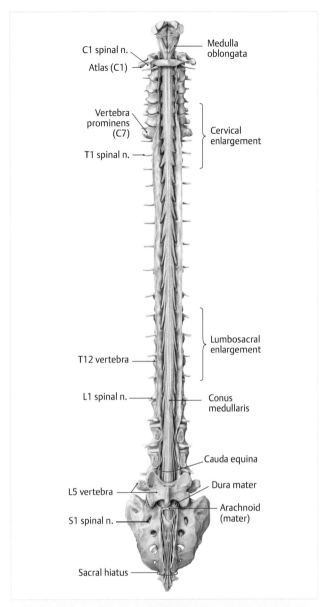

Fig. 10.12 There are two enlargements in the spinal cord, one in the cervical area and the other in the lumbar area. (Reproduced with permission from Schuenke M, Schulte E, Schumacher U. THIEME Atlas of Anatomy Third Edition, Vol 3. © Thieme 2020. Illustrations by Markus Voll and Karl Wesker.)

○ The **posterior intermediate sulcus** divides the **posterior funiculus**. It separates the **fasciculus gracilis** and **fasciculus cuneatus** and is only present at T6 and above. Below T6, the posterior funiculus consists of *only* the fasciculus gracilis.

10.4 Internal Anatomy of the Spinal Cord

10.4.1 Gray Matter

- Cross-sectional observation of the spinal cord shows a butterfly or "H"-shaped central area (**gray matter**) surrounded by myelinated fibers (**white matter**). The area between the "wings" of the butterfly is called the **gray**

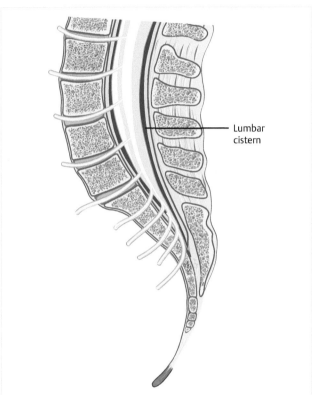

Fig. 10.14 At some point in development, the growth of the vertebral column exceeds that of the spinal cord creating the lumbar cistern.

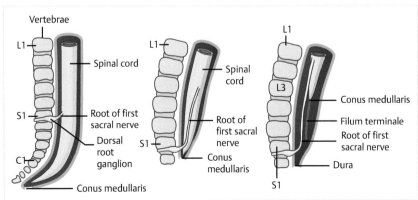

Fig. 10.13 Differential growth of the spinal cord and vertebral column early in development creates a space at the caudal end of the vertebral canal.

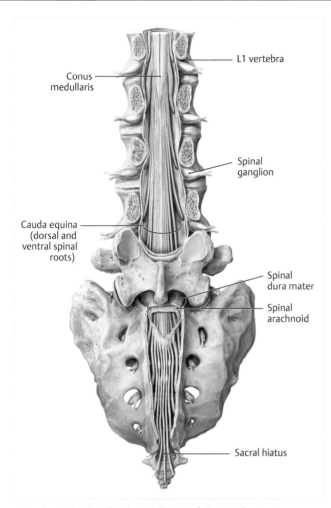

Fig. 10.15 The dorsal and ventral roots of the spinal nerves innervating the lower extremities float in the CSF filled lumbar cistern. Collectively, the roots are called the cauda equina. CSF, cerebrospinal fluid. (Reproduced with permission from Schuenke M, Schulte E, Schumacher U. THIEME Atlas of Anatomy Second Edition, Vol 3. © Thieme 2016. Illustrations by Markus Voll and Karl Wesker.)

L1 vertebra

Conus medullaris

Spinal ganglion

Cauda equina (dorsal and ventral spinal roots)

Spinal dura mater

Spinal arachnoid

Sacral hiatus

commissure. This structure connects the right and left sides of the gray matter. In the center of the gray commissure is a small foramen known as the **central canal** which is continuous throughout the length of the spinal cord. In general, gray matter consists of neuronal cell bodies while white matter is largely composed of axons that collectively form **tracts** (▶ Fig. 10.17).

- The shape and size of the gray matter vary at different spinal cord levels as does the white matter. The lower levels of the spinal cord contain fewer ascending and descending nerve fibers which will alter the ratio of white to gray matter (▶ Fig. 10.18).
- The gray matter is divided into functionally distinct columns: **dorsal horn**, **intermediate column**, **lateral horn**, and **ventral horn** (▶ Fig. 10.19).
  ○ The **dorsal horn** is present at all spinal levels and is comprised of sensory nuclei that receive somatosensory information from the body.
  ○ The **ventral horn** contains motor cell bodies that innervate skeletal muscle.

○ The **intermediate zone** is the area between the dorsal and ventral horn and is continuous with the gray matter that crosses the midline around the central canal. The intermediate zone contains both **interneurons** and **association neurons** that are important for the integration of spinal cord function. Most of the axons projecting from these cell bodies remain in the spinal cord.
○ The **lateral horn** is an extension of the intermediate zone. It contains autonomic cell bodies that innervate viscera and pelvic organs.
○ **Lissauer's tract**, also called the **dorsolateral fasciculus**, is a small bundle of myelinated and unmyelinated axons of sensory neurons that ascend or descend a few spinal cord segments before synapsing. These neurons are primarily involved in transmitting pain and temperature information and synapse on cell bodies located in **Lamina I** (**marginal zone**) and **Lamina II** (**substantia gelatinosa**).

- The gray matter can be mapped based on the distribution of the neurons located in a given area. This pattern of lamination is called **Rexed laminae** (▶ Fig. 10.20). The classification is based on 10 layers (laminae) that groups neurons based on function (▶ Table 10.2).
- In general, Laminae I to IV are concerned with sensory information and make up the dorsal horn. Laminae V and VI deal primarily with proprioception. Lamina VII makes up the intermediate zone and therefore is concerned with relaying information from muscle spindles to the midbrain and cerebellum. Laminae VIII and IV comprise the ventral horn and as such contain mostly motor neurons. Lamina X surrounds the central canal and contains neuroglia.
  ○ **Rexed lamina I**: Also called the **marginal zone**. It is composed of a thin layer that caps the tip of the dorsal horn. Cells in Lamina I primarily respond to noxious and thermal stimuli coming into the dorsal horn via dorsal root fibers. Some of the afferent fibers synapse on cell bodies located in the **posteromarginal nucleus** whose axons cross and ascend as the **lateral spinothalamic tract**.
  ○ **Rexed lamina II**: Contains the **substantia gelatinosa** (**SG**) and responds to noxious stimuli. Many of the neurons in Rexed lamina II receive information from sensory cell bodies in the dorsal root ganglia and project their axons to Rexed laminae III and IV.
  ○ **Rexed laminae III and IV**: Contain the **proper sensory nucleus**. Most of the cell bodies are interneurons that are concerned with proprioception.
  ○ **Rexed lamina IV**: Cells in this layer receive non-noxious information.
  ○ **Rexed lamina V**: This layer is found at the neck of the dorsal horn. Neurons in Lamina V receive information from descending fibers of the **corticospinal** and **rubrospinal tracts**. Axons from cell bodies in this lamina also contribute the **spinothalamic tract**.
  ○ **Rexed lamina VI**: Only present in the cervical and lumbar areas. It receives information from muscle spindles and joint afferents. It also receives afferents from the **corticospinal** and **rubrospinal tracts**.
  ○ **Rexed lamina VII**: Located in the intermediate area of the ventral horn and contains **Clarke's nucleus.** This nucleus receives muscle and tendon afferents. Axons from Clarke's nucleus form the **dorsal spinocerebellar tract**. Other key

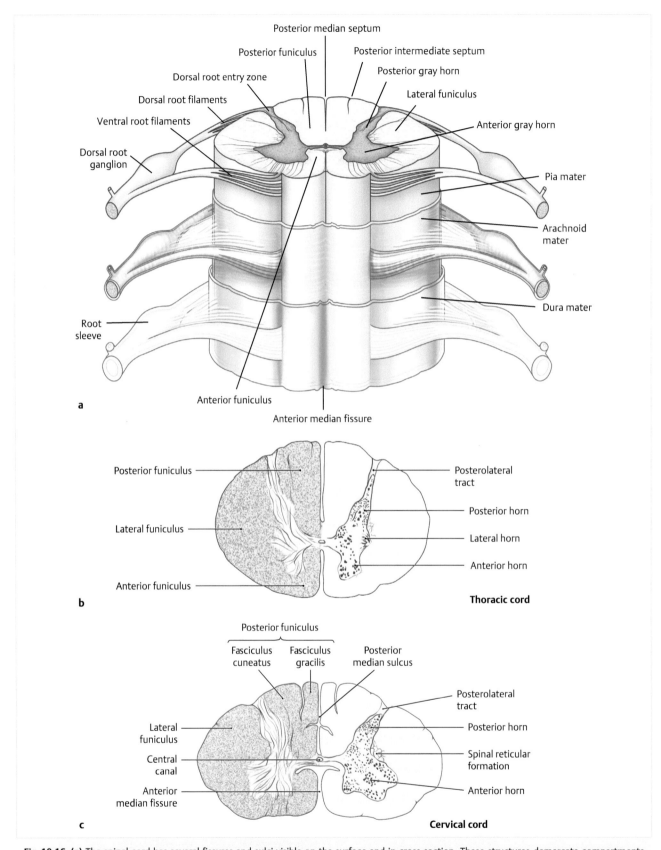

Fig. 10.16 **(a)** The spinal cord has several fissures and sulci visible on the surface and in cross-section. These structures demarcate compartments that contain specific types of neural fibers. **(b)** Cross section of the spinal cord demonstrating compartments (funiculi) along with grey and white matter. **(c)** Cross section of the spinal cord showing compartments within the funiculi (fasiculi) (Fig. 10.16b, c: Reproduced with permission from Schuenke M, Schulte E, Schumacher U. THIEME Atlas of Anatomy Second Edition, Vol 3. © Thieme 2016. Illustrations by Markus Voll and Karl Wesker.)

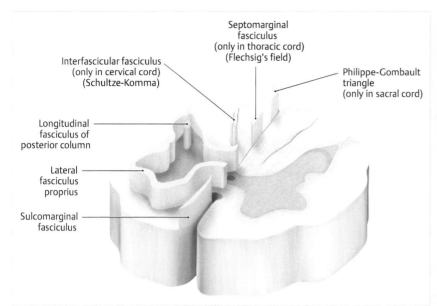

Interfascicular fasciculus
(only in cervical cord)
(Schultze-Komma)

Septomarginal
fasciculus
(only in thoracic cord)
(Flechsig's field)

Philippe-Gombault
triangle
(only in sacral cord)

Longitudinal
fasciculus of
posterior column

Lateral
fasciculus
proprius

Sulcomarginal
fasciculus

Fig. 10.17 When viewed in cross section, the spinal cord appears as an "H"-shaped central area that is known as the gray area. The gray area (cell bodies) is surrounded by white matter which consists of myelinated fibers. (Reproduced with permission from Schuenke M, Schulte E, Schumacher U. THIEME Atlas of Anatomy Second Edition, Vol 3. © Thieme 2016. Illustrations by Markus Voll and Karl Wesker.)

structures found in Lamina VII is the **intermediolateral cell column** (**IML**) which contains **sympathetic preganglionic neurons** (T1–L2) and **parasympathetic neurons** in the sacral spinal cord (S2–S4). Rexed lamina VII also contains many **interneurons**.

○ **Laminae VIII and IX**: Located in the ventral horn of the spinal cord. Motor neurons in this area receive inputs from **descending motor tracts** originating in the cortex and brainstem. They in turn innervate skeletal muscle.

○ **Lamina X**: This lamina consists of the gray matter surrounding the central canal. It consists of somatic and visceral afferents.

10.4.2 White Matter

• The white matter contains both ascending and descending tracts made up of myelinated axons that extend from the cell bodies located in the gray matter.
• Anatomically, it is divided into three main areas known as **funiculi** that are further delineated by their positions: **posterior funiculus**, **anterior funiculus**, and **lateral funiculus** (▶ Fig. 10.21).
• Each funiculus is subdivided into smaller tracts called **fasciculi**.
• The **anterior white commissure** is a bridge formed by crossing myelinated axons that lie ventral to the gray commissure and dorsal to the anterior median fissure. It contains nerve fibers crossing from one side of the spinal cord to the other.
• The **posterior white commissure** is a thin band of white matter that is present at all levels of the spinal cord. It lies dorsal to the gray commissure and ventral to the posterior median sulcus. It contains nerve fibers crossing from one side of the spinal cord to the other.

10.5 Meninges

• The spinal cord is surrounded by the same three meningeal layers as the brain: **dura mater**, **arachnoid membrane,** and **pia mater** (▶ Fig. 10.22 and ▶ Fig. 10.23).

• The **periosteal dural layer** ends at the **foramen magnum** while the **meningeal dural layer** is continuous down to the sacrum (S2) forming the **dural sac**. It attaches to the coccyx via the filum terminale externus.
○ The dura is attached to the foramen magnum and to the vertebrae of the upper cervical region; however, as it extends inferiorly, it is separated from the vertebrae by fat in the **epidural space** (Clinical Correlation Box 10.3 and 10.4). The epidural space also contains the **internal vertebral venous plexus**.
○ The dural layer forming the **dural sac** encloses the entire spinal cord and the **cauda equina**.
○ The dural layer is continuous around the nerve roots and dorsal root ganglia that project laterally from the spinal cord. The nerve roots will eventually join to form a **mixed spinal nerve** (motor and sensory).
○ Shortly after exiting the **intervertebral foramen**, the mixed spinal nerves will branch into dorsal and ventral primary rami. It is at this point that the dural membranes are replaced with connective tissue (**endoneurium, epineurium,** and **perineurium**).
• The arachnoid layer of the spinal cord is also continuous with the arachnoid layer covering the brain. Therefore, it also extends through the foramen magnum and continues inferiorly to S2. The **subarachnoid space** is also present in the spinal cord and is continuous with the subarachnoid space of the brain. Because the two spaces are continuous, some of the CSF in the subarachnoid space of the brain flows inferiorly into the subarachnoid space of the spinal cord and then back up into the subarachnoid space of the brain.
• The innermost meningeal layer is the pia mater. It invests the spinal cord as well as the spinal nerve roots and blood vessels.
○ Bilateral extensions of pia help stabilize the cord within the dural sac. These condensed pial structures separate the dorsal and ventral roots. They are called **denticulate ligaments** due to their "tooth-like" appearance (▶ Fig. 10.23).
○ The filum terminale internus is also a specialized structure derived from pia mater. It can be found internal to the filum terminale externus (dura), which is also known as the

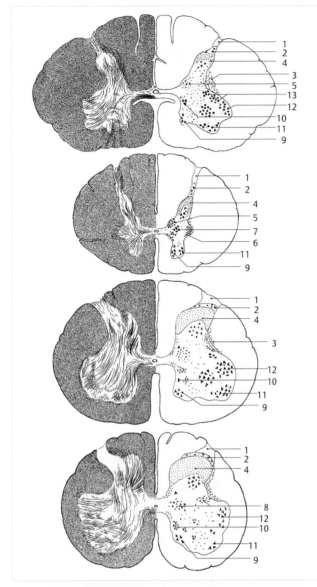

Fig. 10.18 The size and shape of the gray and white matter changes at different levels of the spinal cord. (Reproduced with permission from Kahle W, Frotscher M. Color Atlas of Human Anatomy. Sixth Edition, Vol 3. © Thieme 2011.)

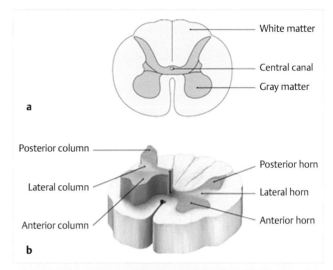

Fig. 10.19 (a,b) The gray matter is divided into functionally distinct columns: dorsal horn (DH), intermediate column (IM), lateral horn (LH), and ventral horn (VH). (Reproduced with permission from Schuenke M, Schulte E, Schumacher U. THIEME Atlas of Anatomy Second Edition, Vol 3. © Thieme 2016. Illustrations by Markus Voll and Karl Wesker.)

coccygeal ligament. The coccygeal ligament anchors the spinal cord to the coccyx and prevents excessive movement.

10.6 Blood Supply to the Spinal Cord

- The blood supply to the spinal cord comes from two main sources, the **vertebral artery** which is a branch of the **subclavian artery** and branches from **segmental** or

radicular arteries such as the **cervical**, **intercostal**, and **lumbar arteries** (▶ Fig. 10.24).

- There are three **longitudinal arteries** that branch off the vertebral artery (▶ Fig. 10.25 and ▶ Fig. 10.26).
  - A single **anterior spinal artery** that runs in the anterior median fissure and supplies the anterior two-thirds of the spinal cord.
  - Paired **posterior spinal arteries** supply the posterior one-third of the spinal cord.
    - The posterior spinal arteries can originate from the vertebral artery or the **posterior inferior cerebellar artery** (**PICA**) which can arise as a branch from the vertebral or basilar arteries.
- Segmental arteries of the vertebral column supply radicular arteries of the spinal cord.
  - In the thoracic and lumbar area, the segmental arteries are the **costocervical**, **intercostal**, and **lumbar arteries**. Radicular branches of the **lateral sacral arteries** supply the spinal cord in the pelvic region. The segmental arteries enter the intervertebral foramina at their respective spinal level where they divide into terminal branches (radicular) that supply the spinal cord.
- Venous drainage closely follows the arterial supply. Anterior and posterior spinal veins along with anterior and posterior radicular veins communicate with the internal venous plexus in the epidural space (▶ Fig. 10.27, ▶ Fig. 10.28, ▶ Fig. 10.29).
  - The veins of the spinal cord and vertebral column are valveless.

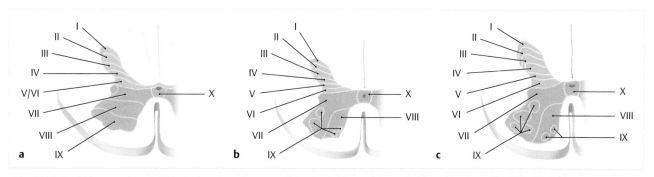

Fig. 10.20 (a-c) The gray area of the spinal cord can be mapped in a lamination pattern called Rexed laminae. (Reproduced with permission from Schuenke M, Schulte E, Schumacher U. THIEME Atlas of Anatomy Second Edition, Vol 3. © Thieme 2016. Illustrations by Markus Voll and Karl Wesker.)

Table 10.2 Rexed laminae classification of spinal cord grey matter

	Spinal Cord Region	Laminae	Nuclei	Function
		I	Marginal nucleus (posterior marginal)	Receive some A delta and C fibers
Alar plate	Dorsal horn	II	Substantia gelatinosa	Receive mainly C fibers Modulate pain and temperature
	Interpret and relay Exteroreceptive Proprioceptive Interoceptive sensation	III–IV	Body of dorsal horn Nucleus proprius (chief sensory nucleus)	Receive A delta and C fibers—pain, temperature; crude touch Second-order neurons Collaterals of proprioceptive
		V–VI	Neck and base of dorsal horn	Receive A delta and C fibers—second-order neurons Receive afferents from viscera Lamina VI receives some proprioceptive from crude touch
	Lateral horn Autonomic function	VII	Intermediolateral nucleus Dorsal nucleus (Clark's nucleus)	Preganglionic autonomic nuclei (GVE) Relay to cerebellum Spinocerebellar
Basal plate	Ventral (anterior) horn	VIII		Modulate motor
	Modulate and execute motor function	IX	Lower motor nuclei Lateral and medial	Initiate motor
		X	Commissure	Surround the central canal

Abbreviation: GVE, general visceral efferent.

Clinical Correlation Box 10.2: Lumbar Puncture

Lumbar puncture (LP) is the withdrawal of CSF from the lumbar cistern. This procedure is a valuable tool for the diagnosis of disorders such as **meningitis, Guillain-Barre syndrome, multiple sclerosis,** or cancers of the brain and spinal cord. Lumbar punctures can also be used to inject drugs into the CSF (▶ Fig. 10.30). The procedure is performed with the patients lying on their side with knees drawn to the chest. Flexion facilitates the insertion of the needle by spreading the **vertebral laminae** and **spinous processes.** A local anesthetic is injected into the lower back to numb the puncture site. A needle is inserted in the midline between the spinous processes of L3 and L4 (or L4 and L5) vertebrae. At these levels, there is no danger of damaging the spinal cord. As the needle passes between the spinous processes it will enter the **ligamentum flavum,** puncture the dura and arachnoid layers, and enter the lumbar cistern. A sample will be removed and sent for analysis. Although done frequently and generally recognized as safe, there are some risks associated with the procedure that include: post–lumbar puncture headache, back pain, and bleeding. In rare cases where the patient has increased cranial pressure due to a brain tumor or space-occupying lesion, it can result in brainstem herniation. A computed tomography (CT) or magnetic resonance imaging (MRI) can be done prior to the procedure to determine if there is a lesion present that may result in increased intracranial pressure.

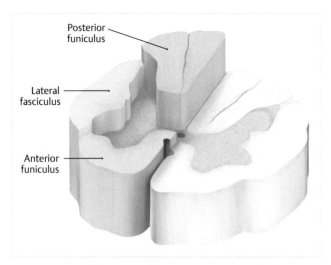

Fig. 10.21 The white matter of the spinal cord is divided into three funiculi. The funiculi are further subdivided into smaller tracts called fasciculi. (Reproduced with permission from Schuenke M, Schulte E, Schumacher U. THIEME Atlas of Anatomy Second Edition, Vol 3. © Thieme 2016. Illustrations by Markus Voll and Karl Wesker.)

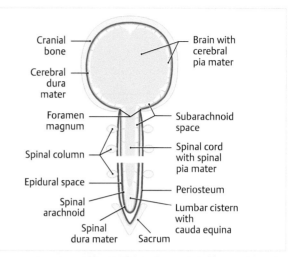

Fig. 10.22 The meningeal coverings of the brain are continuous with the spinal cord. The three layers are (superficial to deep): dura, arachnoid, and pia. (Reproduced with permission from Schuenke M, Schulte E, Schumacher U. THIEME Atlas of Anatomy Second Edition, Vol 3. © Thieme 2016. Illustrations by Markus Voll and Karl Wesker.)

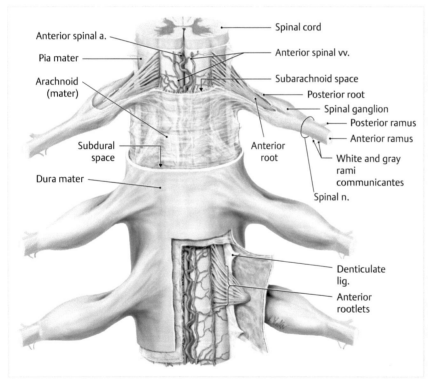

Fig. 10.23 Bilateral extensions of pia (denticulate ligaments) are present between the dorsal and ventral roots. (Reproduced with permission from Gilroy AM, MacPherson BR. Atlas of Anatomy. Third Edition. © Thieme 2016. Illustrations by Markus Voll and Karl Wesker.)

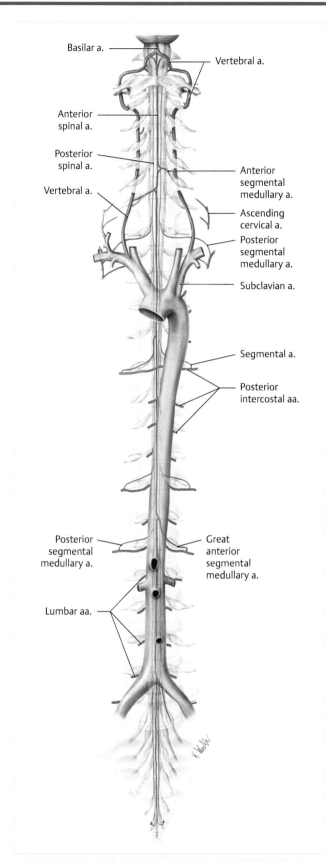

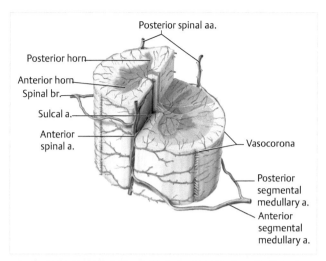

Fig. 10.25 Three longitudinal arteries arise from the vertebral artery. There is a single anterior spinal artery and paired posterior spinal arteries. Segmental arteries supply the radicular arteries of the spinal cord. The segmental arteries are costocervical, intercostal, and lumbar arteries. (Reproduced with permission from Schuenke M, Schulte E, Schumacher U. THIEME Atlas of Anatomy Third Edition, Vol 3. © Thieme 2020. Illustrations by Markus Voll and Karl Wesker.)

Clinical Correlation Box 10.3: Spinal Anesthesia

Spinal anesthesia involves inserting a needle into the **subarachnoid space** (Figs. 1.30 and 10.31). Other names include **spinal block** and **subarachnoid block**. Spinal anesthesia is an effective alternative to **general anesthesia** if the surgical site is located on the **lower extremities, perineum,** or **lower body wall**. The anesthetic is injected directly into the CSF and produces intense **sensory, motor,** and **sympathetic** blocks. Headache is the most common side effect and is likely the result of leakage of CSF through the puncture site. This common side effect is easily treated with the placement of a **blood patch** which involves an injection of autologous blood into the epidural space near the original puncture site. The resulting blood clot will prevent further meningeal leaks.

Clinical Correlation Box 10.4: Epidural Anesthesia

Epidural anesthesia involves the insertion of a needle and a catheter into the epidural space of the lower back. The anesthetic is injected via the catheter and produces pain relief. Epidural anesthesia has become a popular and effective form of anesthesia in childbirth. One of the more common effects of both epidural and spinal anesthesia is **hypotension** which is primarily due to sympathetic blocks from the anesthesia (Figs. 10.30 and 10.31).

Fig. 10.24 Arteries of the spinal cord. The unpaired anterior and paired posterior spinal arteries typically arise from the vertebral arteries. As they descend within the vertebral canal, the spinal arteries are reinforced by anterior and posterior segmental medullary arteries. (Reproduced with permission from Schuenke M, Schulte E, Schumacher U. THIEME Atlas of Anatomy Third Edition, Vol 3. © Thieme 2020. Illustrations by Markus Voll and Karl Wesker.)

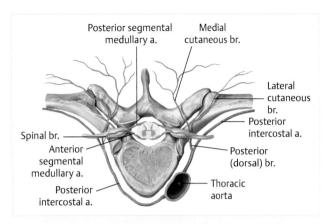

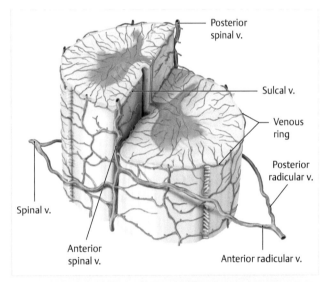

Fig. 10.26 Three longitudinal arteries arise from the vertebral artery. There is a single anterior spinal artery and paired posterior spinal arteries. Segmental arteries supply the radicular arteries of the spinal cord. The segmental arteries are costocervical, intercostal, and lumbar arteries. (Reproduced with permission from Schuenke M, Schulte E, Schumacher U. THIEME Atlas of Anatomy Third Edition, Vol 3. © Thieme 2020. Illustrations by Markus Voll and Karl Wesker.)

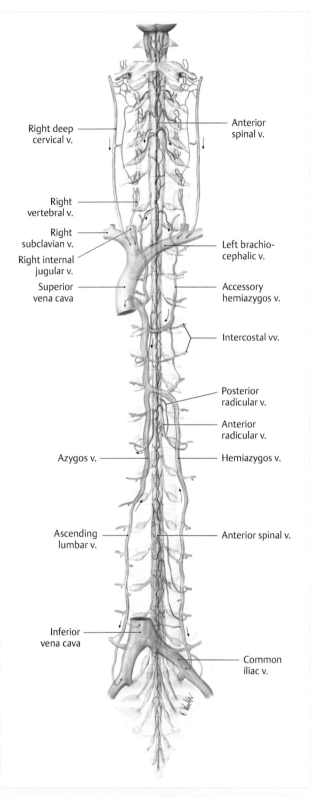

Fig. 10.28 Venous drainage closely follows the arterial supply. The interior of the spinal cord drains via venous plexuses into an anterior and a posterior spinal vein. The radicular and spinal veins connect the veins of the spinal cord with the internal vertebral venous plexus. (Reproduced with permission from Schuenke M, Schulte E, Schumacher U. THIEME Atlas of Anatomy Third Edition, Vol 3. © Thieme 2020. Illustrations by Markus Voll and Karl Wesker.)

Fig. 10.27 Venous drainage closely follows the arterial supply. The interior of the spinal cord drains via venous plexuses into an anterior and a posterior spinal vein. The radicular and spinal veins connect the veins of the spinal cord with the internal vertebral venous plexus. (Reproduced with permission from Schuenke M, Schulte E, Schumacher U. THIEME Atlas of Anatomy Third Edition, Vol 3. © Thieme 2020. Illustrations by Markus Voll and Karl Wesker.)

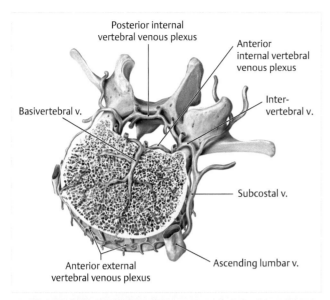

Fig. 10.29 Venous drainage closely follows the arterial supply. The interior of the spinal cord drains via venous plexuses into an anterior and a posterior spinal vein. The radicular and spinal veins connect the veins of the spinal cord with the internal vertebral venous plexus. (Reproduced with permission from Schuenke M, Schulte E, Schumacher U. THIEME Atlas of Anatomy Third Edition, Vol 3. © Thieme 2020. Illustrations by Markus Voll and Karl Wesker.)

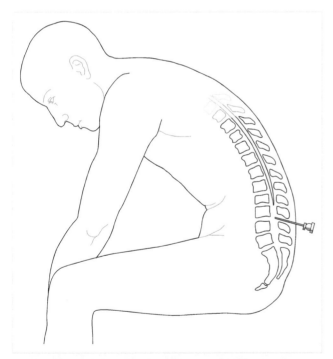

Fig. 10.30 Epidural anesthesia and lumbar anesthesia in preparation for a lumbar puncture. The patient bends far forward to separate the spinous processes of the lumbar spine. The spinal needle is usually introduced between the spinous processes of the L3 and L4 vertebrae. It is advanced through the skin and into the dural sac (lumbar cistern) to obtain a cerebrospinal fluid sample. This procedure has numerous applications, including the diagnosis of meningitis. (Reproduced with permission from Schuenke M, Schulte E, Schumacher U. THIEME Atlas of Anatomy Third Edition, Vol 3. © Thieme 2020. Illustrations by Markus Voll and Karl Wesker.)

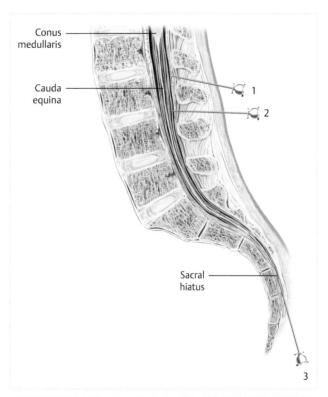

Fig. 10.31 For epidural anesthesia, a catheter is placed in the epidural space without penetrating the dural sac. Lumbar anesthesia is induced by injecting a local anesthetic solution into the dural sac. (Reproduced with permission from Schuenke M, Schulte E, Schumacher U. THIEME Atlas of Anatomy Third Edition, Vol 3. © Thieme 2020. Illustrations by Markus Voll and Karl Wesker.)

Questions and Answers

1. The spinal cord begins at which of the following vertebral levels?
   a) C2
   b) L2
   c) L5
   d) S2
   e) None of the above

Level 2: Moderate

Answer E: None of the above. The spinal cord begins at the level of the pyramidal decussation in the medulla. It also corresponds to the level of the foramen magnum, both of which are superior to the vertebral column so there is no vertebral level. (**A**) C2 is inferior to the beginning of the spinal cord; (**B**) L2 is the end of the spinal cord; (**C**) L5 is below the inferior limit of the spinal cord; (**D**) S2 marks the end of the dural sac, also below the inferior limit of the spinal cord.

2. Which vertebral level is appropriate for accessing CSF from the spinal cord for analysis in an adult?
   a) L1
   b) L4
   c) S2
   d) S5
   e) None of the above

Level 1: Easy

Answer B: Lumber punctures are typically done at the vertebral levels L4/L5. AT this point, you can assume that the needle will be in the lumbar cistern, thus avoiding damage to the spinal cord; **(A)** L1 would be at the level of the spinal cord; **(C)** S2 is approaching the lower limit of the dural sac and therefore the could result in missing the lumbar cistern and **(D)** S5. Would not permit access to the subarachnoid space of the spinal cord.

3. Which of the following structures contains the anterior spinal artery?
   a) Anterior lateral sulcus
   b) Anterior median fissure
   c) Anterior funiculus
   d) Anterior horn

Level 1: Easy

Answer B: Anterior median fissure. **(A)** Anterior lateral sulcus is the point where the ventral rootlets exit the spinal cord. **(C)** Anterior funiculus is the area between the anterior median fissure and the anterolateral sulcus. **(D)** Anterior horn is gray matter.

4. The lateral horn of the gray matter contains which of the following types of neurons?
   a) Motor
   b) Sensory
   c) Autonomic
   d) Interneurons

Level 2: Moderate

Answer C: Autonomic. **(A)** motor neurons are found in the ventral horn. **(B)** sensory neurons are located in the dorsal horn. **(D)** interneurons are located in the intermediate zone. The lateral horn is sometimes considered an extension of the intermediate zone however. The *BEST* answer would be **(C)** autonomic.

5. Which of the following Rexed laminae contains the substantia gelatinosa?
   a) I
   b) II
   c) V
   d) X

Level 1: Easy

Answer B: II. **(A)** RL I is known as the marginal zone. **(C)** RL V receives descending fibers. **(D)** RL X surrounds the central canal.

Unit III

Sensory Systems

11 Anatomical Receptors and Nerve Fibers

Learning Objectives

1. Categorize the somatosensory receptors.
2. Differentiate between phasic and tonic receptors.
3. Describe the sensory modalities associated with somatosensory system.
4. Describe the relationship between the receptive field and receptor density.
5. Differentiate between encapsulated and nonencapsulated receptors.
6. Compare the types of sensory receptors to rate of conduction.
7. Explain the basis for differences in conduction velocity.

11.1 Overview of Anatomical Receptors

The body's ability to adapt to its environment and maintain homeostasis depends on the transmission of sensory input by the peripheral nervous system (PNS). The detection of sensory input occurs through specialized receptive nerve endings, known as **sensory receptors,** found at the terminal ends of afferent (sensory) peripheral nerve fibers. Based on the type of stimulus to which the receptor responds, sensory receptors may be broadly classified as **nociceptors, thermoreceptors, chemoreceptors, photoreceptors,** and **mechanoreceptors**. Each type of receptor plays an integral role in collecting sensory input from the external and internal environment and transmitting the information to the central nervous system (CNS) for conscious and unconscious processing. Sensory receptors that detect sensations of pain, temperature, discriminative touch, pressure, visceral distention, and proprioception are known as **somatosensory receptors** and are broadly distributed within the skin, muscles, joint capsules, and viscera. In comparison, sensory receptors that detect special sensory modalities such as light, smell, taste, and sound are modified neurons or specialized epithelial receptor cells, which exhibit restricted expression to the olfactory epithelium, the retina of the eye, the taste buds of the oral cavity, and the vestibulocochlear apparatus.

This chapter introduces somatosensory stimuli and the types of cutaneous, muscle, joint, and visceral receptors that are responsible for detecting a perceived sensation. Transmission of different somatosensory stimuli follows distinct anatomical sensory pathways to the cerebral cortex and cerebellum. The **ascending somatosensory pathways** of the body and the head are described in Chapters 12 and 13, respectively. The **special sensory pathways** associated with vision, hearing, balance, smell, and taste are described in Chapter 15.

11.1.1 General Properties of Somatosensory Receptors

- The detection of somatic and visceral input from the environment occurs through specialized receptive nerve endings known as **somatosensory receptors,** which are formed by the peripheral axon of **primary (afferent) sensory neurons** (▶ Fig. 11.1).
- The sensory neuron cell body for all somatosensory and visceral receptors is a **pseudounipolar neuron** located in the **dorsal root sensory ganglia** or the **cranial sensory ganglia** associated with CNs V, VII, IX, and X.
- Pseudounipolar neurons possess only a single process that emerges from the ganglion cell body and branches into a **central process** and a **peripheral process.** A synapse does not occur in the sensory ganglion, and the information detected in the periphery passes to the CNS without interruption.

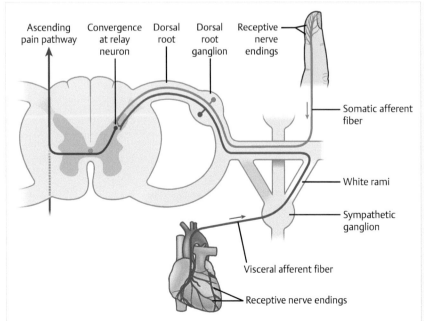

Fig. 11.1 Schematic demonstrating the location of cutaneous and visceral somatosensory receptors and the location of the corresponding primary afferent sensory cell body in the dorsal root ganglia. A simplified path of transmission from the periphery to the spinal cord is shown. Cutaneous receptors convey tactile (mechanosensory), nociceptive, and thermal input from the skin to the CNS. Visceral receptors convey mechanical stretch and nociceptive input from the wall of the viscera to the CNS. The neurons for both types of afferent receptors reside in the dorsal root ganglion (shown) or in some cranial sensory ganglia. Cutaneous sensation follows the spinal nerves while visceral sensory input travels initially from the viscera along autonomic pathways before entering the dorsal horn of the spinal cord. CNS, central nervous system.

Labels in figure: Ascending pain pathway; Convergence at relay neuron; Dorsal root; Dorsal root ganglion; Receptive nerve endings; Somatic afferent fiber; White rami; Sympathetic ganglion; Visceral afferent fiber; Receptive nerve endings

- The **central process** of a pseudounipolar sensory neuron transmits the impulse toward the CNS. The central process of the sensory neuron enters the dorsal root of the spinal nerve or the sensory root of the cranial nerve, and passes to the spinal cord or brainstem, respectively.
  - The **peripheral axonal process** transmits sensory input from the periphery toward the ganglion cell body. The peripheral axon of sensory neurons follows the spinal or cranial nerve to the periphery and terminates as a specific somatosensory receptor that responds to a specific type of stimulus.
- As discussed in Chapter 3, peripheral afferent nerve fibers may be classified based on axonal diameter and transmission speed as **Type I (Aα), Type II (Aβ), Type III (Aδ),** and **Type IV (C)** fibers.
  - Type I, II, and III fibers represent myelinated axons of varying diameters. Unmyelinated afferent fibers that exhibit the smallest axonal diameter comprise group IV. The difference in diameter, myelination, and conduction velocity impacts the speed of sensory transmission and central processing.
- Individual primary afferent sensory neurons respond to specific stimuli based on the properties of the receptor and the type of nerve fiber transmitting the sensory information.
  - Morphological variations, such as axonal diameter, the extent of myelination, receptor location, and the

presence of a connective tissue sheath surrounding the receptor nerve ending (encapsulation), contribute to the functional properties of different somatosensory receptors and serves as the basis for sensory receptor classification.

11.2 Sensory Reception and Transduction

- The process by which receptor stimulation leads to a perceived sensation is similar for all types of sensory receptors (▶ Fig. 11.2).
  - Receptor activation by a specific environmental stimulus initiates **sensory reception** and leads to the conversion of the environmental stimulus into an electrical signal (**generator potential**) through the process of **sensory transduction.** If the generator potential is large enough to exceed threshold an action potential will be generated.
  - Primary sensory afferent fibers of pseudounipolar neurons **transmit** an action potential along a specific somatosensory pathway to precise areas in somatosensory cortex of CNS for **processing** and **interpretation**.
  - The transmission and efficient processing of somatosensory input require that several attributes about receptor activation and transduction be encoded as part of the process. The stimulus components encoded at the time

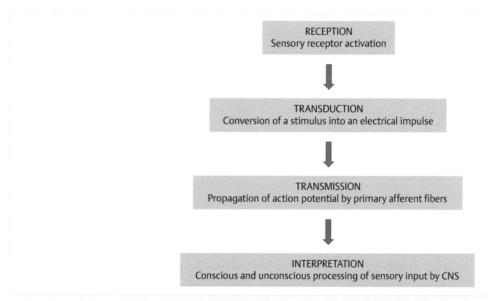

Fig. 11.2 Schematic flowchart demonstrating the four steps of somatosensory processing. Efficient sensory reception, transmission, and perception depend on encoding information about the type of stimulus, the location of the receptive field, the duration of the signal, and the relative intensity of the stimulus. Reception is the first step in the processing of sensation. Sensory input in the form of a stimulus leads to activation of receptors and the conversion of the stimulus into a receptor (generator) potential. A specific receptor will preferentially respond to a specific type of stimulus at a certain threshold. The higher the receptor threshold, the less sensitive the receptor will be to the stimulus. Receptor activation leads to a receptor potential that is graded continuously and dependent on the strength of the stimulus. When the receptor potential exceeds the receptor's signaling threshold, an action potential results. In neurons, the stimulus intensity is coded by the frequency of the action potential so that a stronger stimulus directly correlates with a faster firing rate. The specific area of tissue that responds to the stimulus, and produces a response, corresponds to the sensory neuron's receptive field. The size of the receptive field impacts the accuracy in the ability to precisely detect the location of the stimulus. A smaller receptive field leads to more accuracy in detecting the location of the stimulus. The duration of receptor activation corresponds to the length of time the receptor continues to fire with continued stimulation and depends on the adaptive characteristics of the receptor. Based on the type of stimulus, the transmission of the impulse follows specific sensory pathways to distinct areas in the contralateral (opposite side) cortex, where the stimulus is processed and consciously perceived as a specific sensation, or sensory modality. Sensations are mapped directly from receptors to specific regions of the cortex to give a direct association between the stimulus and the sensory neuron receptor. Perception is the individual's interpretation of the sensation and may vary among individuals due to modulatory effects and cognitive input.

of sensory reception and stimulus transduction includes the following:

– **Stimulus intensity threshold:** Refers to the minimal amount or intensity required by the receptor to generate an action potential. This threshold is referred to as an **adequate stimulus.**

– **Stimulus location or receptive field:** Refers to the specific location where the receptor of the sensory neuron elicits a response when stimulated. The ability to detect the precise location of a stimulus depends on the size of the receptive field.

– **Stimulus duration or adaption:** Refers to the rate at which the receptor adapts to the stimulus and the action potential dissipates.

– **Stimulus (sensory) modality:** Refers to the type of sensation produced in response to activation of a receptor and its sensory neuron by a specific type of stimulus.

• The following section describes each of the encoded sensory attributes in more detail.

11.2.1 Adequate Stimulus

• Each receptor preferentially responds to a specific stimulus and will elicit a response at a specific level or threshold.
• The **minimal stimulus** or **lowest threshold** necessary to generate an action potential is referred to as the **adequate stimulus** and represents the type of stimulus to which the receptor is most sensitive.
• The type of adequate stimulus for a receptor correlates with the sensory modality encoded by the receptor.
• Stimuli such as mechanical deformation, tissue damage, temperature changes, or chemical changes in the environment are adequate to elicit a sensory response and serve as the basis for receptor classification.
  ○ Types of somatosensory receptors include mechanoreceptors, nociceptors, thermoreceptors, and chemoreceptors.
• The **threshold** or intensity of the stimulus necessary to generate an action potential varies for different types of receptors and is known as the **receptor threshold**.
• Information concerning the stimulus intensity is conveyed to the CNS as the frequency of receptor firing and the number of receptors recruited. An intense stimulus causes a rapid firing rate of the receptor, and in some cases, may also initiate action potentials in several adjacent receptors.
• Receptor threshold and intensity serve as a mechanism for further classification. Low threshold (high sensitivity) receptors require only a small or weak stimulus, whereas high threshold (low sensitivity) receptors need intense stimuli to respond.
  ○ Many of the receptors that respond to innocuous tactile input are low threshold receptors, while receptors that only respond to strong or noxious stimuli typically correspond to high threshold receptors.

11.2.2 Receptive Fields

• The ability to discriminate between different points of receptor stimulation is an essential attribute of sensory feedback that is influenced by the location of the receptor, the receptor density of the area, and the size of the receptive field (▶ Fig. 11.3).

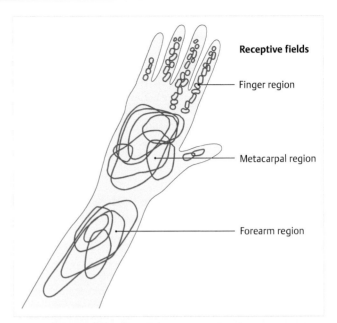

Receptive fields

Finger region

Metacarpal region

Forearm region

Fig. 11.3 Schematic diagram illustrating the difference in the receptive field size supplied by different cortical modules in the upper limb of a primate. Individual receptive fields are depicted by individual red circles with the receptive field size corresponding to the size of the circle. Each receptive field is associated with one cortical module. The receptive field of a sensory neuron represents the area of the body that, when stimulated, leads to receptor activation, and produces a characteristic sensation. Information from sensory receptors in a specific receptive field follows a three-neuron relay chain to terminate in specific regions of the somatosensory cortex for processing. Based on the type of sensory input and location of the receptive field, specific cortical neurons that are arranged in functional columns (cortical modules) receive the information. Due to the topographical organization of the cortex, receptive fields in proximity of the body terminate in adjoining areas of the cortex. The size of the receptive field correlates with the functional requirements of specific regions of the body. Small receptive fields correspond to areas in the body, such as the fingertips, which require fine tactile discrimination and high resolution. One cortical module receives input from a small receptive field. Small receptive fields provide greater acuity and a more localized response. In areas that do not require high specificity, one cortical module supplies a large receptive field. Larger receptive fields such as those depicted in the palm (metacarpal) and forearm region allow for the detection of stimuli over a wider area, but the ability to precisely localize the stimulus is diminished. Because one skin area may be innervated by several neurons, many of the receptive fields overlap. (Reproduced with permission from Schuenke M, Schulte E, Schumacher U. THIEME Atlas of Anatomy Second Edition, Vol 3. © Thieme 2016. Illustrations by Markus Voll and Karl Wesker.)

○ The **receptive field** of a sensory neuron represents the area of tissue that, when stimulated, leads to receptor activation in the region and elicits a characteristic sensation. Therefore, the receptive field provides information about the location of the stimulus and the sensory modality.
○ The neurons associated with the receptors of a specific receptive field are associated with a specific sensory modality and transmit sensory input along particular ascending sensory pathways to terminate in specific regions in somatosensory cortex.
○ The size of the receptive field correlates with the receptor density, the level of receptor sensitivity, and the ability to

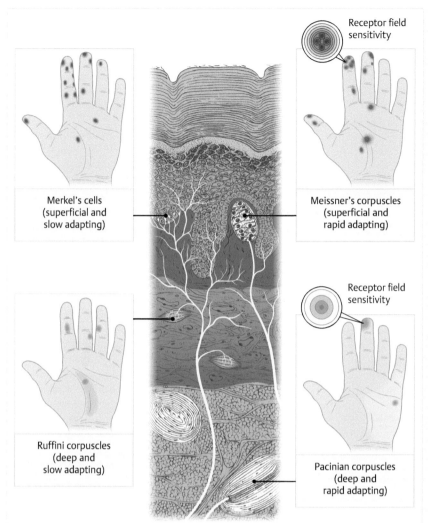

Receptor field
sensitivity

Merkel's cells
(superficial and
slow adapting)

Meissner's corpuscles
(superficial and
rapid adapting)

Receptor field
sensitivity

Ruffini corpuscles
(deep and
slow adapting)

Pacinian corpuscles
(deep and
rapid adapting)

Fig. 11.4 Schematic diagram of cutaneous tactile receptor density, location, and corresponding receptive field size in the skin of the fingertips. Touch receptors vary in density between different areas of the body and within different tissue layers. The four major types of cutaneous (tactile) mechanoreceptors, which include the Merkel's cell, Meissner's corpuscle, Ruffini's corpuscle, and Pacinian corpuscle, are differentially distributed between the superficial and deep layers of the skin. The superficially located Merkel's cell and Meissner's corpuscle exhibit higher receptor density and smaller receptive fields in the fingertips when compared to the Pacinian and Ruffini's corpuscles. The Pacinian and Ruffini's corpuscles also reside in the fingertip but are found in the deep layers of the dermis and hypodermis. These receptors exhibit wider receptive fields and less density. The ability to accurately discern the precise location of a stimulus correlates with the receptor density, receptive field size, as well as the location and function of the receptor. For regions such as the fingertips, which require high resolution and tactile discrimination, the receptive fields are smaller and contain a higher number of superficial receptors that function in fine discriminative touch. The receptors found in deeper regions convey different mechanosensory inputs such as stretch, vibration, and transient pressure, and therefore, exhibit slightly larger receptive fields with fewer receptors scattered throughout the receptive field. The localization of the sensation is less precise and more diffuse.

precisely localize the response. A small receptive field allows more precise localization of stimulus.

○ The location of the receptor correlates with receptor field size and receptor density.

  – Cutaneous receptors that are superficially located exhibit a higher distribution density within a specific area and a more localized or discriminative sensation.

  – In comparison, receptors found in deeper tissue regions such as muscle tissue and joints are widely dispersed, exhibit a broader receptive field, and a less localized sensation (▶ Fig. 11.4).

○ The size of the receptive field and the receptor density vary between different regions of the body and reflect the functional requirements of the region.

○ Areas of the body which exhibit an increase in receptor density and small receptive fields include the face, lips, tongue, oral mucosa, fingertips, and hands. Functionally these areas perform numerous tasks that require a high level of discriminative tactile and proprioceptive input.

11.2.3 Sensory Adaptation

• Most receptors may adjust to prolonged stimulation by decreasing the rate at which it generates an action potential.

The process by which a receptor becomes less sensitive to a continued stimulus is known as **sensory adaptation** and plays an important role in the ability of the sensory system to monitor, adjust, and react to continual changes in the environment.

○ The rate of receptor adaption reflects the duration of how long the receptor encodes the stimulus. This property varies between different types of receptors and allows receptors to be classified as **phasic** or **tonic receptors. Rapid adapting receptors**, or **phasic receptors**, respond quickly to stimuli; however, the sensation rapidly dissipates as the ability of the receptor to generate an action potential diminishes.

  – **Rapidly adapting receptors** detect **moving** or **vibrating stimuli** and provide information about **changes** in the **stimuli intensity**. Rapidly adapting receptors include types of tactile and proprioceptive mechanoreceptors found in skin, muscles, and joints. Several receptors involved in detecting visceral sensation also function as phasic or rapidly adapting receptors.

○ **Slowly adapting** or **tonic receptors** provide input about the continued presence and intensity of the stimulus by sustaining an action potential for the duration of the stimulus.

- **Slow adapting receptors** respond to **static stimuli**, such as constant pressure, and include types of tactile mechanoreceptors, some proprioceptive mechanoreceptors, as well as some nociceptors and visceral receptors.
  - Most tissues, including those in the oral cavity, contain both rapid and slow adapting receptors. The presence of both receptor types alters the rate at which the tissue adapts and responds to sensory input and is an important mechanism to detect changes in the environment and prevent sensory overload.

11.3 Stimulus (Sensory) Modalities

- In the body and head, the cortical processing of sensory input arising from receptors in the skin, muscle, connective tissue, joints, and viscera leads to the perception of somatic sensations or sensory modalities.
- The modalities of somatic sensations include **touch, proprioception, pain**, and **temperature**. Each modality represents a characteristic sensation of a specific stimuli and correlates with a specific type of receptor, its associated afferent fiber, and primary afferent neuron (▶ Table 11.1).
- Sensory modalities may be separated into **submodalities** which further describes the quality of the perceived sensation. Submodalities of touch, proprioception, thermal sensations, and pain are described below and correspond to the stimulus that preferentially activates the receptor.
- **Touch or tactile sensation** refers to the awareness and ability to localize the point of mechanical stimulation. Submodalities of tactile sensations include **crude (light) touch, fine discriminative touch, pressure, vibration**, and **stretch**.
- Activation of tactile receptors occurs through the mechanical displacement of the receptor. The different submodalities of tactile sensation reflect different levels of distortion of the skin and correlate with the stimulation of different types of tactile receptors.
  - **Crude and discriminative touch**: Tactile responses may be described as crude and nondiscriminative touch or as fine, discriminative touch. This difference correlates with the type of receptor and sensory neuron, the receptor location, density, and receptive field size.
    - **Crude touch** receptors only convey the sense of touch and not the location of the stimulus. Crude touch receptors are found throughout the body, including the cornea, dental pulp, mucosa, and viscera.
    - In comparison, **fine, discriminative tactile receptors** enable the ability to distinguish the location of an

applied stimulus to the skin by one or two points. This type of fine, discriminative touch is also known as **two-point discrimination**. The minimal distance that may be detected separately varies between different parts of the body. Areas of the body that functionally require precise tactile discrimination exhibit high receptor density, smaller receptive fields, and smaller distances between two points.
    - **Fine, discriminative tactile receptors** also function to discern the shape, size, and texture of an object by means of touch in the absence of visual input through a process known as **stereognosis.** The ability to perform stereognosis depends on both intact tactile sensory pathways and higher cortical input involving memory of the object.
    - Disruption in discriminative sensory feedback in the regions of the fingertips, oral cavity, hands, and tongue leads to difficulties in coordinating motor responses and an inability to recognize the size, shape, and texture of an object without visual input (**astereognosis**).
  - **Vibration:** Vibratory sense refers to the tactile sensation of a mechanical vibratory movement occurring in the skin, viscera, muscle, joints, or the periosteum of bone. Specific tactile receptors respond to either low- or high-frequency vibrations generated by mechanical stimulation. Low-frequency vibrations produce the sensation of flutter, stroking, or movement, while high-frequency vibrations create the sense of vibration and deep pressure.
  - **Pressure:** Tactile pressure, or deep touch sensations, refers to the perception of a maintained distortion, such as an indentation, or a compressive force applied to the skin, muscle, or viscera. The sensations of deep touch and vibration are important in mediating stability, balance, and bodily movements associated with proprioception.
- **Proprioception** refers to the awareness of **movement** and **position** of the body, limbs, and joints, along with the sensation of **muscle force** and **tension**. The sense of position and movement arises from the mechanical displacement of specific receptors found in tendons, joints, capsules, and muscles.
- **Thermal sensations** range from **hot to warm**, or **cool to cold.** The ability to detect temperature changes is important for homeostatic thermoregulation and as a protective response to excessive temperatures that may cause tissue damage. Each temperature range has a threshold that will trigger the activation of a receptor known as a thermoreceptor.
- **Pain** is a subjective sensation often associated with tissue injury that may involve both physical and emotional discomfort or agony. Different types of receptors, known as nociceptors, respond to noxious stimuli and generate two

Table 11.1 Overview of receptor type, stimulus, and modality

Receptor Type	Adequate Stimulus	Sensory Modality (sensation detected)
Mechanoreceptors	Mechanical displacement Stretch/tissue deformation	Touch (tactile) and conscious proprioception
Thermoreceptors	Temperature change relative to environment/body	Thermal sensations (warm, cool, hot cold)
Nociceptors	Noxious stimuli/Tissue damage	Pain
Chemoreceptors	Chemicals (inflammatory mediators)	Conscious pain or itch*

Note: *Some chemical and proprioceptive sensations are not consciously perceived.

types of nociceptive pain sensations. Submodalities of nociceptive pain include **fast pain** and **slow pain**.

○ **Fast pain**, also known as **first onset (first)** pain, is associated with a well-localized, sharp, pricking, stinging, or stabbing sensation that is of short duration. This type of pain often occurs from mechanical stimuli such as cutting, pinching, or pinpricks, but may also be associated with insect bites, or thermal stimuli such as intense heat. First pain is transmitted rapidly through lightly myelinated nerve fibers to the cortex for conscious processing.

○ **Slow pain,** or **second pain**, is a dull, burning, or aching sensation that is diffuse, poorly localized, and of longer duration. Burning pain is generally caused by inflammation, while aching pain arises from the viscera, or deep subcutaneous structures such as bone, muscles, joints, and connective tissue. Mechanical, thermal, and chemical stimuli associated with swelling, tearing, rupture, ischemia, or inflammation may elicit slow pain. The transmission of second pain occurs slowly through small,

unmyelinated nerve fibers. The fibers follow specific tracts that typically terminate diffusely in regions other than the somatosensory cortex.

11.4 Somatosensory Receptor Classification

Somatosensory receptors may be classified based on function, structure, and location.

11.4.1 Functional Classification

- The type of adequate stimuli to which a receptor responds and elicits a characteristic sensation serves as the basis for receptor classification. Somatosensory receptors may be classified into four functional types: **mechanoreceptors, thermoreceptors, nociceptors,** and **chemoreceptors** (see ▶ Table 11.2).

Table 11.2 Functional receptor classification and sensory modality

Receptor Class	Stimulus	Sensory Modality	Perceived Sensation Submodality
Mechanoreceptor Cutaneous tactile receptors	Mechanical deformation of tissue	Tactile	Crude touch
			Discriminative touch Flutter
			Vibration
			Pressure
			Stretch
Mechanoreceptor Proprioceptive	Mechanical deformation of tissue • Static force maintains position of limb against gravity	Position Pressure	Muscle tension Muscle stretch Joint pressure
Mechanoreceptor Kinesthetic	• Dynamic force applied to muscle, tendon, or joint indicates movement	Stretch Tension	Joint movement Limb position
Mechanoreceptive Visceral receptor	Mechanical deformation of tissue or organ	Stretch	Conscious perception Organ distention/stretch Fullness Pressure
Mechanoreceptor Baroreceptor Visceral receptor	Decrease or increase in arterial blood pressure	Unconscious Visceral reflex	Not consciously perceived
Chemoreceptors Visceral receptor	Decrease O_2 Increase pCO_2 Decrease in pH	Unconscious Visceral reflex	Not consciously perceived
Thermoreceptors	Thermal changes in environment relative to body temperature	Temperature change	Warm/Hot Cool/Cold
Nociceptor • Mechanosensitivenociceptors (high threshold/intense stimuli)	Noxious/intense stimuli associated with mechanical tissue damage Primary trigger: Intense (mechanical)	Perceived as pain	Fast, first pain Sharp (prick/cut)
• Thermosensitive nociceptors (high threshold/extreme temperature)	• Primary trigger: Intense temperatures (above 52 °C or below 15 °C)	Pain	Fast, first pain Sharp (prick/cut)
• Chemical nociceptors	• Primary trigger: Chemical changes due to tissue damage, insect bites, bee stings • Inflammation causing the release of proinflammatory mediators (bradykinin, potassium, serotonin, histamine, prostaglandins)	Pain	Fast, first pain Sharp (prick/cut) Slow, second pain Dull (burn/ache)
• Polymodal nociceptors	• Multiple stimuli (thermal, mechanical, and chemical)	Pain	Slow, second pain Dull (burn/ache)
• Mechano insensitive (silent) (high threshold, normally resistant to mechanical stimuli)	• Activated by inflammation and tissue injury—inflammatory mediators lower threshold stimulus and receptor becomes responsive to mechanical stimuli	Pain	Fast, first pain Sharp (prick/cut) Slow, second pain Dull (burn/ache)

- **Mechanoreceptors**: Respond to mechanical deformation of the skin, muscles, tendons, joint capsules, and viscera. Myelinated and unmyelinated afferent nerve fibers of mechanoreceptors terminate to form three classes of mechanoreceptors: **tactile mechanoreceptors**, **visceral mechanoreceptors**, and **proprioceptors.**
  - A specialized type of visceral mechanoreceptor, known as a **baroreceptor**, monitors arterial blood pressure and acts as pressure receptor. Baroreceptors exhibit a more restricted expression to the cardiovascular system and reside in the wall of the aorta and carotid artery.
  - The nerve fibers associated with the detection of innocuous mechanical stimuli from skin, muscle, tendons, and joints are large diameter, heavily myelinated axons known as large diameter, heavily myelinated axons of **Type Ia (Aα) fibers** and **Type II (Aβ) fibers.** Both types of axons rapidly transmit mechanoreceptive input from several cutaneous mechanoreceptors and proprioceptors to the CNS for processing.
  - Mechanoreceptive signals associated with light (crude) touch and pressure detected from the skin, peritoneum (serosa), mucosa, blood vessels, and organs are conveyed by smaller, lightly myelinated **Type III** (Aδ) and unmyelinated **Type IV** (C) fibers.
- **Thermoreceptors** respond to changes in temperature occurring at the receptive nerve endings found throughout the body. Thermoreceptors, which are important in the homeostatic maintenance of our internal body temperature, are sensitive to warm, hot, cool, and cold stimuli. Thermoreceptors rapidly adapt to temperature changes that vary from the normal skin temperature of 34–36 °C (93–98 °F). Thermal changes within a certain range may be classified as innocuous, while temperature changes above or below those levels are considered noxious stimuli.
  - **Warm (innocuous) receptors** respond to temperatures between 25 °C (77 °F) and 45 °C (113 °F) with maximal stimulation occurring 10 °C above normal skin temperatures. Temperatures above 45 °C (113 °F) are often perceived as pain (heat) due to the activation of a type of noxious high threshold (hot) receptors known as a thermo-nociceptor.
  - **Cold (innocuous) receptors** are more numerous than heat receptors and normally respond to decreases in temperature below the normal skin temperature range of 34 to 36 °C (93–98 °F). Maximal firing occurs about 10 °C below normal skin temperature of 25 °C (77 °F), while skin temperatures below 15 °C (59 °F) stimulate noxious cold receptors. When these thermo-nociceptors become activated, the sensation is one of pain.
  - Thermoreceptors are the free nerve endings of lightly myelinated **Type III, (Aδ),** or **unmyelinated, Type IV (C fibers)** nerve fibers. Typically, the lightly myelinated Aδ fibers convey cool temperature sensations and exhibit faster conduction velocities, whereas unmyelinated C fibers transmit warm sensations at slower conduction speeds. As a result, the time for the body to respond is faster for a cold stimulus and slower for a warm stimulus.
- **Chemoreceptors** associated with the somatosensory system rapidly respond to chemicals released in response to changes in pH, oxygen, and carbon dioxide levels and function as part of unconscious visceral reflex pathways. Chemical stimuli associated with inflammatory mediators produced in response to inflammation from tissue damage are detected by polymodal nociceptors and are often perceived as dull, burning pain.
- **Nociceptors** respond to noxious stimuli characterized as extreme pressure, temperature, and chemical irritants that may cause tissue damage, inflammation, or decreased blood flow (**ischemia**). Activation of nociceptors occurs in response to intense, high threshold stimuli as part of a protective response against further tissue damage and nociceptors are ubiquitously expressed in most tissue, including the skin, connective tissue, joint capsules, muscles, tendons, viscera and serosa, and the periosteum of the bone.
- Nociceptors represent the unencapsulated free nerve ending of either lightly myelinated (**Type III, Aδ**) fibers or unmyelinated axons (**Type IV, C fibers).** Noxious stimuli transmitted by lightly myelinated Aδ fibers pass rapidly to the CNS and generate a fast-onset, localized, sharp pain sensation. Unmyelinated C fibers conduct noxious stimuli slowly toward the CNS, resulting in the sensation of slow, burning, or aching pain.
- Nociceptors are classified based on their sensitivity into noxious mechanical, thermal, and/or chemical stimuli caused by tissue damage and inflammation. There are four classes of nociceptive receptors.
  - **Mechano sensitive nociceptors** represent the receptive nerve endings of nociceptive-specific neurons that respond to extreme pressure, such as cutting or pinching. Lightly myelinated **Type III Aδ** fibers transmit the information from mechano-sensitive nociceptive nerve endings to the CNS for processing.
  - **Thermo sensitive nociceptors** represent high threshold thermal receptors that respond preferentially to intense heat and cold. **Lightly myelinated Type III Aδ** and **unmyelinated Type IV C fibers** convey intense heat (above 45 °C) and intense cold (below 15 °C) to the CNS.
  - **Polymodal nociceptors** respond to noxious chemical, mechanical, or intense thermal stimuli. The transmission of nociceptive input from polymodal nociceptors occurs through **unmyelinated Type IV C fibers** and is perceived as diffuse, dull pain. Polymodal C fibers comprise approximately 70% of all fibers carrying nociceptive input.
  - **Mechano insensitive nociceptors,** also known as **silent nociceptors,** represent the last class of nociceptive nerve endings. **Mechano insensitive receptors** are high threshold receptors that are usually "silent" or unresponsive to mechanical and thermal stimulation. However, in response to tissue inflammation, the **mechano insensitive** nociceptors become sensitized to the noxious chemical mediators produced during the inflammatory response. Sensitization lowers the activation threshold of the receptor causing it to become stimulated at a lower threshold.

11.4.2 Structural Receptor Classification

- The structural and physiological characteristics of receptors, along with the location of the receptors within the tissue, contribute to receptor specificity.

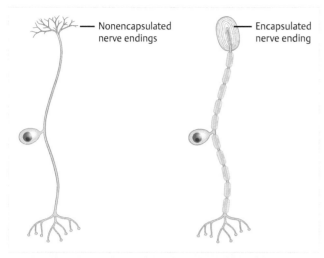

Fig. 11.5 Structural classification of receptors: nonencapsulated and encapsulated receptors. Nonencapsulated receptors transmit nociceptive, thermal, and some mechanosensory input from the skin, viscera, and joints. Encapsulated receptors transmit mechanosensory, proprioceptive, and some thermal input from skin, muscle, joints, and viscera. Nonencapsulated receptors are known as free nerve endings and are not usually named. One exception is the nonencapsulated receptors found in the skin which include Merkel's cell and hair follicle receptors. In comparison, encapsulated receptors are named and include Meissner, Ruffini, Pacinian, Krause end bulbs, muscle spindles, and Golgi tendon organs. Each receptor is associated with the detection of a specific sensory modality and found within specific regions of the tissue.

- Receptors are structurally classified as **encapsulated** or **nonencapsulated** based on the presence or absence of a connective sheath surrounding the receptor nerve ending (▶ Fig. 11.5).
  - Myelinated nerve fibers that terminate as receptors on specific types of tissue, such as collagen fibers or skeletal muscle, are enveloped in a connective tissue capsule, forming an **encapsulated sensory receptor complex**.
    - The connective tissue which encapsulates the nerve ending serves to change the properties of the receptor by filtering and modifying the mechanical stimuli.
    - **Encapsulated nerve endings** are **mechanoreceptors** that detect cutaneous sensations such as discriminative touch, stretch, and vibration, as well as proprioceptive input from muscles and joints.
  - Myelinated and unmyelinated peripheral axons may shed their connective tissue coverings at the receptor nerve ending to terminate as **nonencapsulated receptors** or **free nerve endings**.
    - **Nonencapsulated nerve endings** are broadly distributed throughout the body and represent the most abundant type of sensory nerve ending. Free nerve endings include nociceptors and thermoreceptors that detect sensations of crude touch, tickle, temperature, pain, and itching, as well as two types of cutaneous tactile mechanoreceptors involved in detecting fine, discriminative touch. Nociceptive and thermoreceptor nerve endings convey information through Type III (Aδ) and Type IV C fibers, whereas the free endings associated with cutaneous mechanoreceptors transmit input via Type II Aβ fibers.

11.4.3 Receptor Classification Based on Anatomical Location

Somatosensory receptors found in the skin, muscles, joints, and viscera are responsible for initiating perceived sensations and may be classified based on their anatomical location and source of sensory input as **exteroceptors, proprioceptors**, and **interoceptors.**

- Cutaneous receptors found in the skin may be classified as **exteroceptors** which provide information to the CNS about the external environment.
  - Exteroceptors may be further classified into **protopathic** receptors carrying pain, temperature, and crude touch, and **epicritic** receptors that transmit discriminative tactile sensations.
- **Proprioceptive receptors** associated with muscles, tendons, and ligaments represent encapsulated mechanoreceptors that relay information about body position, movement, and changes in equilibrium. Proprioceptive input is consciously and unconsciously processed in the CNS.
- **Interoceptors** are **visceral receptors** found in viscera and blood vessel walls that monitor the body's internal state and function in unconscious visceral reflexes.

11.4.4 Types of Exteroceptors: Cutaneous Tactile Mechanoreceptors (▶ Table 11.3 and ▶ Table 11.4)

- The skin contains five types of **low threshold, tactile mechanoreceptors** (LTMs) that detect discriminative touch, pressure, vibrations, and stretch. Transmission of epicritic tactile input from the periphery occurs through myelinated Type II Aβ fibers. The fibers carrying fine, discriminative touch and conscious proprioception follow the same pathway to the somatosensory cortex.
- **Tactile mechanoreceptors** are differentially distributed between **glabrous** (hairless) and hairy skin, and may reside superficially in the epidermis and papillary layer of the dermis, or may be located deep within the dermis and subcutaneous connective tissue (▶ Fig. 11.6 and ▶ Fig. 11.7).
- **Superficial cutaneous mechanoreceptors** respond to tactile stimulation associated with discriminative touch and include **Meissner's corpuscles** and **Merkel's cells (discs).**
  - **Merkel's cells (discs)** represent unique, specialized sensory epithelial receptor cells located in the basal layer of the epidermis in both hairy and glabrous skin. Each Merkel's disc synapses with myelinated afferent nerve fibers forming a receptor complex known as a **Merkel neurite complex.**
    - The **Merkel complex** is a **nonencapsulated, low-threshold mechanoreceptor** that slowly adapts to sustained light (discriminative) touch. Merkel's discs facilitate the ability to discern shape, texture, and location of the stimuli (▶ Fig. 11.8).
  - **Meissner's corpuscle** represents an **encapsulated, low-threshold mechanoreceptor** located in the superficial dermal papillae of glabrous skin. Regions such as fingertips, palms, feet, and lips exhibit a high density and

Table 11.3 Summary of encapsulated cutaneous tactile mechanoreceptors

Structural Class: Encapsulated Cutaneous Mechanoreceptors						
Location	Type of Receptors	Primary Afferent Fibers	Stimulus	Sensory Modality	Receptive Field	Adaptation
Superficial Glabrous skin Dermal papillae	**Low threshold Meissner's corpuscle**	Type II (Aβ) fibers	Mechanical Light touch, pressure/ low frequency vibration	Touch: Fine, discriminative (two-point discrimination) flutter	Small	Rapid (phasic)
Deep All skin Reticular dermis Hypodermis Joint capsule Organs	**Low threshold Pacinian corpuscle**	Type II (Aβ) fibers	Mechanical deformation High-frequency vibration	Touch: Vibration, deep pressure	Large	Rapid (phasic)
Deep subcutaneus All skin Reticular dermis Hypodermis Joint capsule Tendons	**Low threshold Ruffini's corpuscle**	Type II (Aβ) fibers	Mechanical deformation stretch	Touch: stretch	Large	Slow (tonic)

Table 11.4 Summary of nonencapsulated cutaneous sensory receptors

Structural Class: Nonencapsulated (Free Nerve Endings) Cutaneous Nociceptors and Thermoreceptors						
Location	Type of Receptors	Primary Afferent Fibers	Stimulus	Sensory Modality	Receptive Field	Adaptation
Superficial; all skin epidermis; dermis	**Low threshold thermoreceptors Warm and cool receptors**	Type III Aδ fibers Type IV (C fibers)	Thermal (innocuous) Minor increases or decreases from normal skin (34–36 °C)	Cool Warm	Variable	Both phasic and tonic
Superficial; all skin epidermis; dermis	**High threshold Thermosensitive nociceptors Hot and cold receptors**	Type III Aδ fibers Type IV (C fibers)	Thermal extreme Below 15 °C Above 45 °C	Cold Hot	Small	Both phasic and tonic
Superficial; all skin epidermis; dermis, joint capsules, muscles	**High threshold Mechanosensitive Nociceptor**	Type III Aδ fibers	(C fibers) Mechanical /tissue damage	Sharp (fast/first) pain	Variable	Rapid
	Polymodal nociceptor (C fiber)	Type IV C fibers	Mechanical; chemical, thermal	Dull/ache/burning (slow/second) pain	Large	Slow (tonic)
Superficial; all skin; dermis joint capsules, ligaments, muscles	**High-threshold mechano-insensitive (silent) nociceptors**	Type IV (C fibers) predominate type	Inflammatory chemical mediators from tissue damage alters stimulus threshold	Diffuse pressure or pain	Large	Slow (tonic)
Structural Class: Nonencapsulated (Free Nerve Endings) Cutaneous Mechanoreceptors						
Location	Type of Receptors	Primary Afferent Fibers	Stimulus	Sensory Modality	Receptive Field	Adaptation
Superficial; all skin; dermis; joint capsules, ligaments, muscles	**Low threshold mechanosensitive**	Type III Aδ fibers Type IV (C fibers)	Mechanical pinch, squeeze pressure	Crude touch; tickle, itch	Large	Slow (tonic)
Superficial; all skin, epidermis	**Low threshold mechanoreceptor Merkel complex—specialized epithelial cells**	Type II (Aβ) fibers	Mechanical, light touch, pressure	Fine, discriminative touch, shape, texture	Small	Slow (tonic)
Deep Reticular dermis Hypodermis Hairy skin	**Low threshold mechanoreceptor Hair follicle receptor**	Type II (Aβ) fibers (primary) Type III Aδ fibers (some)	Mechanical touch; bending of hair	Movement of follicle	Small	Rapid (phasic)

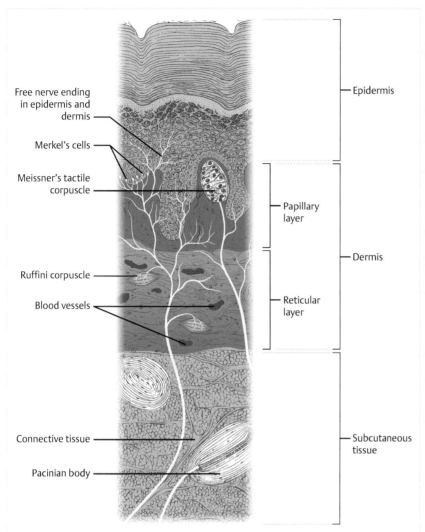

Free nerve ending in epidermis and dermis

Merkel's cells

Meissner's tactile corpuscle

Ruffini corpuscle

Blood vessels

Connective tissue

Pacinian body

Epidermis

Papillary layer

Dermis

Reticular layer

Subcutaneous tissue

Fig. 11.6 Schematic drawing of thick (glabrous) skin from palms and soles illustrating the location of cutaneous tactile mechanoreceptors within the dermis and hypodermis of the connective tissue. Tactile receptors in the superficial layer include free nerve endings, Merkel's disc, a slow-adapting, nonencapsulated mechanoreceptor found in the basal layer of the epidermis, and Meissner's corpuscle, a fast-adapting, encapsulated mechanoreceptor found in the dermal papilla. Merkel's cells and Meissner's corpuscle respond to light discriminative touch. Ruffini's receptor, a slow-adapting, encapsulated receptor, is located in the deeper reticular layer of the dermis. Pacinian receptors are fast-adapting, encapsulated receptors located deep in the connective tissue at the dermal–hypodermal junction. Ruffini's receptor detects heat and stretch in collagenous structures while the Pacinian detects transient deep pressure and high-frequency vibrations. Note the distribution of superficial and deep receptors is of functional importance and allows receptors to work in concert to provide an integrated and refined level of sensation from the outside world.

overlapping pattern of these receptors. Meissner's corpuscles **rapidly adapt** to light tactile stimulation, low-frequency vibration, and function in discriminative touch for glabrous skin (▶ Fig. 11.9).
- Meissner's corpuscle is the only encapsulated, superficial nerve ending that is primarily restricted to areas of glabrous (hairless) skin, such as the palms, soles of feet, and lips.
• **Deep cutaneous tactile receptors** found in the deep dermal and subcutaneous tissue include **follicular hair receptors, Ruffini's end organs (corpuscles),** and **Pacinian corpuscles.** In comparison to Merkel's discs and Meissner's corpuscles, which are tactile receptors confined to only the superficial layers of skin and oral mucosa, the Pacinian corpuscles and Ruffini's corpuscles are found in other regions of the body including viscera and joint capsules.
  ○ **Follicular hair receptors** associated with hairy skin are **nonencapsulated mechanoreceptors** formed by lightly myelinated nerve fibers wrapping around the base of the hair follicle. Follicular receptors **rapidly adapt** in response to **deformations** in the hair follicle and provide discriminative touch for hairy skin.
  ○ **Ruffini's end organs (corpuscles)** are found in the deep connective tissue layers of skin as well as the connective

tissue of ligaments and joint capsules. Depending on their location, the Ruffini's corpuscles may function as cutaneous exteroceptors or proprioceptive receptors.
  – The Ruffini's corpuscles represent **encapsulated, low-threshold mechanoreceptors** that adapt slowly in response to **static stretching** and displacement of the collagen fibers found in the connective tissue.
  – Ruffini's corpuscles serve as the principal receptor in the periodontal ligament surrounding the tooth and provide critical feedback about occlusal bite force and movement of the tooth.
  ○ **Pacinian corpuscles** are large, **encapsulated, low-threshold mechanoreceptors** located in the subcutaneous connective tissue of the skin, periosteum of bone, and some viscera. Pacinian corpuscles rapidly adapt in response to high-frequency vibrations and produce the sensation of deep pressure and vibratory movements.
  ○ **Paciniform corpuscles** reside in joint capsules throughout the body and are structurally similar to the Pacinian corpuscle. Paciniform corpuscles also **rapidly adapt** to deep pressure and vibratory movements associated with joint movement (▶ Fig. 11.10).
• In addition to encapsulated and nonencapsulated mechanoreceptors, the skin also contains numerous

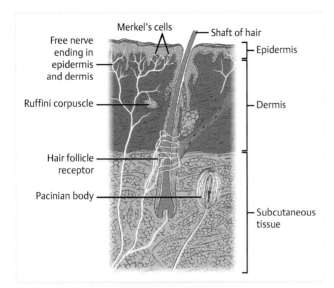

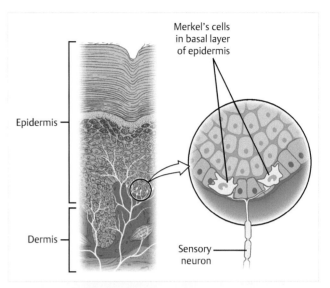

Fig. 11.7 Schematic drawing of thin skin from the scalp demonstrating free nerve endings, hair follicle (root hair) receptors, and other superficial and deep cutaneous tactile mechanoreceptors. The base of the hair follicle receptors resides deep within the skin at the dermal–hypodermal junction but passes through the connective tissue (CT) layers to defined areas of the surface. Hair follicles exhibit as small receptive field and represent nonencapsulated, fast-adapting receptors, which monitor distortion of movement across the body surface. The types of tactile mechanoreceptors found in thin skin are similar to those found in thick skin. A notable exception is Meissner's corpuscle which is found predominantly in hairless, thick skin. All tactile cutaneous mechanoreceptors transmit sensory input by afferent Type II (Aβ) fibers. Free nerve endings conduct sensory impulses along Type III (Aδ) and Type IV (C) fibers.

Fig. 11.8 Merkel complex. Merkel's cells (discs) are unique, specialized epithelial receptor cells located in the basal layer of the epidermis. Each Merkel's cell synapses with a myelinated afferent Aβ fiber to form a mechanoreceptor complex (Merkel complex). Merkel complexes exhibit a high distribution density in regions such as the fingertips, palm, lips, and oral cavity that require a high degree of specificity. Merkel complexes exhibit small receptive fields with defined borders, which allows for accurate localization. Merkel's cell complexes respond to light touch, a sensory modality associated with fine or discriminative touch. Specifically, these mechanoreceptors detect sustained light pressure and fine spatial separation necessary for discerning shape, texture, and two-point discrimination. (according to Andres and von Düring).

nonencapsulated nociceptors and **thermoreceptors** in the superficial and deep layers of the dermal connective tissue. These nonencapsulated free nerve endings transmit protopathic input and function to detect pain, temperature, itch, tickle, and nondiscriminative (crude) touch. Unmyelinated Type IV (C fibers) and lightly myelinated Type III (Aδ) primary afferent fibers convey protopathic information from free nerve endings to the CNS.

11.4.5 Types of Proprioceptive Receptors

- The ability to detect sensory input regarding body position and movement occurs through **proprioceptive** input from the receptors found within the **skeletal muscles, tendons,** and **joint capsules**.
- Striated (skeletal) muscle and tendons contain two types of encapsulated proprioceptors, **muscle spindles,** and **Golgi tendon organs (GTOs)**, which provide information about muscle length and tension (▶ Table 11.5).
- Joint capsules contain three types of encapsulated mechanoreceptors that provide proprioceptive feedback. The receptors include **Golgi-Mazzoni corpuscles** (Golgi end organ), the **Paciniform,** and **Ruffini's corpuscles**.

11.4.6 Muscle Proprioceptors

- Striated (skeletal) muscle tissue is composed of large, contractile muscle fibers known as **extrafusal fibers,** and small encapsulated proprioceptive stretch receptors known as **muscle (neuromuscular) spindles** (▶ Fig. 11.11).
- Muscle spindles which run parallel to extrafusal fibers and are attached to the extrafusal fibers by a connective tissue capsule detect changes in **muscle length** as the extrafusal muscle fibers stretch.
- Each muscle spindle consists of a connective tissue capsule surrounding bundles of 2 to 10 specialized muscle fibers called **intrafusal fibers**. Morphologically, there are two types of intrafusal fibers, **nuclear bag fibers** and **nuclear chain fibers**, which receive afferent (sensory) and efferent (motor) innervations.
- Both types of intrafusal fibers contain contractile elements at their distal ends, and a sensory receptor in the central region of the spindle.
- The intrafusal fibers receive sensory innervation from two afferent terminals known as **annulospiral endings** and **flower spray nerve endings.**
  - **Nuclear bag fibers** consist of both static and dynamic fibers and receive sensory innervation from large myelinated nerve fibers known as **primary muscle spindle afferents (Ia fibers; Aα),** which wrap around the intrafusal fibers and terminate as **annulospiral endings.**

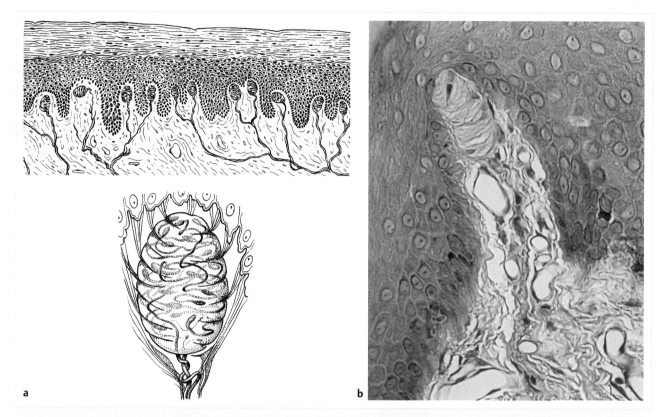

Fig. 11.9 (a, b) Schematic showing the location of Meissner's corpuscle in thick skin. **(a)** Light microscopy of encapsulated Meissner's corpuscles and myelinated Type II Aβ axon in the superficial papillary layer of the dermis; taken from the fingertips (longitudinal section; 40 × magnification; H/E stain). **(b)** Meissner's corpuscle represents a fast-adapting, encapsulated mechanoreceptor located in glabrous (thick) skin. Similar to the Merkel's cell complex, Meissner's corpuscles exhibit a small receptive field and high density in areas requiring discriminative touch such as the fingertips and lips. Meissner's corpuscles detect light pressure, low frequency vibrations (flutter) in addition to fine touch. (▸ Fig. 11.9a: Reproduced with permission from Kahle W, Frotscher M. Color Atlas of Human Anatomy. Sixth Edition, Vol 3. © Thieme 2011.)

– Annulospiral endings become activated as the center of intrafusal muscle fibers begins to stretch and provide information about the rate of length change of the skeletal muscle.

○ The second class of intrafusal fibers, the **nuclear chain fibers,** consists of static fibers that are more resistant to stretch. Nuclear chain fibers receive afferent innervation from two sources: **the primary muscle spindle afferent (Type Ia, Aα)** and the **secondary muscle spindle afferent,** which terminates as a **flower spray ending (Type II, Aβ fibers).**

– **Flower spray endings** respond as the skeletal muscle continues to elongate and monitor the relative change of muscle length.

- The intrafusal fibers also receive motor innervation from efferent fibers that originate from **gamma motor neurons** in the CNS. The efferent nerve fibers terminate to form **motor end plates** along the surface of the intrafusal fibers. Efferent stimulation causes the intrafusal fibers to contract and serve as a mechanism to modulate the length and sensitivity of the intrafusal fiber.
- Muscle spindles function to maintain constant muscle length, provide resistance to stretch as part of a **myotatic reflex** (muscle stretch reflex), and play a role in postural feedback. Muscles involved in fine motor control and postural maintenance contain a higher density of muscle spindles.

11.4.7 Tendon Proprioceptive Receptors

- **GTO**, also known **neurotendinous spindles,** are **encapsulated proprioceptors** located at the boundary between the muscle and tendinous insertion (▸ Fig. 11.12).
- Each GTO is comprised of collagen fibers serially arranged with the extrafusal muscle fibers. Sensory nerve endings of myelinated primary afferent fibers, known as **Type Ib fibers (Aα fibers),** wrap around the collagen fibers of the tendon, and respond to changes in tension as contractile force is applied to the muscle.
- GTOs function to provide information about **muscle tension** as the **muscle contracts** and to mediate **inhibitory tendon reflexes** as a protective mechanism to prevent excessive muscle tension. Feedback from these receptors help to regulate muscle contraction and control force for coordinated motor movements (see Chapter 16).

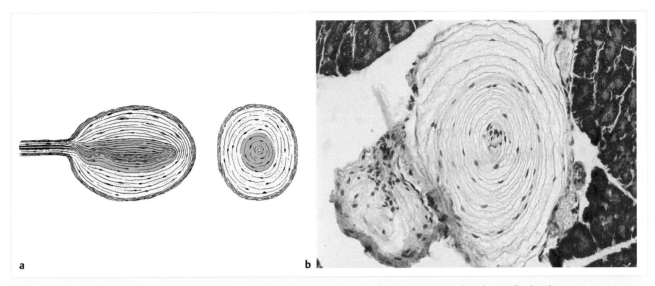

Fig. 11.10 (a,b) Pacinian corpuscle. **(a)** Schematic drawing illustrating the structure of a Pacinian corpuscle in longitudinal and cross section. Image shows a single myelinated axon (Aβ fiber) wrapped circumferentially with glial cells and outer connective tissue sheath giving the cross-sectional cut an onion-like appearance. **(b)** Light microscopy of a Pacinian corpuscle in the wall of the pancreas (longitudinal section; 40 × magnification; H/E stain). Pacinian corpuscles are fast-adapting, encapsulated mechanoreceptors that detect deep pressure and high-frequency vibration. Pacinian corpuscle may be found in some viscera, as illustrated in the micrograph, or in the deep subcutaneous (hypodermis) layer of the skin. Structurally similar receptors are found in joint capsules and the periosteal connective tissue (CT) layer surrounding bone. Pacinian corpuscle and another deep proprioceptor known as Ruffini's corpuscles (not shown) exhibit a large receptive field. (▶ Fig. 11.10a: Modified with permission from Kahle W, Frotscher M. Color Atlas of Human Anatomy. Sixth Edition, Vol 3. © Thieme 2011.)

Table 11.5 Proprioceptive encapsulated muscle receptors

Structural Class: Proprioceptors Encapsulated Mechanoreceptors						
Location	Type of Receptor	Primary Afferent Fiber	Stimulus	Sensory Modality	Receptive Field	Adaptation
Skeletal muscle	Proprioceptors Muscle spindle: Primary afferent Annulospiral ending	Type Ia (Aα)	Mechanical stimulation Onset of muscle stretch	Muscle stretch and velocity	Large	Rapid (phasic) Slow
Skeletal muscle	Proprioceptors Muscle spindle: Secondary afferent Flower spray endings	Type II (Aβ)	Mechanical stimulation Stretch in progress	Muscle stretch	Large	Slow (tonic)
Muscle–tendon insertion	Low threshold mechanoreceptor Golgi tendon organ (GTO)	Type Ib (Aα) fibers	Mechanical stimulation; contraction of muscle	Muscle tension	Large	Slow (tonic)

Note: *Nonencapsulated (free) nerve endings associated with nociceptors and thermoreceptors also located in muscle and joint capsules.

11.4.8 Joint Proprioceptive Receptors (▶ Table 11.6)

- Three types of encapsulated joint receptors are found within the fibrous joint capsule and joint ligaments: Paciniform corpuscle, Ruffini's corpuscle, and Golgi-Mazzoni corpuscles (Golgi end organs).
- Joint receptors provide information about the range of motion and joint position, which occurs in response to mechanical deformation of the receptors found within the capsule and joint ligaments.
- Nociceptive free nerve endings of Aδ fibers (Type III) and C fibers (Type IV) are also widely distributed throughout the joint capsule, muscles, tendons, and ligaments.

- Afferent feedback from joint receptors serves to protect the joint from injury and provide proprioceptive input concerning the position of the joint, which is necessary for modulating movements (▶ Table 11.6).
  - **Paciniform corpuscles,** which are structurally similar to Pacinian corpuscle, reside in the deeper layers of the joint capsule near the articular attachments. The receptor responds to mechanical changes in joint position and provide information about the direction and speed of joint movements.
  - **Ruffini's corpuscles** wrap around the collagen fibers of the superficial capsule and ligaments to provide feedback about joint movements and static joint positions. Stimulation of the receptors occurs by stretch,

Table 11.6 Proprioceptive encapsulated joint receptors

Structural Class: Proprioceptors: Encapsulated Joint Mechanoreceptors						
Location	Type of Receptors	Primary Afferent Fibers	Stimulus	Sensory Modality	Receptive Field	Adaptation
Ligament of joint capsules	High threshold Static mechanoreceptors **Golgi type end organ ending** *also called Golgi-Mazzoni corpuscle	Type II (Aβ) fibers	Activated during extensive range of motion Twisting force	Stretch of capsular ligaments Joint torque	Large	Slow (tonic)
Deep part of capsule of synovial joints Near articular attachments Periosteum of articular attachment Tendons	Low threshold mechanoreceptor **Joint Paciniform corpuscles** *morphologically similar to Pacinian corpuscle	Type II (Aβ)	Dynamic movements activate receptor	Pressure vibratory joint movement Direction and speed of movement	Large	Rapid (phasic)
Superficial Capsule of synovial joints; tendons	Low threshold mechanoreceptor **Joint Ruffini's corpuscle**	Type II (Aβ)	Activated by stretching/ pressure and tactile stimulation	Static joint position conveys pressure and joint angle Changes in intra-articular pressure Direction, amplitude of movement	Large	Slow (tonic)

Note: *Nonencapsulated (free) nerve endings associated with nociceptors and thermoreceptors also located in muscle and joint capsules.

displacement, or physical deformation of the receptor ending. Ruffini's receptors are distributed in superficial areas of the capsule and signal static joint position, changes in intra-articular pressure, direction, amplitude, and velocity of movement.

○ **Golgi-Mazzoni corpuscles** are mechanoreceptors found in joint capsules and ligaments. The receptors detect joint compression during weight-bearing activities and respond as ligaments stretch and twist during joint movement. In the temporomandibular joint (TMJ), the Golgi end organs reside in the superficial layers of the (temporomandibular) lateral ligament which helps to stabilize the capsule.

11.4.9 Visceral Receptors

• Visceral receptors, also known as **interoceptors**, transmit information about the body's internal state from viscera and vessel walls and play an important role in maintaining homeostasis of the internal environment (▶ Table 11.7).
  ○ Functionally, visceral afferent receptors transmit sensations from organs that are perceived consciously such as distention, stretch, nausea, or bloating.
  ○ Visceral receptors also convey unconscious sensations to initiate visceral reflexes in response to changes in CO_2 and O_2 levels, alterations in blood pressure, or acid–base levels.
• Visceral receptors are free nerve endings formed by small myelinated and unmyelinated visceral afferent nerve fibers. The types of receptors include **mechanoreceptors, chemoreceptors,** and **nociceptors.**
  ○ **Mechanoreceptors** found in viscera function to detect changes in distention (stretch) or pressure. Specialized mechanoreceptors, known as **baroreceptors** or

pressoreceptors, are found in the wall of the carotid sinus and aortic arch and specifically monitor blood pressure.
  ○ Peripheral **chemoreceptors**, known as the carotid and aortic bodies, are small clusters of cells found in the carotid artery wall and aortic arch. The chemoreceptors of carotid body monitor changes in pH, CO_2, and O_2 levels, while the aortic body responds only to change in CO_2 and O_2. Changes in CO_2, O_2, and pH trigger afferent fibers to signal a change in ventilation to maintain cardiorespiratory homeostasis.
  ○ Unmyelinated and myelinated **nociceptors** are found throughout visceral organs and may elicit pain in response to decreased blood flow (ischemia), inflammation, or distention.
• Visceral afferent fibers which have their cell bodies in the dorsal root ganglia initially travel from the viscera along autonomic pathways before entering the dorsal horn of the spinal cord (▶ Fig. 11.13).

11.5 Cutaneous Receptors of the Oral Mucosa (▶ Table 11.8)

• The oropharyngeal region exhibits a high number of sensory receptors throughout the facial skin, oral mucosa, periodontal ligament (PDL), muscles, and TMJ. The high receptor density, small receptive field, and the pattern of receptor distribution throughout the orofacial region confer a high level of discrimination, proprioception, and stereognostic input which are critical for modulating oromotor output.

Table 11.7 Visceral receptors

Location in Body	Receptor Class	Type of Receptor	Stimulus	Sensory Modality	Adaptation
Located at bifurcation of internal and external carotid Aorta	Nonencapsulated mechanoreceptors Baroreceptor	Carotid sinus Aortic sinus	Pressure: Decrease or increase in arterial blood pressure	**Unconscious** Visceral reflex	Rapid (phasic)
Wall of internal carotid Wall of aorta	Nonencapsulated Peripheral Chemoreceptor	Carotid body Aortic body	Chemical: Decrease O_2 Increase CO_2 Decrease in pH	**Unconscious** Visceral reflex	Rapid (phasic)
Wall of organs	Nonencapsulated mechanoreceptors	Organ stretch receptors	Mechanical stretch	**Conscious perception** Distention Fullness Stretch	Slow (tonic)
Wall of organs	Encapsulated mechanoreceptors	Pacinian	Mechanical	**Conscious perception** Pressure	Rapid (phasic)
Mucosa of organs	Nonencapsulated nociceptor	Nociceptor	Noxious stimuli Inflammation Chemical	**Conscious perception** Pain Referred pain	Slow (tonic)

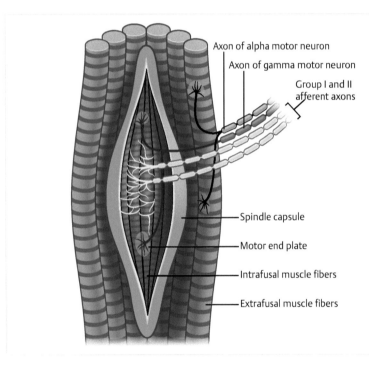

Axon of alpha motor neuron
Axon of gamma motor neuron
Group I and II afferent axons
Spindle capsule
Motor end plate
Intrafusal muscle fibers
Extrafusal muscle fibers

Fig. 11.11 Simplified schematic of a muscle spindle and its nerve supply. Muscle spindles represent encapsulated proprioceptors found in the center of groups of contractile (extrafusal) skeletal muscle fibers. Muscle spindles respond to mechanical deformation and provide conscious and unconscious proprioceptive feedback about active and passive stretching of the skeletal muscle. Muscle spindles contain two types of intrafusal fibers: large, centrally located nuclear bag fibers, and smaller, peripherally located nuclear chain fibers (not labeled). The intrafusal fibers represent specialized sensory organs that are innervated by two types of sensory nerve fibers known as Type Ia (primary annulospiral ending) and Type II (secondary flower spray endings). The muscle spindle is the only sensory receptor with both afferent (sensory) and efferent (motor) innervation. Afferent fibers provide information about the rate (velocity) of the stretch and the extent of the stretch. Efferent Aγ fibers provide innervation to both types of intrafusal fibers and function to regulate the tension of the intrafusal fibers.

- Comparable to the body, each sensory receptor is associated with primary afferent nerve fibers that transmit sensory impulses at a specific speed or conduction velocity toward the CNS. The morphological characteristics of the axon correlate with sensory (modality) information it transmits. The ascending pathway that conveys somatosensory input arising from the face follows a different pathway to the somatosensory cortex than the path followed by the body (see Chapters 12 and 13).

- In general, the mechanoreceptors of the oropharyngeal region are primarily associated with well-myelinated, large-diameter axons, while nociceptors, thermoreceptors, and visceral receptors represent the peripheral terminations of lightly myelinated or unmyelinated nerve fibers with small axonal diameters. The function and role of the orofacial receptors is discussed in Unit II.

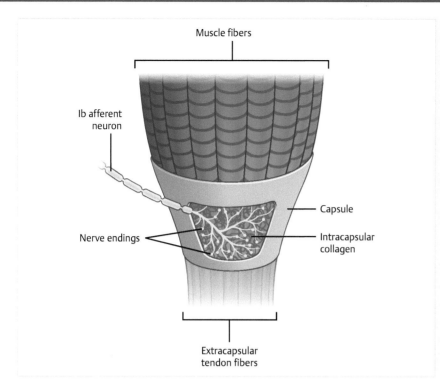

Fig. 11.12 Schematic diagram of the Golgi tendon organ (GTO) and its nerve supply. GTOs are located at the muscle–tendon junction and represent groups of encapsulated collagen fibers (tendons) that attach to skeletal muscle. GTOs are sensory organs involved in proprioception and transmit sensory input via Type Ib fibers. The receptors respond to changes in muscle tension and are highly sensitive to movement. Feedback from these receptors functions to regulate muscle contraction.

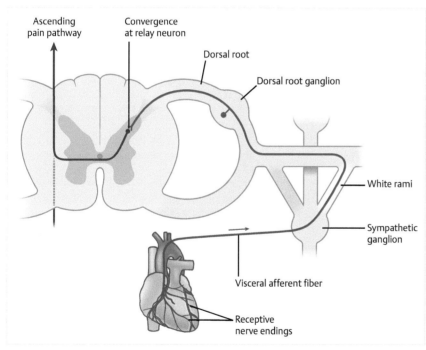

Fig. 11.13 Visceral receptors. A simplified schematic demonstrating the pathway and location of neuron cell bodies in the dorsal root ganglion. Visceral sensory receptors are classified as interoceptors and carry information from the walls of organs, blood vessels, and tissues. Types of receptors include nociceptors, chemoreceptors, and a type of mechanoreceptor known as a baroreceptor. The cell bodies of visceral primary afferent neurons reside in spinal ganglion (depicted) and some cranial ganglia. The mechanoreceptors and nociceptive receptors provide input concerning distention of organs and pain, respectively, which are usually diffusely localized.

Table 11.8 Somatosensory receptors of oral mucosa

Receptor Location	Receptor Type Structural Class of Axon	Sensory Modality	Receptive Field Size** Adaption*
Oral mucosa Temporomandibular joint (TMJ) Periodontal ligament (PDL) Tongue Masticatory muscles	Low threshold Tactile mechanoreceptor Joint receptors Type II (Aβ) – Merkel Meissner Ruffini	Fine, discriminative touch/ stereognosis Conscious proprioception Stretch/ deformation/pressure of TMJ and tooth	Small/SA Small/RA Large/SA
Muscles of mastication Tongue Periodontal ligament	Proprioceptors (low threshold) Muscle spindles of jaw closing muscles Type Ia (Aα) Type II (Aβ) Ruffini Type II (Aβ)	Unconscious and conscious proprioception Muscle stretch Myotatic stretch reflex Deformation/pressure of tooth due to occlusal load (bite force)	Large/SA Large/ both SA/RA
Oral and pharyngeal mucosa Pulp of tooth	Nociceptor/ thermal receptors Free nerve endings: Type III Aδ fibers Type IV C fibers (high threshold) Polymodal nociceptors	Thermal sense—warm, hot, cool, cold Nociceptive pain Fast, sharp, localized pain associated with "first pain" Dull, diffuse slow pain Associated with "second pain"	Small/SA Large/SA
Pharynx and laryngeal mucosa	Visceral receptors mechanical distention Type III Aδ fibers Type IV C fibers	Stretch/distention	Small/SA Large receptive area//SA
Taste receptors of taste buds Fungiform papillae on anterior two-thirds of tongue and some foliate papilla Taste bud of hard and soft palates Circumvallate papillae, foliate papillae on posterior one-third tongue Oropharynx Epiglottis	Gustatory chemoreceptors	Taste	Small/RA

Note: *SA = slow adapting; RA = rapidly adapting; **smaller receptive field; higher receptor density; better discrimination.

Questions and Answers

1. You are asked to examine a biopsied tissue section demonstrating Meissner's Corpuscles. The tissue section may be obtained from which of the following regions?
   a) Skin of forearm
   b) Biceps tendon
   c) Masseter muscle
   d) Fingertips

Level 1: Easy

Answer D: Fingertips. Meissner's corpuscles are sensory receptors found in high density of glabrous (hairless) skin. A biopsy containing these receptors could also come from the palm of the hand, soles of the feet and regions of the oral mucosa. **(A)** The skin of the forearm contains hair follicles and lacks Meissner's corpuscles. **(B)** and **(C)** would contain golgi tendon organs and muscle spindle fibers respectively.

2. A characteristic of a Merkel's receptor complex is that it is _____
   a) fast adapting
   b) innervated by Aδ fibers
   c) an encapsulated receptor
   d) myelinated
   e) found in the dermis

Level 2: Moderate

Answer D: Myelinated. Merkel's cells are specialized epithelial receptor cells found in the epidermis of the skin which form a sensory receptor complex with myelinated Aβ fibers. The receptor complex is non-encapsulated, slow adapting receptor.

3. Group Aα fibers _____
   a) innervate dermis of the skin.
   b) have the smallest fiber diameter.
   c) carry general somatic efferent fibers.
   d) lack myelination.

Level 1: Easy

Answer C: General somatic efferent fibers. Group Aα fibers are myelinated, exhibiting the fastest conduction velocity (70–120 m/sec) and the largest axonal diameter (12–20 μm). Group Aα fibers innervated skeletal muscle fibers (Extrafusal fibers) and carry somatic efferent fibers.

4. The type of encapsulated mechanoreceptor that is involved in a myotactic stretch reflex is the:
   a) Golgi tendon organ.
   b) Ruffini corpuscle.
   c) Pacinian corpuscle.
   d) Muscle spindle.

Level 2: Moderate

Answer D: Muscle spindle. The detection of muscle stretch is mediated through type Ia afferent fibers that innervate the nuclear bag and nuclear chain fibers of a muscle spindle. Muscle spindles monitor changes in muscle length whereas the golgi tendon organ **(A)** which are found in tendons monitor changes in muscle tension as it is transmitted to the tendon. The Ruffini corpuscle detects stretch of collagen fibers **(B)**, not muscle fibers. Pacinian corpuscles **(C)** monitor movement and positional change of joints. During a stretch reflex both the extrafusal muscle fibers and spindle are stretched as the muscle lengthens. The reflex functions to maintain constant length of the muscle.

5. Fast pain is transmitted by _____ fibers
   a) Aβ
   b) Ia
   c) Aδ
   d) C
   e) Ib

Level 1: Easy

Answer C: Aδ fibers are lightly myelinated fibers that transmit stimuli from non-encapsulated nociceptors which is perceived as sharp, fast pain. The myelination aids in the increasing the conduction velocity. Ia fibers **(B)** are afferent fibers associated with annulospiral endings of muscle spindle. Ib fibers **(E)** provide innervation to golgi tendon organs. **(A)** Aβ form the terminal receptive endings for tactile mechanoreceptors. **(D)** C fibers are unmyelinated free nerve endings that transmit nociception slowly due to the lack of myelin. The pain perceived is not well localized and described as dull, diffuse pain.

12 Somatosensory Systems Part I—Somatosensory Pathways of Body

12.1 Overview of Ascending Somatosensory System

- The present chapter describes the three pathways which comprise the ascending somatosensory system for the body: the **anterolateral pathway**, the **dorsal column-medial lemniscus pathway**, and the **spinocerebellar system**. A similar system, known as the trigeminal system, conveys somatosensory input from the head and face and is covered in Chapter 13.

12.1.1 Function of the Somatosensory System

- The somatosensory system is responsible for conveying sensory input concerning the body's external environment, its position, and its internal state from specific peripheral sensory receptors to the central nervous system (CNS). Specific types of mechanoreceptors, thermoreceptors, nociceptors, and chemoreceptors which are found in the skin, joints, muscles, and organs transmit sensory input through **general somatic afferent (GSA) fibers** and **general visceral afferent (GVA) fibers**.
  - **GSA** fibers carry sensory modalities such as touch, vibration, pressure, positional sense, pain, and temperature from the **body (soma)** and head, while **GVA** fibers convey sensations of pain, temperature, stretch, and distention from the **viscera**.
  - GSA and GVA fibers serve as the functional afferent component of spinal nerves. Some cranial nerves also carry these fibers. Specifically, the trigeminal nerve (CN V) carries GSA fibers, while the facial (CN VII), glossopharyngeal (CN IX), and vagus (CN X) carry both GSA and GVA fibers.
- Based on the type of sensory modality transmitted, afferent fibers of the body enter the dorsal root of the spinal cord and ascend along specific sensory pathways to the cortex or cerebellum for conscious and unconscious processing.

12.2 Transmission of Conscious and Unconscious Sensations (▶ Fig. 12.1)

- Although most sensory input is consciously perceived and involves neural processing in the cerebral cortex, some sensory information is unconsciously processed by the cerebellum or may be transmitted to other regions of the CNS as part of a reflexive response and autonomic control.

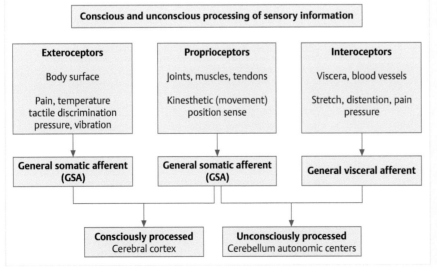

Fig. 12.1 Transmission of conscious and unconscious sensations.

Table 12.1 Overview of ascending somatosensory tracts: conscious and unconscious processing

Conscious Somatosensory Pathways				
Name of Path	Location in Spinal Cord	Receptor	Function of Tract	Termination
Direct anterolateral pathway (aka lateral spinothalamic tract) (neospinothalamic tract)	Anterolateral funiculus Primarily lateral funiculus	Nociceptor; thermoreceptors Lightly myelinated Aδ fibers (Type III)	Mediates sharp localized, pain; cool temperature; itch, crude (light) (nondiscriminative) touch	Conscious cortical processing; immediate awareness of pain Contralateral primary somatosensory cortex via VPL of thalamus
Dorsal column-medial lemniscus	Posterior funiculus	Tactile mechanoreceptors: Meissner, Merkel, Pacinian, Ruffini Proprioceptors: muscle spindles; Golgi tendon organ Aα (Type Ia, Ib) Type II (Aβ)	Mediates tactile two-point discrimination; conscious proprioception regarding limb positions	Conscious cortical processing Contralateral primary somatosensory cortex via VPL of thalamus

Unconscious Somatosensory Pathways				
Name of path	Location in spinal cord	Receptor	Function of tract	Termination
Spinocerebellar tracts	Lateral funiculus	Proprioceptors Muscle spindles Golgi tendon organ Aα (Type Ia, Ib) Type II (Aβ)	Mediates unconscious proprioception necessary for coordination of motor movements; postural maintenance and reflex motor responses	Unconscious processing in ipsilateral cerebellum
Indirect anterolateral pathways (aka anterior spinothalamic, spinomesencephalic, spinoreticular etc.—paleospinothalamic and archispinothalamic)	Anterolateral funiculus Primarily anterior funiculus	Polymodal nociceptors Unmyelinated C fibers	Mediates arousal and the affective/emotional component of pain Dull, diffused, poorly localized pain and crude touch	Unconscious processing Termination of input in regions other than primary somatosensory cortex

Abbreviation: VPL, ventral posterolateral.
Note: Some textbooks consider the anterolateral system or spinothalamic tract to be divided into a lateral and an anterior spinothalamic tracts. The lateral spinothalamic tract is associated with fast pain, whereas anterior spinothalamic tract is associated with slow pain that is poorly localized due to points of termination.

- In general, GSA fibers that arise from exteroceptive and some proprioceptive receptors in the body transmit **conscious** sensations to the cerebral cortex through two principal anatomical pathways (▶ Table 12.1):
  - **Anterolateral system (ALS)**
  - **Dorsal column-medial lemniscus (DCML) pathway**
    - The **ALS** consists of several associated tracts which convey sensations of pain, temperature, itch, and crude (nondiscriminative) touch from nonencapsulated nociceptors, mechanoreceptors, and thermoreceptors found throughout the body. The anterolateral pathway is located in the anterior and lateral funiculi and is important in the discriminative localization of painful stimuli.
    - The **DCML pathway** transmits tactile sensations involving fine, discriminative touch (two-point discrimination), pressure, and vibration, along with conscious proprioceptive input concerning the static position and movement of joints and limbs. Mechanosensory and proprioceptive input is mediated through several types of encapsulated and nonencapsulated mechanoreceptors. The pathway lies in the dorsal column of the spinal cord.

- In addition to these conscious pathways, several ascending pathways transmit **unconscious somatic afferent** information.
  - The **spinocerebellar system,** which includes several paths, conveys unconscious proprioceptive input from encapsulated mechanoreceptors such as muscle spindles and Golgi tendon organs along GSA fibers to the cerebellum. The spinocerebellar pathway plays an important role in maintaining posture while standing or sitting and coordinating motor responses.
  - Several ascending tracts of the ALS, which are also known as **indirect** ALS paths, terminate in regions other than the primary somatosensory cortex and do not reach conscious perception. The indirect ALS pathways convey nociceptive stimulation and play a role in raising the level of awareness of painful stimuli. Components of this pathway are also involved in the affective aspects of processing of painful stimuli as well as modulating pain.

- **Unconscious visceral input** which plays a role in mediating autonomic visceral reflexes is transmitted by **GVA** fibers from visceral receptors to various autonomic control centers throughout the CNS. Sensations associated with viscera are generally unconscious; however, under pathological circumstances, visceral input may produce conscious viscerosomatic sensations, such as pressure or pain which serves as a protective response.
  ○ The conscious perception of painful visceral sensations is often detected in specific regions of the body which differ from the actual source of the visceral stimulus. These painful sensations, known as **referred pain,** are discussed in more detail in **Chapter 14**.

12.2.1 Common Features of the Conscious Somatosensory Pathways (▶ Table 12.2)

- The anterolateral and dorsal column-medial lemniscus pathways follow distinct anatomical routes; however, both ascending pathways share several common attributes:
  ○ Both pathways consist of bundles of axonal tracts that interconnect a chain of three neurons, sequentially arranged as a relay circuit.
  ○ The neurons are referred to as first-, second-, and third-order neurons (▶ Fig. 12.2).
  ○ The sensory neuron cell body is known as the **primary afferent neuron** or **first-order neuron.** The first-order neuron for the somatosensory system of the body resides in the **dorsal root (spinal) ganglia (DRG).** For the region of the head, it resides in cranial sensory ganglia (see Chapters 13 and 14).
    – Morphologically, primary afferent neurons are pseudounipolar neurons with a single peripheral process that terminates as peripheral sensory receptors or on peripheral targets, and a single, centrally projecting process that transmits sensory input toward the CNS. The central process enters the dorsal root of the spinal cord to synapse on second-order neurons.
    – Both the ALS and DCML somatosensory pathways exhibit a somatotopic arrangement of nerve fibers from the point of entry into the spinal cord to the point of termination in the somatosensory cortex (▶ Fig. 12.3, ▶ Table 12.3). The point-to-point connection within the pathway creates a somatotopic map that allows for the specific localization and identification of the stimulus modality.
  ○ The cell bodies of second-order neurons reside in the gray matter on the same **(ipsilateral)** side as the primary afferent neuron; however, the location of the second-order neuron varies according to the type of sensory receptor neuron and sensory modality transmitted.
    – Primary afferent fibers that transmit conscious proprioceptive input and discriminative touch synapse on **second-order mechanoreceptive** and **proprioceptive neurons** in the **medulla,** while those conveying pain, temperature, or crude touch synapse on **nociceptive neurons** in the Rexed lamina of the dorsal horn of the **spinal cord.**

○ Axons of second-order neurons cross the midline **(decussate)** at specific locations and then ascend on the **contralateral** (opposite) side to synapse on **third-order neurons** found in the thalamus.
  – The point of decussation differs between the two paths and has important clinical relevance for determining the point of injury: the **DCML decussates** in the **medulla,** whereas the fibers of the **anterolateral pathway decussate** in the **spinal cord.**
○ Nerve fibers from third-order neurons remain on the contralateral side and project from the ventral posterolateral (VPL) nuclei of the **thalamus** to the **primary somatosensory cortex** so that information entering the CNS on one side is consciously processed by the cerebral cortex of the opposite side.
  – The thalamus serves as a sensory relay station and all sensory information processed in the somatosensory cortex must first synapse in the thalamus before projecting to the cortex.
  – Somatosensory fibers from the thalamus pass through the posterior limb of the internal capsule to terminate in the primary somatosensory cortex.
○ The **primary somatosensory cortex (S1)** is found within the **postcentral gyrus of the parietal lobe** and represents the cortical region responsible for conscious sensory perception. The region of the primary somatosensory cortex is subdivided into four regions known as Brodmann's areas 3a, 3b, 1, and 2 (▶ Fig. 12.4).
○ Thalamocortical projections are somatotopically arranged so that neurons receiving input from the **body** are in the **lateral portion** of the **ventral posterior nucleus (VPL)** of the **thalamus,** while fibers of the **head** are in the **medial part of the ventral nucleus (VPM).**
○ The somatotopic organization of thalamocortical fibers establishes within the primary somatosensory cortex a sensory map of the body and head that reflects a specific point-for-point location of sensory input from specific regions of the body. In the sensory map, the somatotopic arrangement of input from the foot, leg, upper trunk, and face is medial to lateral (▶ Fig. 12.5).
  – The sensory map, also known as **sensory homunculus,** depicts a distorted representation of each body region. The amount presented in the cortical region is proportional to the receptor density. The oral cavity, face, and fingertips have a greater receptor density and so the corresponding cortical region appears larger than other regions.

12.3 Anterolateral System

12.3.1 Functional Overview of the Anterolateral System

- The detection of painful, noxious stimuli or innocuous sensory input, such as thermal changes or nondiscriminative (crude) tactile stimuli, occurs through nonencapsulated nociceptors, thermoreceptors, and mechanoreceptors found throughout the body.

Table 12.2 Comparison of conscious pathways

Structure and Location	Dorsal Column-Medial Lemniscus (DCML)	Anterolateral Spinothalamic Tract
Functional sensory modality	Discriminative fine touch; Vibration Pressure Positional sense (static) Kinesthetic sense (movement)	Nondiscriminative (crude) touch Temperature (hot, cold) Sharp, fast, acute, pricking pain (Aδ fibers) Slow, dull, aching, chronic pain (C fibers)
Type of peripheral sensory receptor	Encapsulated, low-threshold mechanoreceptors (LTM) Meissner, Pacinian, Ruffini (Type II/Aβ), muscle spindle (Type Ia/Aα and II fibers), Golgi tendon organ (Type Ib/Aα)	Nonencapsulated (free nerve endings)
Afferent fiber type	Myelinated Aβ (Type II); Aα (Type Ia, Ib)	Myelinated Aδ; unmyelinated C fibers
First-order neuron/location	Large, pseudounipolar neuron Dorsal root ganglion (DRG)	Small, pseudounipolar neuron Dorsal root ganglion (DRG)
Point of entry to spinal cord	Medial part of dorsal root	Lateral part of dorsal root
Name of primary afferent fiber tracts and location in CNS	Dorsal column of spinal cord Fasciculus gracilis (T6 below) Fasciculus cuneatus (T6 above) Ascends ipsilateral from spinal cord to medulla	Posterolateral tract of spinal cord (tract of Lissauer) Fibers may ascend or descend ipsilaterally 1,2, or 3 levels in the spinal cord before synapsing on second-order neurons.
Second-order neuron/ synapse location	Dorsal column nuclei—lower medulla Multipolar projection neurons • Nucleus gracilis—medially located • Nucleus cuneatus—laterally located	Gray matter of dorsal horn Multipolar projection neurons • Rexed lamina I—receive primarily Aδ • Rexed laminae II and V—receive primarily C fibers
Point of decussation	**Internal arcuate** Lower medulla Collective crossing of all fibers	**Anterior white commissure of spinal cord** Cross at each level of synapse on secondary neurons
Secondary fiber tracts/location	**Forms medial lemniscus tract** Ascends contralateral from lower medulla to thalamus	**Forms anterolateral spinothalamic tract** (part of spinal lemniscus in anterior and lateral funiculus) Ascends from spinal cord entry to contralateral thalamus
Third-order neuron/ Synapse location	**Ventral posterolateral (VPL) nucleus of thalamus—** relay nuclei	**Ventral posterolateral (VPL) nucleus of thalamus**—relay nuclei
Primary termination in cortex	**Primary somatosensory cortex—postcentral gyrus** Brodmann's areas 3a, 3b, 2, and 1	**Primary somatosensory cortex—postcentral gyrus** Brodmann's areas 3a, 3b, 2, and 1
Reflexive response	Monosynaptic muscle stretch reflex Golgi tendon reflex	Polysynaptic withdrawal (pain) reflex
Result of lesion or damage to tract *depends on lesion location	Impairment of proprioception, kinesthesia, and tactile discrimination Result: Sensory ataxia (uncoordinated movements—more pronounced with eyes closed) Deficits in stereognosis (astereognosis)—difficulty recognizing shape and texture **Lesion in spinal cord:** Ipsilateral loss due to injury occurring prior to decussation **Lesion in medulla:** Contralateral loss due to injury occurring after decussation	Diminished crude touch, loss of temperature, itch, tickle sensations Result: Loss of pain (analgesia) and temperature **Lesion in spinal cord or higher:** Contralateral loss due to lesion occurring after fiber decussation

Abbrevviation: CNS, central nervous system.

- Small, lightly myelinated Aδ (Type III) fibers and unmyelinated C (Type IV) fibers of primary sensory neurons transmit the sensations of pain, temperature, itch, and crude touch elicited by receptor stimulation to the ALS in the spinal cord (▶ Table 12.4).
- The **ALS** represents several axonal tracts, including the **spinothalamic**, **spinoreticular**, **spinomesencephalic**, **spinotectal**, and **spinohypothalamic tracts**, that ascend in the contralateral anterolateral quadrant (funiculus) of the white matter of the spinal cord.
- Based on the route followed and the point of termination within the CNS, the tracts are referred to as **direct** or **indirect** anterolateral paths.
  - The **spinothalamic tract**, also known as **neospinothalamic** or lateral spinothalamic tract, follows a **direct path** to the thalamus and somatosensory cortex for

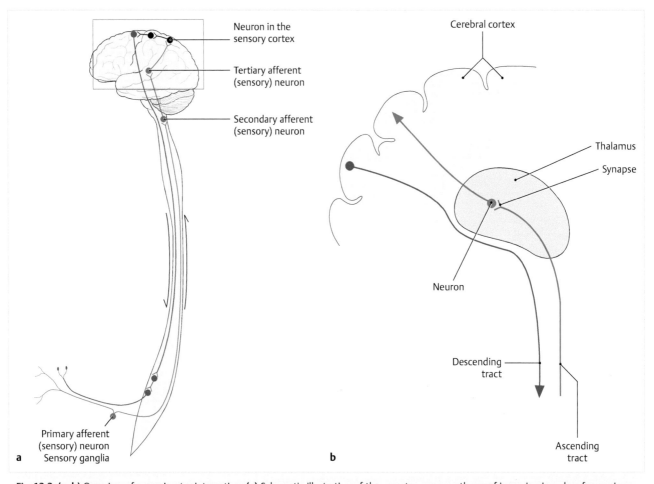

Fig. 12.2 (a, b) Overview of sensorimotor integration. **(a)** Schematic illustration of the somatosensory pathway of incoming impulses from primary (first-order) afferent neurons that form a relay circuit with secondary in the brainstem and tertiary afferent (sensory) neurons. **(b)** The tertiary neurons for most somatosensory pathways reside in the thalamus and terminate on neurons in the somatosensory cortex. Cortical processing is necessary for conscious perception. An interneuron links this with an upper motor neuron in the motor cortex which then descends through the white matter to a lower motor neuron in the spinal cord. The lower motor neuron projects to effector organs. Most descending motor tracts bypass the thalamus. (Reproduced with permission from Schuenke M, Schulte E, Schumacher U. THIEME Atlas of Anatomy Third Edition, Vol 3. © Thieme 2020. Illustrations by Markus Voll and Karl Wesker.)

conscious processing and serves as the principal pathway for the transmission of fast, sharp, localized pain and cool temperature sensations. Approximately 15% of nociceptive input follows the direct pathway and ascends primarily in the contralateral **lateral funiculus** of the spinal cord.

○ In comparison, the **anterior spinothalamic, spinoreticular, spinotectal**, and **spinomesencephalic tracts,** along with several other minor pathways, encompass the paleospinothalamic and archispinothalamic tracts. These tracts follow an **indirect path** to the cortex. Many of the indirect fiber tracts project from second-order neurons in the spinal cord and ascend in the contralateral **anterior funiculus** to nuclei in the reticular formation of the brainstem before ascending to the intralaminar thalamic nuclei, limbic system, or hypothalamus. The indirect path transmits approximately 85% of nociceptive input to the following regions:

– Input to the **reticular formation** and **intralaminar thalamic nuclei** functions in the arousal and awareness of nociceptive stimuli.

– Projections to the **hypothalamus** and **limbic system** play a role in integrating autonomic activity and reflexes with nociceptive input and function in the emotional processing associated with painful experiences.

– Some fibers of the indirect paths project to the **periaqueductal gray** and play a role in the modulation and inhibition of pain.

– The indirect paths that terminate in the insular and cingulate gyrus of the cortex mediate slow, dull, poorly localized pain and provide an affective and emotional component to painful stimuli.

• Two notable differences between the conscious and unconscious ALS pathways are that the direct tract is a **contralateral** pathway, which exhibits a somatotopic pattern, whereas the indirect path provides **bilateral** input and does not exhibit somatotopic organization.

• A comparison of both routes is shown in ▶ Table 12.5.

• Both the Aδ fibers (Type III) and unmyelinated C fibers (Type IV) enter the **lateral division** of the **dorsal root** of the spinal cord. The fibers may ascend or descend one or two spinal

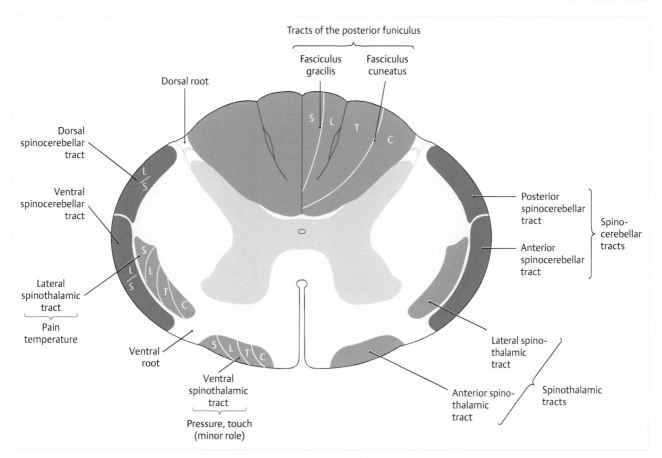

Fig. 12.3 The location of the ascending somatosensory tracts. Transverse section through the spinal cord. The tracts of the anterolateral and dorsal column-medial lemniscus (DCML) systems exhibit a somatotopic arrangement of nerve fibers from the point of entry to the point of termination. The ALS transmits pain, temperature, and crude (nondiscriminative light) touch, whereas the DCML transmits fine (discriminative) touch and conscious proprioception. The spinocerebellar tracts carry unconscious proprioception to the cerebellum. An example of the somatotopic arrangement of the input into the fasciculi gracilis and the cuneatus of the dorsal column (posterior column) is illustrated. (Modified with permission from Schuenke M, Schulte E, Schumacher U. THIEME Atlas of Anatomy Second Edition, Vol 3. © Thieme 2016. Illustrations by Markus Voll and Karl Wesker.)

Table 12.3 Ascending tracts of the spinal cord

	Tract	Location	Function		Neurons
1	Anterior spinothalamic tract	Anterior funiculus	Pathway for crude touch and pressure sensation		1st afferent neurons located in spinal ganglia; contain 2nd neurons and cross in the anterior commissure
2	Lateral spinothalamic tract	Anterior and lateral funiculus	Pathway for pain, temperature, tickle, itch, and sexual sensation		
3	Anterior spinocerebellar tract	Lateral funiculus	Pathway for unconscious coordination of motor activities (unconscious proprioception, automatic processes, e.g., jogging, riding a bike) to the cerebellum		Projection (2nd) neurons receive proprioceptive signals from 1st afferent fibers originating at the 1st neurons of spinal ganglia
4	Posterior spinocerebellar tract				
5	Fasciculus cuneatus	Posterior funiculus	Pathway for position senses (conscious proprioception) and fine cutaneous sensation (touch, vibration, fine pressure sense, two-point discrimination)	Conveys information from upper limb (not present below T3)	Cell bodies of 1st neuron located in spinal ganglion; pass uncrossed to the dorsal column nuclei
6	Fasciculus gracilis			Conveys information from lower limb	

Source: Reproduced with permission from Gilroy AM, MacPherson BR, Ross LM. Atlas of Anatomy. Second Edition. © Thieme 2017. Illustrations by Markus Voll and Karl Wesker.

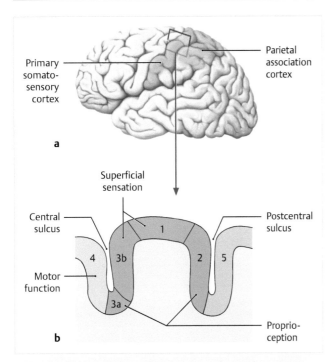

Fig. 12.4 **(a)** Primary somatosensory cortex and parietal association cortex are shown; left lateral view. **(a)** The primary somatosensory cortex (S1) lies within the postcentral gyrus of the parietal lobe. **(b)** The four Brodmann's areas within the cortex that receive somatosensory input are numbered in the sectional view. The parietal association cortex receives information from both sides of the body, whereas the primary somatosensory cortex receives input from the contralateral head and body. The perioral region is the exception and is represented bilaterally. (Reproduced with permission from Schuenke M, Schulte E, Schumacher U. THIEME Atlas of Anatomy Second Edition, Vol 3. © Thieme 2016. Illustrations by Markus Voll and Karl Wesker.)

cord segments in the axonal tract known as the **dorsolateral fasciculus (tract of Lissauer)** before entering the gray matter of the dorsal horn to synapse on **second-order neurons** associated with specific **Rexed laminae** of the **dorsal horn** (▶ Fig. 12.6)**.**

- In general, the sensory modality transmitted by the Aδ and C fibers correlates with the site of the synapse of the second-order neurons and whether the nerve fiber contributes to the direct or indirect pathway of the ALS.

• **Secondary afferent fibers** of the direct and indirect pathways ascend together in the **anterolateral column** of the white matter as the **spinal lemniscus** but terminate on third- order neurons in different regions of the brainstem and thalamus as described in the following sections (▶ Fig. 12.7).

12.3.2 Direct Path of Anterolateral Pathway (▶ Fig. 12.8, ▶ Table 12.6)

• Thinly myelinated Aδ fibers which conduct sensations of crude touch, temperature (cold), and sharp, acute pain from nonencapsulated mechanoreceptors and nociceptors synapse either directly or indirectly on second-order neurons found in the **posteromarginal nucleus (Lamina I)**, the **substantia gelatinosa (Lamina II)**, and deeper, in **Lamina V** of the dorsal horn.

- Aδ fibers carrying nociceptive input from mechanosensitive and thermo-sensitive nociceptors synapse primarily on second-order projection neurons in Lamina I. A few collaterals may synapse on interneurons in Laminae I and II before projecting second-order neurons in nucleus proprius (Laminae IV to VI).
- Non-noxious and mechanoreceptive inputs associated with crude touch synapse in Lamina V, with a few collateral

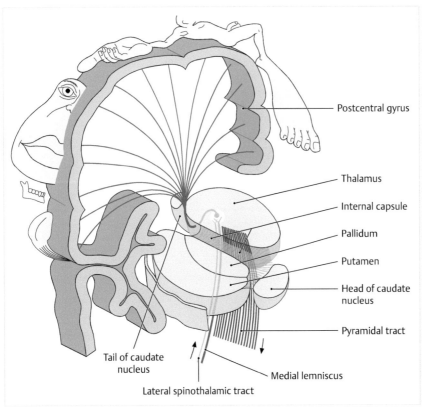

Postcentral gyrus

Thalamus

Internal capsule

Pallidum

Putamen

Head of caudate nucleus

Pyramidal tract

Tail of caudate nucleus

Medial lemniscus

Lateral spinothalamic tract

Fig. 12.5 The somatotopic representation of the body and face in the primary somatosensory cortex (anterior view of right postcentral gyrus). Somatosensory information originating from each body region projects to a specific cortical area of the postcentral gyrus and creates a topographical map depicted as the sensory homunculus. Within this sensory map, the foot, leg, upper trunk, and face exhibit a medial to a lateral arrangement. The cortical body regions are not proportionate to their actual size but in proportion to the receptor density. Note the axons of the sensory neurons ascending from the thalamus travel side by side with the axons forming the pyramidal tract (red) in the posterior limb of the internal capsule. (Reproduced with permission from Schuenke M, Schulte E, Schumacher U. THIEME Atlas of Anatomy Second Edition, Vol 3. © Thieme 2016. Illustrations by Markus Voll and Karl Wesker.)

Table 12.4 Summary of receptors for anterolateral pathway

Nerve Type Sensory Receptor	Letter	Roman Numeral	Modality	Location	Primary Pathway	Conduction Velocity	Axon Diameter
Lightly myelinated free nerve endings: • Nociceptors (intense mechanical/ mechano-thermal) • Thermoreceptor • Hair follicle mechanoreceptor • Visceral receptors	Aδ	Type III	Sharp fast pain Cold	Skin Visceral walls	Direct ALS Lateral funiculus (neospinothalamic)	5–30 m/sec	Small 2–5 μm
Unmyelinated Free nerve endings • Nociceptor (include polymodal) • Thermoreceptors • Visceral receptors	C fiber	Type IV	Dull, slow pain Warm Crude touch	Skin Muscles Joints Viscera	Indirect ALS Anterior funiculus (paleospinothalamic) (archispinothalamic)	Slow 0.5–2 m/sec	Small <1.5 μm

Abbreviation: ALS, anterolateral system.

branches synapsing first on interneurons in the proper sensory nucleus in Lamina III.

- In addition to contributing to ascending pathways, Aδ fibers form intersegmental spinal reflexes such as the **nociceptive (withdrawal) reflex.** The withdrawal reflex is considered a **polysynaptic reflex arch** since the Aδ fibers synapse on interneurons at several spinal levels. The interneurons in turn send fibers to somatic motor neurons in the ventral horn (Lamina IX) to elicit the reflexive motor response (see Chapter 15 for details).

- Axons from second-order neurons **decussate** in the **anterior white commissure** of the spinal cord and ascend contralaterally in the lateral funiculus as the **lateral spinothalamic tract** of the ALS. The lateral spinothalamic tract follows a direct path to the thalamus and is also known as **neospinothalamic tract**.
  - Ascending fibers exhibit a somatotopic arrangement such that fibers from the **lumbosacral** region ascend in the **lateral** (most external) part of the spinothalamic tract, while fibers from the **thoracocervical** spinal segments ascend in the **medial** portion of the tract.
  - The somatotopic organizations is of clinical significance when considering the region first affected by compression lesions of the spinal cord.

- Contralateral afferent fibers of the **spinothalamic tract** project directly to the thalamus and synapse on third-order neurons in the **VPL nucleus** of the thalamus.
  - A few collateral branches from the spinothalamic tract project to other thalamic nuclei, including the intralaminar thalamic nuclei and mediodorsal nuclei. These fibers along with fibers of indirect pathway convey the emotional aspects of noxious stimuli and terminate in the insular cortex and anterior cingulate gyrus of the cerebral cortex.

- Third-order axons project somatotopically through the **posterior limb** of the **internal thalamic capsule** to terminate in the **primary somatosensory cortex (S1)** in the postcentral gyrus (Brodmann's areas 3a, 3b, 2, and 1).
  - Pain and temperature sensations conveyed by the direct lateral spinothalamic tract to the primary somatosensory

cortex are well localized, and the pain is perceived as sharp, pricking, and of short duration.

12.3.3 Indirect Pathways of the Anterolateral System

- Unmyelinated, polymodal (wide-dynamic range), nociceptive C fibers which primarily respond to high intensity mechanical, thermal, or chemical stimuli primarily contribute to the indirect anterolateral pathway.
  - The indirect paths are also known as the **paleospinothalamic** and **archispinothalamic tracts**, and encompass several multisynaptic pathways, including the anterior spinothalamic, the spinomesencephalic, the spinotectal, and the spinoreticular tracts.
  - The different paths ascend to higher brain regions in the anterior funiculus, adjacent to the lateral spinothalamic tract in the anterolateral quadrant.
  - Each tract synapses at different locations and functions to modulate pain, integrate autonomic and reflexive movements, and provide the affective and emotional component to pain. The pathways are briefly described below and summarized in ▶ Table 12.7.

- **Anterior spinothalamic tract**
  - The anterior spinothalamic tract is part of the paleospinothalmic tract.
  - Unmyelinated C fibers of first-order neurons carrying nociceptive, crude touch, and warm temperature sensations primarily synapse on second-order neurons in Lamina II (substantia gelatinosa). The second-order neurons may synapse diffusely in Laminae III to VII.
  - Afferent fibers decussate in the anterior commissure and ascend bilaterally in the anterior funiculus of the anterolateral quadrant.
  - The majority of the afferent fibers ascending in the anterior paleospinothalamic and archispinothalamic tract projects to the intralaminar nuclei of the thalamus;

Table 12.5 Comparative summary of the direct and indirect anterolateral pathways

	Direct ALS Pathway (Conscious)	Indirect ALS Pathway (Unconscious)
Name of pathways	Direct path—conveys 15% of nociceptive input One path recognized **Neospinothalamic** (lateral spinothalamic) Secondary afferents project: • Directly to thalamus (VPL)	Indirect path—conveys 85% of nociceptive input Two paths recognized **Paleospinothalamic** Secondary afferents project to intralmainar thalamic nuclei via anterior spinothalamic Secondary afferents project to reticular formation → intralaminar thalamic nuclei via: • Spinoreticular • Spinomesencephalic • Spinotectal **Archiospinothalamic** Secondary afferents projects to: • Medullary reticular formation • Periaqueductal gray
Receptor	Nonencapsulated, mechanical nociceptor Thermal nociceptors	Nonencapsulated, polymodal nociceptor (respond to chemical, mechanical, thermal)
Types of fibers	Thinly myelinated Aδ fibers	Polymodal unmyelinated C fibers
Stimuli	Intense mechanical, mechanothermal stimuli occurring at initial point of injury	Chemical, mechanical, and thermal stimuli resulting from inflammation or tissue damage following injury
Sensory modality	Fast, sharp, acute, localized sensations Pain Crude touch Cold	Slow, dull, chronic, poorly localized sensations Pain Some crude touch Warm
First-order neurons	Dorsal root ganglia	Dorsal root ganglia
Entry zone to spinal cord	Lateral division of dorsal root	Lateral division of dorsal root
Tract of primary afferent fibers	Dorsolateral tract of Lissauer	Dorsolateral tract of Lissauer
Second-order neurons	Rexed laminae I and V some Lamina II	Rexed lamina II—diffuse synaptic connections to laminae III, V, and VI–VIII
Point of decussation	Anterior white commissure of spinal cord (contralateral input)	Anterior white commissure of spinal cord for crossed contains also uncrossed (bilateral input—crossed and uncrossed)
Ascending tract in spinal cord	Anterolateral column in spinal lemniscus: Somatotopic arrangement of fibers in tract: lumbosacral fibers lie lateral thoracocervical fibers lie medial	Anterolateral column in spinal lemniscus
Third-order neurons	Contralateral thalamic VPL nuclei	• Periaqueductal gray • Superior colliculus of tectum • Spinal cord reticular formation • Medullary reticular formation • Mesencephalic reticular formation • Intralaminar nuclei of thalamus May project to higher centers
Termination point	Primary somatosensory cortex of postcentral gyrus (Brodmann's areas 3b, 3a, 1, and 2) *Receives input from VPL of thalamus *Somatotopic organization	Intralaminar thalamic nuclei → cortex Limbic • Insular cortex • Anterior cingulate gyrus Hypothalamus *Receive input from third-order neurons and intralaminar nuclei *No somatotopic organization
Function	Conscious processing and precise localization/intensity of stimuli, integration of input	• Affective-motivational processing (fear, anger, depression) • Increased alertness to painful stimuli • Pain modulation • Reflex to turn toward stimuli • Autonomic and reflexive responses

Abbreviations: ALS, anterolateral system; VPL, ventral posterolateral.

Table 12.6 Summary of the direct anterolateral pathway: conscious path

Direct Pathway (Pathway Name) Location in Spinal Cord	Fiber Type	Location of First-Order Neurons	Location of Second-Order Neurons Rexed Laminae	Termination	Function
Neospinothalamic tract/ Anterolateral spinothalamic tract Located: Anterolateral funiculus of spinal cord	Thinly myelinated Aδ fiber Thermal (cool), some crude touch Sharp, acute pain	Dorsal root ganglia	Synapse on second-order neurons Laminae I and V (some II) Decussate anterior white commissure Ascend in contralateral anterolateral funiculus of spinal cord	Ventral posterolateral nucleus of thalamus → primary somatosensory cortex Brodmann's areas 3, 2, and 1 Somatotopically arranged	Conscious processing and precise localization/intensity of stimuli Perceived sensations well localized, sharp, short duration

Table 12.7 Summary of indirect pathways of anterolateral system: unconscious path

Indirect Pathway (Pathway Name) Located in Anterolateral Funiculus	Fiber Type	Location of First-Order Neuron	Location of Second-Order Neuron Dorsal Horn (Rexed Laminae)	Termination *Multisynapses	Pathway Function
Spinothalamic (anterior) *Crossed and uncrossed	Polymodal unmyelinated C fibers	Dorsal root ganglion	Lamina II interneurons → Laminae IV–VII	Intralaminar nucleus of thalamus → insula and cingulate gyrus →secondary somatosensory cortex	Processing of emotional aspects of pain Perception of diffuse, poorly localized, chronic sensations: Pain (slow, dull) Warm temperatures Crude touch
Spinoreticular *Primarily uncrossed fibers	Polymodal unmyelinated C fibers	Dorsal root ganglion	Lamina II interneurons → Laminae IV–VII	Medullary and pontine reticular formation → intralaminar nucleus of thalamus	Increased alertness to painful stimuli
Spinomesencephalic *Crossed and uncrossed fibers	Polymodal unmyelinated C fibers	Dorsal root ganglion	Laminae II and V; some interneurons of II → Laminae IV–VII	Periaqueductal gray (of midbrain tegmentum)	Feedback to regulate pain from spinal cord; involved in descending pain modulation/inhibition via descending fibers
Spinotectal tract	Polymodal unmyelinated C fibers	Dorsal root ganglion	Lamina I and some II → Laminae IV–VII	Superior colliculus of tectum→ visual reflex pathway	Facilitates reflexive movement of head/eyes toward stimuli
Spinohypothalamic tract	Polymodal unmyelinated C fibers	Dorsal root ganglion	Laminae II and IV–VII	Hypothalamus	Autonomic and reflexive response associated with GSA and GVA input

Abbreviations: GSA, general somatic afferent; GVA, general visceral afferent.
Note: *Collaterals from direct (spinothalamic) pathway also contribute to indirect pathway.

however, some fibers also project to periaqueductal gray, mesencephalic reticular formation, and other locations.

  ○ Fibers project from the intralaminar nuclei to terminate in the insula and rostral cingulate gyrus. The diffuse termination of nociceptive input to the cerebral cortex allows for the continued perception of pain following damage to the primary somatosensory cortex and contributes to the poor localization of painful stimuli.

- **Spinomesencephalic tract**
  ○ Primary afferent C fibers that contribute to the **spinomesencephalic tract** synapse on second-order neurons found primarily in Lamina II. Diffuse projections from Lamina II end in Laminae IV to VII.

  ○ Secondary afferent fibers decussate in the anterior commissure and ascend as the **spinomesencephalic tract** (► Fig. 12.9).

  ○ Fibers of the spinomesencephalic tract divide into two groups: one group of fibers projects to the **superior colliculus of the midbrain tectum** to form the **spinotectal tract**, while the remaining fibers of the **spinomesencephalic tract** project to the **periaqueductal region of the midbrain.**

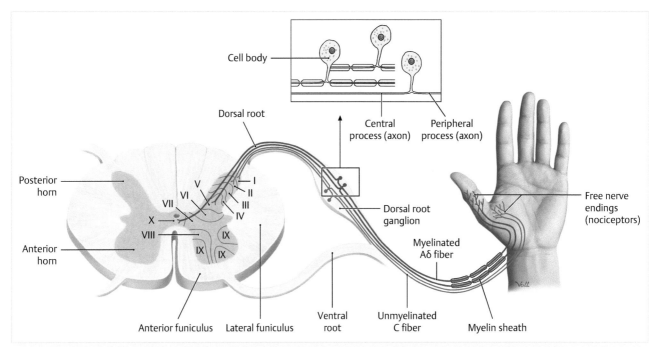

Fig. 12.6 Transmission of somatic pain conduction through the ALS. (Adapted from Lorke.)
Several types of noxious stimuli, including mechanical, chemical, and thermal input can activate peripheral nociceptors and alert the body of potential tissue damage. The transmission of somatic pain impulses occurs from the trunk and limbs by myelinated Aδ fibers and unmyelinated C fibers. The fiber diameter and the extent of myelination determine the speed of signal transmission. The cell bodies (pseudounipolar neurons) of these primary afferent nerve fibers reside in the dorsal root ganglion. The primary afferent axons enter the lateral part of the dorsal axons to synapse on second-order neurons in the Rexed lamina I, II, or V. After synapsing, the afferent fibers carrying nociceptive input decussate and follow one of the anterolateral pathways located in the anterior and lateral funiculi of the spinal cord and ascend to higher brain centers. Secondary axons associated with Aδ fibers ascend in the lateral funiculus and comprise the direct (neospinothalamic) lateral spinothalamic tract. The direct path terminates in the somatosensory cortex and consciously processes sharp, well-localized pain and cool temperatures. Secondary afferents associated with unmyelinated C fibers ascend in the anterior funiculus and convey crude touch and slow, dull pain. Input carried by C fibers follow the indirect pathways and terminate in other higher brain regions. ALS, anterolateral system. (Reproduced with permission from Schuenke M, Schulte E, Schumacher U. THIEME Atlas of Anatomy Second Edition, Vol 3. © Thieme 2016. Illustrations by Markus Voll and Karl Wesker.)

○ The **spinotectal tract** elicits a reflexive action to orient the head and eyes toward the painful stimuli, whereas the **spinomesencephalic tract** plays a role in modulating pain. The mechanisms of pain modulation are covered in Chapter 14.

- **Spinoreticular tract**
  ○ The spinoreticular tract, which transmits poorly localized, dull, aching pain, alerts the body and increases its awareness of painful stimuli.
  ○ Polymodal C fibers of the indirect **spinoreticular tract** initially synapse on interneurons in Lamina II (substantia gelatinosa) and then terminate on second-order neurons found in Rexed laminae IV to VII. Secondary afferent fibers ascend **bilaterally** in the ALS as the **spinoreticular tract**.
  ○ The fibers of the spinoreticular tract synapse on **third-order neurons** in the **reticular formation** of the medulla and pons. The **reticular formation** is a set of interconnected nuclei that are located throughout the brainstem and mediate several functions, including **arousal** and increased **attention.**
  ○ Fibers from the medullary-pontine reticular formation send axons, known as **reticulothalamic fibers,** to terminate mainly in the **intralaminar thalamic nuclei** (central lateral thalamic nucleus).
  ○ The intralaminar nuclei, which also receive some collateral fibers from the anterior spinothalamic tract, send axons to areas associated with the cortical limbic system, specifically the insular cortex and the anterior cingulate gyrus.

- **Spinohypothalamic tract**
  ○ The fibers of the spinohypothalamic tract project to the hypothalamus. The hypothalamus functions to integrate autonomic and reflexive responses associated with painful stimuli.

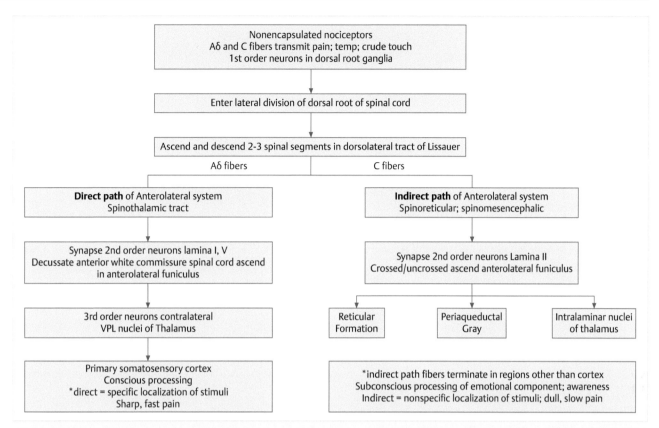

Fig. 12.7 Schematic comparison of the direct and indirect nociceptive pathways of the ALS. The direct and indirect paths of the ALS both contain first-order neurons in the dorsal root ganglion that enter the lateral part of the dorsal horn and may ascend or descend two to three levels in Lissauer's tract before synapsing on second-order neurons in the Rexed lamina I, II, or V. Afferent fibers decussate at the point of synapse and then ascend in the lateral and anterior funiculi of the spinal cord to terminate in different areas of the CNS. Points of termination include the primary somatosensory cortex, insular cortex, hypothalamus, thalamus, periaqueductal gray, and reticular formation. The direct path exhibits a somatotopic arrangement and ascends contralaterally to terminate primarily in the primary somatosensory cortex. Conversely, the indirect path provides bilateral input to the intralaminar thalamus which projects to diffuse areas of the cortex and results in a poorly localized sense of pain. Additional fibers that follow the indirect path terminate in higher brain regions that play a role in the emotional processing and modulation of pain. Differences in the types of afferent fibers, the pathway followed, and the points of termination reflect differences in the ability to precisely localize stimuli and whether the pain perceived is sharp or dull. ALS, anterolateral system; CNS, central nervous system.

Clinical Correlation Box 12.1: Lesions of the Anterolateral System

- Damage to the spinal cord may result from numerous causes and depending on the location of the lesion may impact one or more sensory and motor tracts. In general damage to the ALS may occur due to lateral compression injuries of the spinal cord such as that associated with tumors in the surrounding meninges (**meningioma**), or from tumors originating within the spinal cord. Expansion of the central canal, a disease, known as **syringomyelia**, may also impact the ALS. Expansion of the central cord will compress secondary afferent fibers as they decussate in the anterior white commissure.
  - Lesions compressing one side of the spinal cord will result in contralateral loss of pain and temperature one to two levels below the level of the lesions.
  - Lesions occurring due to expansion of the central canal (Syringomyelia) and subsequent destruction of the anterior white commissure fibers will result in bilateral loss of pain and temperature at the level of the lesions.
- The Aδ fibers (fast pain) of the direct path enter the dorsal horn along with the C fibers which mediate slow pain. The secondary

afferent fibers of both paths ascend together through the spinal cord. However, the two paths diverge from each other in the brainstem. Fast pain ascends in the spinothalamic tract which is laterally located in the brainstem, whereas slow pain fibers, which follow the indirect route to the reticular formation, ascends more medially. Clinically, the divergence of the direct and indirect paths impacts the type of pain lost because of a brainstem lesion. The region of the brainstem which contains sensory and motor nuclei of the head may also be affected and contribute to the clinical picture. The path for somatosensory input from the head follows a comparable route and will be discussed in Chapter 13.
  - Lateral compression in the spinal cord results in a contralateral loss of fast and slow pain in the region caudal to the injury. In comparison, lateral compression or damage to the brainstem will cause a contralateral loss or decreased sensitivity of fast pain which travels in the anterolateral region of the spinal cord, but slow pain which projects medially to the reticular formation will remain intact.

12.4 Dorsal Column-Medial Lemniscus (DCML) Pathway

12.4.1 Functional Overview of DCML

- The DCML transmits mechanoreceptive and proprioceptive sensations from tactile mechanoreceptors, muscle spindles, and Golgi tendon organs to the primary somatosensory cortex for conscious processing.
- The DCML pathway permits the ability to discriminate between two closely spaced mechanical stimuli (**two-point discrimination**), the capability to distinguish between shapes and textures of objects (**stereognosis**), and functions to provide conscious awareness and feedback about body position during dynamic movements (**kinesthetic**) and at rest (**static proprioception).**
- Proprioceptive and mechanoreceptive neurons associated with the DCML propagate sensory input from tactile mechanoreceptors, joint receptors, muscle spindles, and Golgi tendon organs, through myelinated Aβ (Type II) fibers, Type Ia fibers, and Type IIb afferent fibers, respectively (▶ Table 12.8).

12.4.2 DCML Pathway (▶ Fig. 12.10, ▶ Table 12.8)

- The cell bodies of first-order proprioceptive and mechanoreceptive sensory neurons reside in the dorsal root ganglia at all levels. Large, myelinated fibers (Type II, Aβ fiber; Type Ia; and Type IIb, Aα fiber) of primary afferent neurons project from peripheral receptors and enter the medial part of the dorsal root of the spinal cord in a somatotopic arrangement.
- Most of these primary afferent fibers coalesce to form **fasciculi (tracts)** which ascend **ipsilaterally** within the **dorsal column (funiculus)** of the spinal cord to synapse on **second-order neurons** found in the **dorsal column nuclei** of the **caudal medulla**.
  - Type Ia and Type IIb afferent fibers that arise from muscle spindles and Golgi tendon organs, respectively, enter the gray matter of the spinal cord, project to Rexed lamina IX, and synapse on motor neurons as part of monosynaptic reflexive responses. These reflexes include the **myotatic stretch reflex** involving muscle spindles and the **inhibitory stretch reflex** (or **Golgi tendon reflex**). These reflexes work cooperatively to control muscle length, tone, and tension (see Chapter 16).
  - Other collateral branches carry proprioceptive fibers and enter the dorsal horn to synapse on interneurons in the **proper sensory nucleus** (**Rexed laminae III and IV**) or on neurons in **Clarke's nucleus** (**Rexed lamina VII**). Postsynaptic proprioceptive input joins ascending fibers of the dorsal column. Some of the fibers may project to the cerebellum as the **dorsal spinocerebellar tract** for unconscious processing of proprioceptive input.
- Based on the vertebral level at which the afferent fibers enter the spinal cord, the dorsal column (funiculus) may consist of two fasciculi (tracts).

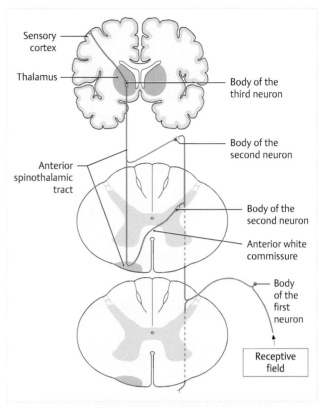

Fig. 12.8 The conscious spinothalamic tracts and their central connections. Afferent fibers of the anterolateral system (ALS) pathways travel in the lateral and anterior funiculi (shown) and represent a three-neuron relay chain that serves as the main pathway for transmitting conscious pain, temperature, and crude touch from the trunk and limbs. Secondary afferent fibers decussate and then ascend to contralateral neurons in the ventral posterolateral (VPL) of the thalamus and the primary somatosensory cortex for conscious processing. The primary somatosensory cortex plays an important role in the conscious perception of pain, along with determining the intensity and the specific location of painful stimuli. Additional collateral paths of ALS that travel in the indirect spinothalamic tracts also provide input to other higher brain regions (not shown) that function in modulation and mediate visceral, autonomic, and emotional reactions to pain. (Reproduced with permission from Schuenke M, Schulte E, Schumacher U. THIEME Atlas of Anatomy Second Edition, Vol 3. © Thieme 2016. Illustrations by Markus Voll and Karl Wesker.)

  - In the **lower portion of the cord (below T6)**, the dorsal columns on each side consist of a single fiber tract known as the **gracile fasciculus**. Fibers in the gracile fasciculus enter from the lower limb and trunk to ascend in the medial portion of the dorsal column.
  - In the region **above the sixth thoracic (T6) level**, primary afferent fibers that originate from the upper limb and all cervical levels form another ascending tract, the **cuneate fasciculus.** The cuneate fasciculus ascends within the dorsal column lateral to the gracile fasciculus.
  - The somatotopic arrangement of fibers as they ascend within the gracile and cuneate fasciculi of the dorsal column is clinically important when considering lesions of the spinal cord.
- Fibers of the gracile and cuneate fasciculi synapse ipsilaterally in the caudal medulla on second-order neurons

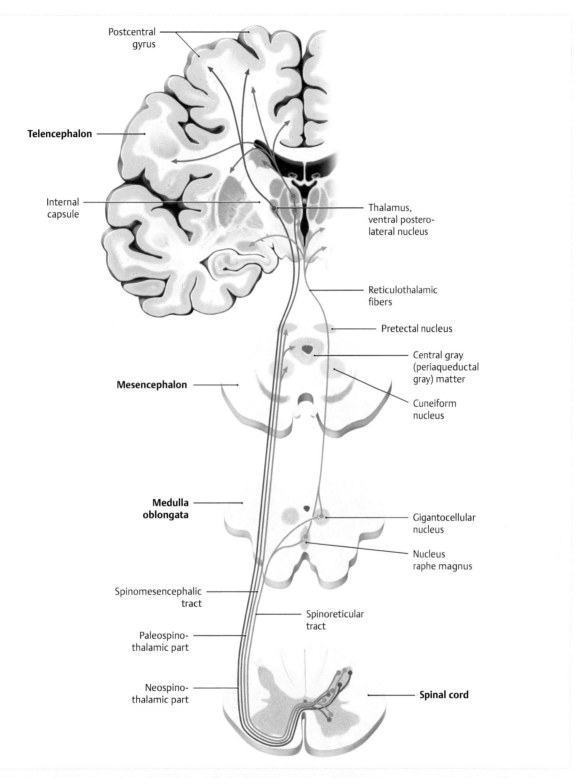

Postcentral gyrus

Telencephalon

Internal capsule

Thalamus, ventral postero-lateral nucleus

Reticulothalamic fibers

Pretectal nucleus

Central gray (periaqueductal gray) matter

Mesencephalon

Cuneiform nucleus

Medulla oblongata

Gigantocellular nucleus

Nucleus raphe magnus

Spinomesencephalic tract

Spinoreticular tract

Paleospino-thalamic part

Neospino-thalamic part

Spinal cord

Fig. 12.9 Ascending pain pathways from the trunk and limbs. Collectively, the tracts that convey pain, temperature, and crude touch from the body are also known as the anterolateral system and encompass several multisynaptic tracts. The anterolateral system includes the direct neospinothalamic tract as well as several indirect paths. The direct path projects through the lateral funiculus to the contralateral VPL of the thalamus and terminates in the primary somatosensory cortex for conscious processing, while the indirect paths terminate in other cortical areas or subcortical regions. The indirect paths are also known as the paleospinothalamic and archispinothalamic tracts. Afferent fibers of the indirect paleospinothalamic tract travel in the anterior funiculus with the direct fibers of the lateral spinothalamic tract to the thalamus, where the fibers of the indirect path synapse in the intralaminar nuclei and then project to diffuse cortical regions including the insula and cingulate gyrus. The nociceptive input from the indirect paleospinothalamic tract is perceived as dull, poorly localized pain. The archispinothalamic path includes spinomesencephalic, spinoreticular, and several smaller pathways that follow the direct pathway a short distance before terminating in the reticular formation (gigantocellular and nucleus raphe of reticular formation are shown), the periaqueductal gray area of the brainstem, the hypothalamus, or the limbic system. These pathways modulate pain, integrate autonomic and reflexive movements, and provide the affective and emotional component to pain. VPL, ventral posterolateral. (Reproduced with permission from Schuenke M, Schulte E, Schumacher U. THIEME Atlas of Anatomy Second Edition, Vol 3. © Thieme 2016. Illustrations by Markus Voll and Karl Wesker.)

Table 12.8 Summary of receptors for dorsal column-medial lemniscus pathway

Nerve Type Sensory Axon	Modality	Receptor	Location	Roman Numeral	Letter	Conduction Velocity	Axon Diameter
Myelinated, low threshold Encapsulated Proprioceptor Kinesthetic	Muscle stretch Detects movement	Muscle spindle (neuromuscular spindle) Annulospiral ending	Muscle	Type Ia	Aα	Fast 70–120 m/sec	Large 12–20 μm
Myelinated, low threshold Encapsulated Proprioceptor	Muscle tension Static position	Golgi tendon organ (neurotendinous spindle)	Joints Tendons	Type Ib	Aα	Fast 70–120 m/sec	Large 12–20 μm
Myelinated, low threshold Encapsulated mechanoreceptor	Vibratory movement Stretch Discriminative touch Stereognosis Pressure Static position Stretch of muscle	Pacinian Ruffini Meissner Merkel Muscle spindle Flower spray ending	Skin Joints Muscle Viscera	Type II	Aβ	Fast 30–70 m/sec	Medium 6–12 μm

of the **nucleus gracilis** and **nucleus cuneatus**, respectively. Collectively, both nuclei comprise the **dorsal column nuclei**.

- The second-order axons, referred to as **internal arcuate fibers,** decussate to form the **medial lemniscus** (ribbon), a **contralateral axonal tract**, which ascends through the brainstem. Fibers in the medial lemniscus ascend contralaterally to synapse on **third-order neurons** in the **VPL nucleus** of the **thalamus.**

- Fibers from VPL neurons project through the **posterior limb** of the **internal capsule** of the thalamus to terminate principally in the **primary somatosensory cortex** found in the **postcentral gyrus** of the **parietal lobe.**
- Mechanosensory input from the thalamus and primary somatosensory cortex may also project through **cortical association neurons** to the **secondary somatosensory cortex** and **posterior parietal cortex.**

Clinical Correlation Box 12.2: Lesion of the Dorsal Column-Medial Lemniscus Path

Lesions may occur at any point as fibers in the dorsal column and medial lemniscus ascend to the cortex. Lesions affecting the dorsal column will vary based on the level at which they occur in the spinal cord but will be ipsilateral to the side of the lesions. Lesions involving the medial lemniscus will result in contralateral sensory deficits because of the decussation of the fibers in the lower medulla.

The **fasciculus gracilis**, which is found at all levels of the spinal cord, carries information from the **lower body, limbs,** and T6–T12.

- Lesions will result in an ipsilateral loss of fine touch, pressure, and vibratory sensation, and conscious proprioception from the lower body and limbs at the level of the lesions; Sensory ataxia is also common due to loss of proprioceptive input to the lower limbs.

The **fasciculus cuneatus,** which is found at levels **T6–C2,** carries tactile and conscious proprioceptive information from the upper body and upper extremity.

- Lesions will result in an ipsilateral loss of fine touch, pressure and vibratory sensation, and conscious proprioception from the lower body and limbs at the level of the lesion and below.

The **medial lemniscus** is formed by secondary afferent fibers arising from the dorsal column nuclei. The fibers decussate as the internal arcuate fibers in the lower medulla and continue to ascend medially within the brainstem.

- Lesions or a tumor compressing the dorsal column at any point above the decussation will result in the **contralateral** loss of two-point discrimination and conscious proprioceptive input. Sensory ataxia and an inability to detect the shape and texture (astereognosis), along with swaying of the body when standing with closed eyes (**Romberg's test**), are hallmark features.

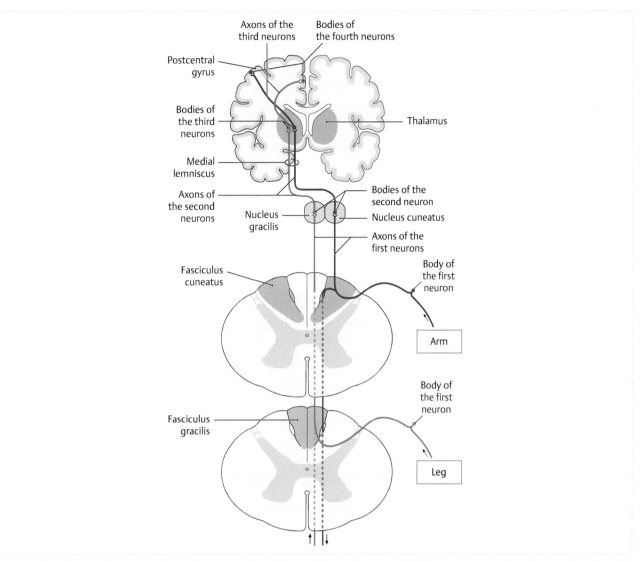

Fig. 12.10 Fasciculi gracilis and cuneatus and their central connections. The dorsal column-medial lemniscus represents primarily a three-neuron relay chain that serves as the main pathway for transmitting conscious proprioceptive input and discriminative touch from the trunk and limbs to contralateral neurons in the ventral posterolateral (VPL) of the thalamus and the primary somatosensory cortex for conscious processing. Primary afferent fibers arise from pseudounipolar neurons in the dorsal root ganglion, enter the dorsal horn of the spinal cord, and ascend ipsilaterally in the fasciculi gracilis and cuneatus of the dorsal column to synapse in the nuclei gracilis and cuneatus in the medulla. Decussation occurs at the level of the synapse in the medulla. The secondary afferents form the medial lemniscus. (Reproduced with permission from Schuenke M, Schulte E, Schumacher U. THIEME Atlas of Anatomy Second Edition, Vol 3. © Thieme 2016. Illustrations by Markus Voll and Karl Wesker.)

Table 12.9 Comparison of spinocerebellar pathways

Pathway	Receptors	Modality	First-Order Neuron	Second-Order Neuron	Location of Pathway in Spinal Cord	Terminate	Function
Dorsal (posterior) spinocerebellar	Muscle spindles (Type Ia) Golgi tendon organs (Type Ib) Joint receptors (Aβ, Type II)	Unconscious proprioception of lower limb and trunk (C8–L3) *Fibers below L3 must ascend and then synapse in nucleus dorsalis	Dorsal root ganglion	Synapse on dorsal horn—nucleus dorsalis/Clarke's nucleus	Lateral funiculus Uncrossed path	Ipsilateral cerebellum	Conveys input about individual muscle movement Postural maintenance Smooth coordination of motor movements
Cuneocerebellar	Muscle spindles (Type Ia) Golgi tendon organs (Type Ib) Joint receptors (Aβ, Type II)	Unconscious proprioception of upper extremity and neck (C2–T6)	Dorsal root ganglion	Synapse on accessory cuneate nucleus	Lateral funiculus Uncrossed path	Ipsilateral cerebellum	Provides input from upper limb Smooth coordination of motor movements
Ventral (anterior) spinocerebellar	Muscle spindles (Type Ia) Golgi tendon organs (Type Ib) Joint receptors (Aβ, Type II)	Unconscious proprioception of lower extremity (L1–L3)	Dorsal root ganglion	Synapse on doral horn intermediate gray column	Lateral funiculus Double crossed path	Ipsilateral cerebellum	Mediate reflex activity Provide input about the level of activity of spinal cord interneurons for proper coordination of motor movements

12.5 Spinocerebellar System (▶ Table 12.9)

- Most proprioceptive information from Golgi tendon organs, muscle spindles, and joint receptors is not transmitted to the cerebral cortex for conscious processing, but rather is transmitted directly to the **cerebellum** via the ascending **spinocerebellar pathways**.
- The pathways include the **dorsal spinocerebellar tract**, the **cuneocerebellar tract**, the **ventral spinocerebellar tract**, and the **rostral spinocerebellar tract** (▶ Table 12.9).
  - The dorsal spinocerebellar and ventral spinocerebellar tracts convey unconscious proprioceptive input from the lower extremity, while the cuneocerebellar and rostral spinocerebellar tracts convey input from the upper limb and neck.
  - Collectively, these tracts relay information concerning muscle tone, tension, length, and limb position to the cerebellum. Based on incoming signals the cerebellum functions to maintain posture, coordinate movement, and regulate muscle tone (see Chapter 17).
- Several notable differences exist between the unconscious spinocerebellar pathways and the conscious proprioceptive pathways.
  - The **unconscious** spinocerebellar pathways terminate in the **cerebellum** and represent a **two-neuron relay path**: consisting

of first-order neurons found in the dorsal root ganglia and second-order neurons found in the spinal cord or medulla.
  - In comparison, the **conscious** sensory pathways involve a **three-neuron chain** and terminate in the **cerebral cortex**.
  - The dorsal spinocerebellar, cuneocerebellar, and rostral spinocerebellar pathways represent **uncrossed tracts**. The primary afferent fibers synapse on second-order neurons but do not decussate. Fibers ascend ipsilaterally to terminate on the same side of the cerebellum from which the primary fibers entered. The ventral spinocerebellar tract also processes sensory input on the **ipsilateral side** of the cerebellum. However, fibers in the ventral pathway **decussate twice** such that information that enters on one side of the spinal cord terminates in the cerebellum on the same side of the origin.
    - In comparison, **conscious proprioceptive pathways decussate** resulting in **contralateral** processing of the information in the cerebral cortex.
  - In general, cerebellar lesions produce an ipsilateral loss, whereas cerebral lesions result in contralateral deficits.
- An overview of the spinocerebellar pathways involved in mediating unconscious proprioception is depicted in ▶ Fig. 12.11 and ▶ Fig. 12.12. A detailed description of each path is provided in Chapter 17.

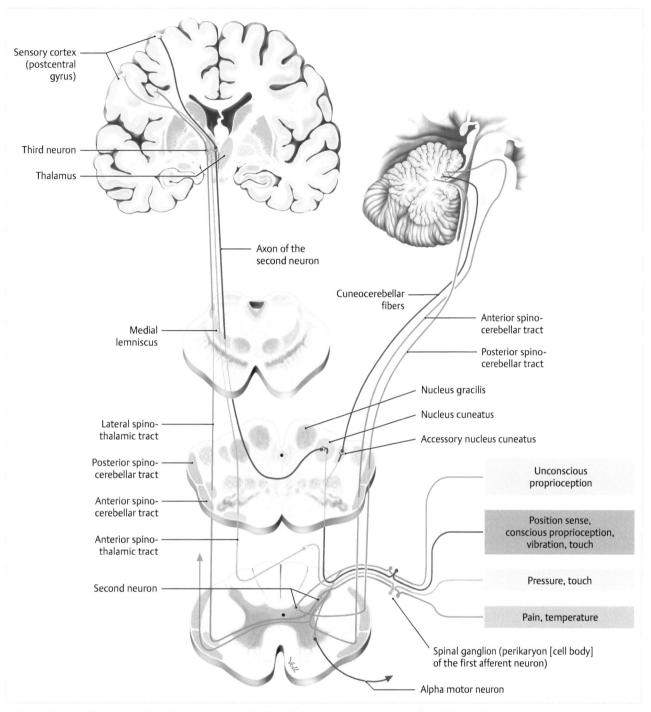

Fig. 12.11 A simplified schematic of the conscious and unconscious somatosensory pathways. Stimuli generate impulses in various receptors in the periphery of the body which are transmitted to the cerebrum and cerebellum along the sensory (afferent) pathways or tracts as shown. (Reproduced with permission from Schuenke M, Schulte E, Schumacher U. THIEME Atlas of Anatomy Second Edition, Vol 3. © Thieme 2016. Illustrations by Markus Voll and Karl Wesker.)

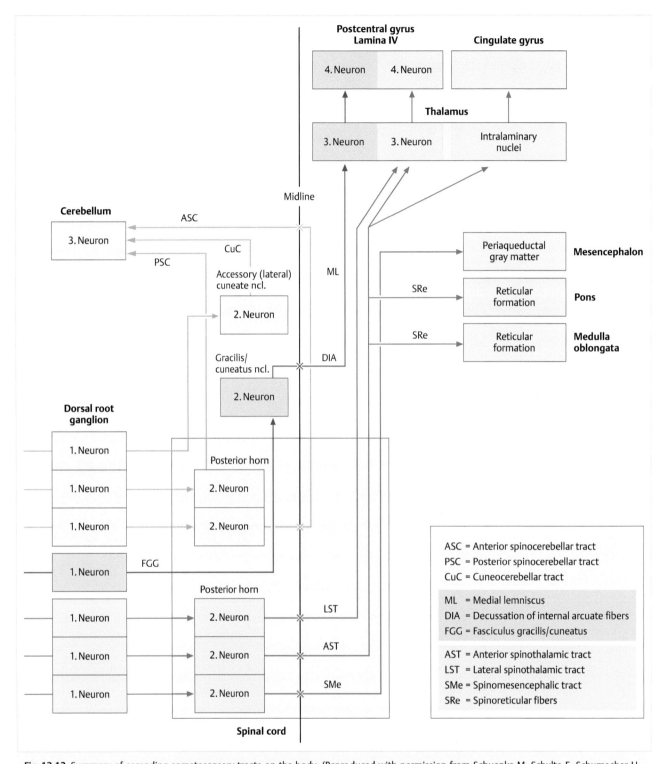

Fig. 12.12 Summary of ascending somatosensory tracts on the body. (Reproduced with permission from Schuenke M, Schulte E, Schumacher U. THIEME Atlas of Anatomy Second Edition, Vol 3. © Thieme 2016. Illustrations by Markus Voll and Karl Wesker.)

Questions and Answers

1. The tract which carries tactile, discriminative, pressure, and vibration sensations along with conscious proprioception for the upper body is the _____.
   a) fasciculus cuneatus
   b) cuneocerebellar tract
   c) dorsal spinocerebellar tract
   d) fasciculus gracilis

Level 1: Easy

Answer A: The fasciculus cuneatus transmits the sensory modalities of tactile and conscious proprioception for the region corresponding to the T6 thoracic and cervical levels. The fasciculus gracilis (**D**) transmits the same information for the lower body. The dorsal spinocerebellar (**C**) and cuneocerebellar (**B**) tracts convey unconscious proprioception for the lower and upper body, respectively. The dorsal spinocerebellar carries proprioceptive input from the lower body (S5–T1), while the cuneocerebellar carries input from C8–C2. Both fibers of the tract project to the cerebellum via the inferior peduncle.

2. The sensory fibers associated with the transmission of sharp, fast pain that travel in the direct spinothalamic tract are the _____.
   a) Aδ fibers
   b) Aβ fibers
   c) Aα (Type Ia) fibers
   d) C fibers

Level 1: Easy

Answer A: The Aδ fibers are lightly myelinated fibers that are primarily associated with the spinothalamic tract and mediate sharp fast pain. The fibers are associated with free nerve endings and synapse in Laminae I and II of the spinal cord. (**C**) Heavily myelinated Aα (Type Ia) fibers and Aβ fibers (**B**) convey proprioceptive and discriminative tactile sensations. C fibers (**D**) transmit pain and temperature, but usually follow the indirect ALS paths, which project in a diffuse manner to the cerebral cortex and are therefore associated with diffuse, poorly localized painful sensations.

3. The first-order neurons of ventral spinocerebellar tract _____.
   a) reside in the dorsal root ganglia at all spinal levels
   b) ascend in the tract of Lissauer
   c) decussate to form the medial lemniscus
   d) enter the dorsal root through medial portion

Level 2: Moderate

Answer D: The first-order neurons of the ventral spinocerebellar tract are proprioceptive neurons that send Aβ fibers to enter the spinal cord through the medial part of the dorsal root. The fibers, which carry unconscious proprioceptive input from Golgi tendon organs and muscle spindles, enter at L5–T12 and synapse on spinal border cells before decussating to ascend in the ventral spinocerebellar tract in the anterior funiculus. (**A**) Small, unmyelinated C fibers and lightly myelinated Aδ fibers from the primary afferent neurons enter through the lateral portion of the dorsal root. The tract of Lissauer (**B**) contains ipsilateral Aδ and C fibers that will synapse on second-order neurons in the dorsal horn. These fibers contribute to the spinothalamic tract. The first-order neurons are found in the ganglia at spinal levels L1–S2, and not distributed throughout all levels. (**C**) The secondary afferent fibers of the dorsal column decussate to form medial lemniscus.

4. The tract which conveys nociceptive input from the contralateral side of the body is the _____.
   a) fasciculus cuneatus
   b) tract of Lissauer
   c) spinothalamic tract
   d) dorsal spinocerebellar tract

Level 2: Moderate

Answer C: The spinothalamic tract conveys nociceptive information from the *contralateral* body. The fibers carried in the spinothalamic tract decussates immediately after synapsing of second-order neurons in the dorsal horn and the sensation of pain is processed and perceived by the contralateral side of the primary somatosensory cortex. The nociceptive fibers in the tract of Lissauer (**B**) are primary afferent fibers that have not synapsed on second-order neurons and have not decussated at the anterior white commissure. Therefore, the tract of Lissauer is associated with ipsilateral nociceptive fibers. The other tracts convey other sensory modalities. (**A**) Fasciculus cuneatus transmits tactile and proprioceptive input from the head and trunk (T6–C1) while the (**D**) the dorsal spinocerebellar tract carries proprioceptive input from the lower limbs and trunk (S5–T1).

5. A recent magnetic resonance imaging (MRI) of your 46-year-old patient reveals *lateral* compression from a meningioma pressing on the right side of the spinal cord at the level of the umbilicus (T10). Based on the location of the lesion, which of the following symptoms will your patient most likely experience.
   a) Left side loss of vibratory and positional sensation in the right leg
   b) Left side loss of pain, temperature, and crude touch below T10
   c) Right side loss of tactile discrimination in the left foot
   d) Right side loss of proprioceptive input from muscle spindles

Level 3: Difficult

Answer B: There will be contralateral (left side) loss of pain and temperature below T10. Lateral compression of the spinal cord will primarily impact the anterolateral tract, which carries pain and temperature from the contralateral side of the body. Fibers decussate at the level of the synapse on the second-order neurons. A loss of vibratory sensation (**A**), tactile discrimination (**C**), and proprioceptive (**D**) input will most likely not occur. Epicritic sensations travel in the fasciculus gracilis of the dorsal (posterior) column which is not in the vicinity of the meningioma. The fibers of the dorsal column in the spinal cord (T10) will ascend ipsilaterally to synapse in second-order neurons in the caudal medulla. Decussation of fasciculus gracilis occurs in the medulla.

13 Somatosensory Systems Part II—Somatosensory Pathways of Head

1. Describe peripheral and central distribution of the trigeminal nerve.
2. Describe the two pathways that mediate orofacial sensations.
3. Compare the similarities and differences between the pain and temperature path of the face to that of the body.
4. Compare the tactile mechanosensory and proprioceptive path of the face to that of the body.
5. Explain the location of the first-order neurons for facial proprioception.
6. Explain the path for GSA input from facial, glossopharyngeal, and vagus nerves.
7. Compare the path for GSA to that of GVA path. Include in your comparison the cranial nerves involved, the location of the cell bodies for the first- and second-order neurons.
8. Describe the sensory modalities carried by trigeminal, facial, glossopharyngeal, and vagus.
9. Describe the sensory receptors involved in detecting stimuli for the trigeminal sensory system.

13.1 Overview of Somatosensory Innervation of the Head

The transmission of somatosensory sensations from the head, face, and oral cavity to the central nervous system (CNS) for conscious and unconscious processing follows comparable pathways to that of the body.

The **anterolateral, dorsal column-medial lemniscus,** and **spinocerebellar pathways** discussed in Chapter 12 mediate the somatosensory transmission from the body to the CNS. These paths are analogous to the **trigeminal nerve pathways** which convey pain, temperature, touch, and proprioception from the anterior head, face, and oral cavity.

The **trigeminal (CN V), facial (CN VII), glossopharyngeal (CN IX)**, and **vagus (CN X)** nerves convey general somatic afferent (GSA) sensations from cutaneous structures and mucous membranes of the head. Somatosensory input from the cranial region follows two principal pathways to the cortex for conscious processing: a **ventral** and **dorsal trigeminothalamic tract (DTT) (trigeminal lemniscus)**, which comprise the trigeminal sensory system. In addition to somatosensory input, **general visceral afferent (GVA)** sensations from blood vessels, glands, and mucous membranes are carried by the **facial (CN VII), glossopharyngeal (CN IX)**, and **vagus (CN X)** nerves and mediate unconscious, reflexive activity. The present chapter summarizes the components of the trigeminal sensory system and reviews the general somatosensory and viscerosensory pathways followed by CNs V, VII, IX, and X.

13.1.1 General Organization of the Trigeminal System

- Analogous to the organizational pattern of the somatosensory path of the body, the afferent fibers of the head utilize a three-neuron relay chain to transmit sensory input from peripheral receptors to the CNS (▶ Table 13.1).
- Within the CNS, craniofacial somatosensory afferent fibers follow similar routes to that of the body and contribute to one of three pathways (▶ Table 13.2) (▶ Fig. 13.1):
  - Sensory fibers serve as the afferent limb for somatic and autonomic reflex activity.
  - Afferent fibers follow distinct pathways and project to contralateral ventral posteromedial (VPM) nuclei of the thalamus and the somatosensory cortex for conscious perception and localization of stimulus.
  - Afferent fibers project to reticular formation and alternative thalamic nuclei for sensory arousal, emotional processing, and modulation of somatosensory input.

13.1.2 Trigeminal Nerve Distribution

- The trigeminal nerve, which is the largest of the 12 cranial nerves, consists of a small motor root and a large sensory root. The motor and sensory roots of the trigeminal nerve enter and exit the brainstem at the level of the mid-pons (▶ Table 13.3).
  - **Motor Root**
    - The small motor root of the trigeminal nerve provides efferent (motor) innervation to the muscles of mastication, and four smaller muscles. The function of these muscles and the nerve path are discussed in Chapter 20. The cell bodies for the motor neurons are found in the **motor nucleus of V (trigeminal motor nucleus)** within the pons.
  - **Sensory Root**
    - The large trigeminal sensory root contains an aggregation of GSA fibers which is formed by the convergence of the three principal divisions of the trigeminal nerve. The three principal divisions are the

Table 13.1 General comparison of three-neuron sensory system for body and head

	Location in Body	Location in Head*
First-order neuron	Dorsal root ganglia	Cranial sensory ganglia
Second-order neuron	Spinal cord and medulla	Brainstem and cervical spinal cord (C2)
Third-order neuron	VPL nuclei thalamus	VPM nuclei thalamus

Abbreviations: VPL, ventral posterolateral; VPM, ventral posteromedial.
Note: *Unconscious proprioceptive input is not included in chart.

Table 13.2 Comparison of trigeminal and spinal somatosensory pathways

Trigeminal Somatosensory System					
Modality and Fiber Type	**First-Order Neurons**	**Second-Order Nucleus**	**Anatomical Path to Thalamus**	**Third Order**	**Termination in Cortex**
Protopathic Pain/temperature/crude touch to head (Aδ and C fibers)	Trigeminal (semilunar) ganglion	Spinal trigeminal nucleus	Contralateral ventral trigeminothalamic tract (VTT)	Contralateral ventral posteromedial (VPM) of thalamus	Primary somatosensory cortex
Epicritic Fine tactile, two-point discrimination, vibration/pressure (Aβ Type II fibers)	Trigeminal (semilunar) ganglion	Main/chief sensory nucleus (principal/pontine nucleus)	Contralateral VTT Ipsilateral dorsal trigeminothalamic tract (DTT)	Contralateral VPM of thalamus Ipsilateral VPM of thalamus	Primary somatosensory cortex
Unconscious proprioception (Aα fibers Type Ia and Aβ Type II)	Mesencephalic nucleus in rostral pons of central nervous system (CNS)	*Monosynaptic reflex with motor nucleus V **Few project to main sensory nucleus, spinal trigeminal nucleus, cerebellum, hypoglossal motor, and nucleus ambiguus	* Some secondary fibers from main sensory DTT *Most fibers terminate in cerebellum via trigeminocerebellar tract and don't project to cortex	Few ipsilateral fibers to VPM of thalamus	Primary somatosensory cortex *Most secondary fibers terminate in cerebellum or motor nucleus
Spinal Somatosensory Systems					
Modality and fiber type	**First-order neurons**	**Second-Order Nucleus**	**Anatomical Path to Thalamus**	**Third-Order Nucleus**	**Termination**
Protopathic Pain/temperature/crude touch to head (Aδ and C fibers)	Dorsal root ganglion	Dorsal horn Rexed laminae I and II (substantia gelatinosa)	Direct anterolateral path: Spinothalamic (neospinothalamic) tract	Contralateral VPL of thalamus	Primary somatosensory cortex
Epicritic Fine tactile discrimination, vibration/pressure proprioception (Aα fibers Type Ia and Aβ Type II fibers)	Dorsal root ganglion	Dorsal column nuclei (gracilis and cuneatus nuclei)	Medial lemniscus	Contralateral VPL of thalamus	Primary somatosensory cortex
Unconscious proprioception (Aα fibers Type Ia and Aβ Type II fibers)	Dorsal root ganglion	Clarke's nucleus and accessory cuneatus nucleus	Spinocerebellar tracts Terminate in cerebellum	Not applicable	Not applicable

Abbreviations: VPL, ventral posterolateral; VPM, ventral posteromedial.
Note: As a result of incoming sensory information and descending input, modulation of synaptic transmission may occur at first-, second-, or third-order relay stations.

ophthalmic (V1), maxillary (V2), and **mandibular (V3) divisions** (▶ Fig. 13.2).

- Each of the three divisions divides extensively to give rise to peripheral nerve fibers which innervate well-defined territories of the anterior face and orofacial region (▶ Table 13.4).
- The cutaneous sensory innervation of the face follows the distribution pattern for CNs V1, V2, and V3, and results in a dermatome pattern that exhibits defined borders with little overlap of cutaneous sensations (▶ Fig. 13.3a–c)

- The dermatomes of the head, like that of the spinal nerves, have clinical relevance regarding the diagnosis of certain diseases. Symptoms such as rash or pain that follow a dermatome may indicate the involvement

of the related nerve root (see Clinical Correlation Box 13.1).

- The primary afferent fibers which comprise the **ophthalmic (CN V1)**, **maxillary (CN V2)**, and **mandibular (CN V3)** divisions pass from the periphery and enter the skull through three specific foramina: the **superior orbital fissure, foramen rotundum**, and **foramen ovale,** respectively (▶ Fig. 13.4).

- In the middle cranial fossa, the ophthalmic (CN V1) and maxillary (CN V2) divisions pass through the **cavernous venous sinus,** accompanied by the **trochlear nerve (CN IV),** the **oculomotor nerve (CN III),** the **abducens nerve (CN VI)** and the sympathetic fibers associated with the internal carotid artery (ICA). The proximity of the structures within the sinus puts the nerves at risk for compression

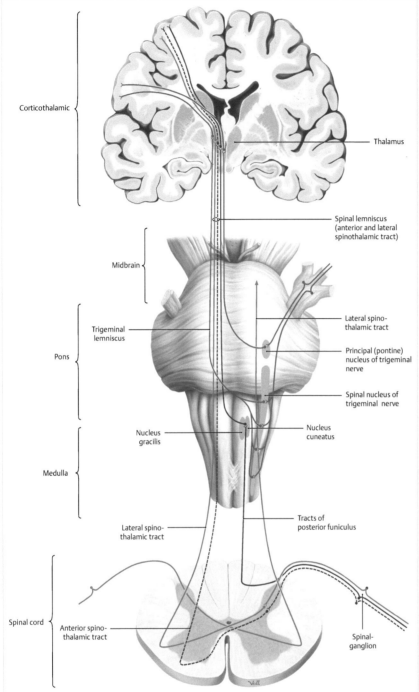

Corticothalamic

Thalamus

Spinal lemniscus
(anterior and lateral
spinothalamic tract)

Midbrain

Trigeminal
lemniscus

Lateral spino-
thalamic tract

Pons

Principal (pontine)
nucleus of trigeminal
nerve

Spinal nucleus of
trigeminal nerve

Nucleus
cuneatus

Nucleus
gracilis

Medulla

Tracts of
posterior funiculus

Lateral spino-
thalamic tract

Spinal cord

Anterior spino-
thalamic tract

Spinal-
ganglion

Fig. 13.1 Principal ascending somatosensory paths of body and head. Protopathic and epicritic sensations for body and head follow a three-neuron relay chain. Primary afferent neurons reside in dorsal root or trigeminal sensory ganglia, and synapse on second-order neurons in the spinal cord or brainstem. Third-order neurons reside in specific thalamic nuclei and project to primary somatosensory cortex (S1). The ascending somatosensory pathways of the body and head decussate at different points, but travel in close proximity through the brainstem and may be susceptible to damage. (Reproduced with permission from Schuenke M, Schulte E, Schumacher U. THIEME Atlas of Anatomy. Second Edition, Vol 3. © Thieme 2016. Illustrations by Markus Voll and Karl Wesker.)

injuries due to infections or thrombosis occurring within the sinus. The mandibular division which passes outside the sinus is usually spared (Clinical Correlation Box 13.2) (▶ Fig. 13.5a, b).

- The three divisions, which carry the peripheral axonal processes of primary afferent (GSA) neurons, converge in the middle cranial fossa and enter a large peripheral sensory ganglion known as the **trigeminal ganglion.**

Table 13.3 Overview of trigeminal motor and sensory components

Fiber Type	Distribution /Function	General Overview of Path
Efferent fibers (SVE) Branchial motor component	Motor to muscles of mastication: Masseter, temporalis, pterygoids, mylohyoid, anterior digastric, tensor tympani, tensor veli palatini	• Motor branch emerges from the motor nucleus of V in the pons • SVE fibers pass inferior to CN V sensory ganglia (trigeminal ganglia) • Follows the mandibular division (V3)
Afferent fibers (GSA) General somatic afferent	Sensory input for anterior face, scalp, and oral cavity **Protopathic:** Nociceptive Thermal Crude touch **Epicritic** Conscious proprioception Proprioceptive • Vibration • Pressure • Stretch • Joint position • Joint movement Mechanoreceptive • Fine, tactile (two-point discrimination)	Peripheral nerve fibers from ophthalmic (V1), maxillary (V2), mandibular (V3) Location of first-order cell bodies: • Trigeminal ganglion • Mesencephalic nucleus *Part of trigeminal nuclear complex Sensory root fibers enter the pons and project to trigeminal nuclear complex

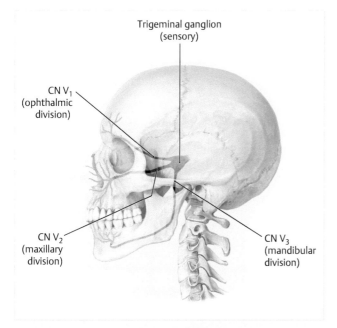

Trigeminal ganglion (sensory)

CN V₁ (ophthalmic division)

CN V₂ (maxillary division)

CN V₃ (mandibular division)

Fig. 13.2 Trigeminal nerve divisions and distribution. Left lateral view. (Reproduced with permission from Schuenke M, Schulte E, Schumacher U. THIEME Atlas of Anatomy Third Edition, Vol 3. © Thieme 2020. Illustrations by Markus Voll and Karl Wesker.)

Clinical Correlation Box 13.1: Herpetic Infections of the Trigeminal Ganglia

- The peripheral sensory nervous system is the primary target of the **herpes simplex virus (HSV)** infections. During a primary infection, the virus may undergo retrograde axonal transport along nerves to the neuronal cell bodies in the sensory ganglia and establish chronic latency. The trigeminal nerve and ganglia are principal targets of HSV and reactivation causes recurrent HSV infections. Outbreaks are often associated with cold sores, facial herpetic lesions, or corneal infections. The pattern of recurrence tends to follow the dermatome of the primary infection; however, because of the involvement of the sensory ganglia, a recurring infection may become associated with another dermatome.

- The **varicella-zoster virus** that causes chickenpox is another example of a herpes virus that may remain dormant in nerve ganglia. Reactivation of the virus leads to shingles also known as herpes zoster, which is associated with a painful rash and blisters along a defined dermatome. Although often associated with the trunk, it can also develop on the face, mouth, and around the eyes. The complication associated with shingles developing in the orofacial region is an ipsilateral loss of sensation on the affected side or the development of postherpetic neuralgia, which is hallmarked by sharp, burning pain along the affected dermatome.

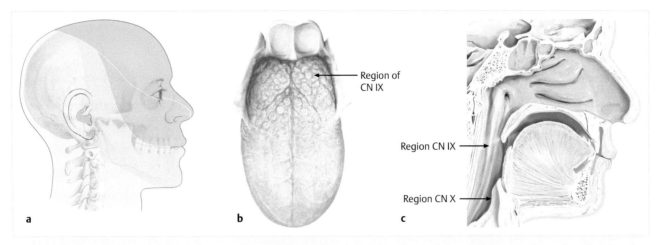

Fig. 13.3 Somatosensory nerve distribution pattern of trigeminal nerve (CN V). Right lateral view of trigeminal divisions. The trigeminal nerve is the major sensory nerve of the face. It has three major divisions that convey general somatic afferent (GSA) sensation of touch, pain, and proprioception from the face (a) and select mucosa (b, c). Each division exhibits a distinct dermatome distribution pattern with little cutaneous overlap and is of clinical relevance regarding diagnosis. Mandibular nerve shown in yellow (a, b, c); maxillary division in green (a, c); ophthalmic division in blue (a, c). Additional shading for GSA distribution from CN VII, CN IX, and CN X shown in region of ear. (Modified with permission from Schuenke M, Schulte E, Schumacher U. THIEME Atlas of Anatomy Third Edition, Vol 3. © Thieme 2020. Illustrations by Markus Voll and Karl Wesker.)

Clinical Correlation Box 13.2: Trigeminal Neuropathy Due to Pathology of Cavernous Sinus

Tumors, aneurysms of the ICA, venous thrombosis, or the spread of infection in the cavernous sinus, may lead to compression and subsequent trigeminal neuropathy of the sensory nerve branches of ophthalmic and maxillary divisions, as they pass through the cavernous sinus to exit the skull. The resulting neuropathy will follow the trigeminal dermatome and may manifest as cutaneous sensory loss, or in some cases, as sharp intermittent pain associated with trigeminal neuralgia. Compression of the oculomotor, trochlear, and abducens nerve may also occur due to their shared route through the cavernous sinus, leading to weakness or paralysis of extraocular eye muscles (ophthalmoplegia). Horner's syndrome associated with damage to sympathetic fibers may also be manifested. Typical signs include decreased pupil size, a drooping eyelid (partial ptosis), and decreased sweating of the face on the affected side.

13.1.3 Trigeminal Ganglia

- The trigeminal ganglion, also known as the **semilunar ganglion** or **Gasserian ganglion,** is housed in a small depression (**Meckel's cave**) in the petrous temporal bone, just lateral to cavernous sinus (see ▶ Fig. 13.5a).
- The trigeminal ganglion represents a functional equivalent to the dorsal root ganglion and contains most of the first-order pseudounipolar neuron cell bodies that convey GSA fibers for the head, face, and intraoral region.
  - The ganglion contains the pseudounipolar cell bodies of the first-order (GSA) neurons associated with protopathic

(pain, temperature) and epicritic (discriminative tactile, pressure, vibration) sensations.
- There is one notable exception to the types of primary sensory neurons located within the trigeminal ganglia. The primary afferent neurons that transmit proprioceptive information from the masticatory jaw-closing muscles, tongue, periodontal ligament, and extraocular eye muscles lie within the **mesencephalic trigeminal nucleus** of the midbrain.
- The peripheral axons which carry proprioceptive input for the trigeminal divisions (CN V1–V3) enter the skull and bypass the trigeminal ganglion to enter the pons.
- The presence of first-order sensory neurons in the CNS rather than the peripheral nervous system (PNS) is unique to the mesencephalic nucleus. All other first-order sensory neurons of the head and body reside within the PNS in cranial sensory ganglia (CNs V, VII, IX, and X) or the dorsal root ganglia.

13.2 Trigeminal Nuclear Complex

- The central axonal processes of GSA neurons enter the brainstem at the level of the pons as the sensory root and project to the **trigeminal nuclear (sensory) complex**—a cluster of three sensory nuclei that extends from the midbrain to upper cervical region of the spinal cord (▶ Fig. 13.6, ▶ Table 13.5).
- The three sensory nuclei of the **trigeminal nuclear complex** include the following:
  - **Spinal trigeminal nucleus (STN)**
  - **Main (chief, principal, pontine) sensory nucleus of V**
  - **Mesencephalic nucleus of V**
- Each nucleus receives specific types of sensory input from peripheral receptors and then transmits the sensory information along specific ascending pathways for conscious and unconscious processing.

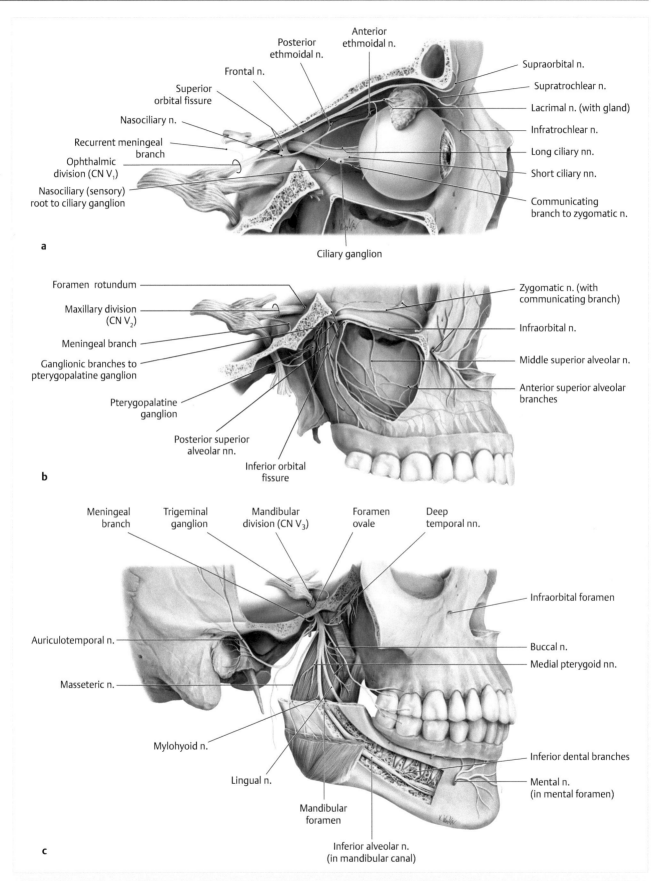

Fig. 13.4 Peripheral course of the trigeminal nerve divisions. Right lateral views. **(a)** Partially open right orbit showing ophthalmic division (CN V1). **(b)** Partially opened right maxillary sinus showing maxillary division (CN V2). **(c)** Partially opened mandible with middle cranial fossa windowed showing mandibular division (CN V3). (Reproduced with permission from Schuenke M, Schulte E, Schumacher U. THIEME Atlas of Anatomy Third Edition, Vol 3. © Thieme 2020. Illustrations by Markus Voll and Karl Wesker.)

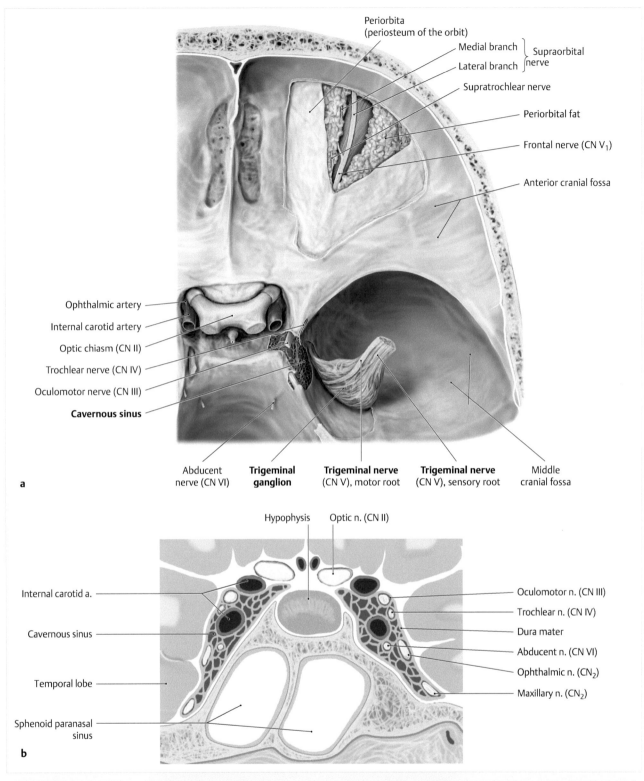

Fig. 13.5 **(a)** Intracavernous course of cranial nerves that enter the orbit. Anterior and middle cranial fossa on right side, superior view. The lateral and superior wall opened. The trigeminal ganglion has been retracted laterally; the orbit roof removed. The oculomotor (CN III), trochlear (CN IV), and abducens (CN IX), which innervate the ocular muscles, enter the cavernous sinus and lie in close proximity with ophthalmic (CN V1) and maxillary (CN V2) divisions of the trigeminal nerve. **(b)** Cavernous sinus, coronal section through middle cranial fossa. Anterior view, coronal section, showing the relationship of the cranial nerves within the cavernous sinus to the hypophysis, optic nerve (CN II), and internal carotid artery. Sympathetic fibers travel with the internal carotid artery as they pass through the sinus. (▶ Fig. 13.5a: Reproduced with permission from Schuenke M, Schulte E, Schumacher U. THIEME Atlas of Anatomy Third Edition, Vol 3. © Thieme 2020. Illustrations by Markus Voll and Karl Wesker. ▶ Fig. 13.5b: Reproduced with permission from Gilroy AM, MacPherson BR, Ross LM. Atlas of Anatomy. Second Edition. © Thieme 2012. Illustrations by Markus Voll and Karl Wesker.)

Table 13.4 Distribution of three sensory divisions of trigeminal nerve (CNV)

	Ophthalmic (V1)	Maxillary (V2)	Mandibular (V3)
Region of sensory distribution	Innervates forehead, upper eyelid, cornea (thus the corneal reflex), conjunctiva, dorsum of the nose, and dura of some of the anterior cranial fossa	Supplies upper lip, lateral and posterior portions of nose, upper cheek, anterior temple, mucosa of nose, upper jaw, upper teeth, roof of mouth, and dura of part of the middle cranial fossa	Supplies lower lip, chin, posterior cheek, temple, mucosa of lower part of mouth, anterior two-thirds of the tongue, and portions of the dura of anterior and middle cranial fossae
Peripheral path to central nervous system (CNS)	• Peripheral afferent fibers enter the cranium through superior orbital fissure • Lies in lateral wall of cavernous sinus • Passes through trigeminal ganglia (no synapse) • Primary afferent fibers enter the pons	• Peripheral afferent fibers enter the cranium through the foramen rotundum • Travels through the inferior part of the cavernous sinus • Passes through the trigeminal ganglion (no synapse) • Primary afferent fibers enter the pons	• Peripheral afferent fibers enter the cranium through the foramen ovale • Passes outside (posterolateral) to the cavernous sinus • Passes through the trigeminal ganglion (no synapse) • Primary afferent fibers enter the pons

13.2.1 Components of Trigeminal Sensory Nuclear Complex

Spinal Trigeminal Nucleus

- The **spinal trigeminal nucleus** is the largest nuclei of the trigeminal system and extends from the caudal region of the pons to the upper cervical levels (C2) of the spinal cord, where it merges with the Rexed lamina (marginal zone, substantia gelatinosa) in the dorsal horn gray matter.
- The **spinal trigeminal nucleus** contains second-order neurons and is the only cranial nerve nucleus to process **thermal** and **nociceptive input** from the ipsilateral part of the face. It receives crude touch, thermal, and noxious stimuli from all three trigeminal divisions, as well as the facial (CN VII), glossopharyngeal (CN IX), and vagus (CN X) nerves.
- The spinal trigeminal nucleus is further divided rostrocaudally into three subnuclei: the **pars oralis, pars interpolaris**, and **pars caudalis** (▶ Table 13.6).
- Nociceptive and temperature sensations conveyed by central axons of primary afferent neurons descend from the trigeminal ganglia to the ipsilateral spinal trigeminal nucleus via the **spinal (descending) trigeminal tract.** Protopathic sensation carried by primary afferent fibers of CNs VII, IX, and X enter at different levels of the brainstem and follow the spinal trigeminal tract to the spinal trigeminal nucleus.
- **Primary afferent fibers** synapse **ipsilaterally** in the **spinal trigeminal nucleus** in a rostrocaudal somatotopic pattern.
  - The somatotopic distribution reflects the segmental organization of the trigeminal spinal nucleus and corresponds to a concentric semicircular pattern (**Sölder lines**) of sensory distribution on the face. Therefore, the axons from the **central orofacial (perioral) region** synapse in the **rostral portion of the nucleus**, whereas peripheral axons from the **lateral facial region** project to the **caudal portion of the spinal trigeminal nucleus** (▶ Fig. 13.7a, b) (Clinical Correlation Box 13.3).

- The spinal trigeminal nucleus is similar in function to Rexed laminae I, II, and IV, which process protopathic input for the anterolateral (spinothalamic) system (Clinical Correlation Box 13.4).

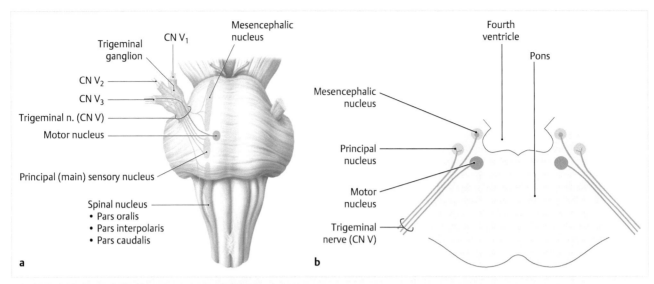

Fig. 13.6 Trigeminal nerve nuclei. Anterior view of brainstem (**a**). Superior view; cross section through the pons (**b**). Primary afferent neurons of the trigeminal nerve divisions convey general somatic afferent (GSA) sensations (touch, pain, proprioception) to the central nervous system (CNS). The central axons of the primary afferent neurons enter the mid-pons as the sensory root and synapse in three brainstem nuclei, which comprise the trigeminal nuclear complex. The nuclei include the spinal trigeminal nucleus, which conveys nociceptive and thermal sensations; the main sensory nucleus, which transmits discriminative touch and conscious proprioception; and the mesencephalic, nucleus which carries unconscious proprioception from the jaw. Special visceral efferent fibers carried by the mandibular division (CN V3) arise from lower motor neurons in the trigeminal motor nucleus and exit the pons as a small motor root. (Reproduced with permission from Schuenke M, Schulte E, Schumacher U. THIEME Atlas of Anatomy Third Edition, Vol 3. © Thieme 2020. Illustrations by Markus Voll and Karl Wesker.)

Table 13.5 Summary of trigeminal sensory nuclear complex

Trigeminal Sensory Nuclei	Location of Nuclei	Type of Neuron in Nuclei	Sensory Modality Transmitted	Analogous Location for Second-Order Nuclei for Body
Spinal trigeminal nucleus: Three parts: • Pars oralis • Pars interpolaris • Pars caudalis	Caudal part of pons to level C2 of spinal cord	Second-order neuron	Nonencapsulated nociceptive receptors Polymodal mechano-nociceptive Protopathic sensations (pain, temperature, crude touch, itch)	Rexed laminae I, II, and V in dorsal horn of spinal cord
Main (chief, principal) sensory nucleus of V	Mid-pons	Second-order neuron	Encapsulated and nonencapsulated mechanosensory receptors: Epicritic sensations (tactile discrimination, pressure, vibration, stretch)	Dorsal column nuclei of medulla: • Cuneate nucleus • Gracilis nucleus
Mesencephalic nucleus of V	Rostral pons to rostral midbrain	First-order neurons	Encapsulated proprioceptors and mechanosensory receptors: • Proprioceptive input from mechanoreceptors in teeth, temporomandibular joint (TMJ); periodontal ligament (PDL); gingiva • Muscle spindles of jaw closing masticatory muscles • Extraocular and facial muscles	Not applicable Mesencephalic Nucleus unique to trigeminal system **In the body second-order neurons involved in transmitting unconscious proprioceptive input reside in: • Accessory cuneate nucleus • Clarke's nucleus

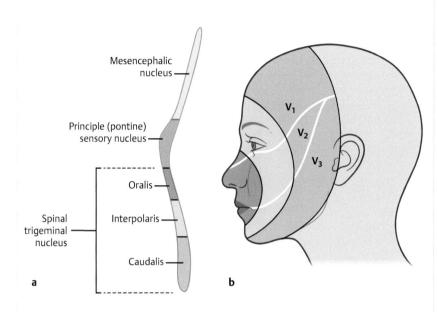

Fig. 13.7 **(a)** Segmental organization of the subnuclei in the spinal trigeminal nucleus. Pain and temperature sensations terminate in a rostrocaudal somatotopic distribution pattern. Cranial parts of the nucleus receive input from the center of the face, and more caudal subnuclei receive axons from the peripheral face. The somatotopic arrangement corresponds to an "onion-skin" pattern of three semicircular rings on the face (also known as Sölder lines). **(b)** Segmental and divisional distribution patterns of trigeminal nerve. Lesions to specific subnuclei of the spinal trigeminal nucleus may lead to sensory deficits that follow a characteristic "onion-skin" pattern (Sölder lines) corresponding to semicircular zones radiating from the center of the face toward the periphery (shaded rings). Because of the segmental arrangement, lesions in pars caudalis may cause peripheral deficits in protopathic sensations with central sparing of the perioral region. In comparison, lesions involving damage to a specific peripheral nerve division produce sensory deficits that follow the dermatome distribution of CN V1, CN V2, and CN V3.

Table 13.6 Spinal trigeminal subnuclei

Subnuclei	Location	Function
Pars oralis	Most rostral subnucleus; fuses with chief sensory nucleus	Integrate nociceptive input in the teeth, oral mucosa, and PDL; receives crude touch
Pars interpolaris	Middle region of spinal trigeminal nucleus Transition zone between interpolaris and caudalis important in processing deep pain	Processes deep tissue pain from the TMJ, PDL, gingiva, masticatory muscles as well as integrating nociceptive input from orofacial and dental regions; receives crude touch
Pars caudalis (medullary dorsal horn)	Superior to the substantia gelatinosa of dorsal horn; referred to as **medullary dorsal horn**	Principal site for processing pain and temperature (protopathic) sensations from the face and orofacial region

Abbreviations: PDL, periodontal ligament; TMJ, temporomandibular joint.

Clinical Correlation Box 13.4: Trigeminal Neuralgia (Tic Douloureux)

Trigeminal neuralgia or Tic douloureux manifests as short durations of an intermittent severe, stabbing pain on one side (unilateral) of the face and usually involves the maxillary (CN V2) or mandibular (CN V3) divisions of the trigeminal nerve. There is no loss of sensory or motor function, and pain follows the dermatome distribution pattern. Trigeminal neuralgia may be idiopathic but is often caused by vascular compression of trigeminal nerve root. Additional causes include demyelination of axons carrying protopathic sensations, neoplastic growths, or posttraumatic nerve lesions. Several terminal sensory branches of the mandibular division are at risk during dental procedures, and damage to the nerve can result in trigeminal neuralgia.

Main (Chief or Principal) Sensory Nucleus of CN V

- The main (chief) sensory nucleus of CN V resides in the middle of the pons, adjacent to the entering sensory root fibers, and just lateral to motor nucleus of CN V. The nucleus contains second-order neurons that mediate conscious proprioception, stereognosis, discriminative fine touch, and oral mechanical sensations received from all three trigeminal nerve divisions.
- There are two divisions of the main sensory nucleus: **dorsomedial** and **ventrolateral divisions**. The dorsomedial comprises approximately one-third of the nucleus and receives oral mechanosensory and conscious proprioceptive input from the teeth and oral cavity. The ventrolateral division is larger and receives epicritic input from all three divisions. Secondary afferents arising from each division follows a different ascending path.

- Lesions of the main sensory nucleus occur in the mid-pons and often affect the motor nucleus of V and the entering sensory root fibers on the ipsilateral side due to their proximity. Symptoms may include loss of pain, temperature, and touch over the ipsilateral face and ipsilateral masticatory muscle paralysis. Unilateral muscle paralysis results in reduced bite force and jaw deviation to the injured side (see Chapter 20, **Fig. 20.6**).
- The main sensory nucleus is similar in function to the dorsal column nuclei (nucleus gracilis and nucleus cuneatus) associated with the dorsal column-medial lemniscus system of the body.

Mesencephalic Nucleus of V

- The **mesencephalic nucleus of V** lies near the periaqueductal gray in the floor of the fourth ventricle and extends from the rostral pons to the caudal midbrain.
- The nucleus contains first-order pseudounipolar sensory neurons that mediate unconscious proprioceptive input from muscle spindles in the jaw-closing muscles, as well as mechanoreceptive input originating from mechanoreceptors in the periodontal ligament fibers surrounding the teeth and gingiva. The neurons which mediate proprioceptive input from the tongue, extraocular, and facial muscles may also reside in the mesencephalic nucleus.
- The mesencephalic nucleus receives peripheral primary afferent axons that enter the pons, ascends in the **mesencephalic trigeminal tract,** and passes through the nucleus without synapsing.
- In the body, the second-order neurons comprising Clarke's nucleus and the accessory cuneate nucleus serve a comparable function to the mesencephalic nucleus. Each nucleus provides input to the cerebellum for unconscious processing and plays a role in the coordination of movement and reflex activity.

13.3 Trigeminal Somatosensory Pathways (▶ Fig. 13.8) (▶ Table 13.7)

13.3.1 Central Ascending Pathways: Protopathic Sensations of the Face (▶ Table 13.8)

The **spinal trigeminal pathway** carries contralateral **protopathic information** from the head and face and is functionally comparable to the **spinothalamic** tract in the body.

- Small diameter, lightly myelinated Aδ and unmyelinated C fibers from primary sensory neurons in the trigeminal ganglion enter the pons through the sensory root of CN V.
- Primary afferent fibers from all three trigeminal divisions initially descend in an axonal tract known as the **spinal trigeminal tract (spinal tract of CN V)** to reach the **spinal trigeminal nucleus.**
- Most of the primary afferent nociceptive fibers enter the **spinal trigeminal nucleus** and synapse on second-order neurons in the **pars caudalis**.

- Secondary afferent fibers arising from the spinal trigeminal subnuclei **decussate** at the midline and ascend as a bilateral crossed path. Fibers follow one of two routes: **ventral trigeminothalamic tract (VTT)** or **trigeminoreticular path**.
- The **VTT** is comparable to the **spinothalamic tract of the ALS** and is important in the discriminative localization of painful stimuli.
  - The secondary afferents that originate from the spinal trigeminal nucleus and follow the contralateral VTT transmit input from mostly Aδ fibers.
  - Aδ fibers convey sensations of crude touch, temperature, and well-localized, sharp, acute pain.
- Contralateral afferent·fibers of the VTT ascend and synapse on third-order neurons in the contralateral **VPM nucleus** of the **thalamus.**
  - Third-order axons project somatotopically through the **posterior limb of the internal capsule** to terminate in the orofacial region of the **primary somatosensory cortex** (S1) in the postcentral gyrus.
- Fibers following the **trigeminoreticular (trigeminal reticular) path** are comparable to those protopathic fibers in the body which follow the **indirect spinoreticular path** of the anterolateral system.
  - Secondary afferents that arise from spinal trigeminal nucleus and follow the **trigeminoreticular tract** carry nociceptive input from mainly **C fibers.**
  - The trigeminoreticular tract transmits poorly localized, dull aching pain and functions to increase awareness of painful stimuli.
- Fibers from the **trigeminoreticular path** follow in close association with VTT but project secondary afferent fibers to the **reticular formation, periaqueductal gray**, and **intralaminar thalamic nuclei.** The axons of the intralaminar nuclei project diffusely to the cortex, terminating in the insular and cingulate gyrus.
- The termination and processing of nociceptive fibers from the VTT and trigeminoreticular tract occur in different regions of the cortex. As a result, specific lesions to the somatosensory cortex result in diminished pain perception rather than a complete loss of nociceptive sensations.
  - Typically lesions to the primary somatosensory (S1) cortex result in the loss of perception and localization of fast, sharp pain. However, the awareness and perception of dull, aching pain persist due to the termination of trigeminoreticular fibers to other cortical connections.
- The path for protopathic sensations is outlined in ▶ Table 13.8 and summarized in ▶ Fig. 13.8 and ▶ Fig. 13.9.

13.3.2 Central Ascending Pathways: Epicritic Sensations for the Face (▶ Table 13.9)

The **main sensory trigeminal pathway** carries **epicritic sensations** and ascends bilaterally as crossed and uncrossed paths. It is functionally similar to the **medial lemniscus pathway** of the body.

- Low-threshold mechanoreceptors such as Ruffini's corpuscles, Meissner's corpuscles, and Merkel's cell transduce conscious proprioceptive, stereognostic, and

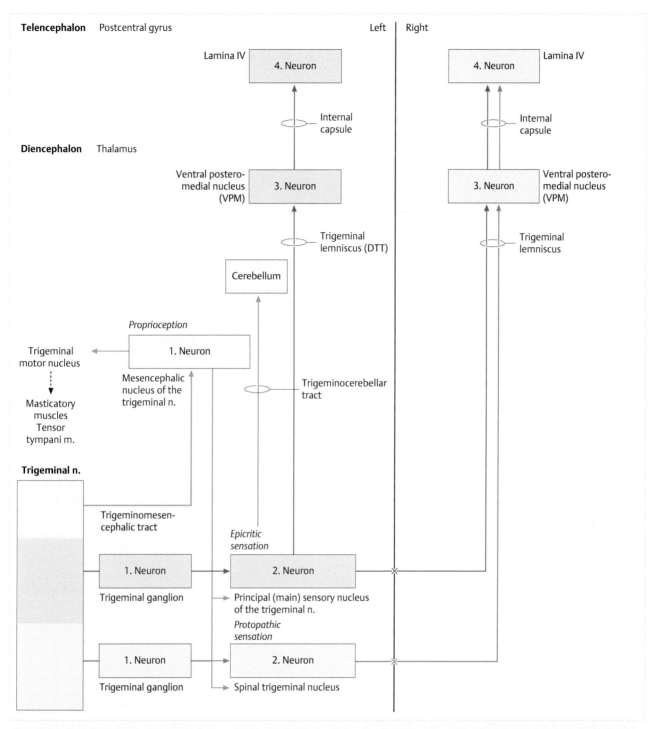

Fig. 13.8 Schematic summary of trigeminal sensory pathways. Cell bodies for nociceptive, thermal, and fine discriminative touch are located in the trigeminal ganglion. Secondary afferent fibers that arise from the spinal trigeminal nucleus and main sensory nucleus decussate to ascend in the contralateral trigeminal lemniscus (VTT) to the contralateral ventral posteromedial (VPM) nucleus of the thalamus. Some secondary afferent fibers from the main sensory nucleus remain ipsilateral and ascend in the dorsal trigeminothalamic tract (DTT) to synapse in the ipsilateral VPM nucleus of the thalamus. The third-order (thalamic) neurons terminate in the primary somatosensory cortex (S1). Cell bodies for unconscious proprioceptive input reside in the mesencephalic nucleus and contribute primarily to reflex activity. Fibers from the mesencephalic nucleus may also contribute to the trigeminocerebellar tract. Nociceptive input following the trigeminoreticular path to terminate in other regions of the cortex is not shown. Protopathic pathways (blue), epicritic (pink), and unconscious proprioceptive (green) are shown. (Reproduced with permission from Schuenke M, Schulte E, Schumacher U. THIEME Atlas of Anatomy. Second Edition, Vol 3. © Thieme 2016. Illustrations by Markus Voll and Karl Wesker.)

Table 13.7 Summary of major ascending pathways of trigeminal system

Trigeminal Sensory Nuclear Complex			
Trigeminal nuclei	Spinal nucleus of V (second order) • Pars oralis • Pars interpolaris • Pars caudalis	Main sensory nucleus of V (second order) (*aka: pontine trigeminal, chief, principal nucleus)	Mesencephalic nucleus of V (*unique—first-order neurons)
Functional component and pathway	Protopathic sensations of orofacial skin and oral mucosa Pathway for pain, temperature, crude touch	Epicritic sensation of orofacial skin and oral mucosa Pathway for fine tactile discrimination and conscious proprioception (pressure, vibration)	Proprioceptive input Muscle of muscle spindles in jaw-closing muscles and mechanoreceptors of PDL, TMJ, gingiva, tongue Pathway for unconscious proprioception
Territory of trigeminal	All three divisions transmit from: Skin, mucosa, gingiva, PDL, TMJ, and eye	All three divisions transmit from: Skin, mucosa, teeth, gingiva, PDL, and eye	Received primarily from V2 and V3: V1 carries some proprioceptive from extraocular eye muscles
Principal ascending tract	Second afferents → Contralateral ventral trigeminothalamic tract (VTT) → VPM → S1	1. Ipsilateral dorsal trigeminothalamic tract (DTT) 2. Contralateral VTT to form trigeminal lemniscus	Monosynaptic reflex to trigeminal motor nucleus
Alternative routes	Trigeminoreticular tract Unconscious processing of pain via collateral of VTT → may terminate in reticular formation, periaqueductal gray, and intralaminar thalamic nuclei	Chief sensory nucleus provides reflexive input to cranial nerve motor nuclei (VII, XII) to mediate reflexes and coordinate movements	Trigeminocerebellar tract Unconscious processing of jaw position via mesencephalic nucleus → to cerebellum via superior peduncle Project from chief sensory nucleus and spinal trigeminal nucleus → to terminate in ipsilateral cerebellum—enter cerebellum via inferior peduncles

Abbreviations: PDL, periodontal ligament; TMJ, temporomandibular joint.
*Epicritic fibers join protopathic fibers in ventral trigeminothalamic tract at level of pons Collectively fibers ascend as trigeminal lemniscus which is near of medial lemniscus

discriminative tactile sensations from the ophthalmic (CN V1), maxillary (CN V2), and mandibular (CN V3) divisions.
- Large myelinated primary afferent Aβ (Type II) fibers from first-order mechanosensory neurons in the trigeminal ganglion enter the pons through the sensory root of CN V, and synapse on second-order neurons in the **main sensory nucleus of V** (principal or chief sensory nucleus of V).
- Afferent fibers from second-order neurons in the main sensory nucleus of V may either **decussate** and follow the **contralateral VTT** or remain **ipsilateral** and ascend in the **DTT.**
  ○ Most secondary afferent fibers that carry conscious mechanoreceptive sensations from the three trigeminal divisions arise from the ventrolateral part of the nucleus, cross the midline, and join the protopathic fibers in the **contralateral VTT,** at the level of the pons.
  ○ Collectively, the **protopathic** and **epicritic fibers** traveling in the **VTT** ascend together as the **trigeminal lemniscus** to synapse on the **contralateral VPM** nucleus of the thalamus. The trigeminal lemniscus ascends in close association with the medial lemniscus pathway. Both are susceptible to damage during their course through the pons and midbrain.
  ○ The remaining secondary afferents which arise from the dorsomedial division of the main sensory nucleus of V carry mechanosensory input from the region of the **oral cavity**. These fibers remain ipsilateral and follow the **DTT**

to synapse on third-order neurons in the **ipsilateral VPM** nucleus of the thalamus.
- The **VPM** receives **bilateral input** from the **main sensory nucleus**. The axons of third-order neurons ascending from the **contralateral** and **ipsilateral VPM nuclei** pass through the **posterior limb of the internal capsule** and project to the **orofacial area** of the **primary somatosensory cortex.**
- The path for epicritic sensations is outlined in ▶ Table 13.9 and summarized in ▶ Fig. 13.8 and ▶ Fig. 13.9.

13.3.3 Central Ascending Pathways: Unconscious Proprioception from the Orofacial Region (▶ Table 13.10)

The principal pathways associated with mesencephalic nucleus mediate reflex activities involved in controlling bite force, jaw position, and stability or transmit unconscious proprioceptive input to the cerebellum.
- Muscle spindles found in the masticatory jaw-closing muscles, along with mechanoreceptors in the periodontal ligament of the teeth and gingiva, transduce unconscious proprioceptive input from the maxillary and mandibular nerves to the mesencephalic nucleus. Additional input from the muscles of the face, tongue, and eye may also project to the nucleus.

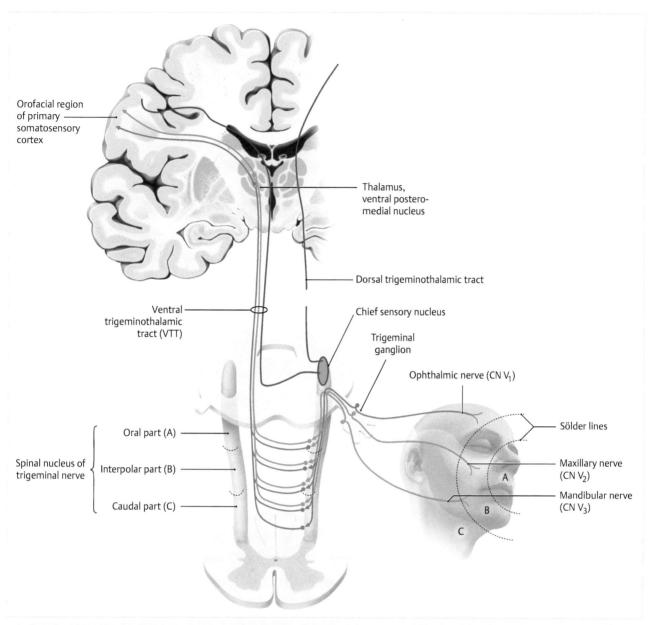

Fig. 13.9 Summary of protopathic and epicritic sensory pathways for the trigeminal nerve. Primary afferent fibers carrying nociceptive and thermal input from CN V1, CN V2, and CN V3 descend ipsilaterally in the spinal trigeminal tract to synapse in the spinal trigeminal nucleus. Note the somatotopic organization of this nuclear region: The perioral region **(A)** is cranial and the occipital regions **(B)** are caudal. Fine discriminative touch and conscious proprioceptive input concerning pressure and vibratory sensations synapse somatotopically in the chief (main) sensory nucleus. Secondary afferents from the main (chief) sensory nucleus may follow either ventral trigeminothalamic tract (VTT) or dorsal trigeminothalamic tract (DTT) and project bilaterally to ventral posteromedial (VPM) thalamic nuclei. The VTT carries epicritic and protopathic sensations to contralateral VPM thalamic nuclei. The DTT transmits only epicritic sensation from the dorsal part of the main sensory nucleus to the ipsilateral VPM thalamic nuclei. Unconscious proprioception and the mesencephalic nucleus are not shown. (Reproduced with permission from Schuenke M, Schulte E, Schumacher U. THIEME Atlas of Anatomy Third Edition, Vol 3. © Thieme 2020. Illustrations by Markus Voll and Karl Wesker.)

- Large myelinated Aα (Type Ia) and Aβ (Type II) fibers, which represent the peripheral afferent fibers of first-order proprioceptive neurons, enter the pons through the trigeminal nerve root and then ascend as a group of axons in the **mesencephalic trigeminal tract** to the **mesencephalic nucleus**.
- The central axons of proprioceptive primary afferent fibers pass through the mesencephalic nucleus without synapsing and then project to several possible locations:

  ○ **Motor nucleus of CN V** in the mid-pons.
  ○ **Masticatory central pattern generators (CPGs)** in the pontine reticular formation.
  ○ **Spinal trigeminal nucleus.**
  ○ **Chief sensory nucleus.**
- Most of the proprioceptive central axons passing through the mesencephalic nucleus synapse directly on the **motor nucleus of V** to elicit a **myotatic stretch reflex** also known as the jaw jerk reflex (see Clinical Correlation Box 13.6).

Table 13.8 Summary of central path for orofacial protopathic sensations

Central Path: Protopathic Sensations of Trigeminal		
Peripheral Input from Primary Afferents	**Trigeminal Nuclear Complex**	**Central Ascending Path**
Modality Pain/temperature/crude touch/itch from skin/mucosa/oral cavity for all three division **Receptors:** • Nonencapsulated nociceptive receptors • Polymodal mechano-nociceptive receptors **Fibers:** Thinly myelinated Aδ fibers (Type III) Unmyelinated C fibers (Type IV) *Additional GSA input from skin/mucosa of CNs VII, IX, and X; upper cervical regions (C1–C3)	**Spinal nucleus of V** (second-order neurons) **Brainstem location** Caudal part of pons to C2 of spinal cord Region joins Rexed laminae I, II, and V in dorsal horn of spinal cord Comprised of **three subnuclei** arranged rostral to caudal—receive somatotopic input from specific regions Each subnuclei contains nociceptive specific and wide dynamic range (WDR) secondary afferent neurons **Three parts of subnuclei:** **Pars oralis** • Integrates nociceptive input from oral cavity and dental structures (perioral region) **Pars oralis input:** • PDL, teeth, pulp **Pars interpolaris** • Involved in processing deep tissue pain from the TMJ, masticatory muscles as well as integrating nociceptive input from orofacial and dental regions **Pars interpolaris input:** • TMJ masticatory muscles • Oral mucosa • Dental pulp **Pars caudalis** • Principal site for processing pain and temperature from face and orofacial region **Pars caudalis input:** • Skin from V1, V2, and V3, external ear from VII, IX, and X • Oral mucosa of oral cavity and oropharynx	**Primary route conscious perception of pain via contralateral ventral trigeminothalamic tract** 1. Secondary afferent fibers **decussate** and form the **ventral trigeminothalamic tract** (VTT) • Joined by fibers from chief (main) sensory nucleus of V at the level of pons to form **trigeminal lemniscus** • Secondary fibers synapse on third-order neurons in **contralateral VPM nuclei of thalamus** • Third-order fibers pass through **posterior internal capsules** • **Thalamocortical fibers** project to orofacial area of primary somatosensory cortex **Unconscious emotional processing of pain via trigeminoreticular pathway** 2. Unmyelinated C (pain) fibers ascend as trigeminoreticular fibers in VTT and may project to: • **Mesencephalic reticular formation** • **Periaqueductal gray** • **Intralaminar thalamus**, then **insular cortex** for pain modulation and emotional processing of pain **Additional input for reflexes** • **Corneal reflex** Secondary afferents from spinal trigeminal nucleus project bilaterally to facial motor nucleus to elicit consensual blink reflex • **Lacrimal reflex** Secondary afferents from spinal trigeminal nucleus project to superior salivatory nucleus. Preganglionic fibers follow greater petrosal nerve of CN VII and postganglionic fibers follow branches of V2 and then V1 lacrimal nerve to lacrimal gland. Lacrimation often occurs with corneal reflex.

Abbreviations: GSA, general somatic afferent; PDL, periodontal ligament; TMJ, temporomandibular joint.

- Fibers projecting the **masticatory CPGs** aid in modulating rhythmic chewing and bite force (see Chapter 22).
- Central axons from the mesencephalic nucleus project to the trigeminal nuclei and synapse on second-order neurons in the pars oralis, the interpolaris of the **spinal trigeminal nucleus,** or the neurons in the **main sensory nucleus,** before following the **trigeminocerebellar path** or ascending in the **trigeminothalamic tracts.**
  - The fibers carrying **ipsilateral unconscious proprioceptive** information from the temporomandibular joint (TMJ) and jaw muscles follow the **trigeminocerebellar path** and pass through the ipsilateral inferior cerebellar peduncle to terminate in the cerebellum.
  - The **trigeminocerebellar pathway** functions to correct for motor error and coordinate jaw movements. It is similar to the **spinocerebellar tracts** in the body.
- Some of the proprioceptive input concerning jaw activity passes from the mesencephalic nucleus to synapse on the dorsal part of the **main sensory nucleus**. Secondary afferents ascend in the **DTT** to the **ipsilateral VPM nuclei** of the thalamus. Third-order neurons pass fibers to the **orofacial area of the somatosensory cortex** for the conscious processing of proprioceptive input needed for sensorimotor feedback.
- The path for proprioceptive input is outlined in ▶ Table 13.10 and summarized in ▶ Fig. 13.8.

Table 13.9 Summary of central path for orofacial conscious proprioception and discriminative touch

Central Pathway Epicritic Sensations for Trigeminal		
Peripheral Input from Primary Afferents	Trigeminal Nuclear Complex	Central Path
Modality: Tactile, fine (two-point) discrimination, pressure, and vibration associated with conscious proprioception, stretch, and stereognostic input for all three divisions **Receptors:** Encapsulated and nonencapsulated mechanosensory receptors: Mechanoreceptors located in the mucosa and face (V1, V2, V3) Mechanoreceptors located in teeth, TMJ, periodontium (V2, V3) **Fibers:** Large diameter, myelinated Type II Aβ fibers *Additional GSA input from skin/mucosa of CNs VII, IX, and X	**Chief (main/pontine) sensory nucleus of V** (contains second-order neurons) **Brainstem location** Mid-pons—lateral to motor nucleus of V	**Primary routes for conscious processing of mechanosensation:** Central axons of epicritic primary afferents synapse on second-order neurons from the chief sensory nucleus and follow either a crossed and uncrossed **path** to somatosensory cortex: **Mechanosensation of face** 1. Secondary afferent fibers **decussate** and join the **contralateral ventral trigeminothalamic tract** to form trigeminal lemniscus • Secondary afferent synapse on third-order neurons in contralateral **VPM nuclei of thalamus** • Fibers pass through **the posterior limb of internal capsule** and project to **orofacial area of primary somatosensory orofacial cortex (S1)** *VTT carrying both epicritic and protopathic fibers is referred to as trigeminal lemniscus. **Mechanosensation to teeth** and **oral cavity** 2. Secondary afferent fibers from oral and dental tissue remain **ipsilateral** from **dorsal trigeminothalamic tract** • Secondary afferent fibers synapse on third-order neurons in **ipsilateral VPM nuclei of thalamus** → • Third-order neurons pass through the posterior limb of internal capsule to **ipsilateral** orofacial region of **somatosensory orofacial cortex (S1)** **Additional input for reflexes:** **Mechanosensory salivary reflex** Secondary afferents project to **nucleus tractus solitarius** (NTS) and then to **salivatory nucleus** for salivary reflex

Abbreviations: GSA, general somatic afferent; TMJ, temporomandibular joint; VPM, ventral posteromedial.

Clinical Correlation Box 13.5: Lesions of the Trigeminal Somatosensory Pathways

Lesions resulting from trauma, tumors, hemorrhage, or infarctions may occur at any point along the trigeminothalamic tracts as the fibers ascend to the thalamus and cortex. The clinical symptoms resulting from central lesions in the trigeminothalamic tracts depend on the site and extent of the injury. Frequently, adjacent paths such as the medial lemniscus or anterolateral spinothalamic tract are also damaged due to their proximity (▶ Table 13.11) (▶ Fig. 13.11).

The VTT transmits protopathic and epicritic sensations from the spinal trigeminal nucleus and main sensory nucleus of V. Lesions affecting the VTT will be contralateral to the side of the lesion because of decussation of secondary fibers in the medulla and pons. Clinical symptoms may involve only a loss of pain and temperature if the lesion occurs in the medulla or caudal pons. Discriminative tactile sensations may also be lost on the contralateral side if the lesion occurs after the secondary afferent fibers from the main sensory nucleus join the VTT. Discriminative touch and conscious proprioception may still be present on the ipsilateral side due to the preservation of the ipsilateral dorsal trigeminothalamic tract.

13.4 Sensory Contributions from Facial, Glossopharyngeal, and Vagus Nerves

13.4.1 GSA Input from Facial, Glossopharyngeal, and Vagus Cranial Nerves (▶ Table 13.12)

• In addition to the trigeminal nerve, a small amount of nociceptive sensory input is relayed from the region of the external ear, posterior one-third of the tongue, pharynx, and larynx by the **facial (CN VII), glossopharyngeal (CN IX)**, and **vagus (CN X)** nerves, respectively. The general path followed is described below and the details are summarized in ▶ Table 13.12.
• The cell bodies of the primary afferent neurons for CNs VII, IX, and X reside in the specific sensory ganglia associated with each cranial nerve: the **geniculate ganglion of CN VII, the petrosal (inferior)** and **superior ganglion of CN IX,** and the **nodose (inferior) ganglion** and **jugular (superior vagal) ganglion of CN X**.
• The primary afferent fibers of the CNs VII, IX, and X, which carry primarily nociceptive GSA input from peripheral

Table 13.10 Summary of central paths of orofacial unconscious proprioception

Central Pathway: Unconscious Proprioception for Trigeminal		
Peripheral Input from Primary Afferent	**Trigeminal Nuclear Complex**	**Central Path**
Modality Proprioception—position/movement for V2 and V3 **Receptors:** **Encapsulated proprioceptors:** Muscle spindles masticatory jaw closing muscles and tongue **Mechanoreceptors** Ruffini receptors in periodontal ligament (PDL), gingiva, and palate **Fibers** Large diameter, myelinated Aα (Ia) and Type II Aβ	**Mesencephalic nucleus** (first-order neurons) **Brainstem location:** Rostral pons to rostral midbrain	**Primary path for unconscious proprioception:** Central axons of primary afferents from the mesencephalic nucleus project to neurons in four primary locations: **Monosynaptic reflex:** **1. Motor nucleus of V**—receives bilateral input from majority of primary afferent fibers and forms protective (monosynaptic) jaw reflex (see Chapter 22) **Function:** Control bite force and mediate proprioceptive reflexes for jaw opening **Unconscious modulation of** **2. Central pattern generator** (CPG)* in pontine reticular formation sends inhibitory and excitatory input to LMNs in motor nucleus of CNs V, VII, and XII **Function:** Based on proprioceptive input from jaw, tongue, and perioral muscles during feeding and speech, the CPG modulates bite forces, rhythmic chew patterns, and oromotor behaviors (see Chapter 22) **3. Spinal trigeminal** and **chief sensory nucleus ->** secondary afferents ascend to the **cerebellum** via **trigeminocerebellar** path **Function:** Unconscious feedback to cerebellum about positional information for jaw; serves to correct motor error and coordinate jaw movement **Conscious proprioceptive input:** **4. Main sensory nucleus** –>secondary afferents ascend in **dorsal trigeminothalamic tract** (DTT) → VPM —>somatosensory cortex **Function:** Provide conscious proprioception about jaw activity to mediate sensorimotor feedback from cortex

Abbreviations: LMN, lower motor neuron; VPM, ventral posteromedial.
Note: *CPGs represent groups of inhibitory and excitatory interneurons in the brainstem reticular formation which project to cranial motor nuclei and generate rhythmic movement patterns involved in mastication, swallowing, speech, and respiration (see Chapter 22).

Table 13.11 Lesions of the trigeminal somatosensory pathway

Location of Lesion	Pathway/Structures Involved	Functional Loss
Cortical /subcortical	Lesions to third-order thalamocortical fibers terminating in primary somatosensory cortex of postcentral gyrus of the parietal lobe	Contralateral loss of sensory input to area will result in complete sensory deficit in discriminative touch and proprioception but diminished perception of pain and temperature sensations due multiple nociceptive inputs to cortical regions. Deficits may manifest as paresthesia (tingling) and numbness. Motor deficits and motor control may also occur due to somatosensory input to motor cortex. Specific deficits depend on the location of lesion within cortex relative to somatotopic organization of fiber termination from body and head.
Thalamus (ventral posterior nuclei)	Complete lesion in secondary afferent fibers terminating on third-order neurons in VPM and VPL	Contralateral loss of all sensations (hemianesthesia) in body and head—loss of light touch, conscious proprioception, two-point discrimination and vibration, and pain and temperature (complete). Thalamus serves as the gateway for conscious processing.
Rostral pons (mediolateral)	Partial lesion of ascending VTT from chief sensory nucleus; medial lemniscus	Contralateral loss/decreased tactile sensation for body and face Pain and temperature spared
Rostral pons (lateral)	Partial lesion of VTT from spinal trigeminal nucleus prior to input from chief sensory nucleus Lateral spinothalamic	Pain and temperature to contralateral face and body Tactile perception spared
Mid-pons	Motor and chief sensory nucleus; pars oralis of spinal trigeminal nucleus and entering sensory and motor root fibers	Ipsilateral loss of tactile sensation to face; ipsilateral loss of motor to masticatory muscles and jaw jerk, ipsilateral loss of pain and temperature to face. Contralateral loss of pain/temperature and tactile to body.
Mid-lower pons	Spinal trigeminal nucleus; descending spinal trigeminal tract; lateral spinothalamic tract	Ipsilateral loss of pain/temperature to face; contralateral loss of pain/temperature to body
Lateral medulla or lateral caudal pons	Spinal trigeminal nucleus and ipsilateral spinothalamic tract	Ipsilateral loss of pain and temperature of face and contralateral loss of pain and temperature of body

Abbreviations: VPL, ventral posterolateral; VPM, ventral posteromedial; VTT, ventral trigeminothalamic tract.
Notes: *Additional deficits that may occur if there is damage to pathways or nuclei located in the proximity of the lesion are not listed.
**Clinically, it is important to recognize the point of entry of primary afferents, the type of information conveyed along the path, and the level at which decussation occurs.
***Lesions occurring before the point of decussation lead to ipsilateral lesions, while lesions occurring distal to (after) the point of decussation lead to contralateral lesions.

Table 13.12 Summary of GSA contributions from CNs V, VII, IX, and X

	Trigeminal (CN V)	Facial (CN VII)	Glossopharyngeal (CN IX)	Vagus (CN X)
Modality	Pain/temperature/crude touch, tactile discrimination/pressure /proprioception	Aδ and C fibers carry pain and temperature /crude touch Some Aβ fibers carry discriminative tactile input	Aδ and C fibers carry pain and temperature/ crude touch Some Aβ fibers carry discriminative tactile input	Aδ and C fibers carry pain and temperature/crude touch Some Aβ fibers carry discriminative tactile input
GSA region innervated	* Principal GSA input for head Face, eye, oral and nasal cavities, meninges	Skin behind ear, auditory canal	Tympanic membrane; auditory tube posterior one-third of tongue, upper pharynx	Posterior ear, external auditory canal, and dura Tympanic membrane, external auditory canal, dura, lower pharynx, epiglottis, larynx
First-order neuron	Trigeminal ganglion (pain/temperature/tactile/pressure) Mesencephalic nucleus (proprioceptive)	Geniculate ganglion (GSA)	Superior ganglion of CN IX (GSA)	Jugular (superior) ganglion of CN X (GSA)
Path of primary afferents	Spinal tract of CN V Mesencephalic tract (proprioceptive)	Spinal tract of CN V	Spinal tract of CN V	Spinal tract of CN V
Second-order neurons	Spinal trigeminal nucleus Main sensory nucleus	Spinal trigeminal nucleus *Some fibers—main sensory nucleus	Spinal trigeminal nucleus *Some fibers—main sensory nucleus	Spinal trigeminal nucleus *Some fibers—main sensory nucleus
Path of secondary afferents	Decussate Primarily ascend ventral trigeminothalamic tract (VTT)* Ventral and dorsal trigeminothalamic (DTT)	Decussate Ascend VTT	Decussate Ascend VTT	Decussate Ascend VTT
Third-order neurons	VPM thalamus	VPM thalamus	VPM thalamus	VPM thalamus
Terminate	Primary somatosensory cortex face Brodmann's areas 3, 2, and 1	Primary somatosensory cortex face Brodmann's areas 3, 2, and 1	Primary somatosensory cortex face Brodmann's areas 3, 2, and 1	Primary somatosensory cortex face Brodmann's areas 3, 2, and 1

Abbreviations: GSA, general somatic afferent; VPM, ventral posteromedial.

nociceptors, pass through their respective ganglia without synapsing and follow the **spinal trigeminal tract** to synapse on second-order neurons in the caudal (**subnucleus caudalis/par caudalis**) region of the **spinal trigeminal nucleus**. The primary afferent fibers exhibit a rostrocaudal somatotopic arrangement within pars caudalis as described above.

- Fibers of secondary axons decussate and ascend in the **VTT** to synapse on third-order neurons located in the **contralateral VPM nucleus** of the thalamus.
- Fibers project to the primary somatosensory cortex to allow for the specific localization of painful sensations.

13.4.2 Reflexes Associated with CNs V, VII, IX, and X (▶ Table 13.13)

- Reflexes are rapid, predictable, and involuntary motor responses elicited by afferent general somatic (GSA) or general visceral (GVA) stimulation. Similar to the spinal nerves in the body, the cranial nerves play a role in mediating somatic and autonomic reflexive actions that serve as a protective response.

- Reflexes in the body and head require an afferent signal (**afferent limb**) and an effector (motor) response (**efferent limb**). The number of synapses occurring between the sensory and motor neuron dictates the complexity of the reflex.
  - A simple reflex (simple reflex arc), also known as a **monosynaptic reflex**, involves an afferent fiber synapsing directly on efferent motor neurons to elicit a response. The **myotatic reflex**, also known as the **muscle-tendon** or **muscle stretch reflex**, is an example of a monosynaptic reflex mediated by Type Ia afferent fibers of muscle spindles synapsing directly on efferent motor neurons. This type of reflex is found in the body and head.
    - In the head, the **masseteric (jaw jerk) (jaw-closing) reflex** is a myotatic stretch reflex important in determining jaw position and is often tested to assess trigeminal nerve function when other signs of trigeminal nerve damage exist.
    - Both the afferent and efferent limbs of the jaw jerk reflex occur through the mandibular division of the trigeminal nerve (CN V3) (▶ Fig. 13.10). The afferent fibers originate from the mesencephalic nucleus and synapse directly on lower motor neurons (LMNs) in the motor nucleus of V to elicit contraction of jaw-closing muscles. The normal jerk

Table 13.13 Reflexes mediated through trigeminal nuclei

	Location of Sensory Neurons	Afferent Limb (GSA) and Path	Location of Motor Neurons	Efferent Limb (SVE) and Path	Protective Function
Gag reflex Polysynaptic reflex	Inferior ganglion of CN IX (GVA) and superior ganglion of CN IX (GSA) **May occur by either contribution or both GVA serves as the primary contributor	Glossopharyngeal (CN IX) projects to: • Spinal trigeminal nucleus • Nucleus tract of solitarius • Secondary afferent fibers from sensory nuclei project bilaterally to nucleus ambiguus	Nucleus ambiguus	Vagus (CN X) to muscle in pharynx Ipsilateral to nucleus ambiguus = direct elevation Contralateral input to nucleus ambiguus results in consensual elevation	Prevent chocking or swallowing hazardous items *Stimulation of one side of palate results in consensual elevation of both sides of palate Causes expulsion of item
Corneal reflex Polysynaptic reflex	Trigeminal ganglion	Ophthalmic (CN V1) → spinal trigeminal nucleus *A few fibers may project to chief sensory of CN V but not principal path →project bilaterally to facial motor nucleus	Facial motor nucleus	Facial (CN VII) to facial muscles around eye (orbicularis oculi) Ipsilateral to motor CN VII = direct closure Contralateral input to motor CN VII—indirect closure (consensual)	Protect eye against foreign objects *Stimulation of one eye results in consensual closure of both eyes **Reopening of eye involves input to oculomotor nucleus and CN III and is a secondary part of the response
Lacrimal reflex	Trigeminal ganglion	Ophthalmic (CN V1) Spinal trigeminal nucleus Secondary afferents project bilaterally to superior salivatory nucleus	Superior salivatory nucleus of CN VII	Greater petrosal of CN VII provides (GVE) parasympathetic innervation; postganglionic fibers accompany CN V1 to lacrimal gland in eye	Protective tearing reflex to cleanse eye of debris *Usually occurs along with the corneal reflex
Jaw jerk reflex Monosynaptic reflex	Mesencephalic nucleus	Mandibular (CN V3) afferents of muscle spindles *Monosynaptic—direct bilateral input to motor nucleus	Trigeminal motor nucleus	Mandibular (CN V3) to masticatory muscles	Prevents excessive stretch and provides joint stability during movement

Abbreviations: GSA, general somatic afferent; GSE, general somatic efferent; SVE, special visceral efferent; GVA, general visceral afferent.
Notes: *SVE = special visceral efferent fibers—efferent motor fibers which innervate skeletal muscle derived from pharyngeal arches (equivalent to GSE).
**GVA fibers of CN IX may also elicit gag reflex; however, stimulation through GVA is mediated through nucleus solitarius.
***Reflexes are subject to modulation leading to suppression or amplification of effect response.

response is of small amplitude and hard to detect; however, the reflex may become exaggerated and is important in the diagnosis of **pseudobulbar palsy** (upper motor neuron [UMN] paralysis) affecting the trigeminal motor pathway (Clinical Correlation Box 13.6).

○ More complex reflex arcs are known as polysynaptic reflex pathways and require one or more interneurons to connect the afferent sensory neuron to the motor neuron. The nociceptive (withdrawal) reflex and jaw-opening reflex are examples of polysynaptic reflexes triggered by painful or mechanical stimuli (see Chapter 22 for reflex pathways of head).

• GSA input from CNs V, VII, IX, and X mediates several cranial reflexes through the trigeminal nuclei, including the **gag, corneal, lacrimal**, and **jaw jerk reflexes**. These reflexes are summarized in ▶ Table 13.13 and covered in detail in Chapter 22.

Clinical Correlation Box 13.6: Hyperactive Jaw Jerk Reflex

Tapping the mandible while the jaw is slightly open activates muscle spindles in the jaw-closing muscles as the muscles begin to stretch. Stretching of muscle spindles results in slight contraction of the masticatory muscles and jaw closure due to stimulation of the efferent neurons in the motor nucleus of V. Visual observation of the jerk response is normally not evident and considered to be absent. However, in a positive response, the stretch of the muscle spindles elicits a brisk upward motion of the jaw. This forceful upwards (hyperactive) jerk of the jaw may be indicative of damage to descending corticobulbar tracts or UMNs in the cerebral cortex (▶ Fig. 13.10a–c).

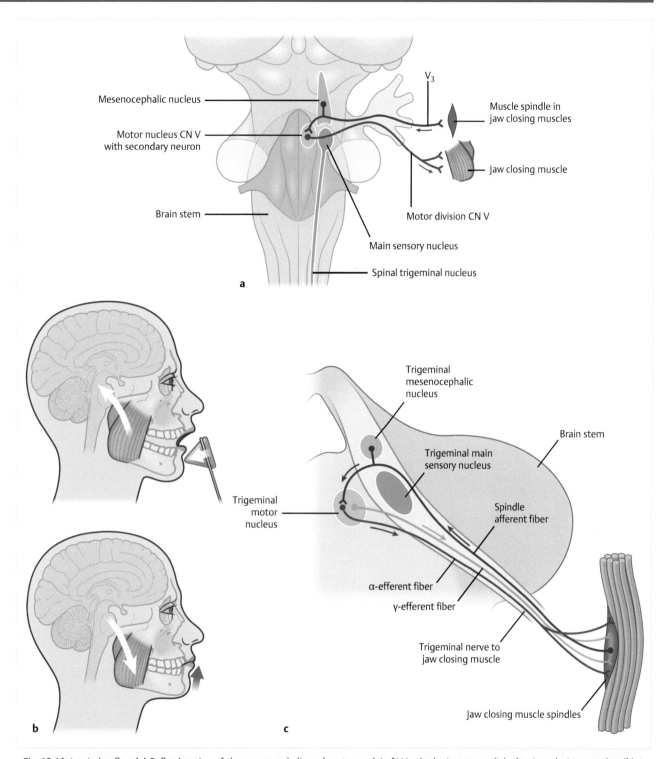

Fig. 13.10 Jaw jerk reflex. **(a)** Reflex location of the mesencephalic and motor nuclei of V in the brainstem are linked to jaw-closing muscles. **(b)** A downward tap of the mandible while the jaw is slightly open activates muscle spindles as the masticatory muscles stretch. In response to stretching, the Type Ia primary afferent fibers of the mesencephalic nucleus transmit impulses directly to lower motor neurons (LMNs) in the motor nucleus of V. Stimulation of motor neurons leads to a brisk, partial upward jerk of the lower jaw as jaw-closing muscles contract. The normal jerk response is of small amplitude and hard to detect; however, a forceful upward (hyperreflexia) jerk suggests damage to descending trigeminal motor path or upper motor neurons in the cortex. **(c)** First-order sensory neurons reside in the mesencephalic nucleus and primary afferent fibers (blue) pass through the nucleus to synapse directly on LMNs in the trigeminal motor nucleus (motor nucleus of V). Efferent fibers (red) elicit skeletal muscle contraction.

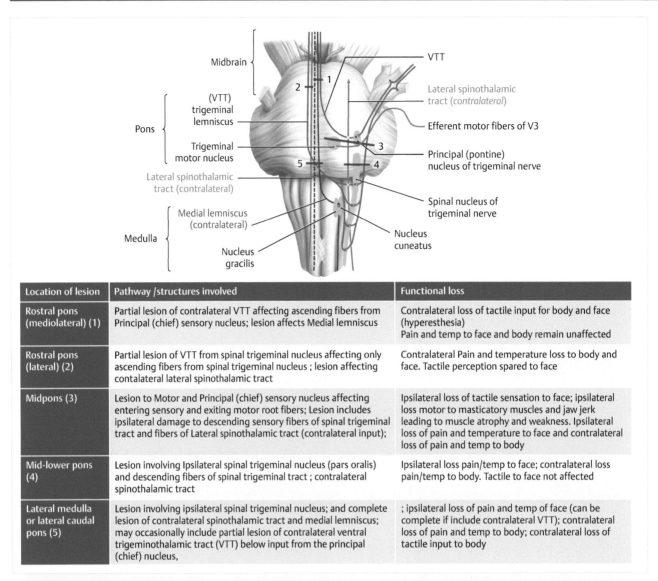

Location of lesion	Pathway /structures involved	Functional loss
Rostral pons (mediolateral) (1)	Partial lesion of contralateral VTT affecting ascending fibers from Principal (chief) sensory nucleus; lesion affects Medial lemniscus	Contralateral loss of tactile input for body and face (hyperesthesia) Pain and temp to face and body remain unaffected
Rostral pons (lateral) (2)	Partial lesion of VTT from spinal trigeminal nucleus affecting only ascending fibers from spinal trigeminal nucleus ; lesion affecting contalateral lateral spinothalamic tract	Contralateral Pain and temperature loss to body and face. Tactile perception spared to face
Midpons (3)	Lesion to Motor and Principal (chief) sensory nucleus affecting entering sensory and exiting motor root fibers; Lesion includes ipsilateral damage to descending sensory fibers of spinal trigeminal tract and fibers of Lateral spinothalamic tract (contralateral input);	Ipsilateral loss of tactile sensation to face; ipsilateral loss motor to masticatory muscles and jaw jerk leading to muscle atrophy and weakness. Ipsilateral loss of pain and temperature to face and contralateral loss of pain and temp to body
Mid-lower pons (4)	Lesion involving Ipsilateral spinal trigeminal nucleus (pars oralis) and descending fibers of spinal trigeminal tract ; contralateral spinothalamic tract	Ipsilateral loss pain/temp to face; contralateral loss pain/temp to body. Tactile to face not affected
Lateral medulla or lateral caudal pons (5)	Lesion involving ipsilateral spinal trigeminal nucleus; and complete lesion of contralateral spinothalamic tract and medial lemniscus; may occasionally include partial lesion of contralateral ventral trigeminothalamic tract (VTT) below input from the principal (chief) nucleus,	; ipsilateral loss of pain and temp of face (can be complete if include contralateral VTT); contralateral loss of pain and temp to body; contralateral loss of tactile input to body

Fig. 13.11 Lesions of trigeminal somatosensory pathways. The clinical symptoms resulting from central lesions of the trigeminothalamc tracts depend on the site and extent of the injury. Frequently, adjacent paths such as the medial lemniscus or anterolateral spinothalamic tract may also be damaged. (Modified with permission from Schuenke M, Schulte E, Schumacher U. THIEME Atlas of Anatomy Third Edition, Vol 3. © Thieme 2020. Illustrations by Markus Voll and Karl Wesker.)

13.4.3 Viscerosensory (GVA) Input from Cranial Nerves VII, IX, and X (▶ Table 13.14)

- In addition to GSA fibers, the **facial (CN VII), glossopharyngeal (CN IX), and vagus (CN X)** also carry **GVA** fibers and transmit conscious and unconscious visceral sensations from visceral receptors found in the oropharyngeal mucosa, glands, and blood vessels.
  - The trigeminal nerve does not carry GVA fibers.
- The viscerosensory information transmitted by the facial, glossopharyngeal, and vagus nerves follows a different path than the somatosensory trigeminal system, and primarily mediates protective unconscious somatic and autonomic reflexes involved in swallowing, coughing, and blood pressure maintenance (▶ Table 13.14).

- The cell bodies of the primary GVA fibers reside along the sensory neurons that transmit somatosensory (GSA) and taste (SVA) sensation in the sensory ganglia of CNs VII, IX, and X. The pathway for taste sensation initially follows the GVA pathway and is covered in Chapter 15.
- Central processes of the primary GVA afferent fibers enter the **solitary tract (tract of solitarius)**, a compact bundle of axons that extends through the posterolateral medulla to the caudal region of the pons.
- The solitary tract is surrounded by sensory nuclei forming a column of gray matter known as the **solitary nucleus (nucleus tract of solitarius, NTS)**. The caudal part of the solitary nucleus serves as the principal visceral sensory nucleus of the brainstem.
- GVA fibers from the solitary tract synapse on second-order neurons in the solitary nucleus (NTS) before projecting to higher regions of the CNS to mediate regulatory function.

Table 13.14 GVA input from cranial nerves VII, IX, and X

Cranial Nerve	Receptor	Receptor Location	Modality	Primary Sensory Neurons	Tract	Path	Reflex Activity
Facial (GVA) Nervus intermedius	Polymodal nociceptor Mechanoreceptors	Mucous membranes of posterior palate, nasopharynx	Tactile stimulation Chemical irritation	Geniculate ganglion	Solitary tract	Primary afferent fibers terminate in nucleus solitarius	Not associated with specific reflex
Glossopharyngeal (GVA) (CN IX)	Tactile mechanoreceptors Polymodal nociceptors Chemoreceptors Baroreceptors	Mucous membranes of posterior one-third of tongue, pharynx Carotid sinus/body	Conscious sensations of mucosa in oropharynx Detect changes in blood CO_2; detect changes in arterial pressure	Petrosal (inferior) ganglion	Solitary tract	Primary afferent fibers terminate in nucleus solitarius	Carotid sinus reflex (baroreflex) Carotid body reflex (chemoreceptor reflex)
Vagus (GVA) (CN X)	Mechanoreceptors Polymodal nociceptors Chemoreceptors Baroreceptors	Mucous membranes of larynx, epiglottis, Aorta Pulmonary	Respond to stimulation of laryngeal and tracheal mucosa Detect changes in blood CO_2; increase in pressure/stretch in vessel wall	Nodose (inferior) ganglion	Solitary tract	Primary afferent fibers terminate in nucleus solitarius	Cough Swallow Reflex Aortic body (chemoreflex) Aortic sinus (baroreflex)

Abbreviation: GVA, general visceral afferent.

Questions and Answers

1. The ventral trigeminothalamic tract (VTT) carries what type of sensory information?
   a) Mechanosensory input from the teeth
   b) Discriminative tactile sensations from the oral mucosa
   c) Mechanosensory information from the gingiva
   d) Discriminative touch from the skin of lip

Level 2: Moderate

Answer D: The VTT carries epicritic sensations arising from the contralateral face, as well as pain, temperature, and crude touch from the contralateral face. The two fiber paths together are referred to as the trigeminal lemniscus. The fibers of the main (chief) sensory nucleus decussate to join the protopathic fibers in the VTT at the level of mid-pons. The primary afferent fibers from all three trigeminal divisions transmit tactile, vibratory, and positional input from the face, and synapse on neurons in the ventral part of the main (chief) sensory nucleus. In comparison, epicritic sensations arising from the oral cavity travel via maxillary and mandibular divisions to synapse in the dorsal region of the chief sensory nucleus. These fibers remain ipsilateral and ascend via the DTT. Discriminative and mechanosensory inputs from the teeth (**A**), oral mucosa (**B**), and gingiva (**C**) follow the DTT to the ipsilateral VPM.

2. A 67-year-old woman exhibits a decrease in pain and temperature loss on the left side of her face, from the forehead to her lower jaw, with central sparing of nose and mouth. The onion-skin pattern of sensory loss suggests the lesion is located in which of the following locations.
   a) Left main sensory nucleus
   b) Left pars caudalis
   c) Right pars interpolaris
   d) Right pars oralis
   e) Left mesencephalic nucleus

Level 2: Moderate

Answer B: The pattern of protopathic sensory loss to the lateral side of the face suggests the lesion occurred in the left pars caudalis. Fibers carrying pain and temperature enter through the trigeminal ganglion and then descend ipsilaterally in the spinal trigeminal tract to terminate on second-order neurons in the spinal trigeminal nucleus. The spinal trigeminal nucleus extends from the pons to the cervical spinal cord. The nucleus consists of three components: the pars oralis, pars interpolaris, and pars caudalis which are oriented rostral to caudal along the longitudinal axis of the brainstem. The majority of the protopathic fibers synapse in the pars caudalis. The spinal trigeminal nucleus exhibits a somatotopic arrangement; the central area of the face, including the nose and oral cavity, is represented rostrally and the lateral face caudally. The right pars interpolaris (C) and right pars oralis (D) receive protopathic sensations from the right side of the face. Damage to the rostral part of the nucleus would also be associated with loss of pain and temperature to the central region of the face. The secondary afferent fibers of the spinal trigeminal nucleus decussate after synapsing in the nucleus and travel in the ventral trigeminothalamic tract. (A) Discriminative tactile and vibratory sensations from the left side of the face synapse on the ipsilateral main (chief) sensory nucleus. (E) The left mesencephalic nucleus contains cell bodies of the primary afferent fibers carrying unconscious proprioception from masticatory muscles and the TMJ and would not result in protopathic sensory loss.

3. Which of the following type of myelinated sensory fibers travels in both the spinal trigeminal tract and the tract of Lissauer?
   a) Type Ia (Aα)
   b) Type II (Aβ)
   c) Type III (Aδ)
   d) Type Ib (Aα)

Level 1: Easy

Answer C: Both the spinal trigeminal tract and the tract of Lissauer (dorsolateral tract) contain Type III (Aδ) fibers (C) and unmyelinated C fibers that carry pain, temperature, and crude touch. The tracts are considered to be analogous tracts. The spinal trigeminal tract extends from the caudal pons to C2 of the spinal cord. The tract of Lissauer represents axons of dorsal root fibers located near the dorsal column. The fibers of the tract project up or down one or two spinal segments before entering the gray matter. This tract is found throughout the spinal cord and is usually spared, along with the dorsal column, during occlusion of the vertebral artery. Proprioceptive input follows Type Ia fibers (A) from muscle spindles, and Type Ib (D) from Golgi tendon organs. Type II afferent fibers (B) carry tactile mechanosensory input. These fibers enter the medial aspect of the dorsal root in the spinal cord or enter the pons to synapse in the main (chief) sensory nucleus of V and do not travel in these tracts.

4. The tract that carries unconscious proprioceptive input from muscle spindles of the jaw-closing muscles is the
   _____ tract.
   a) posterior spinocerebellar
   b) trigeminoreticular
   c) cuneocerebellar
   d) trigeminocerebellar

Level 1: Easy

Answer D: The trigeminocerebellar tract carries unconscious proprioceptive input from the muscle spindles of the jaw-closing muscles and pressure receptors in the TMJ. The posterior spinocerebellar (C8–L2) (A) and cuneocerebellar (C2–T7) (C) tracts carry unconscious proprioception from the muscle spindles, GTO, and pressure receptors in the lower limb, trunk, and

upper limb. The two spinocerebellar tracts are comparable to the trigeminocerebellar tract. The trigeminoreticular tract (B) carries nociceptive input from free nerve endings associated with unmyelinated C fibers to the reticular formation, periaqueductal gray, and the limbic portion of the cortex. The input is perceived as dull, diffuse pain.

5. A 14-year-old patient developed a fever and a progressively severe headache following a dental infection. Her left eyelid began to droop (partial ptosis) 2 days ago. She has some swelling behind the eye, and the pupil size (miosis) is reduced. A clinical examination reveals altered facial sensations on the left side in the area around the eye and cheek and loss of the corneal reflex. The left eye is turned in medially toward the nose and she is unable to abduct the eye during the examination. The magnetic resonance imaging (MRI) reveals a cavernous sinus thrombosis on the left side that is most likely related to the dental infection. The compression of each of the following nerves may lead to the symptoms described EXCEPT one. Which one is the exception?
   a) Abducens, CN VI
   b) Postganglionic sympathetic fibers
   c) Ophthalmic division of trigeminal (CN V1)
   d) Mandibular division of the trigeminal (CN V3)
   e) Maxillary division of the trigeminal (CN V2)

Level 2: Moderate

Answer D: The mandibular division is the exception. The CN V3 division passes outside the wall of the cavernous sinus. All other nerves listed as choices pass through the cavernous sinus.

The abducens (CN VI), along with trochlear (CN IV) and oculomotor nerves (CN III), passes through the cavernous sinus to enter the orbit. The nerves supply the extraocular muscles. The compression of the abducens nerve leads to medial adduction of the eye due to the unopposed action of the medial rectus muscle. The medial rectus is innervated by the oculomotor nerve (CN III). As compression increases, the oculomotor nerve (CN III) and trochlear nerve (CN IV) may eventually become involved. The compression of the abducens is an early sign of ophthalmoplegia (paralysis of the eye muscles) that often accompanies cavernous sinus thrombosis. CN V1 (C) and CN V2 (E) also pass through the sinus and compression may lead to diminished tactile and protopathic sensations in the face. Trigeminal neuralgia (intermittent, sharp pain) associated with damage may also occur in some cases. The compression of the CN V1 division leads to the loss of the afferent limb of the corneal reflex. (B) Postganglionic sympathetic fibers that target the eye travel with internal carotid and also pass through the sinus. Sympathetic fibers enter the superior orbital fissure and travel with the long ciliary fibers of the nasociliary nerve (CN V1). The compression of sympathetic fibers leads to small pupil size and ptosis. The sympathetic fibers, along with the oculomotor (CN III) nerve, contribute to elevation and retraction of the eyelid.

14 Pain

Learning Objectives

1. State the definition of pain.
2. What is nociceptive pain? Identify subtypes.
3. What is neuropathic pain? Identify subtypes.
4. How does nociceptive and neuropathic pain differ?
5. Identify pain receptors and afferents.
6. What are the neural processes involved in the physiology of pain?
7. Discuss mechanisms involved in pain modulation.
8. Describe descending pain pathways for pain modulation.
9. Identify the differences between acute and chronic pain.
10. Discuss central sensitization and neuroplasticity.

14.1 Overview of Pain

Pain can be defined as an unpleasant sensory or emotional experience that is associated with real or potential tissue damage. It is a complex modality that is both a symptom and a perception. It is also essential for survival. Although most sensory input is informational, pain is protective. Nociceptive (noxious) stimuli trigger behavioral processes that protect tissue from damage and are often associated with behavioral changes directed at preventing further damage. Additionally, pain perception can be influenced by past experiences and is therefore highly variable and not necessarily proportional to the extent of tissue damage.

At the cellular level, pain is described as **nociceptive** (Latin for *nocere*, "to hurt") meaning that it is noxious or potentially damaging. **Noxious stimuli** activate receptors (**nociceptors**) that will then initiate an **action potential** (**AP**) in pain nerve fibers. The impulse is transmitted by nerve fibers into the spinal cord and eventually to the brain via ascending sensory tracts. Ultimately, the signal that began from the activation of nociceptors in the peripheral nervous system is interpreted as pain by the cerebral cortex. One caveat to the several well-documented pain pathways is the observation that the intensity of pain is not necessarily a direct function of the activation of pain receptors. Pain transmission can be modulated such that endogenous analgesia is produced resulting in a percep-

tion of decreased pain intensity. Conversely, pain can also be exaggerated or perceived as originating from a different source. The endogenous analgesia mechanism was initially suggested based on anecdotal accounts by physicians treating soldiers on the battlefield, and is now the basis for modern-day pharmaceutical pain control using opioids.

14.2 Classification of Pain

- Pain can be classified as **nociceptive** or **neuropathic** (▶ Table 14.1).
  - **Nociceptive**: Pain evoked as a result of stimulation of pain receptors.
    - **Somatic**: Pain caused by damage to skin, muscles, joints, or bone. Pain is described as sharp and localized.
    - **Visceral**: Pain caused by damage/disease involving viscera, e.g., stomach, heart, or gastrointestinal (GI) tract. Pain is described as vague, diffuse, and difficult to localize. Visceral pain can ultimately involve the body wall at which point it becomes somatic and therefore well localized.
    - **Referred**: Pain of visceral origin that appears to originate from somatic structures. There are several hypotheses proposed to explain **referred pain** (▶ Fig. 14.1a). The **convergence theory** suggests that referred pain is due to the **convergence** (synapsing) of visceral and somatic afferents on the same sensory neurons in the dorsal horn of spinal cord. This mechanism involves sensory information from both visceral and somatic structures entering the spinal cord at approximately the same level. Typically, visceral and somatic afferents synapse on specific/separate second-order neurons. There are circumstances where collaterals from visceral afferents will synapse on somatic second-order neurons. If visceral afferents synapse on a somatic second-order sensory neuron, which typically receives somatic information, the visceral sensory information is ultimately interpreted as somatic (▶ Fig. 14.1b). A second hypothesis, the **common dermatome** principle, states that referred pain originating from a structure can refer to a different structure that developed from the same **dermatome**

Table 14.1 Pain classification

Classification	Etiology	Examples	Description
Nociceptive	Caused by stimulation of pain receptors	Somatic	Pain caused by damage to skin, muscles, joints, and bone
		Visceral	Pain caused by damage to viscera (stomach, intestines, bladder)
		Referred	Originates in viscera but perceived as somatic
Neuropathic	Results from abnormal signaling or dysfunction of nociceptive neurons	Phantom limb	Pain experienced after amputation; may involve somatosensory memory or central sensitization
		Peripheral neuropathy	Degeneration of distal nerves
		Central pain syndrome	Caused by injury to central pain pathway in spinal cord or thalamus

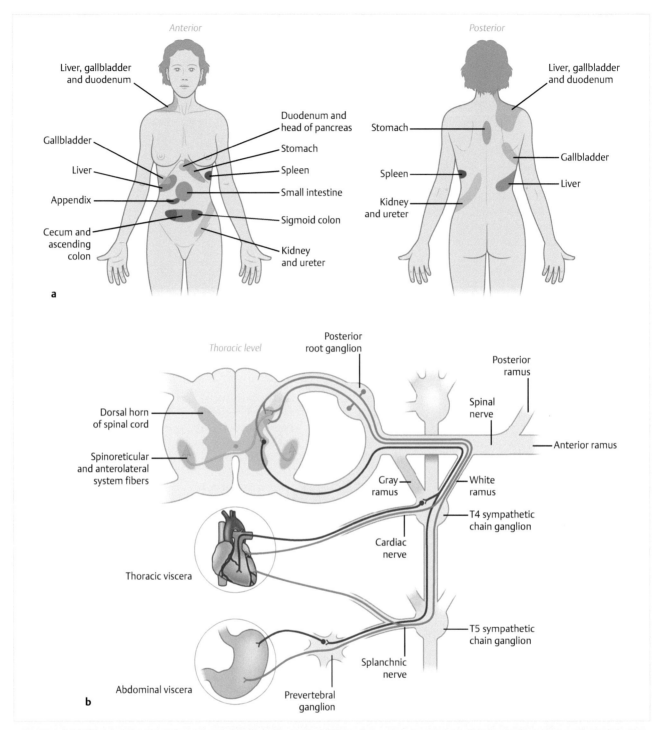

Fig. 14.1 **(a)** Referred pain occurs when visceral pain is perceived as originating from somatic structures. **(b)** Convergence theory of referred pain. Nociceptive (and non-nociceptive information) can converge on the same second-order neuron from different parts of the body.

(Continued)

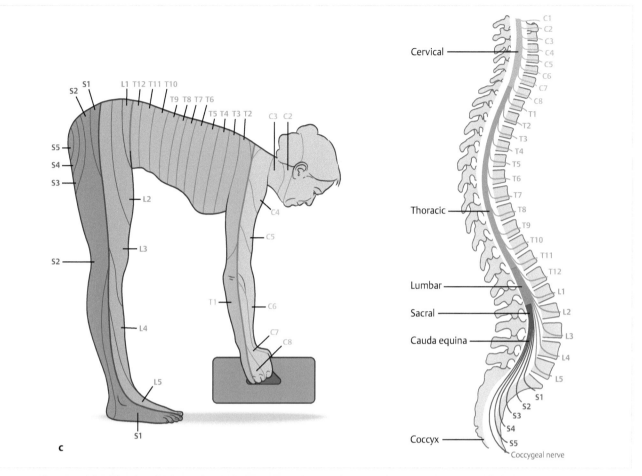

Fig. 14.1 (*Continued*) **(c)** The common dermatome hypothesis states that pain from a structure can "refer" to a different structure that developed from the same dermatome.

(▶ Fig. 14.1c). Both hypotheses can explain **angina** (cardiac pain) localizing to the left shoulder/arm (▶ Fig. 14.2).

○ **Neuropathic**: Pain resulting from abnormal signaling due to injury or dysfunction of peripheral nociceptive neurons. The deficit may involve peripheral nerves or central nervous system (CNS) pathways. Pain is often poorly localized. This disorder can be caused by **compression**, **transection**, **ischemia**, and **infiltration**. Neuropathic pain can be acute or chronic and **intractable**.

– **Phantom limb:** Painful sensations experienced after amputation of extremities. Reported to be as high as 70% among amputees in the first week post surgery. Pain is typically intermittent and described as shooting, stabbing, throbbing, and burning and may subside over time. The etiology of this disorder is unclear. The "pain" is thought to be originating from the CNS and the cause is proposed as somatosensory "memory" or **central sensitization**. Other factors believed to be involved in the phenomena are: the formation of scar tissue at the site of amputation, development of neuromas, and damaged nerve endings. Treatment is often unsuccessful.

– **Peripheral neuropathy:** A degeneration of distal nerves common in several diseases. Pain is described as burning, often involving the toes and feet. Diabetes mellitus is one of the most common causes of peripheral neuropathy.

– **Central pain syndrome:** This disorder is due to injury to central pain pathways that include sensory pathways in the spinal cord and the thalamus. Common sources of lesions include: **infarction**, **hemorrhage**, **abscesses**, **tumors,** and **trauma**. The intensity of the pain ranges from mild to excruciating. The pain is often constant and significantly impacts the patient's quality of life. The mechanisms involved in central pain syndrome are poorly understood at this time. Treatment is not universally effective and typically does not eliminate pain.

14.3 Pain Receptors and Afferents

Nociceptors are unspecialized receptors that are activated by noxious stimuli.

• These pain receptors transduce stimuli into receptor potentials that in turn initiate afferent **AP** (see Chapter 4).
• Nociceptors take origin from sensory neurons in the dorsal root ganglion or in the trigeminal ganglion.
  ○ Sensory neurons (pseudounipolar) have a single axon and a **central** (**CP**) and **peripheral** (**PP**) **axonal process** (see Chapter 3).

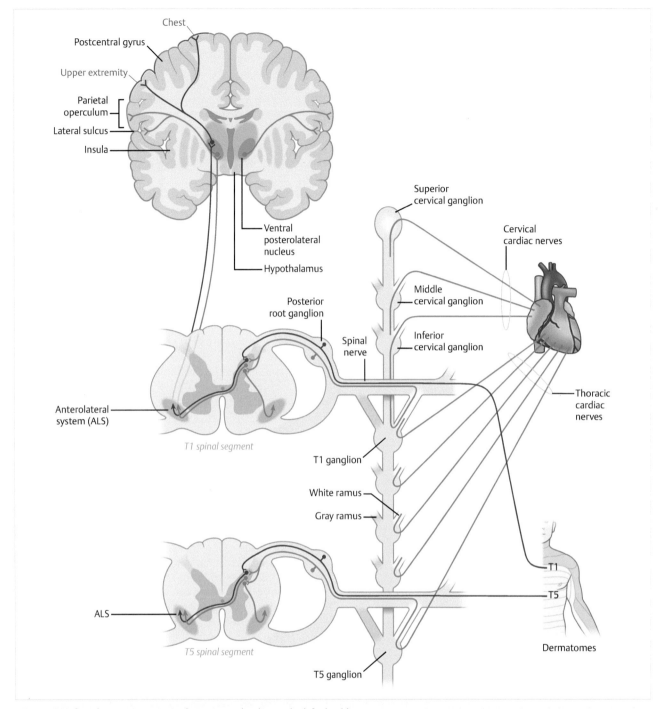

Fig. 14.2 Referred pain in angina. Cardiac pain can localize to the left shoulder.

- The CP enters the CNS while the PP extends into the periphery.
- Nociceptors are also called **free nerve endings** (see Chapter 11).
  - They are unspecialized and unmyelinated or lightly myelinated.
  - Nociceptors can be categorized by the properties of the axon fibers that they associate with:
    - Aδ fibers

      - Respond to intense mechanical or mechanothermal stimuli
      - Myelinated
      - Large diameter
      - Fast conduction (20 m/sec)
      - Carry fast, sharp pain sensation
    - C fibers
      - Respond to thermal, mechanical, and chemical stimuli
      - Unmyelinated
      - Small diameter

- Slow conduction (2 m/sec)
- Carry delayed, slow pain sensation

14.4 Physiology of Pain

- There are four neural processes involved in the physiology of pain: **transduction**, **transmission**, **modulation**, and **perception**. The situations that may result in the initiation of these processes may include:
  - Inflammation (neuritis).
  - Injury to the nerves or nerve endings (disc prolapse).
  - Nerve invasion by cancer (neural plexus involvement).
  - Injury to structures that process neural information (spinal cord, thalamus or cortical areas).
  - Abnormal activity in neural pathways (phantom pain).
- **Transduction** involves the activation of nociceptors in peripheral tissues. Chemical mediators released in response to tissue damage modulate free nerve endings resulting in activation. These molecules sensitize the receptors and facilitate the conversion of the stimulus into an AP.
  - Three types of stimuli can activate pain receptors: mechanical, heat, and chemical.
  - Noxious stimuli results in the release of chemical mediators such as **prostaglandins**, **bradykinins**, **substance P**, **potassium**, and **histamine**.
  - Chemical mediators sensitize/stimulate the nociceptors to the noxious stimuli.
    - Generation of an AP and subsequent pain impulse require an exchange of sodium and potassium ions (polarization and repolarization) in the nerve cell membrane (see Chapter 4).
- **Transmission** occurs when the nociceptive stimulus is carried from the periphery into the CNS.
  - The pain impulse is taken into the CNS via the peripheral process of the sensory neuron whose cell body is located in the dorsal root ganglion (DRG).
  - The central process of the sensory neuron enters the dorsal horn of the spinal cord and synapses on second-order cell bodies located in Rexed lamina (RL) I (see Chapter 10). Fibers from the second-order neurons cross and ascend in the spinal cord. These fibers combine to form the **neospinothalamic tract,** which also constitutes the **lateral spinothalamic tract (LST).** The LST projects to the thalamus.
    - This tract is involved in the immediate awareness of pain as well as localization.
  - A number of both αδ and C fibers synapse on cell bodies located in RL II (substantia gelatinosa) and then project to second-order neurons located in RL IV–VI (**nucleus proprius**). Most of these axons cross and ascend in the anterior region of the spinal cord and are thus called the **anterior spinothalamic tract (AST)**. The AST is part of the **paleospinothalamic tract** which also projects to the thalamus. Additionally, the paleospinothalamic tract includes nerve fibers that project to other structures and are known as the **spinorecticular tract**, the **spinomesencephalic tract,** and the **spinotectal tract** (**tectum**).

- These fibers are involved in the emotional response to pain.
    - The spinoreticular tract (spinal cord to reticular formation) is thought to be responsible for the affective components of pain including depression, fear, and anger.
    - The spinomesencephalic and spinotectal pathways (spinal cord to midbrain) are involved in the central modulation of pain and various reflex reactions to pain including "alerting" reactions.
  - The **anterolateral system/tract** (**ALS**) is composed of the anterior and lateral spinothalamic tracts.
  - The oldest of the ascending pain pathways is the **archispinothalamic tract**. In this pathway, the first-order sensory neurons synapse in RL II (SG) and ascend to laminae IV–VII. From these RL, the fibers ascend and descend to ultimately make their way to the **medullary reticular formation-periaqueductal gray** (**MRF-PAG**) area. Some fibers will continue toward the thalamus and send collaterals to the hypothalamus and limbic nuclei.
    - These fibers are involved in the visceral, emotional, and autonomic response to pain.
- Both anecdotal and experimental observations support the concept of **endogenous pain modulatory mechanisms**. Although it has been shown that there are several modulatory pathways, three major regulatory mechanisms play a significant role in the inhibition of pain in humans: **segmental inhibition, endogenous opioid system,** and **descending inhibitory tracts** (see Section 14.5).
- It is commonly accepted that there are differences between the reality of a painful stimulus and the individuals' response to it. **Pain perception** involves much more than just the neural impulse. This phenomenon reflects the complex neural loops involved in pain transmission as well as the recognition that there is a demonstrable psychological component to pain. Emotional aspects of pain are most apparent in individuals experiencing chronic pain but are also important in the treatment of acute pain.
  - The emotional response to pain involves cortical and subcortical structures that include the **limbic system**, the **anterior cingulate gyrus,** and part of the **prefrontal cortex**. Studies have shown that in cancer patients a frontal lobotomy can completely block the affective aspects of pain. These patients can recognize and feel pain but report that it doesn't "bother" them.
  - Factors known to be involved in the perception of acute and chronic pain are:
    - *Context*: The situation in which an individual experiences pain has a profound influence on perception, e.g., pain perceived in battle is not proportional to the extent of the wounds.
    - *Attention*: Focusing attention on pain makes the pain worse. Distracting patients is highly effective in reducing pain. Burn patients report excruciating pain during therapy even opioids are given, however, if distracted with video or virtual reality, they report a fraction of the pain.
    - *Anxiety*: Treating a patient for fear, anxiety, and loss of control has been shown to decrease pain and reduce analgesic use.

– *Memory*: Patients who experienced low levels of pain remember it as being worse than originally reported.
– *Expectations*: Patients' expectations of how much pain they should feel can influence how much pain they feel and their response to treatment. Cultural influences can also influence expectations and thus pain perception. The **placebo effect** is also influenced by the patients' expectations.
– *Beliefs and coping*: Psychosocial issues such as coping skills, tendency to "catastrophize," self-efficacy, and what patients "believe" about their pain can impact how much pain they feel and how it affects them.

14.5 Mechanisms of Pain Modulation

14.5.1 Endogenous Opioids

The effect of **opioids** on pain modulation is well documented. These peptides directly inhibit ascending transmission of noxious stimuli from the dorsal horn of the spinal cord and activate descending pain control circuits from the midbrain to the dorsal horn of the spinal cord. In addition to analgesia, opiates are involved in a diverse array of homeostatic functions including the cardiovascular system, thermoregulation, neuroendocrine activity, learning, and memory.

• Opioid peptides and their receptors are distributed throughout the CNS.
• Three classes of **opioid receptors** have been identified: **μ-mu, δ-delta,** and **κ-kappa**.
• Three classes of **opioid peptides** are known to interact with the opioid receptors: **endorphins**, **enkephalins,** and **dynorphins**.
  ○ Enkephalins are considered the ligands for δ receptors.
  ○ β endorphins bind μ receptors.
  ○ Dynorphins are the ligand for κ receptors.
• Opioid peptides modulate nociceptive information by:
  ○ Blocking neurotransmitter release by inhibiting Ca⁺ influx into the presynaptic terminal.
  ○ Opening K⁺ channels which hyperpolarizes neurons and inhibits spike activity.

14.5.2 Segmental Inhibition

The **gate theory** of pain control was proposed by Melzack and Wall in 1965. Today's version is somewhat different but the theory remains valid. The model is based on the premise that noxious information carried on Aδ and C fibers can be blocked by activating larger Aβ touch fibers (▶ Fig. 14.3).

• Activation of the small diameter fibers (Aδ and C) terminating in the SG transmits noxious stimuli by inhibiting the SG inhibitory interneuron and activating the second-order neuron of the spinothalamic tract (STT) which keeps the gate "open."
• Rubbing the injured area stimulates the touch Aβ fibers which in turn activates the inhibitory interneuron. The inhibitory interneuron prevents the activation of the endogenous peptide analgesic system via presynaptic inhibition of the Aδ/C fibers. Thus, rubbing "closes" the gate.

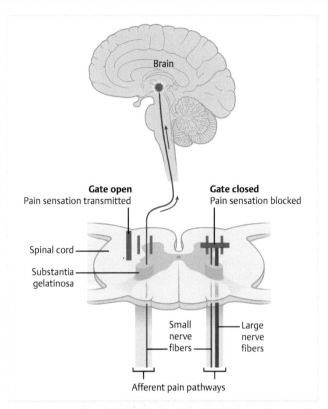

Fig. 14.3 Gate theory of pain control. Noxious information carried on small pain fibers can be blocked by activating larger nonpain fibers.

• The "gate theory" of pain modulation is the basis of **transcutaneous electrical nerve stimulation** (**TENS**).

14.6 Descending Pathways of Pain Modulation

Pain can be modulated by descending pathways with in the CNS. Norepinephrine and serotonin are the principal neurotransmitters involved in descending inhibition. This system is described in detail below.

• These pathways are polysynaptic and project from cerebral nuclei and subcortical structures to the dorsal horn of the spinal cord.
• Ascending pathways carry the stimulus from the dorsal horn to the cortex where it will be interpreted as pain.
• Descending pathways modulate/inhibit nociception at the level of the dorsal horn by blocking the transmission of the nociceptive signal.

14.6.1 Overview of Pain Modulation

Pain information from the body is carried on the spinothalamic tract in the spinal cord (▶ Fig. 14.4).

• Nociceptive information is picked up by peripheral receptors and transmitted into the spinal cord by a sensory neuron located in the dorsal root ganglia. The central process of the

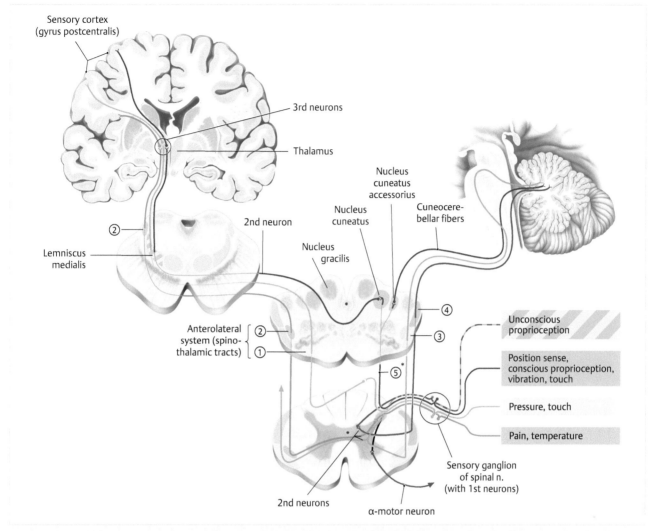

Fig. 14.4 Pain information is carried on ascending fibers known as the spinothalamic tract. (Reproduced with permission from Schuenke M, Schulte E, Schumacher U. THIEME Atlas of Anatomy Third Edition, Vol 3. © Thieme 2020. Illustrations by Markus Voll and Karl Wesker.)

sensory neuron carries the noxious information into the dorsal horn where it will synapse on second-order neurons located in superficial laminae.

- Axons from second-order neurons run in the *direct* (**spinothalamic**) pathway or the *indirect* (**spinoreticular**) pathway.
  - In the direct pathway, fibers synapse on the contralateral thalamus and send collaterals to the reticular formation.
  - In the indirect pathway, fibers project to the reticular formation (**spinoreticular**) and send collaterals to the thalamus or as the **spinomesencephalic**, **spinotectal,** or **spinohypothalamic** fibers to brainstem nuclei.

14.6.2 Pathways

The periaqueductal gray (PAG) of the midbrain receives inputs from ascending pain pathways (neospinothalamic, paleospinothalamic, and archispinothalamic) as well as from multiple areas in the brain including the **hypothalamus**, **amygdala**, **insula**, **orbitofrontal cortex,** and **anterior cingulate cortex**

among others. Upon stimulation, the neurons in the PAG project to the **nucleus raphe magnus** (**NRM**) located in the medulla or the **locus coeruleus** in the pons.

- The pathway from the NRM is often called the **serotonin pathway** due to the large number of serotonergic neurons found there (▶ Fig. 14.5).
  - The axons of the **serotonergic neurons** in the NRM project to the dorsal horn of the spinal cord and synapse on **enkephalinergic interneurons** and activate them by secreting serotonin (▶ Fig. 14.6).
  - Enkephalinergic interneurons in the dorsal horn synapse on both first-order neurons and second-order neurons of the STT.
    – Opiate receptors are located on the presynaptic first-order neuron located in laminae I and II (SG).
    – **Enkephalin** secreted by the dorsal horn interneurons inhibits the release of substance P and glutamate from the central process of the first-order neuron by binding to the opiate receptors.

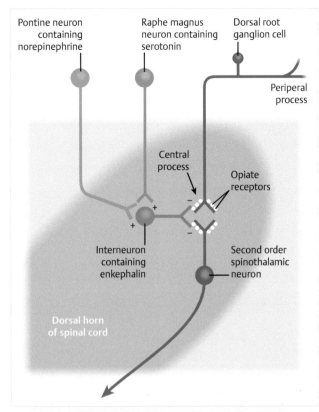

Fig. 14.5 Serotonin pathway of pain modulation. Besides the ascending pathways that carry pain sensation to the primary somatosensory cortex, there are also descending pathways that have the ability to suppress pain impulses.

- Enkephalins released from the interneurons can also activate postsynaptic opiate receptors on the second-order neuron. This activation results in hyperpolarization resulting in inhibition.
- The end result is disruption of the transmission of the pain stimulus from the first-order neuron to the second-order neuron. This in turn will prevent the stimulus from ascending in the STT.
- Pain modulation from the **locus coeruleus** (**LC**) is referred to as the **noradrenergic pathway**. Noradrenergic neurons residing within the LC project their axons to the dorsal horn of the spinal cord (▶ Fig. 14.5).
  ○ The noradrenergic neurons synapse on enkephalinergic neurons in the dorsal horn and activate them by secreting norepinephrine (NE) (▶ Fig. 14.6).
    - The activated enkephalinergic neurons secrete enkephalins and inhibit transmission of the pain stimulus in the same manner as that described in the pathway from the NRM.

14.7 Acute versus Chronic Pain

- **Acute pain** is limited and confined to the affected area. It is considered to have a biological purpose in that it provides a "warning" that an injury has occurred.

- Acute pain can activate the sympathetic arm of the autonomic system resulting in the "fight or flight" behaviors including increased heart and respiratory rates.
- Somatic, visceral, and referred pain are types of acute pain.
- **Chronic pain** is prolonged pain lasting well beyond the expected normal healing time.
  ○ Chronic pain can be continuous or intermittent.
  ○ It is more complex than acute pain and more difficult to manage. The etiology is often unclear.
  ○ Patients with chronic pain may not display the same behaviors and clinical presentations as those with acute pain. Autonomic responses may be absent.
  ○ Research now points to **central sensitization** and **neuroplasticity** as mechanisms involved in the development of chronic pain.

14.8 Differences in Pain Perception

- Sex based: Studies have shown that women report pain with greater frequency than men as well as exhibit lower thresholds and tolerance to painful stimuli than men. The mechanisms underlying these observations are unclear but hormones and differing brain patterns have been suggested to play a role.
- Children: Although not extensively studied, there is data that shows that lack of analgesia for pain induces "rewiring" in pathways resulting in alterations in pain perception during subsequent painful experiences (central sensitization). Children also experience chronic pain syndromes.
- Elderly: The effects of aging on pain perception are not clear. It has been shown that older adults rely more on C fibers and therefore more likely to describe pain as "burning" rather than "sharp or pricking" (A fibers). There is no evidence to suggest that pain intensity decreases with age.

14.8.1 Central Sensitization and Neuroplasticity

Central sensitization refers to enhanced neuronal function and circuitry in pain pathways. In addition to enhanced activity, there is a concomitant reduction in inhibition. The phenomenon of central sensitization is a reflection of the **neuroplasticity** of the nervous system, particularly the somatosensory system. Nociceptive pain is a protective process involving reflex withdrawal activity and complex behavioral strategies that prevent further contact with the stimulus. However, in many pathologies, pain no longer becomes protective.

- Clinically, abnormal pain conditions can be described as:
  ○ **Allodynia**: Caused by normally innocuous stimuli
  ○ **Hyperalgesia**: Exaggerated and prolonged response to noxious stimuli
  ○ **Secondary hyperalgesia**: Spreads beyond the site of injury

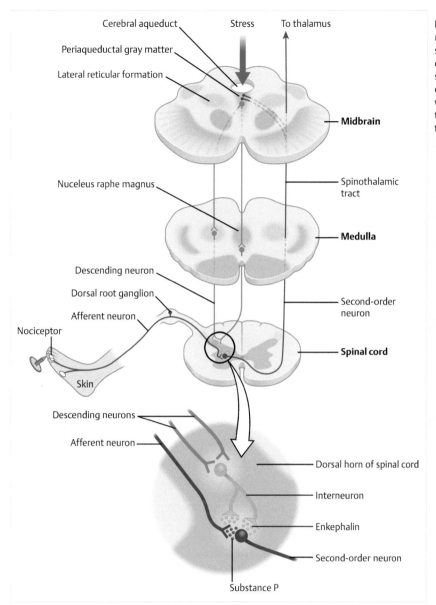

Fig. 14.6 Serotonergic neurons from the nucleus raphe magnus project to the dorsal horn of the spinal cord. These neurons synapse on enkephalnergic neurons and activate by secreting serotonin. The activated enkephalnergic neurons secrete enkephalin which binds to opiate receptors, thus inhibiting the transmission of pain in the spinothalamic tract.

- Enhanced function of neurons and circuits are due to increases in membrane excitability, synaptic efficiency, and reduced inhibition.
- Neurons in the dorsal horn exhibit the development or increase in spontaneous activity, a reduction in threshold for activation from peripheral stimuli, increased responses to supra-threshold stimulation, and increase in receptive fields.
- Two pathways thought to be involved include: First, **chronification** of nociceptive pain which involves **neuroplastic** changes and peripheral sensitization and second, a more psychological explanation involving elevated stress, anxiety, sleeplessness, and decreased pain thresholds.
- Central sensitization differs mechanistically from **peripheral sensitization**.
  - Peripheral sensitization involves a reduction in threshold and an amplification in responsiveness of nociceptors.
  - Central sensitization involves novel inputs to normal nociceptive pathways. In other words, the pathways can be activated by signals that ordinarily would not activate them. It is also typically represented by increased pain hypersensitivity in noninflamed tissues by altered responses to normal inputs and increased pain sensitivity long after the stimulus is removed.
- Pain associated with central sensitization is a result of alteration to properties of CNS neurons and is not dependent on the presence, intensity, or duration of peripheral stimuli.
- Pain is generated due to changes in the CNS neurons that then alters the response to sensory inputs or even the presence of sensory inputs. Chronic pain associated with some conditions, e.g., fibromyalgia and phantom pain, is thought to be the result of central sensitization. Persistent pain stimulation results in **maldynia** (maladaptive pain) which hypersensitizes neurons to stimuli and induces "rewiring" of neural pathways. Studies in neuropathic pain have demonstrated reorganization of cortical somatotropic maps in both motor and sensory areas, increase in activity in

nociceptive areas and nociceptive activity in cortical areas not typically involved in pain pathways, and even neural degeneration.

Neuroplasticity refers to the ability of the nervous system to alter its anatomy and physiology under both normal and pathological conditions. These neuronal changes occur in response to the environment which includes other cells, neurotransmitters, growth factors, and stimuli. Research has shown that the nervous system is not static as originally thought. Neural plasticity is essential for normal brain and circuit development as well as for playing a significant role in learned behavior and repair after injuries. The human body has developed specific pathways for transmitting pain information. This helps to recognize potentially damaging events and allows one to make adjustments that will prevent and/or limit damage. However, **neuroplastic** changes can affect the transmission of pain in a negative way resulting in **maladaptive behavior**. Neuroplasticity can be consequence of chronic pain, it can contribute to the development of chronic pain, and it can be involved in the maintenance of pain symptoms.

- The nervous system can become sensitized peripherally and centrally. Hyperalgesia and allodynia brought on by sensitization are thought to contribute to the production of chronic pain.
- Neuroplastic changes can be induced by disease. Pathologies have been shown to produce adaptive changes to single molecules, synapses, cellular function, and circuit activity. These changes can affect and influence the transmission and interpretation of pain signals.
- Sensory stimuli can continue to interact with neural systems that have been modified by past inputs or events. The altered component of the nervous system can be influenced by "memory" of past events. It is thought that **neural memory** may explain sensory perceptions seen in the amputation of extremities (phantom pain).

Reference

1. Melzack R, Wall PD. Pain mechanisms: a new theory. Science. 1965 Nov 19;150(3699):971-9

Questions and Answers

1. Phantom limb is thought to be the result of which of the following conditions?
   a) Hypocondriasis
   b) Central sensitization
   c) Convergence
   d) Nociceptive pain

Level 1: Easy
Answer B: Central sensitization. **(A)** Hypochondriasis is an excessive preoccupation with one's health. **(C)** Convergence is the theory behind referred pain. **(D)** Phantom pain is a category of neuropathic pain. Nociceptors are not being activated.

2. Which of the following tracts is involved in the immediate awareness of pain and localization?
   a) Paleospinothalamic
   b) Archispinothalamic
   c) Neospinothalamic
   d) Anterior spinothalamic

Level 1: Easy
Answer C. Neospinothalamic. **(A)** Paleospinothalamic is involved in the emotional response to pain. **(B)** Archispinothalamic is involved in the visceral autonomic response to pain. **(D)** Anterior spinothalamic is part of the paleospinothalamic tract.

3. The gate theory of inhibition is based on the "blocking" the transmission of impulses by the activation of α which of the following fiber types?
   a) Aα
   b) Aδ
   c) Aβ
   d) C

Level 1: Easy
Answer C: Aβ activation closes the "gate" and prevents transmission of impulses on Aδ and C fibers. **(A)** Aα fibers carry proprioception. **(B)** Aδ fibers carry fast pain. **(D)** C fibers carry fast pain.

4. Which of the following molecules are secreted by neurons located in the nucleus raphe magnus?
   a) Norepinephrine
   b) Seratonin
   c) Substance P
   d) Glutamate

Level 1: Easy
Answer B: Seratonin. **(A)** Norepinephrine is secreted by neurons in the locus coeruleus. **(C)** Substance P is secreted by dorsal horn neurons. **(D)** Glutamate is secreted by dorsal horn neurons.

5. The periaqueductal gray (PAG) receives input from which of the following structures?
   a) Dorsal column-medial lemniscus tract
   b) Amygdala
   c) Chief sensory nucleus of CNV
   d) Mesencephalic nucleus of V

Level 3: Hard
Answer B: Amygdala. **(A)** The DC-ML carries proprioceptive information from body. **(C)** Chief sensory nucleus of V carries proprioceptive information from face. **(D)** Mesencephalic nucleus of V carries proprioceptive information from the jaw.

15 Special Senses

Learning Objectives

1. Identify the cranial nerves carrying SVA fibers.
2. Identify the cranial nerves carrying SSA fibers.
3. Identify the ganglia associated with SVA and SSA cranial nerves.
4. Identify the specialized receptors for the SVA and SSA afferents.
5. Discuss the olfactory pathway and associated structures.
6. Discuss the visual pathway and associated structures.
7. Discuss the gustatory pathway and associated structures.
8. Discuss the vestibular pathway and associated structures.
9. Discuss the auditory pathway and associated structures.

15.1 Special Visceral Afferents (SVA) (▶ Table 15.1)

15.1.1 CN I

CN I contains *only* SVA fibers that function in the sense of smell or **olfaction**. The olfactory system develops from the **embryonic nasal placode** and consists of the **olfactory epithelium, olfactory bulb,** and **tract**, as well as the olfactory associated cortical areas, sometimes called the **rhinencephalon** (▶ Fig. 15.1).

- Specialized receptors of the olfactory system are stimulated by chemicals that generate odors (**odorants**). Odorants must be drawn into the nasal cavity in order to activate the sensory neurons.
- **Olfactory receptors** (**ORs**) are present on the **cilia** of sensory neurons within the olfactory epithelium.
  - ORs are **G-protein coupled receptors** that bind odorants. Binding of the odorant to the receptor activates the G-protein. Activation of the G-protein receptor ultimately generates an action potential (AP) via second messenger systems. The olfactory signal is then transduced to the brain via the olfactory nerve.

Table 15.1 Special senses

Cranial Nerve	Types of Fibers	Function
I	SVA	Olfaction
VII	SVA	Taste—anterior two-third of tongue, hard and soft palates
IX	SVA	Taste—posterior one-third of tongue
V	SVA	Taste—epiglottis
II	SSA	Vision
VIII	SSA	Hearing
	SSA	Balance

Abbreviations: SSA, special somatic afferent; SVA, special visceral afferent.

- The **bipolar olfactory neurons**, along with their processes, are located in specialized epithelium (**olfactory epithelium**) in the roof of the superior concha of the nasal cavity, beneath the cribriform plate (▶ Fig. 15.2).
  - The first-order bipolar neurons have a single **dendrite** that communicates with the **olfactory mucosa** as **olfactory knobs**. The olfactory knob or terminal end of the dendrite has cilia that are embedded in the apical mucosa.
    - A single, unmyelinated axon arises from the opposite end of the olfactory neurons. The axons are SVA fibers that transmit olfactory sensation. They form bundles that collectively create CN I.
    - Unlike most sensory systems, the first-order neurons of CN I do not reside in a sensory ganglion.
    - Sensory neurons are replaced when aged or damaged via differentiation of basal cells that reside near the lamina propria.
- The **olfactory threads** (SVA fibers) pass through the small openings in the **cribriform plate** of the **ethmoid bone** and terminate in the ipsilateral **olfactory bulb** where the second-order neurons and interneurons are located (▶ Fig. 15.3).
  - The olfactory bulb consists of **mitral cells** (primary projection neurons), **granule cells** (interneurons), and **tufted cells** (projection neurons).
  - The olfactory bulb constitutes an enlargement of the rostral aspect of the olfactory tract. The olfactory tract extending from the olfactory bulb represents the axons of the second-order neurons (mitral and tufted cells) (▶ Fig. 15.4).
- The olfactory tract projects to the olfactory associated areas of the cortex (rhinencephalon).
  - In man, most of the second-order neurons project to the **lateral olfactory area**, which consists of the **uncus** and the **hippocampal gyrus**. Other projections include the medial aspect of the frontal lobe where connections to the limbic system are responsible for emotional responses to odors (▶ Fig. 15.5).
- See Clinical Correlation Box 15.1.

Clinical Correlation Box 15.1: Anosmia

Anosmia or loss of smell can occur from trauma, inflammation, rhinitis, and aging. One of the chief complaints in individuals who suffer from anosmia is the complete or altered loss of taste. In severe head injuries the olfactory bulbs can be torn away from the olfactory nerves. Depending on the etiology, loss of smell can be transient or permanent. Treatment includes resolution of underlying condition with medication or surgery if there is an anatomic abnormality. In some instances, anosmia resolves on its own.

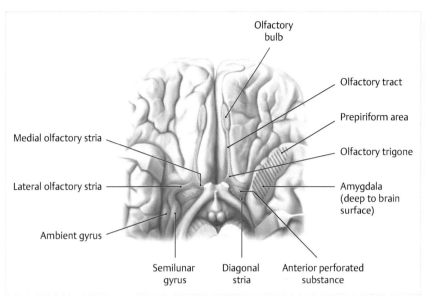

Fig. 15.1 The olfactory system consists of the olfactory epithelium, the olfactory bulb and tract as well as the olfactory related cortical areas. (Reproduced with permission from Schuenke M, Schulte E, Schumacher U. THIEME Atlas of Anatomy Third Edition, Vol 3. © Thieme 2020. Illustrations by Markus Voll and Karl Wesker.)

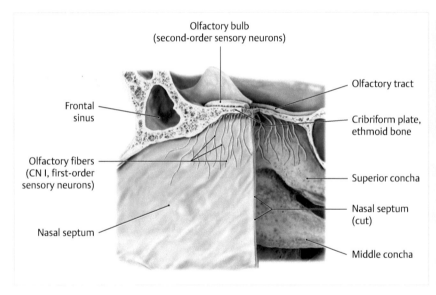

Fig. 15.2 Fiber bundles in the olfactory mucosa pass from the nasal cavity through the cribriform plate of the ethmoid bone into the anterior cranial fossa, where they synapse in the olfactory bulb. (Reproduced with permission from Schuenke M, Schulte E, Schumacher U. THIEME Atlas of Anatomy Third Edition, Vol 3. © Thieme 2020. Illustrations by Markus Voll and Karl Wesker.)

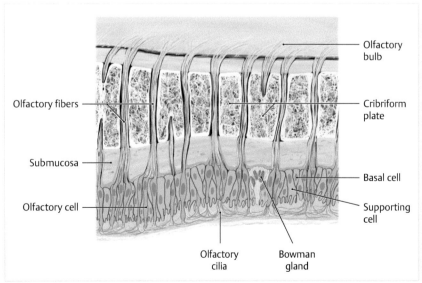

Fig. 15.3 The SVA fibers pass through the openings of the cribriform plate and terminate on the olfactory bulb. SVA, special visceral afferent. (Reproduced with permission from Schuenke M, Schulte E, Schumacher U. THIEME Atlas of Anatomy Third Edition, Vol 3. © Thieme 2020. Illustrations by Markus Voll and Karl Wesker.)

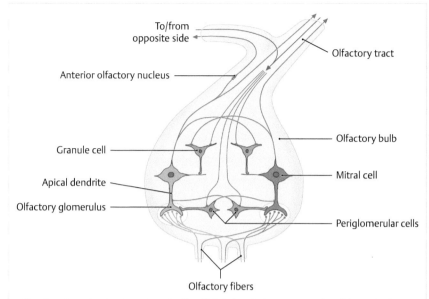

Fig. 15.4 Specialized neurons in the olfactory bulb, called mitral cells, form apical dendrites that receive synaptic contact from the axons of thousands of primary sensory cells. The dendrite and the synapses make up the olfactory glomeruli. Axons from sensory cells with the same receptor protein form glomeruli with only one or a small number of mitral cells. The basal axons of the mitral cells form the olfactory tract. The axons that run in the olfactory tract not only project primarily to the olfactory cortex but are also distributed to other nuclei in the central nervous system. (Reproduced with permission from Baker EW. Anatomy for Dental Medicine. Second Edition. © Thieme 2015. Illustrations by Markus Voll and Karl Wesker.)

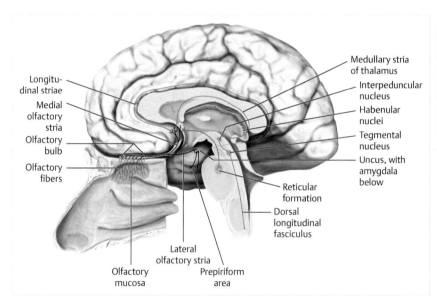

Fig. 15.5 The olfactory tract projects to the olfactory associated areas of the cortex (rhinencephalon). In man, most of the second-order neurons project to the lateral olfactory area which includes the uncus and the hippocampal gyrus. (Reproduced with permission from Baker EW. Anatomy for Dental Medicine. Second Edition. © Thieme 2015. Illustrations by Markus Voll and Karl Wesker.)

15.1.2 CN VII

The SVA fibers in CN VII carry taste sensation from the anterior two-thirds of the tongue as well as the hard and soft palates (▶ Fig. 15.6). The five taste sensations are: sweet, bitter, salty, sour, and umami (Japanese word for *pleasant*).

- Afferent fibers transmit sensory information from chemoreceptors in the tongue.
- The chemoreceptors (taste receptor cells) lie within the taste buds (**fungiform**) of the tongue (see Chapters 9 and 19).
  - Salivary fluid containing dissolved substances enters the taste bud through a **taste pore** and bathes the microvilli associated with the taste receptor cells.
  - Taste receptor cells have a limited lifespan and are replaced every 1 to 2 weeks by the differentiation of basal cells that migrate from the surrounding epithelium.

- The generation of APs from taste signals involves several methods depending on the type of taste sensation.
  - These processes include ligand-gated and G-protein coupled mechanisms among others.
- Taste buds communicate with peripheral processes from the first-order pseudounipolar neurons (▶ Fig. 15.7). These afferent fibers run with the lingual nerve and then chorda tympani to the sensory cell body located in the geniculate ganglion.
- The central process of the first-order neuron emerges from the geniculate ganglion and enters the facial canal. They eventually enter the brainstem as part of the **nervous intermedius**. The fibers then join the rostral part of the **solitary tract** to synapse on second-order neurons in the **solitary nucleus** (▶ Fig. 15.8a, b).
- Axons from the cell bodies in the solitary nucleus will ascend both ipsilaterally and contralaterally to the ventral

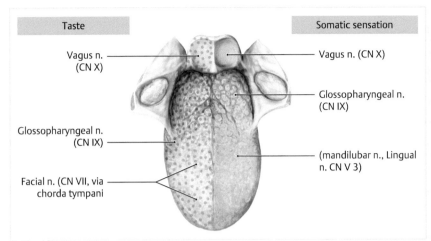

| Taste | Somatic sensation |

Vagus n.
(CN X)

Glossopharyngeal n.
(CN IX)

Facial n. (CN VII, via
chorda tympani

Vagus n. (CN X)

Glossopharyngeal n.
(CN IX)

(mandilubar n., Lingual
n. CN V 3)

Fig. 15.6 SVA fibers carried in CN VII carry taste sensation from the anterior two-thirds of the tongue and the palate. SVA, special visceral afferent. (Reproduced with permission from Schuenke M, Schulte E, Schumacher U. THIEME Atlas of Anatomy Third Edition, Vol 3. © Thieme 2020. Illustrations by Markus Voll and Karl Wesker.)

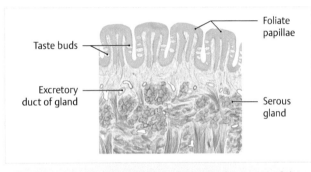

Foliate
papillae

Taste buds

Excretory
duct of gland

Serous
gland

Fig. 15.7 Taste buds communicate with peripheral processes of the first-order pseudounipolar neurons. These afferents run in the lingual nerve and chorda tympani. (Reproduced with permission from Schuenke M, Schulte E, Schumacher U. THIEME Atlas of Anatomy Third Edition, Vol 3. © Thieme 2020. Illustrations by Markus Voll and Karl Wesker.)

posteromedial (**VPM**) of the thalamus where they synapse on third-order neurons.
- The axons of third-order neurons project via the posterior limb of the internal capsule to the area of the cortex responsible for taste.
  - The **primary gustatory cortex** is located in the **frontoparietal operculum** and the **anterior insula**. It should be noted that there is significant variation between species and the exact location in humans continues to be investigated.

15.1.3 CN IX

The SVA fibers of CN IX carry taste sensation from the posterior one-third (**circumvallate** and **foliate papilla**) on the tongue (**Fig. 14.6**). These afferent fibers transmit special sensory information from chemoreceptors in the tongue. The chemoreceptors initiate an AP that is transmitted into the central nervous system (CNS) for interpretation (see section **CN VII**).
- The first-order neurons carrying taste information are located in the **inferior ganglion** of the glossopharyngeal

nerve, which is located in a depression in the lower border of the **petrous part of the temporal bone**.
- The peripheral processes run with the trunk of the glossopharyngeal nerve from the posterior one-third of the tongue to the inferior ganglion via pharyngeal branches.
- The central processes of the first-order neurons exit the ganglion and pass through the jugular foramen to enter the brainstem via the glossopharyngeal root. The SVA fibers ascend in the **tractus solitarius** and terminate on second-order neurons in the rostral **solitary nucleus** (▶ Fig. 15.8a, b).
- The second-order neurons located in the solitary nucleus project bilaterally to the VPM of the thalamus and terminate on third-order neurons.
- Axons from the third-order neurons of the thalamus project to the gustatory cortex of the somatosensory strip (parietal lobe) via the posterior limb of the internal capsule.

15.1.4 CN X

SVA fibers of the vagus nerve carry taste information from chemoreceptors of taste buds on the epiglottis (▶ Fig. 15.6).
- The SVA pseudounipolar neurons are located in the inferior ganglion (**nodose**) of the vagus nerve, which lies just inferior to the foramen magnum.
- The peripheral processes of the first-order neurons course with the internal branch of the superior laryngeal nerve and terminate in the taste buds.
- The central processes of the first-order neurons exit the ganglion and pass through the jugular foramen to enter the brainstem along with other vagal branches. The SVA fibers ascend in the tractus solitarius and terminate on second-order neurons in the rostral solitary nucleus (▶ Fig. 15.8a, b).
- The second-order neurons located in the solitary nucleus project bilaterally to the VPM of the thalamus and terminate on third-order neurons.
- Axons from the third-order neurons of the thalamus project to the gustatory cortex of the somatosensory strip (parietal lobe) via the posterior limb of the internal capsule.

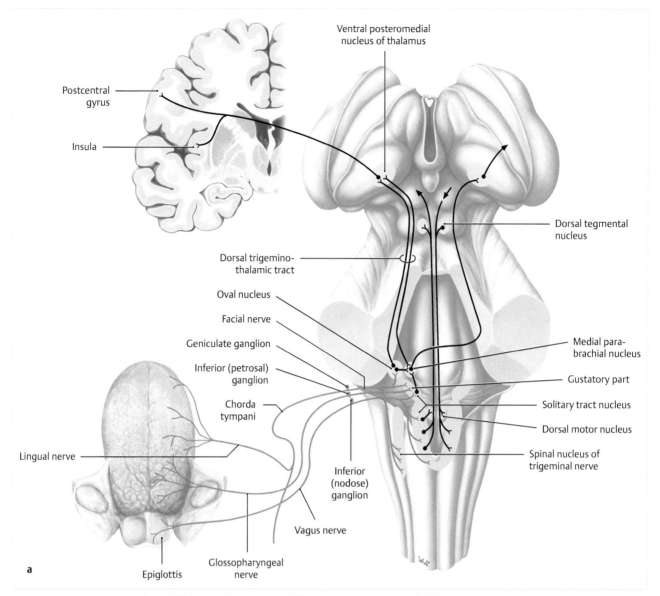

Fig. 15.8 (a) The central processes of the first-order neurons emerge from the geniculate ganglion and join the solitary tract. These afferent fibers project to the solitary nucleus and eventually the VPM of the thalamus before synapsing in the gustatory cortex.

(*Continued*)

15.2 Special Somatic Afferents (SSA) (▶ Table 15.1)

15.2.1 CN II

CN II has only SSA fibers that convey the special sense of vision. The paired optic nerves are extensions of the forebrain (diencephalon) and are therefore are covered with cranial meninges and contain a cerebrospinal fluid (CSF) filled subarachnoid space. The photons of light entering the eye are converted to electrical signals that activate the photoreceptors of the retina.

- **Rods** and **cones** are the photoreceptors of the eye. They process and integrate sensory information. These light sensitive receptors are the first-order neurons in the visual pathway.
  - Cones are responsible for vision in daylight. There is lower sensitivity than with dim/night vision but the resolution is greater.
  - Rods are specialized for night vision. Loss of rods results in loss of night and peripheral vision.
- Cell bodies of second-order bipolar neurons are found in the retina.
  - A light stimulus changes the membrane potential of the bipolar cell.
  - They transmit visual input to multipolar third-order neurons also found in the retina (▶ Fig. 15.9).
- Third-order neurons of the **retinal ganglion** project unmyelinated axons that converge at the optic disc and enter the posterior aspect of the sclera. These axons become

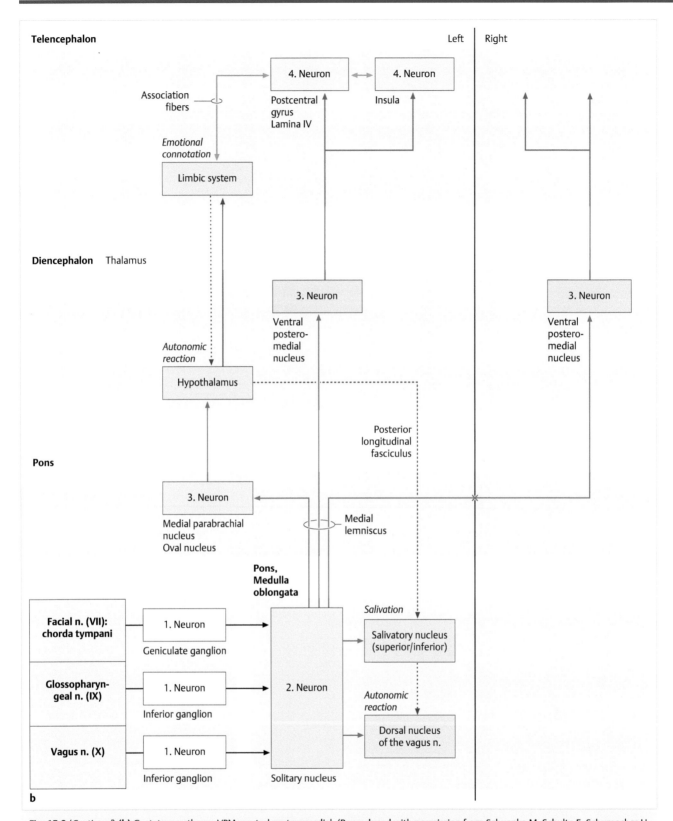

Fig. 15.8 (*Continued*) (**b**) Gustatory pathway. VPM, ventral posteromedial. (Reproduced with permission from Schuenke M, Schulte E, Schumacher U. THIEME Atlas of Anatomy. Third Edition, Vol 3. © Thieme 2020. Illustrations by Markus Voll and Karl Wesker.)

myelinated just deep to the optic disc and form the **optic nerve** (▶ Fig. 15.10).

- The optic nerve passes posteromedially in the orbit, exiting the **optic canal** and entering the **middle cranial fossa**.
- Once inside the middle cranial fossa, the right and left optic nerves join to form the **optic chiasm** (▶ Fig. 15.11). Here some of the fibers (medial half) decussate and eventually join uncrossed fibers (temporal half) to form the **optic tract**.
  - Fibers from right halves of both retinas form the **right optic tract** and those from the left halves form the **left optic tract** (▶ Fig. 15.12).

  - Crossing of the fibers is necessary for **binocular vision** and **depth perception**.
- The axons of the ganglion cells running in each optic tract curve around the **cerebral peduncle** and terminate in visual input centers of the brain (▶ Fig. 15.13).
- Visual input areas of brain include:
  - **Lateral geniculate nucleus**: Thalamic relay station for vision
    - Cell bodies in lateral geniculate nucleus project to visual cortex of occipital lobe.
  - **Superior colliculus**: Mesencephalic relay station for vision
  - **Pretectal area**: Mesencephalic region associated with autonomic reflexes
  - Hypothalamus
- See Clinical Correlation Box 15.2.

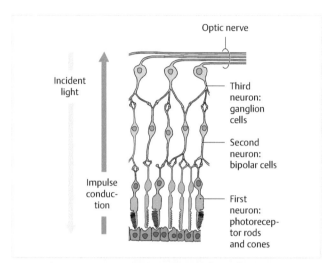

Fig. 15.9 Visual pathway. Rods and cones of the eye are the first-order neurons of the visual pathway. Second- and third-order neurons are located in the retina. Light is processed by the first-order neurons which stimulate the second-order neurons. Visual input is then transmitted to third-order neurons which ultimately form the optic nerve. (Reproduced with permission from Schuenke M, Schulte E, Schumacher U. THIEME Atlas of Anatomy. Third Edition, Vol 3. © Thieme 2020. Illustrations by Markus Voll and Karl Wesker.)

Clinical Correlation Box 15.2: Pupillary Light Reflex

The **pupillary light reflex** controls the diameter of the pupil. The pupil responds to light conditions by contracting or dilating and also permits both pupils to react in unison (direct and consensual). This reflex requires CN II, CN III, and brainstem connections. Light exposure to the pupil stimulates photoreceptors and the retinal ganglion cells whose axons project via the optic nerve to the pretectal nucleus. Pretectal neurons project to the Edinger-Westphal nucleus bilaterally. The preganglionic fibers of the parasympathetic nucleus project to the ciliary ganglion. Postganglionic fibers of the ganglion innervate the pupillary constrictor muscle. Thus, light that is directed in one eye (direct) results in the constriction of both pupils (consensual). A lesion of CN II results in an unresponsive reaction in both eyes when the stimulus is directed at the eye on the same side as the lesion. When light is shined in the unaffected eye, both pupils will constrict. A lesion of CN III results in lack of ipsilateral pupil constriction on the affected side when light is directed at either eye.

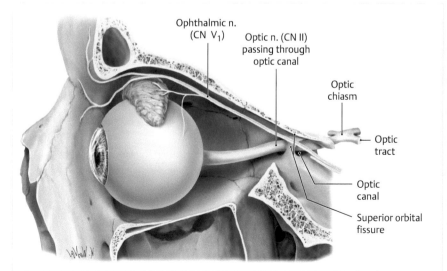

Fig. 15.10 The optic nerve passes from the eyeball through the optic canal into the middle cranial fossa. (Reproduced with permission from Schuenke M, Schulte E, Schumacher U. THIEME Atlas of Anatomy Third Edition, Vol 3. © Thieme 2020. Illustrations by Markus Voll and Karl Wesker.)

15.2.2 CN VIII

CN VIII is a special sensory (SSA) nerve for hearing and equilibrium. It consists of two separate nerves that are enclosed within a connective tissue sheath, the **vestibular nerve** (position sense and balance) and the **cochlear nerve** (hearing). Both nerves transmit SSA information from specialized mechanoreceptors called **hair cells**. The vestibulocochlear nerve emerges from the junction of the pons and medulla and enters the internal acoustic meatus where it separates into the two separate nerves.

• Auditory system (▸ Fig. 15.14)

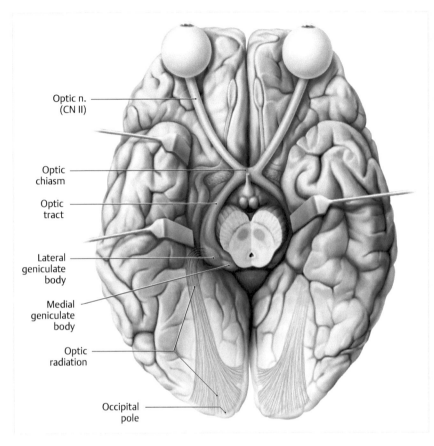

Optic n.
(CN II)

Optic
chiasm

Optic
tract

Lateral
geniculate
body

Medial
geniculate
body

Optic
radiation

Occipital
pole

Fig. 15.11 The two optic nerves join below the base of the diencephalon to form the optic chiasm, before dividing into the two optic tracts. Each of these tracts divides into a lateral and medial root. Many retinal cell ganglion axons cross the midline to the contralateral side of the brain in the optic chiasm. (Reproduced with permission from Schuenke M, Schulte E, Schumacher U. THIEME Atlas of Anatomy Third Edition, Vol 3. © Thieme 2020. Illustrations by Markus Voll and Karl Wesker.)

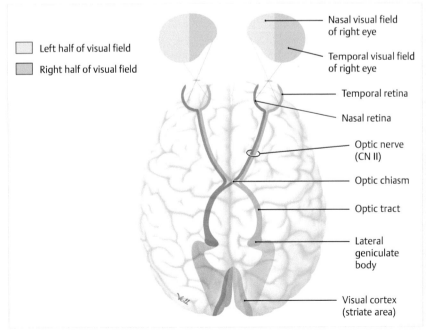

Left half of visual field

Right half of visual field

Nasal visual field
of right eye

Temporal visual field
of right eye

Temporal retina

Nasal retina

Optic nerve
(CN II)

Optic chiasm

Optic tract

Lateral
geniculate
body

Visual cortex
(striate area)

Fig. 15.12 Representation of each visual field in the contralateral visual cortex. The light rays in the nasal part of each visual field are projected to the temporal half of the retina, and those from the temporal part are projected to the nasal half. Because of this arrangement, the left half of the visual field projects to the visual cortex of the right occipital pole, and the right half projects to the visual cortex of the left occipital pole. (Reproduced with permission from Schuenke M, Schulte E, Schumacher U. THIEME Atlas of Anatomy Third Edition, Vol 3. © Thieme 2020. Illustrations by Markus Voll and Karl Wesker.)

○ The outer ear transmits air pressure waves to the tympanic membrane (▶ Fig. 15.15). The middle ear conducts pressure through the three bony **ossicles** (**malleus, stapes,** and **incus**) from the **tympanic membrane** to the **oval window**

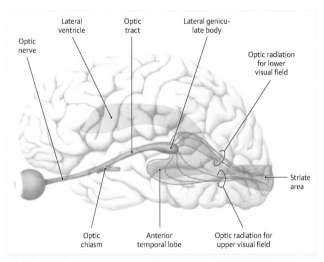

Fig. 15.13 Fibers of the optic tract curve around the cerebral peduncle and terminate in the visual input centers of the brain. (Reproduced with permission from Baker EW. Anatomy for Dental Medicine. Second Edition. © Thieme 2015. Illustrations by Markus Voll and Karl Wesker.)

(▶ Fig. 15.16a, b). The inner ear then conducts waves through a fluid medium along the **organ of Corti**, initiating impulses in the hair cells (▶ Fig. 15.17). The impulses are ultimately transmitted to the **auditory cortex** where they are interpreted as sound.

○ Cell bodies of the first-order sensory bipolar neurons are located within the **cochlear** (**spiral**) **ganglion**.

○ The peripheral processes of the first-order neurons terminate in the organ of Corti, which contains specialized receptors that transduce sound waves into electrical impulses. The spiral ganglia and the organ of Corti are found in the cochlea of the inner ear (▶ Fig. 15.18).

○ The central processes of the first-order sensory neurons travel with the vestibular nerve and terminate in the ipsilateral cochlear nuclei located at the junction of the pons and medulla.

○ Second-order neurons within the cochlear nucleus project their axons rostrally to terminate in the ipsilateral and contralateral **superior olivary nucleus**. Most the outputs from the superior olivary nucleus join the **lateral lemniscus** and terminate in the **inferior colliculus**.

○ All afferents from the inferior colliculus synapse in the **medial geniculate body** (nucleus) of the thalamus.

○ Thalamic projections from the auditory pathway reach the **primary auditory cortex** (**superior temporal gyrus**) via the internal capsule (Clinical correlation Box 15.3 and 15.4) (▶ Fig. 15.19).

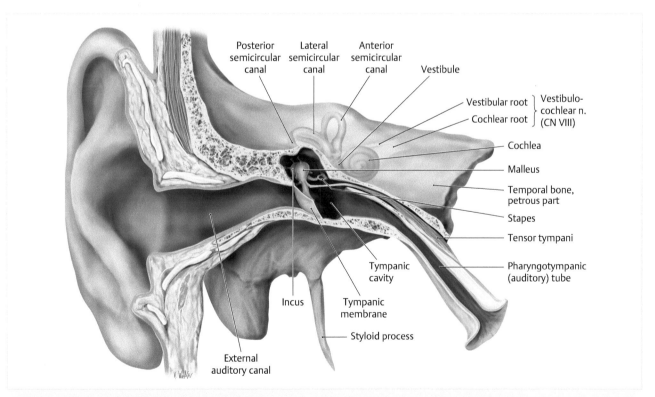

Fig. 15.14 Overview. Coronal section through right ear, anterior view. (Reproduced with permission from Schuenke M, Schulte E, Schumacher U. THIEME Atlas of Anatomy Third Edition, Vol 3. © Thieme 2020. Illustrations by Markus Voll and Karl Wesker.)

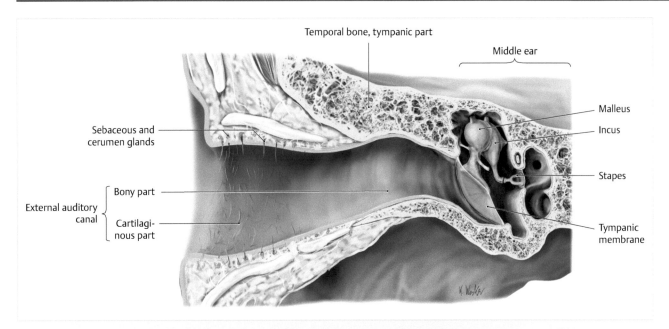

Fig. 15.15 External auditory canal be introduced into a straightened canal. Coronal section through right ear, anterior view. The tympanic membrane separates the external auditory canal from the tympanic cavity (middle ear). The outer third of the auditory canal is cartilaginous, and the inner two-thirds are osseous (tympanic part of temporal bone). (Reproduced with permission from Schuenke M, Schulte E, Schumacher U. THIEME Atlas of Anatomy Third Edition, Vol 3. © Thieme 2020. Illustrations by Markus Voll and Karl Wesker.)

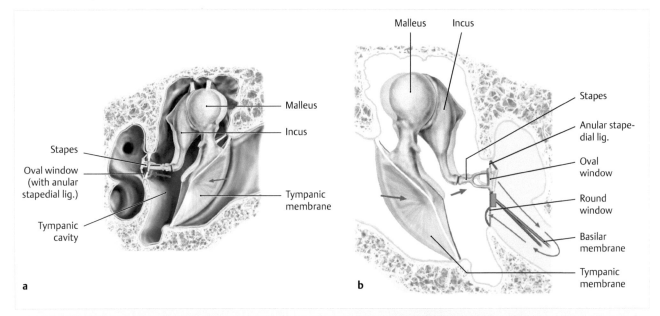

Fig. 15.16 (a) Auditory ossicles. Left ear. The ossicular chain consists of three small bones that establish an articular connection between the tympanic membrane and the oval window. (b) Bones of the ossicular chain. Medial view of the left ossicular chain. (Reproduced with permission from Schuenke M, Schulte E, Schumacher U. THIEME Atlas of Anatomy Third Edition, Vol 3. © Thieme 2020. Illustrations by Markus Voll and Karl Wesker.)

Clinical Correlation Box 15.3: Tinnitus

Tinnitus is ringing in the ears when there is no noise present. This condition can be acute or chronic. The CDC reports that as many as 15% of Americans experience some form of tinnitus. Ringing in the ears is symptomatic of an underlying condition rather than a condition itself. Treatment is geared toward resolving the underlying condition that is causing the tinnitus.

Clinical Correlation Box 15.4: Injuries of the Vestibulocochlear Nerve

Although the vestibular and cochlear nerves are separate entities, peripheral lesions often cause concurrent clinical symptoms because of their unique relationship. Lesions of CN VIII can cause tinnitus, vertigo, and hearing loss in patients.

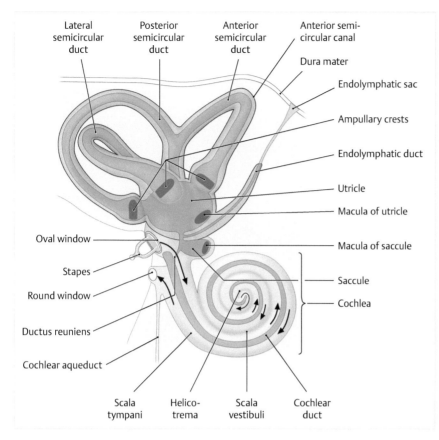

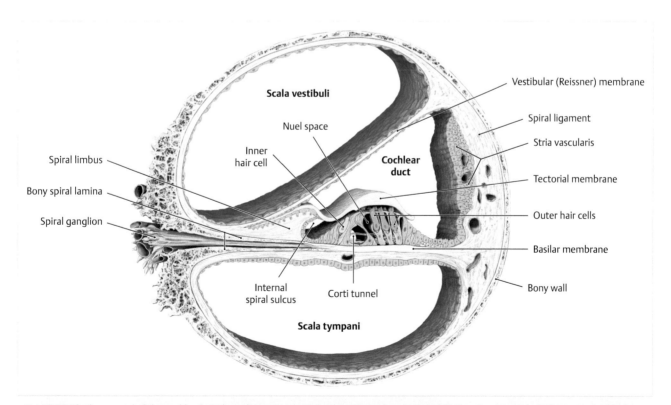

Fig. 15.17 The inner ear, embedded within the petrous part of the temporal bone, is formed by a membranous labyrinth, which floats within a similarly shaped bony labyrinth, loosely attached by connective tissue fibers. Membranous labyrinth (blue): The membranous labyrinth is filled with endolymph. This endolymphatic space (blue) communicates with the endolymphatic sac, an epidural pouch on the posterior surface of the petrous bone, via the endolymphatic duct. (Reproduced with permission from Schuenke M, Schulte E, Schumacher U. THIEME Atlas of Anatomy Third Edition, Vol 3. © Thieme 2020. Illustrations by Markus Voll and Karl Wesker.)

Fig. 15.18 The bony canal of the cochlea (spiral canal) is approximately 30 to 35 mm long in the adult. It makes two and a half turns around its bony axis, the modiolus, which is permeated by branched cavities and contains the spiral ganglion. The base of the cochlea is directed toward the internal acoustic meatus. A cross section through the cochlear canal displays three membranous compartments arranged in three levels. The upper and lower compartments, the scala vestibuli and scala tympani, each contain perilymph; the middle level, the cochlear duct (scala media), contains endolymph. The perilymphatic spaces are interconnected at the apex by the helicotrema, and the endolymphatic space ends blindly at the apex. The cochlear duct, which is triangular in cross section, is separated from the scala vestibuli by the vestibular membrane and from the scala tympani by the basilar membrane. (Reproduced with permission from Schuenke M, Schulte E, Schumacher U. THIEME Atlas of Anatomy Third Edition, Vol 3. © Thieme 2020. Illustrations by Markus Voll and Karl Wesker.)

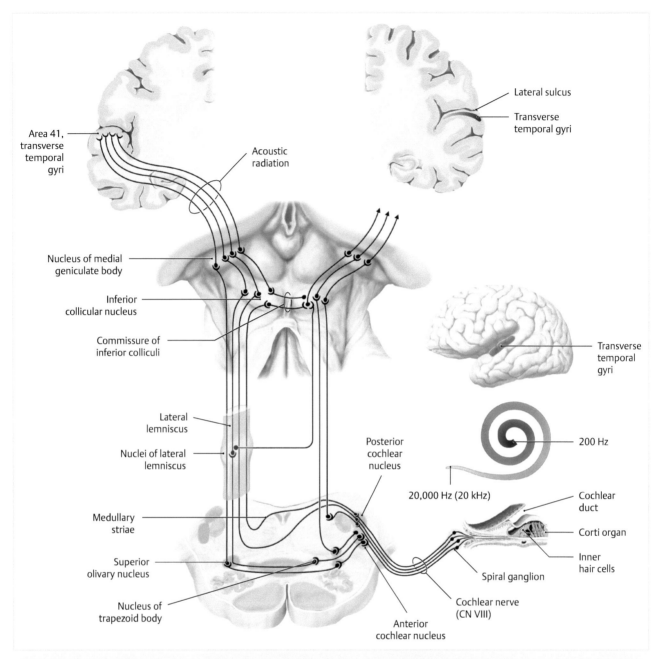

Fig. 15.19 Afferent auditory pathway of the left ear. The receptors of the auditory pathway are the inner hair cells of the organ of Corti. Because they lack neural processes, they are called secondary sensory cells. They are located in the cochlear duct of the basilar membrane and are studded with stereocilia, which are exposed to shearing forces from the tectorial membrane in response to a traveling wave. This causes bowing of the stereocilia. These bowing movements act as a stimulus to evoke cascades of neural signals. Dendritic processes of the bipolar neurons in the spiral ganglion pick up the stimulus. The bipolar neurons then transmit impulses via their axons, which are collected to form the cochlear nerve, to the anterior and posterior cochlear nuclei. In these nuclei the signals are relayed to the second neuron of the auditory pathway. Information from the cochlear nuclei is then transmitted via four to six nuclei to the primary auditory cortex, where the auditory information is consciously perceived (analogous to the visual cortex). (Reproduced with permission from Schuenke M, Schulte E, Schumacher U. THIEME Atlas of Anatomy Third Edition, Vol 3. © Thieme 2020. Illustrations by Markus Voll and Karl Wesker.)

- The vestibular system
  - The vestibular system of the inner ear is concerned with equilibrium. The vestibular organs are located in the **membranous labyrinth** found within the vestibule (**saccule** and **utricle**) and in the ducts within the **semicircular canals** (▶ Fig. 15.20). The receptive organs (**macula** in the **saccule** and the **cristae** in the **semicircular canals**) contain hair cells that release neurotransmitters upon stimulation (bending of cilia). The nerve fibers of the vestibular nerve have contact with the hair cells of the macula and cristae.
  - Cell bodies of the first-order bipolar neurons are located in the **vestibular ganglion of Scarpa** found at the distal end of the internal auditory meatus.

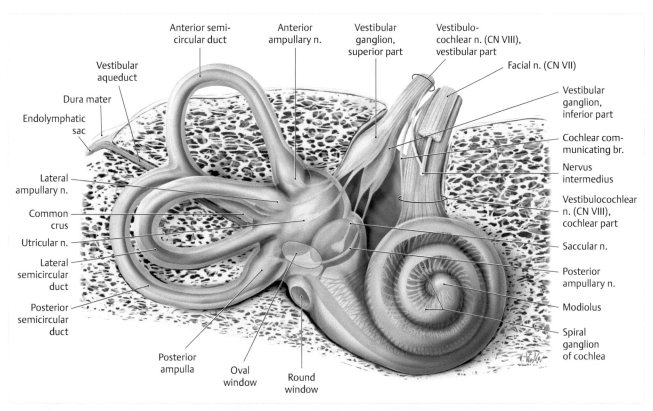

Fig. 15.20 Innervation of the membranous labyrinth. Right ear, anterior view. The vestibulocochlear nerve (CN VIII) transmits afferent impulses from the inner ear to the brainstem through the internal acoustic meatus. The vestibulocochlear nerve is divided into the vestibular and cochlear nerves. (Reproduced with permission from Schuenke M, Schulte E, Schumacher U. THIEME Atlas of Anatomy Third Edition, Vol 3. © Thieme 2020. Illustrations by Markus Voll and Karl Wesker.)

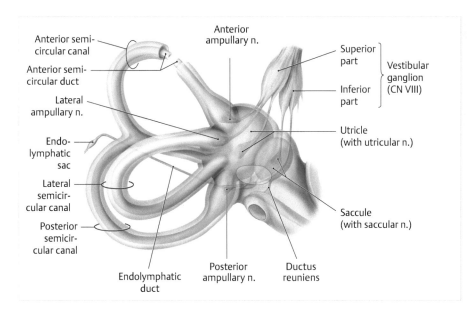

Fig. 15.21 Vestibular apparatus. Right lateral view. (Reproduced with permission from Schuenke M, Schulte E, Schumacher U. THIEME Atlas of Anatomy Third Edition, Vol 3. © Thieme 2020. Illustrations by Markus Voll and Karl Wesker.)

○ The peripheral processes of the first-order sensory neurons terminate in the specialized receptors of the **cristae** in the **ampullae** of the **semicircular canal** and the **maculae** of the **utricle** and **saccule**, both of which are located in the petrous temporal bone (▶ Fig. 15.21).

○ The central processes of the sensory neurons enter the brainstem and synapse on second-order neurons in the **vestibular nuclear complex** or the **cerebellum**.

– The vestibular nuclear complex consists of four nuclei (**superior**, **lateral**, **medial**, and **inferior**) found beneath

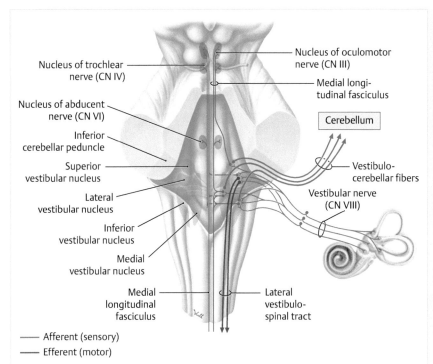

Nucleus of trochlear nerve (CN IV)

Nucleus of abducent nerve (CN VI)

Inferior cerebellar peduncle

Superior vestibular nucleus

Lateral vestibular nucleus

Inferior vestibular nucleus

Medial vestibular nucleus

Medial longitudinal fasciculus

Nucleus of oculomotor nerve (CN III)

Medial longitudinal fasciculus

Cerebellum

Vestibulo-cerebellar fibers

Vestibular nerve (CN VIII)

Lateral vestibulo-spinal tract

—— Afferent (sensory)
—— Efferent (motor)

Fig. 15.22 Vestibular nuclei: topographic organization and central connections. Four nuclei are distinguished: Superior vestibular nucleus, lateral vestibular nucleus, medial vestibular nucleus, and inferior vestibular nucleus. (Reproduced with permission from Schuenke M, Schulte E, Schumacher U. THIEME Atlas of Anatomy Third Edition, Vol 3. © Thieme 2020. Illustrations by Markus Voll and Karl Wesker.)

the floor of the fourth ventricle in the medulla and pons (▶ Fig. 15.22).
  – CN VIII is unique in that it is the only cranial nerve to have first-order neurons directly project to the cerebellum.
  ○ The main projections from the vestibulonuclear complex including the spinal cord (head and body position), to the three extraocular motor nuclei (CNs III, IV, and VI controlling eye movement), to the thalamus that then projects to the cortex (conscious perception of movement) (▶ Fig. 15.23) and to the cerebellum (postural adjustments) (▶ Fig. 15.24).
• Ascending and descending vestibular tracts

○ Projections from superior and medial nuclei ascend in the **medial longitudinal fasciculus** (**MLF**) to the **oculomotor nuclei** (CNs III, IV, and VI).
○ The **lateral vestibulospinal tract** descends ipsilaterally to the sacral cord.
  – This pathway helps to walk upright.
○ The **medial vestibulospinal tract** descends bilaterally in the MLF to thoracic spinal levels.
  – Affects head movements and helps to integrate eye and head movements.
○ **Cerebellar afferents** come from the medial and inferior vestibular nuclei.

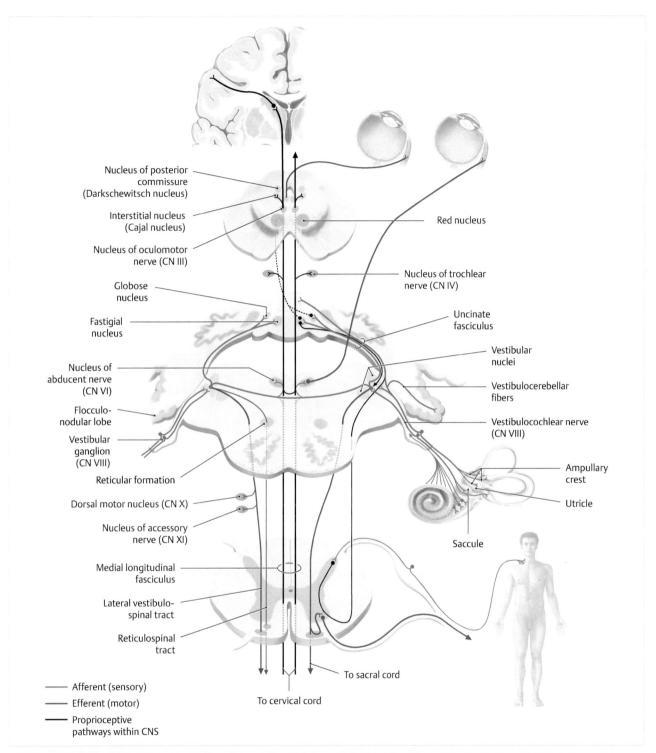

Nucleus of posterior commissure (Darkschewitsch nucleus)

Interstitial nucleus (Cajal nucleus)

Nucleus of oculomotor nerve (CN III)

Globose nucleus

Fastigial nucleus

Nucleus of abducent nerve (CN VI)

Flocculo-nodular lobe

Vestibular ganglion (CN VIII)

Reticular formation

Dorsal motor nucleus (CN X)

Nucleus of accessory nerve (CN XI)

Medial longitudinal fasciculus

Lateral vestibulo-spinal tract

Reticulospinal tract

Red nucleus

Nucleus of trochlear nerve (CN IV)

Uncinate fasciculus

Vestibular nuclei

Vestibulocerebellar fibers

Vestibulocochlear nerve (CN VIII)

Ampullary crest

Utricle

Saccule

To sacral cord

To cervical cord

Afferent (sensory)

Efferent (motor)

Proprioceptive pathways within CNS

Fig. 15.23 Main projections from the vestibulonuclear complex includes: spinal cord, extraocular nuclei (CNs III, IV, and VI), thalamus, and cerebellum. (Reproduced with permission from Schuenke M, Schulte E, Schumacher U. THIEME Atlas of Anatomy Third Edition, Vol 3. © Thieme 2020. Illustrations by Markus Voll and Karl Wesker.)

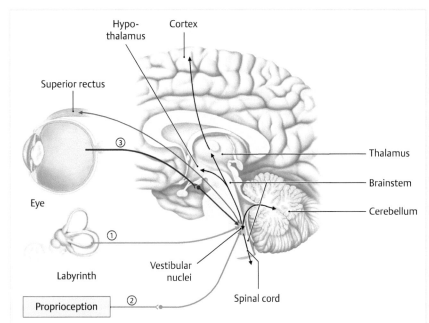

Superior rectus

Eye

Labyrinth

Proprioception

Hypo-thalamus

Cortex

Vestibular nuclei

Thalamus

Brainstem

Cerebellum

Spinal cord

Fig. 15.24 Role of the vestibular nuclei in the maintenance of balance. The vestibular nuclei receive afferent input from the vestibular system ①, proprioceptive system ② (position sense, muscles, and joints), and visual system ③. They then distribute efferent fibers to nuclei that control the motor systems important for balance. These nuclei are located in the: A. Spinal cord (motor support). B. Cerebellum (fine control of motor function). C. Brainstem (oculomotor nuclei for oculomotor function). D. Efferents from the vestibular nuclei are also distributed to the following regions: Thalamus and cortex (spatial sense) and Hypothalamus (autonomic regulation: vomiting in response to vertigo). Note: Acute failure of the vestibular system is manifested by rotary vertigo. (Reproduced with permission from Schuenke M, Schulte E, Schumacher U. THIEME Atlas of Anatomy Third Edition, Vol 3. © Thieme 2020. Illustrations by Markus Voll and Karl Wesker.)

Questions and Answers

1. First-order neurons for taste carried on chorda tympani are located in which of the following structures?
   a) Geniculate ganglion
   b) Submandibular ganglion
   c) Solitary nucleus
   d) VPM of the thalamus

Level 2: Medium

Answer A: Geniculate ganglion. **(B)** Submandibular for the auditory system ganglion is a parasympathetic ganglion, **(C)** solitary nucleus is where second order neurons are located, and **(D)** VPM of the thalamus is where third order neurons in the pathway are located.

2. Which of the following cranial nerves carry SVA fibers from the epiglottis?
   a) CN VII
   b) CN IX
   c) CN X
   d) All of the above

Level 1: Easy

Answer C: CN X carries SVA fibers from the epiglottis via the internal branch of the superior laryngeal nerve; **(A)** CN VII carries SVA fibers from the anterior 2/3 of the tongue via chorda tympani; **(B)** CN IX carries SVA from the posterior 1/3 of the tongue, **(D)** cannot be D as A and B are incorrect.

3. The receptive organ for the vestibular system is:
   a) Utricle
   b) Cristae
   c) Saccule
   d) Organ of corti

Level 2: Medium

Answer B: Cristae is the receptive organ for the vestibular system; **(A)** utricle is a space in the membranous labyrinth in the middle ear; **(C)** Saccule is a membranous labyrinth in the inner ear; **(D)** the organ or Corti is a receptive organ for the auditory system.

4. Second order neurons in the auditory system project to which of the following structures?
   a) Spiral ganglion
   b) Superior temporal gyrus
   c) Superior olivary nucleus
   d) Ganglion of Scarpa

Level 2: Medium

Answer C. Superior olivary nucleus; **(A)** Spiral ganglion is where first order neurons for the auditory system are located; **(B)** Superior temporal gyrus is part of the cortex and is the end of the pathway; **(D)** ganglion of Scarpa's where first order neurons of the vestibular system are located.

5. The peripheral processes of the first order SVA neurons for CN IX terminate in which of the following structures?
   a) Chemoreceptors in the tongue
   b) Tractus solitarius
   c) Solitary nucleus
   d) Petrous ganglion

Level 2: Medium

Answer A: Chemoreceptors in the posterior tongue; **(B)** tractus solitarius contains central processes from first order neurons; **(C)** Solitary nucleus is where second order neurons are located; **(D)** Petrous ganglion is where the cell bodies of first order neurons are located.

Unit IV

Motor Systems

16 Direct Activation Pathways

16.1 Overview of Direct Motor Pathways

Motor control is a complex system composed of several individual components that together produce movement. These include motor neurons, descending motor pathways and associated cortical areas, basal ganglia, and cerebellum. Pathways that are directly responsible for the voluntary activity of the muscles of the head, neck, and limbs are referred to as the **direct activation pathway**. The direct motor pathway is monosynaptic. Cortical **upper motor neuron** (**UMN**) project to and synapses on a **lower motor neuron** (**LMN**) located in the brainstem and spinal cord. Fibers from cortical neurons connect the UMN, LMN, and the skeletal muscle they innervate forming the descending pathways. The **corticobulbar tract** involves cortical UMNs that project to cranial nerve motor nuclei (LMN) in the brainstem. The **corticospinal tract** consists of UMN in the cortex projecting to the ventral gray matter of the spinal cord where the LMN cell bodies are located. The axons of LMNs synapse on skeletal muscle to initiate movement. Although not part of the direct motor pathways, the **basal ganglia** and **cerebellum** have profound regulatory influence on movement (see Chapter 17). Other descending pathways involved in movement but not originating in the cortex and involving multiple synapses are the **rubrospinal tract**, the **tectospinal tract**, **reticulospinal tract,** and the **vestibulospinal tract** (see Chapter 17). These four **indirect pathways** originate in brainstem nuclei. In addition to movement, motor pathways are important components of **reflex pathways**. Reflexes are involuntary (efferent) responses to sensory (afferent) input.

16.2 Motor Neurons

- UMN (**pyramidal cells**) reside within the cerebral cortex. There are four specific cortical areas where the corticospinal and corticobulbar tracts originate (▶ Fig. 16.1).
  ○ Precentral gyrus (primary motor cortex)
    – Located in **frontal lobe**.
    – Receives input from the thalamus, supplemental motor area, cingulate gyrus, and primary somatosensory gyrus (postcentral gyrus).
    – Involved in the execution of voluntary movements.
  ○ Postcentral gyrus (primary somatosensory cortex)
    – Located in the **parietal lobe**.
    – Some fibers from the dorsal column medial lemniscus tract in the dorsal column carry proprioceptive and tactile input to the primary motor and premotor cortex.
  ○ Supplemental motor areas (SMA)
    – Located in medial aspect of frontal lobe, rostral to precentral gyrus.
    – Involved in programming complex sequences of movements and coordinating bilateral movement.
  ○ Premotor cortex (PMC)
    – Located in frontal lobe, rostral to precentral gyrus.
    – Mediates the selection of movements by utilizing information from other areas of the cortex.
- The precentral gyrus is **somatotopically** organized.
  ○ Stimulation of motor neurons in a specific area of the primary motor cortex results in the contraction of specific muscles. In other words, there is a direct relationship between areas of the motor cortex and regions of the body creating a cortical map, known as a **homunculus** (▶ Fig. 16.2).

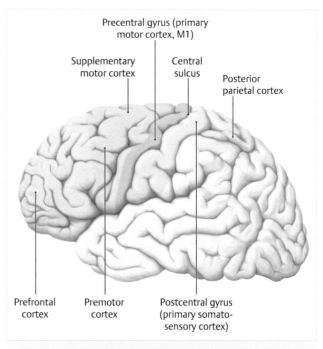

Fig. 16.1 Sensory and motor systems. The sensory system and motor system are so functionally interrelated they may be described as one (sensorimotor system). Cortical areas of the sensorimotor system. Lateral view of the left hemisphere. (Reproduced with permission from Schuenke M, Schulte E, Schumacher U. THIEME Atlas of Anatomy Third Edition, Vol 3. © Thieme 2020. Illustrations by Markus Voll and Karl Wesker.)

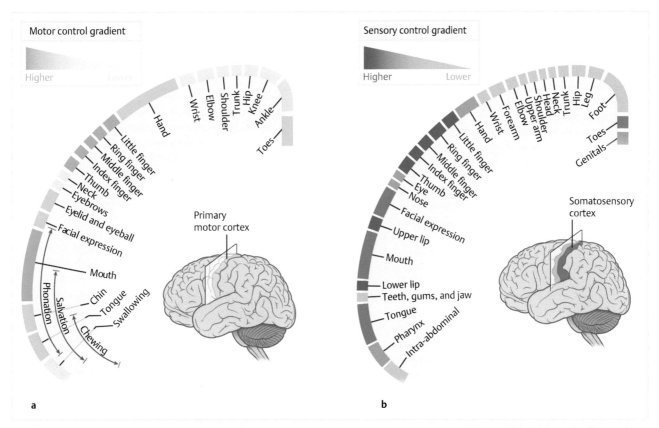

Fig. 16.2 **(a)** Motor homunculus. **(b)** Sensory homunculus. The relationship between the motor cortex and the rest of the body can be illustrated by the homunculus. This cortical map represents the area of the brain that is responsible for motor function in the rest of the body, as well as the relative number of motor units as seen by the proportions of the structures.

- ○ The proportions of the **motor homunculus** represent the relative number of motor units involved in control of that particular region. Thus, the homunculus indicates the amount of fine motor control in a given area. For example, the hands, face, and tongue are depicted as being quite large compared to the trunk.
- UMN cells in the cortex project to LMN in the brainstem and spinal cord (▶ Fig. 16.3).
  - ○ The axons of the UMNs that innervate cranial nerve nuclei (LMN) exit the pathway at the appropriate level forming the **corticobulbar tract**.
  - ○ The remainder of the axons continue through the pyramids. Most will cross or **decussate** forming the **decussation of the pyramids.** All will enter the spinal cord as the **corticospinal tract.**
  - ○ LMNs are the target of UMN.
    - – Axons of UMN terminate directly on LMN *or* on **interneurons**, which in turn will synapse on LMN.
- LMN initiates skeletal muscle contraction.
  - ○ LMN cell bodies are found within the gray matter of the cranial nerve nuclei in the brainstem and the ventral horn of the spinal cord.
  - ○ Their axons exit the gray matter/nuclei and innervate skeletal muscle via peripheral nerves or cranial nerves.

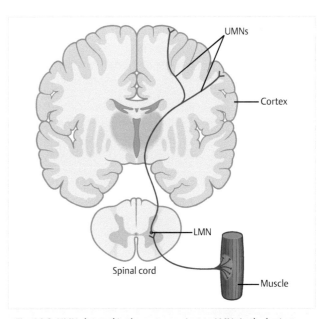

Fig. 16.3 UMNs located in the cortex project to LMNs in the brainstem and spinal cord. LMN, lower motor neuron; UMN, upper motor neuron.

– Not all cranial nerves have LMN components. Some cranial nerves contain only sensory fibers (CNs I, II, and VIII).
  ○ LMNs are somatotopically arranged (▶ Fig. 16.4).
• Skeletal muscles receive innervation from a **motor pool**.
  ○ A motor pool consists of all α-motor neurons that innervate a single muscle.
  ○ Each α-motor neuron within a motor pool sends an efferent (motor) axon toward the periphery, which branches to form synapses called **neuromuscular**

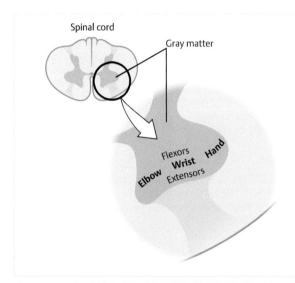

Fig. 16.4 LMNs in the brainstem and spinal cord are also somatotopically positioned. LMN, lower motor neuron.

junctions (**NMJs**) on specific groups of individual muscle fibers.
  ○ Innervation is achieved by release of a neurotransmitter (**acetylcholine**) that is released from the axon of the LMN. Receptors present in the membrane of the plasma membrane of the muscle fiber bind the acetylcholine, which will facilitate the transmission of the impulse resulting in contraction of the muscle fiber.
• The group of individual muscle fibers innervated by a single α-motor neuron and its efferent axon constitutes a **motor unit**. An action potential generated by a motor neuron results in the simultaneous contraction of all muscle fibers in the motor unit.
• There are three different types of motor units (▶ Table 16.1).
  ○ **S or slow-twitch**
    – Produces small amounts of force over prolonged periods of time.
  ○ **FF or fast-twitch**
    – Produces large amounts of force for short periods of time.
  ○ **FR or fast-twitch, fatigue resistant**
    – Produces moderate amounts of force that can be sustained for moderate amounts of time.
• Any given muscle contains multiple types of motor units that are interspersed throughout different regions of the muscle and provides a selective level of motor unit activation and control. Difference in motor unit fiber distribution reflects difference in muscle function.
• The relative proportion of a specific type of motor unit along with the innervation ratio (motor unit size), the motor unit distribution within a muscle, and the overall number of motor units found in a muscle varies between different muscles and reflects muscle function.

Table 16.1 Classification of motor neurons

Motor Unit Classification	Size of Motor Neuron	Activation Threshold of Neuron	Type of Muscle Fibers	Contraction (Twitch) Speed	Contractile Force of Muscle Fiber	Resistance to Fatigue
Type I	Small neuron Discharge at slower rates	Low threshold—responds to weak stimulus Recruited first	Type I fibers—slow oxidative, fatigue resistant Small fibers with high amount of mitochondria Myosin isoform MHC-β	Slow twitch	Low tension Remain tonically active during movements requiring sustained activation	Fatigue resistant
Type IIa	Intermediate neuron Discharge at intermediate rates	Intermediate threshold—requires higher stimulus than Type I	Type II fibers; fast oxidative/glycolytic, fatigue resistant Moderate fiber size Moderate glycogen and mitochondria Myosin isoform MHC-IIa	Moderate Fast twitch	Moderate amount of force	Fatigue resistant
Type IIb	Large neuron Discharge at faster rates	High activation threshold—requires strong stimulus Recruited last	Type IIx fibers Fast glycolytic, fatigue quickly Large fiber size High glycogen Myosin isoform MHC IIx/b	Fastest twitch	High Maximal contractile force	Fatigue easily

16.3 Corticospinal Tract

- Multiple cortical areas contribute to motor control of the head and the rest of the body.
- The axons of the UMN in the cortex project to both the spinal cord and brainstem.
- There are three major descending motor tracts that innervate skeletal muscles of the head and body (▶ Fig. 16.5).
  ○ Lateral corticospinal tract
    – Predominantly controls muscles of the limbs.
  ○ Anterior (ventral) corticospinal tract
    – Controls girdle and axial muscles.
  ○ Corticobulbar tract
    – Innervates muscles of the head.
- The axons of cortical UMNs exit the subcortical white matter and form the **corona radiata** (▶ Fig. 16.6).

  ○ The corona radiata also contains ascending **thalamocortical axons**.
  ○ The corona radiata eventually forms the **internal capsule**.
- Thus, the internal capsule contains the same axons of the corona radiata (▶ Fig. 16.7).
  ○ It is flanked by the basal ganglia and the thalamus.
  ○ The internal capsule is made up of an **anterior** and a **posterior limb**.
    – The **genu** is between the two limbs and therefore connects the anterior and posterior limbs.
    – The descending fibers from the motor cortex primarily run in the posterior limb.
- The motor fibers continue to descend through the brainstem (▶ Fig. 16.8a). As they approach the **crus cerebri** (the anterior portion of the **cerebral peduncle**) (▶ Fig. 16.8b), they reorganize such that the fibers associated with the head

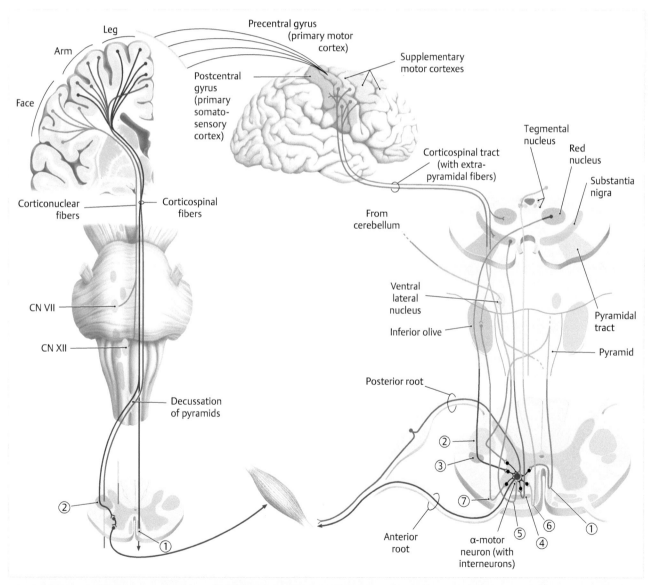

Fig. 16.5 Motor pathways. Descending tracts. (Reproduced with permission from Schuenke M, Schulte E, Schumacher U. THIEME Atlas of Anatomy Third Edition, Vol 3. © Thieme 2020. Illustrations by Markus Voll and Karl Wesker.)

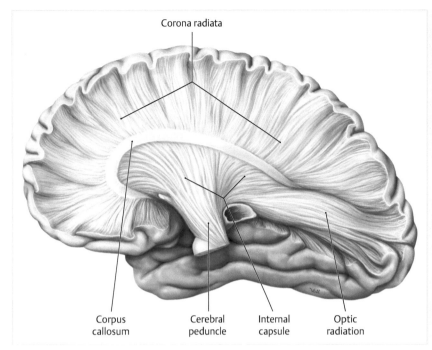

Corona radiata

Corpus callosum

Cerebral peduncle

Internal capsule

Optic radiation

Fig. 16.6 Axons of the UMNs form the corona radiata and eventually forms the internal capsule. UMN, upper motor neuron. (Reproduced with permission from Schuenke M, Schulte E, Schumacher U. THIEME Atlas of Anatomy Second Edition, Vol 3. © Thieme 2016. Illustrations by Markus Voll and Karl Wesker.)

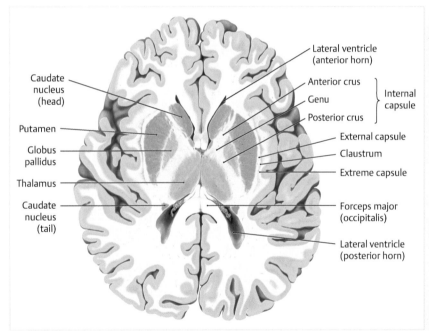

Caudate nucleus (head)

Putamen

Globus pallidus

Thalamus

Caudate nucleus (tail)

Lateral ventricle (anterior horn)

Anterior crus
Genu
Posterior crus
} Internal capsule

External capsule

Claustrum

Extreme capsule

Forceps major (occipitalis)

Lateral ventricle (posterior horn)

Fig. 16.7 The internal capsule contains the same axons as the corona radiata. (Reproduced with permission from Schuenke M, Schulte E, Schumacher U. THIEME Atlas of Anatomy Third Edition, Vol 3. © Thieme 2020. Illustrations by Markus Voll and Karl Wesker.)

are more medial (corticobulbar) and those associated with the legs are more lateral (corticospinal). The fibers that will innervate the upper limbs are in between (corticospinal).

- As the fibers approach the lower brainstem (medulla), the corticospinal and corticobulbar fibers form the **medullary pyramids** (▶ Fig. 16.9a, b).
  - Corticobulbar fibers leave the **pyramids** along the entire length of the medulla to terminate in the **medullary reticular formation** and cranial **nerve nuclei**.
- When the corticospinal fibers approach the spinal cord, most will cross in the midline to form the **pyramidal decussation.**
  - From the decussation, the corticospinal tract continues into the spinal cord (▶ Fig. 16.10a, b).

- Approximately 85% of the corticospinal fibers will cross as the **lateral corticospinal tract**. They descend in the **lateral funiculus** of the spinal cord and will ultimately innervate the more distal musculature.
- The remaining 15% of corticospinal fibers that descend uncrossed are called the **anterior (ventral) corticospinal tract**. These fibers run in the **anterior funiculus** of the spinal cord and will innervate the more proximal musculature.
  - Most of the fibers of the anterior corticospinal tract will decussate in the spinal cord via the anterior white commissure and then synapse on the ventral horn of the gray matter.

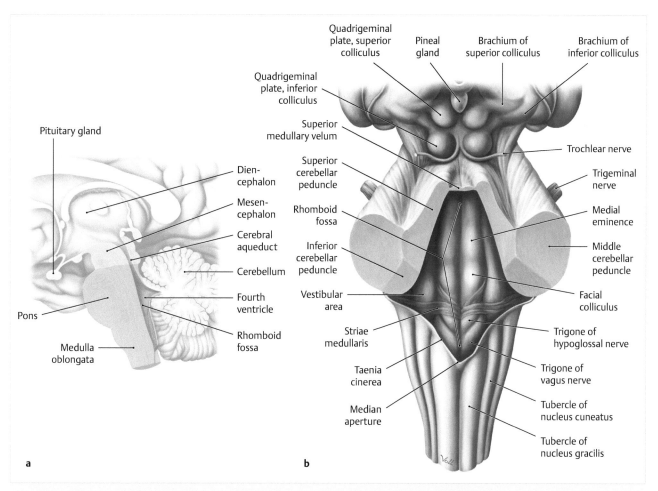

Fig. 16.8 (a) Division of the brainstem into levels: Midsagittal section: The brainstem is divided macroscopically into three levels, with the bulge of the pons marking the boundary lines between the parts: (A) Mesencephalon (midbrain). (B) Pons. (C) Medulla oblongata. The three levels are easily distinguished from one another by gross visual inspection, although they are not differentiated in a functional sense. The functional organization of the brainstem is determined chiefly by the arrangement of the cranial nerve nuclei. Given the close proximity of nuclei and large fiber tracts in this region, even a small lesion of the brainstem (e.g., hemorrhage, tumor) may lead to extensive and complex alterations of sensorimotor function. **(b)** After exiting the internal capsule, the motor fibers descend through the brainstem. (Reproduced with permission from Schuenke M, Schulte E, Schumacher U. THIEME Atlas of Anatomy Third Edition, Vol 3. © Thieme 2020. Illustrations by Markus Voll and Karl Wesker.)

- The majority of the corticospinal fibers will terminate on interneurons rather than directly on motor neurons in the **ventral horn** of the spinal cord (► Fig. 16.11).
- There are functional differences between the different components of corticospinal tract.
  - The lateral corticospinal tract innervates the cervical and lumbar part of the spinal cord and controls fine movements of the extremities.
  - The anterior corticospinal tract mediates postural mechanisms.
  - Some fibers from the corticospinal tract project to the dorsal horn in order to modulate sensory information that travels to the cortex.

16.4 Corticobulbar Tract

- The corticobulbar tract originates from the lateral aspect of the primary motor cortex (► Fig. 16.12).

- Cortical neurons from the parietal area represent the UMNs that target cranial nerve motor nuclei, which are the LMNs.
- The axons of the UMN travel through the corona radiata, internal capsule, crus cerebri of the midbrain, and the medullary pyramids in a similar trajectory to corticospinal fibers.
- The UMN of the corticobulbar tract will synapse directly on motor neurons or indirectly on interneurons of the reticular formation.
- This system is responsible for motor control of the muscles of facial expression, eye movements, movements of the tongue, and elevation and depression of the mandible.
- One of the unique aspects of the corticobulbar system is how it innervates some of its targets.
  - Like the corticospinal tract, most cranial nerve motor nuclei are innervated *bilaterally.*
  - Exceptions to this phenomenon include:
    - Contralateral innervation of the ventral motor neurons of CN VII that control the facial muscles below the eye.

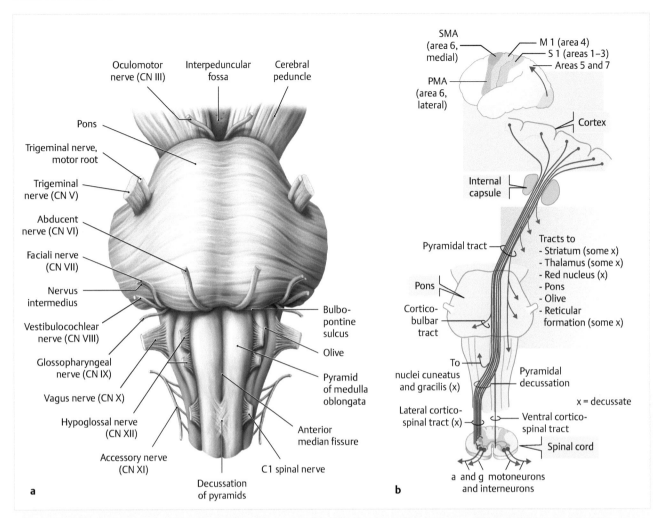

Fig. 16.9 (a) The descending motor fibers form the medullary pyramids at the lower end of the brainstem. **(b)** Most of the corticospinal fibers cross as they near the spinal cord forming the pyramidal decussation. Corticobulbar fibers exit the pyramids along the length of the medulla. (Fig. 16.9a: Reproduced with permission from Schuenke M, Schulte E, Schumacher U. THIEME Atlas of Anatomy. Second Edition, Vol 3. © Thieme 2016. Illustrations by Markus Voll and Karl Wesker. Fig. 16.9b: Modified with permission from Silbernagl S, Despopoulos A. Color Atlas of Physiology. Sixth Edition. © Thieme 2009.)

– Contralateral innervation of the hypoglossal nucleus (CN XII), which innervates the genioglossus.

16.4.1 Lesions of the Corticobulbar Tract

As previously indicated, most of the innervation of cranial nerve motor nuclei from the cortex is bilateral. Therefore, a lesion that occurs between the cortex and the cranial nerve nuclei will not result in paralysis of the muscles of the face and head.

- In the case of the face (CN VII), the area above the eyes would only experience mild weakness, if anything, due to the bilateral innervation. However, the area below the eyes receives unilateral innervation, so marked weakness or paralysis would be evident. Furthermore, the input is contralateral so that muscles of facial expression below the

eyes and protrusion of the tongue would be affected on the side contralateral to the lesion (▶ Fig. 16.13).

- Clinical symptoms of a CN XII lesion are also dependent on whether or not the lesion involves UMNs or LMNs (▶ Fig. 16.14a, b). A **supranuclear lesion** (UMN) lesion of CN XII would result in deviation of the tongue on protrusion to the side opposite to the lesion.
  ○ CN XII innervates the genioglossus, which is responsible for protrusion of the tongue.
  ○ Knocking out the fibers (lesion) projecting to the motor nucleus of CN XII (UMN) will produce **contralateral** deficits. The tongue protrudes to the side *opposite* to the lesion because it is unopposed.
  ○ Knocking out CN XII at the level of the nucleus or distally (LMN) would result in **ipsilateral** deficits. In an LMN lesion, the tongue will deviate to the *same* side as the lesion because it is unopposed.

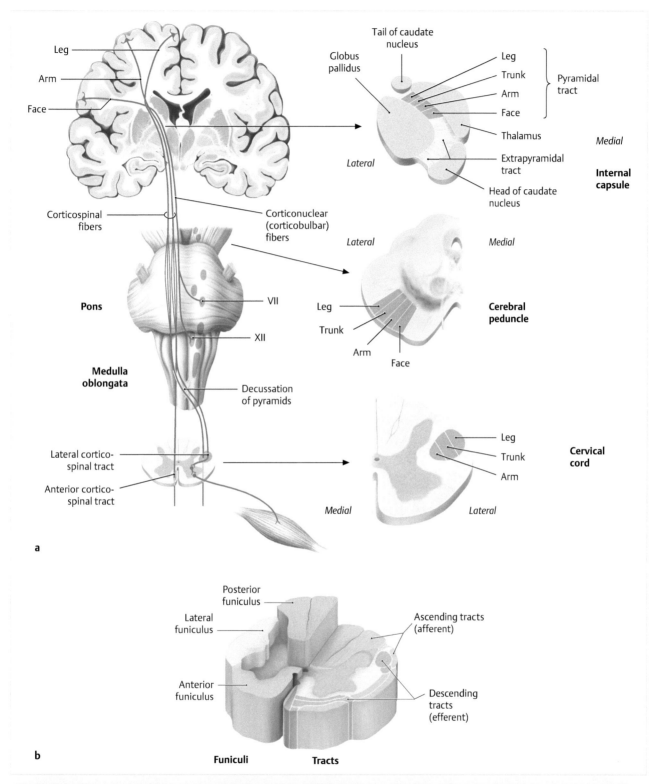

Fig. 16.10 **(a)** The corticospinal tract continues into the spinal cord. **(b)** The majority of the fibers will cross as the lateral corticospinal tract. They descend in the lateral funiculus and will innervate the more distal muscles. (Reproduced with permission from Schuenke M, Schulte E, Schumacher U. THIEME Atlas of Anatomy Third Edition, Vol 3. © Thieme 2020. Illustrations by Markus Voll and Karl Wesker.)

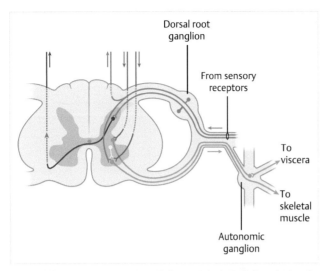

Fig. 16.11 Corticospinal fibers will descend to the spinal cord where they synapse on interneurons or motor neurons.

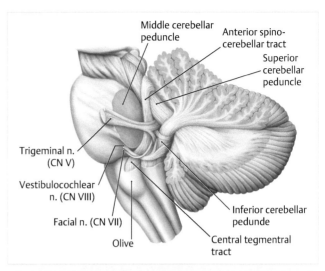

Fig. 16.12 The corticobulbar tract originates from the lateral aspect of the motor cortex. (Reproduced with permission from Schuenke M, Schulte E, Schumacher U. THIEME Atlas of Anatomy Third Edition, Vol 3. © Thieme 2020. Illustrations by Markus Voll and Karl Wesker.)

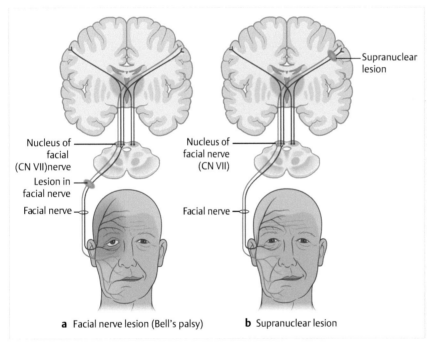

a Facial nerve lesion (Bell's palsy)   **b** Supranuclear lesion

Fig. 16.13 (a) LMN lesion. (b) UMN lesion. Most of the cranial nerve nuclei are bilaterally innervated (right and left cortices) so a lesion occurring between the cortex and the nuclei (UMN) will not result in paralysis. One exception to that rule is CN VII. In the face, the area above the eyes is bilaterally innervated, so a lesion would result in mild weakness, if anything. However, the area below the eyes in unilaterally innervated, so the same lesion would cause marked weakness or paralysis. Additionally, the unilateral innervation is contralateral, so the effect would be seen on the side of the face opposite to the lesion (lesion right side = paralysis left side) LMN, lower motor neuron; UMN, upper motor neuron.

16.5 Disorders of the Motor System

Damage or disease of the motor system can cause unique symptoms and challenges for patients depending on the type of motor neuron that is involved. Damage can involve the motor cell bodies or their axons. Both UMN and LMN damage produces characteristic symptoms that allow clinicians to determine the type of disorder the patient is experiencing (Clinical Correlation Box 16.1 and 16.2) (▶ Table 16.2).

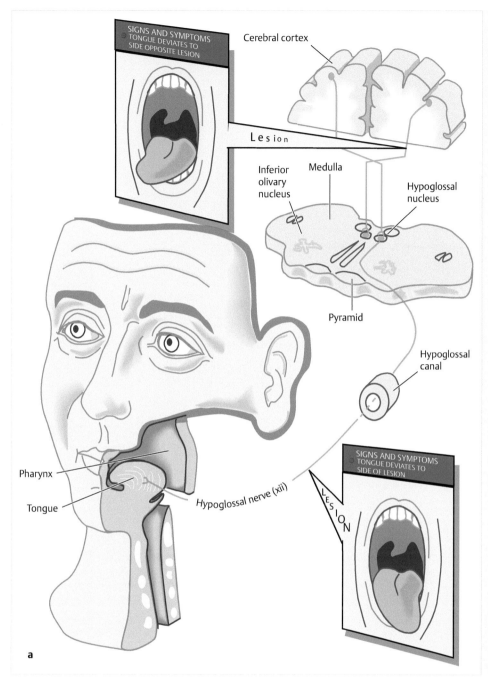

SIGNS AND SYMPTOMS
TONGUE DEVIATES TO
SIDE OPPOSITE LESION

Cerebral cortex

Lesion

Inferior olivary nucleus

Medulla

Hypoglossal nucleus

Pyramid

Hypoglossal canal

SIGNS AND SYMPTOMS
TONGUE DEVIATES TO
SIDE OF LESION

LESION

Pharynx

Tongue

Hypoglossal nerve (xii)

a

Fig. 16.14 (a) Clinical symptoms of a lesion in CN XII is dependent on whether or not the lesion involves UMNs or LMNs. (▶ Fig. 16.14a: Reproduced with permission from Alberstone CD, Benzel EC, Najm IM, et al. Anatomic Basis of Neurologic Diagnosis. © Thieme 2009.)

(*Continued*)

Clinical Correlation Box 16.1: Brown Sequard Syndrome

Brown Sequard syndrome is a spinal cord lesion that results from a **hemisection** injury to the spinal cord (▶ Fig. 16.16). This results in interruption of the lateral corticospinal tract, lateral spinothalamic tract, and posterior column. Clinical presentation includes a spastic weak leg with intact reflexes and a strong leg with loss of pain and temperature. The motor fibers of the corticospinal tract cross at the decussation of the pyramids. Thus, damage to the corticospinal tract on one side produces ipsilateral weakness below the lesion with UMN and LMN signs. Common causes of spinal cord hemisection include trauma, herniated disks, and degenerative disease of the vertebral column.

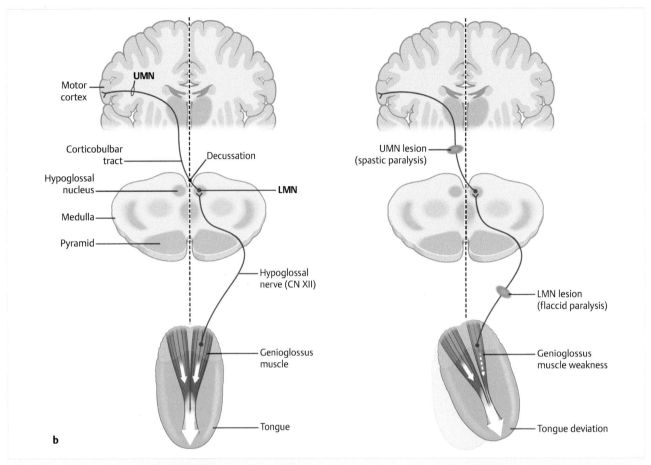

Fig. 16.14 (*Continued*) **(b)** A UMN lesion would result in contralateral deviation of the tongue (opposite the lesion) while an LMN lesion would result in ipsilateral deficits (same side as the lesion). LMN, lower motor neuron; UMN, upper motor neuron.

Clinical Correlation Box 16.2: Myasthenia Gravis

Myasthenia gravis (MG) is a chronic autoimmune disease that results in weakness of skeletal muscles. The hallmark characteristic of this disorder is muscle weakness that becomes more severe with increased activity and shows improvement with rest. MG pathology is due to antibody-mediated blocking of acetylcholine receptors at the neuromuscular junction. In these individuals, autoantibodies form against the postsynaptic receptors involved in neuromuscular transmission. The result is inefficient transmission of the impulse from the motor neuron to the muscle fiber. When this failure occurs in enough muscle fibers, it can manifest clinically. The ocular and bulbar muscles are most frequently involved and are often the most severe. One of the greatest concerns with this disease is if respiratory muscles become involved it can lead to respiratory failure. MG is a disorder that has been studied extensively and is clearly defined. It is also very well managed. Therapy includes anticholinesterase drugs as well as immunotherapy. Thymectomy is often performed if acetylcholine receptor antibodies are present.

Table 16.2 Symptoms of UMN and LMN syndromes

Upper Motor Neuron Syndrome	Lower Motor Neuron Syndrome
Reflex activity absent	Paralysis
Spasticity	Paresis
Hyporeflexia	Areflexia
Clonus	Hypotonia
Babinski sign	Atrophy
	Fasciculations
	Fibrillations

Abbreviations: LMN: lower motor neuron; UMN: upper motor neuron.

16.5.1 Upper Motor Neuron Syndrome

Damage to UMNs is common because of the large surface area they occupy in the cortex and because the pathways run for significant distances, that is, cortex to lower end of the spinal cord. Lesions occurring anywhere along the pathway result in a disorder known as *upper motor neuron syndrome.*
- Damage to the motor cortex or internal capsule results in immediate muscle **flaccidity** on the contralateral face and body.
  ○ This phenomenon will be most severe in the limbs.

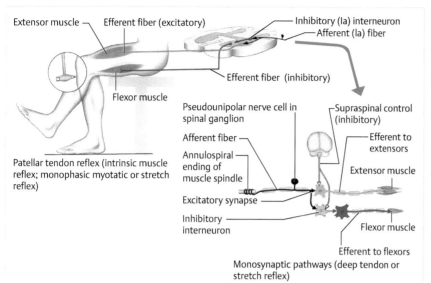

Extensor muscle — Efferent fiber (excitatory) — Inhibitory (Ia) interneuron — Afferent (Ia) fiber — Efferent fiber (inhibitory) — Flexor muscle

Patellar tendon reflex (intrinsic muscle reflex; monophasic myotatic or stretch reflex)

Pseudounipolar nerve cell in spinal ganglion — Afferent fiber — Annulospiral ending of muscle spindle — Excitatory synapse — Inhibitory interneuron — Supraspinal control (inhibitory) — Efferent to extensors — Extensor muscle — Flexor muscle — Efferent to flexors

Monosynaptic pathways (deep tendon or stretch reflex)

Fig. 16.15 A spinal reflex involves both afferent and efferent fibers in that sensory input results in efferent output. (Modified with permission from Rohkamm R, ed. Color Atlas of Neurology. Second Edition. © Thieme 2014.)

- The initial **hypotonia** is also known as **spinal shock** (**Clinical correlation Box 16.3**).
  - After several days, spinal cord circuits may regain function.
- **Reflex activity** on the affected side is absent.
- Trunk muscles may be functional due to bilateral innervation from the corticospinal pathway.
- Classic patterns of UMN syndrome are as follows:
  - **Babinski sign**
    - The normal response to stroking the sole of the foot is flexion of the great toe as well as the other toes. UMN damage results in the extension of the great toe and fanning of the other toes upon stroking the sole of the foot. A similar response is present in infants prior to the development of the corticospinal pathway. Children from birth to 2 years of age will display this plantar response due to the underdeveloped motor pathways.
  - **Spasticity**
    - Increased muscle tone and *hyper-reactive stretch reflexes*. Extensive UMN damage can be accompanied by rigidity, likely due to the removal of inhibitory influences.
  - **Hyporeflexia**
    - Deceased superficial reflexes such as the corneal reflex, superficial abdominal reflex, and cremasteric reflex in males.
  - **Clonus**
    - Oscillatory motor response to muscle stretching.

16.5.2 Lower Motor Neuron Syndrome

Damage to the motor neurons of the spinal cord and brainstem are called **lower motor neuron syndrome**. Damage may occur to the cell bodies or their axons.
- Classic patterns of lower motor neuron damage include:
  - Paralysis
    - Loss of movement in affected muscles.
  - Paresis
    - Weakness of affected muscles.
  - Areflexia
    - Loss of reflexes.
  - Hypotonia
    - Loss of muscle tone in affected muscles.
  - Atrophy
    - Appears later due to disuse and denervation.
  - **Fasciculations** and **fibrillations** may be present. Fasciculations are due to abnormal activity in the damaged motor neuron. Fibrillations are the result of changes in excitability of the denervated motor neuron.

16.6 Spinal Reflexes

A spinal reflex involves efferent output in response to afferent input (▶ Fig. 16.15). Reflexes range from simple such as the stretch reflex to more complicated activities like walking movements. Therefore, all reflexes involve a motor neuron and a sensory neuron and except for a few circumstances, interneurons as well.

- The **stretch reflex** is a **myotactic reflex**. It is one of the simplest of reflexes involving two neurons and one synapse. The afferent limb of the reflex is an afferent fiber from a sensory neuron in the **dorsal root ganglia**. Its peripheral process is associated with a **muscle spindle**. The central process of the sensory neuron synapses on a motor neuron within the spinal cord. Activation of the motor neuron will cause the muscle to contract.
  - One of the major roles of the myotactic reflex is to maintain posture. If an individual is standing upright and loses balance, the muscles in the limbs are stretched, activating the **reflex arc** to counteract the swaying.
  - The myotactic reflex is a clinically important reflex as it is the basis for the **knee-jerk reflex**. By tapping the patellar tendon, the reflex movement of the extensor muscles of the thigh occurs, thereby extending the lower leg. This is also known as a **deep tendon reflex** and, if absent, can indicate an interruption in the corticospinal pathway.

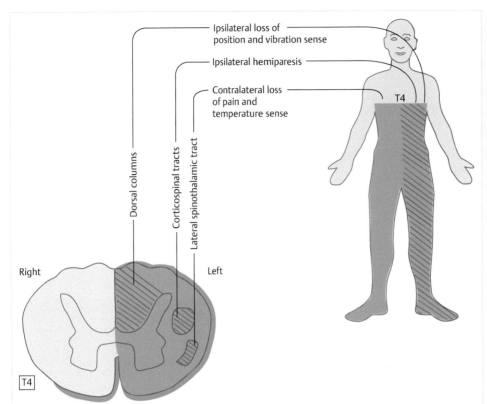

Fig. 16.16 Brown Sequard syndrome is a condition that is caused by injury to the spinal cord resulting in a hemisection. The result is damage to the corticospinal tract, spinothalamic tract, and posterior column. Clinical presentation includes: affected (weak) leg with intact reflexes and unaffected (strong) leg with loss of pain and temperature. (Reproduced with permission from Alberstone CD, Benzel EC, Najm IM, et al. Anatomic Basis of Neurologic Diagnosis. © Thieme 2009.)

- **Hyporeflexia** is an absent or diminished reflex response and can indicate an issue with one of the components in the two-neuron reflex.
- **Hyperreflexia** is an overreaction and repeated (**clonic**) response. It usually indicates a problem with the corticospinal tract or other descending pathways that influences the reflex arc.
- The **flexor reflex** is initiated by a cutaneous receptor and involves the entire limb. This reflex is also called the **withdrawal reflex**, which is illustrated by a painful stimulus and a subsequent withdrawal from that stimulus by **flexion**.
  - Typically, only nociceptor (pain) receptors can initiate this reflex.
  - Reflex involves entire limb, so pathway encompasses several spinal segments.
- **Crossed extension reflex** is a compensatory reflex that results in support of the body during a flexion reflex. In other words, activation of the flexion reflex on one side of the body which results in flexion of a group of muscles in one limb is always accompanied by contraction of the extensors of the limb on the other side of the body.
  - This activity provides support for the body and prevents a loss of balance.
  - Afferents activated from the flexion reflex innervate an interneuron that sends its axon across the midline to the contralateral spinal cord. Here, it excites a motor neuron that innervates extensor muscles of the opposite leg. The extensors act as contralateral antagonists.
  - This crossed effect allows balance and body posture to be maintained.

- **Autogenic reflex/Golgi tendon reflex** is thought to have a protective function by regulating motor unit activity. It most likely also plays an important role in normal function by spreading work more evenly across the entire muscle, thus making motor units more efficient.
  - The **Golgi tendon organ (GTO)** is located at the junction of the tendon and the muscle.
  - When tension is applied to a muscle, afferents innervating the GTO are activated.
  - The central process of the afferent neuron synapses on an interneuron that then makes an inhibitory synapse on the motor neuron that innervates the same muscle that is sending the afferent signal.
  - This reflex results in a decrease or cessation of the muscle contraction.

Clinical Correlation Box 16.3: Spinal Shock

Spinal shock refers to the pathophysiologic condition that occurs following a transection of the spinal cord resulting in temporary loss or diminished spinal reflex activity below the level of injury. Spinal shock is commonly associated with trauma and is typically immediate. In some instances, loss of reflex activity may be seen above the lesion. The period of spinal shock varies from days to weeks. The end of the phase is marked by abnormal corticospinal reflexes such as Babinski's sign or exaggerated muscle spindle reflex arcs. Reflexes may never return in areas that are severely damaged by the trauma.

Questions and Answers

1. Which of the following structures contributes proprioceptive information to the corticospinal tract?
   a) Precentral gyrus
   b) Postcentral gyrus
   c) Frontal lobe
   d) Supplemental motor cortex

Level 2: Medium

Answer B: The postcentral gyrus is also called the primary somatosensory cortex. It provided proprioceptive information via the dorsal column-medial lemniscus pathway; **(A)** precentral gyrus is the primary motor cortex; **(C)** the precentral gyrus, **(D)** the supplemental motor area and the premotor cortex are all found in the frontal lobe. None of these areas provide sensory information.

2. In terms of the motor homunculus, which of the following areas represent the origin of the corticobulbar tract?
   a) Parietal lobe
   b) Frontal lobe
   c) Temporal lobe
   d) Occipital lobe

Level 1: Easy

Answer B: Frontal lobe; **(A)** Parietal, **(C)** Temporal and **(D)** Ooccipital lobes are not involved in the motor activity.

3. Descending motor fibers that form the decussation of the pyramids are called:
   a) Corticobulbar tract
   b) Ventral corticospinal tract
   c) Lateral corticospinal tract
   d) Anterior funiculus tract

Level 1: Easy

Answer C: Lateral corticospinal tract; **(A)** Fibers from Corticobulbar tract exit the pyramids to innervate the head; **(B)**

Ventral corticospinal tract descends into the spinal cord uncrossed; **(D)** Anterior funiculus is made up of descending motor fibers from the ventral corticospinal tract within the spinal cord.

4. Patient A presents with a lesion of the right lateral corticospinal tract at L2. Which of the following signs would be present?
   a) Negative Clonus
   b) Negative Babinski sign
   c) Contralateral spastic paralysis
   d) Ipsilateral hypertonia

Level 3: Difficult

Answer D: Ipsilateral hypertonia. Lesions of the corticospinal tract results in ipsilateral UMN symptoms, which includes hypertonia; **(A)** Clonus would be positive ipsilaterally; **(B)** Ipsilateral positive Babinski sign would be present; **(C)** Spastic paralysis would be present but it would be *ipsilateral.*

5. Patient B suffered a stroke. Among other issues, when asked to protrude her tongue, it deviates to the right side. There is no muscle atrophy. Fasciculations are absent. What type of lesion does Patient B suffer from?
   a) UMN right side
   b) UMN left side
   c) LMN right side
   d) LMN left side.

Level 3: Difficult

Answer B: UMN left side. Lack of muscle atrophy and fasciculations with deviation of the tongue indicates UMN damage. Symptoms in an UMN syndrome are contralateral to the lesion. Patients' tongue deviates to the right so lesion occurred on the left side; **(A)** would be ipsilateral; **(C)** and **(D)** answers are incorrect because symptoms indicate and UMN lesion.

17 Indirect Activation Pathways

17.1 Overview of Indirect Influences on Movement

Historically, the corticospinal and corticobulbar tracts were considered to be part of the **pyramidal system** because their fibers run in the medullary pyramids. More recently, the **pyramidal/extrapyramidal** nomenclature has been dropped in favor of more descriptive terms such as **direct** (corticospinal and corticobulbar) and **indirect activation pathways** in the motor system. Physiologically, the corticospinal and corticobulbar are **monosynaptic**; an upper motor neuron (UMN) projects and synapses on a lower motor neuron (LMN) which in turn innervates skeletal muscle. Thus, they directly control voluntary motor activity. However, there are numerous other **polysynaptic pathways** that also influence movement, which were referred to as the **extrapyramidal system.** For the purposes of this discussion, theses tracts will be identified as indirect pathways. In the indirect system, neuronal activity also begins in the cortex and then project to structures such as the **basal ganglia**, **brainstem nuclei,** and **cerebellum** before synapsing on LMN (▶ Fig. 17.1). The role of the indirect pathways is to modify or influence neural impulses originating in the cerebral cortex. These pathways include the **rubrospinal**, **reticulospinal, vestibulospinal,** and **tectospinal** tracts as well as the basal ganglia and cerebellum (▶ Table 17.1).

17.2 Brainstem Nuclei and Tracts

The brainstem houses several nuclei that are important in movement. UMN in the cortex directly influences spinal cord circuits by synapsing on LMN in the ventral horn of the spinal cord or by synapsing on cranial nerve motor nuclei in the brainstem. Indirectly, some cortical neurons influence movement via polysynaptic pathways involving the **red nucleus**, **vestibular nuclei**, **reticular nuclei,** and from neurons located in the **superior colliculus** of the midbrain. These nuclei are associated with descending motor tracts that influence movement (▶ Fig. 17.2).

17.2.1 Rubrospinal Tract

- The **rubrospinal tract** (**RST**) originates from the **red nucleus** (**RN**) of the midbrain (▶ Fig. 17.3).
- The red nucleus receives input from the motor cortex and the cerebellum.
  - Its function is to facilitate control of motor neurons supplying flexors and inhibiting motor neurons supplying extensors of the upper extremity.
- The rubrospinal tract represents an alternative to the corticospinal tract by which motor commands can be sent to the spinal cord.
  - The rubrospinal tract decussates immediately after leaving the RN and descends in the spinal cord.
    - It can be found running lateral to the corticospinal tract.
- The rubrospinal tract is more prominent in species that use limbs for locomotion. In humans, the tract is primarily directed to cervical levels in the spinal cord and its size is somewhat diminished. In lower species, it continues into the lumbar area.

17.2.2 Reticulospinal Tract

The **reticular formation** forms the core of the brainstem. It extends from the caudal medulla and continues rostrally to include the midbrain. There are two **reticulospinal tracts** originating from the reticular formation: the *lateral*, which arises from the medulla, and the *medial*, which originates from the pons (▶ Fig. 17.4).

- Functionally, these tracts are involved in preparatory and movement related activities, postural control, and some autonomic responses.
- The reticulospinal tract is a major alternative to the corticospinal tract. It allows cortical neurons to control motor function by projecting to the reticular formation.
- It receives input from the cortex, cerebellum, vestibular system, auditory system, somatosensory system, and other brainstem nuclei.
- Pathways are generally bilateral and have large numbers of fibers projecting to axial and proximal muscles.
- Collectively, the reticulospinal tract regulates the sensitivity of the flexor response so that only noxious stimuli will elicit a response. Damage will result in innocuous stimuli such as a gentle touch to cause a reflex response.
- Individually, the medial and lateral tracts have opposing actions.
  - The **medial reticulospinal tract** facilitates cortical and voluntary movement and increases muscle tone.
  - The **lateral reticulospinal tract** inhibits cortical and voluntary movement and reduces muscle tone.
  - Both tracts exit at all spinal levels.

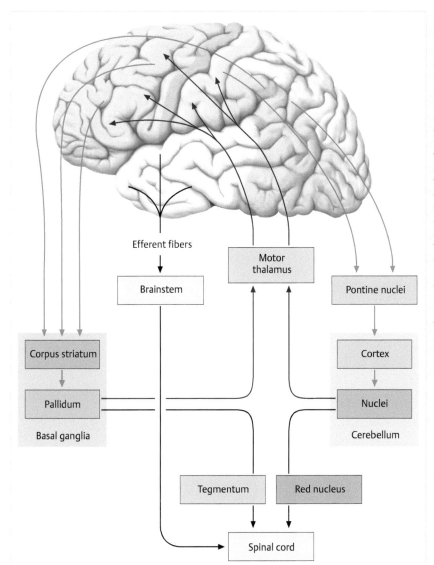

Fig. 17.1 Connections of the cortex with the basal ganglia and cerebellum: programming of complex movements. The pyramidal motor system (the primary motor cortex and the pyramidal tract arising from it) is assisted by the basal ganglia and cerebellum in the planning and programming of complex movements. While afferent fibers of the motor nuclei (green) project directly to the basal ganglia (left) without synapsing, the cerebellum is indirectly controlled via pontine nuclei. The motor thalamus provides a feedback loop for both structures. The efferent fibers of the basal nuclei and cerebellum are distributed to lower structures including the spinal cord. The importance of the basal ganglia and cerebellum in voluntary movements can be appreciated by noting the effects of lesions in these structures. Although diseases of the basal ganglia impair the initiation and execution of movements (e.g., in Parkinson's disease), cerebellar lesions are characterized by uncoordinated movements (e.g., the reeling movements of inebriation caused by a temporary toxic insult to the cerebellum). (Reproduced with permission from Schuenke M, Schulte E, Schumacher U. THIEME Atlas of Anatomy. Second Edition, Vol 3. © Thieme 2016. Illustrations by Markus Voll and Karl Wesker.)

Table 17.1 Polysynaptic pathways from brainstem

Tract	Origin	
Rubrospinal tract	Red nucleus of midbrain	Stimulates flexors and inhibits extensors of the upper limb
Reticulospinal tract	Reticular nuclei of brainstem	Inhibit and facilitates cortical voluntary movement; increase or reduces muscle tone
Vestibulospinal tract	Vestibular nuclei of brainstem	Balance and posture; coordination of head and eye muscles
Tectospinal tract	Superior colliculus of midbrain	Involved in reflex responses of the head to visual stimuli

17.2.3 Vestibulospinal Tract

The **vestibulospinal tract** originates in two vestibular nuclei located beneath the floor of the fourth ventricle in the brainstem. Both tracts convey neural impulses from the labyrinth of the inner ear to the spinal cord (▸ Fig. 17.5).

- The **medial vestibulospinal tract** originates from the **medial vestibular nucleus**.
  - Projects as the descending **medial longitudinal fasciculus**.
  - Primarily reaches cervical levels (T6 and above).
  - Stabilizes head muscles.
  - Important for coordination of head and eye muscles.
  - Plays an important role in the maintenance of posture and balance.

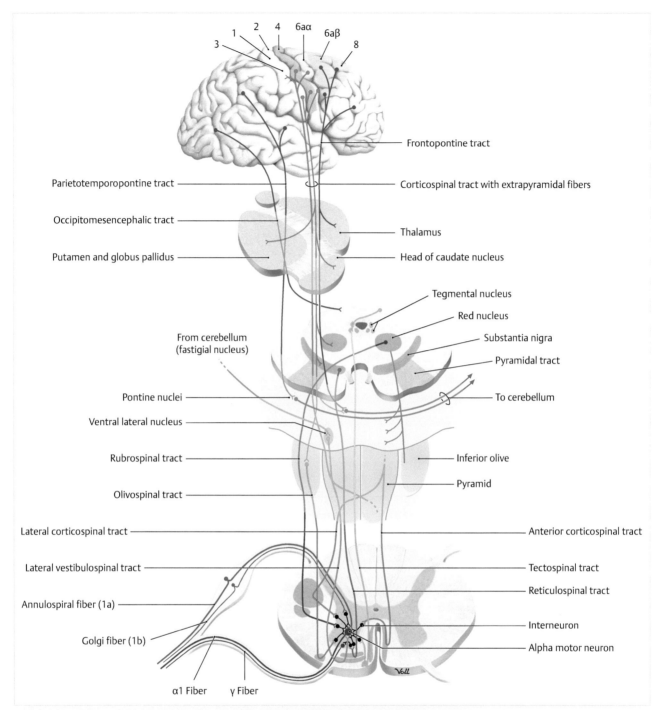

Fig. 17.2 Descending tracts of the extrapyramidal motor system. The neurons of origin of the descending tracts of the extrapyramidal motor system* arise from a heterogeneous group of nuclei that includes the basal ganglia (putamen, globus pallidus, and caudate nucleus), the red nucleus, the substantia nigra, and even the motor cortical areas. The following descending tracts are part of the extrapyramidal motor system: (A) Rubrospinal tract, (B) Olivospinal tract, (C) Vestibulospinal tract, (D) Reticulospinal tract, (E) Tectospinal tract. These long descending tracts terminate on interneurons which then form synapses onto alpha and gamma motor neurons, which they control. Besides these long descending motor tracts, the motor neurons additionally receive sensory input. All impulses in these pathways are integrated by the alpha motor neuron and modulate its activity, thereby affecting muscular contractions. The functional integrity of the alpha motor neuron is tested clinically by reflex testing. (Reproduced with permission from Schuenke M, Schulte E, Schumacher U. THIEME Atlas of Anatomy. Second Edition, Vol 3. © Thieme 2016. Illustrations by Markus Voll and Karl Wesker.)

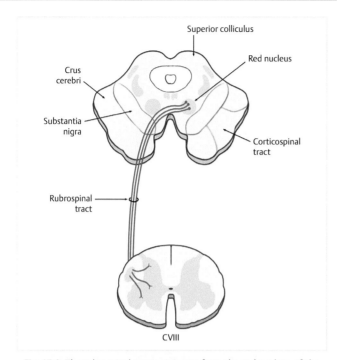

Fig. 17.3 The rubrospinal tract originates from the red nucleus of the midbrain. It receives input from the motor cortex and the cerebellum. It facilitates control of motor neurons supplying flexors of the upper extremity (among other functions). (Reproduced with permission from Alberstone CD, Benzel EC, Najm IM, et al. Anatomic Basis of Neurologic Diagnosis. © Thieme 2009.)

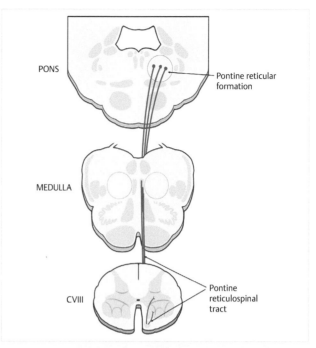

Fig. 17.4 The reticulospinal tract originates from the reticular formation of the midbrain. Functionally, this tract is involved in preparatory and movement related activities, postural control, and some autonomic responses. (Reproduced with permission from Alberstone CD, Benzel EC, Najm IM, et al. Anatomic Basis of Neurologic Diagnosis. © Thieme 2009.)

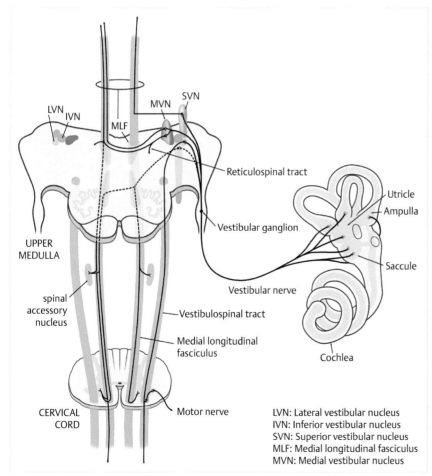

Fig. 17.5 The vestibulospinal tract originates from vestibular nuclei in the floor of the fourth ventricle. This tract conveys neural impulses from the inner ear to the spinal cord. It is involved in the maintenance of balance and posture. (Reproduced with permission from Alberstone CD, Benzel EC, Najm IM, et al. Anatomic Basis of Neurologic Diagnosis. © Thieme 2009.)

LVN: Lateral vestibular nucleus
IVN: Inferior vestibular nucleus
SVN: Superior vestibular nucleus
MLF: Medial longitudinal fasciculus
MVN: Medial vestibular nucleus

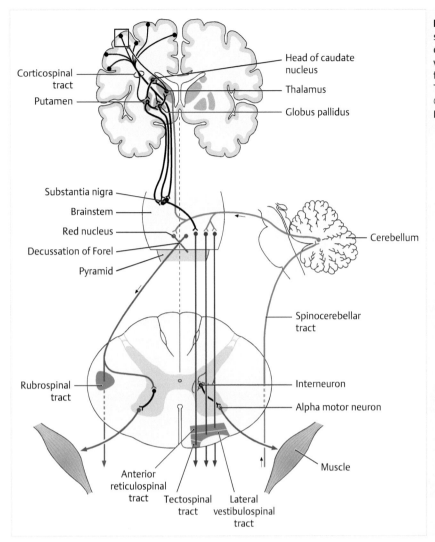

Corticospinal tract
Putamen
Head of caudate nucleus
Thalamus
Globus pallidus
Substantia nigra
Brainstem
Red nucleus
Decussation of Forel
Pyramid
Cerebellum
Spinocerebellar tract
Rubrospinal tract
Interneuron
Alpha motor neuron
Anterior reticulospinal tract
Tectospinal tract
Lateral vestibulospinal tract
Muscle

Fig. 17.6 The tectospinal tract originates in the superior colliculus of the midbrain. Although not entirely certain, it is thought to be involved in visual responses. (Reproduced with permission from Schuenke M, Schulte E, Schumacher U. THIEME Atlas of Anatomy. Third Edition, Vol 3. © Thieme 2020. Illustrations by Markus Voll and Karl Wesker.)

- The **lateral vestibulospinal tract** originates from the **lateral vestibular nucleus**.
  - Projects as **ventrolateral funiculus** of the spinal cord.
  - Projects to all levels of the spinal cord.
  - Activates extensor motor neurons.
  - Plays an important role in maintenance of posture and balance.
    - Facilitates extensors of the neck, back, and extremities. It is inhibitory to flexors.

17.2.4 Tectospinal Tract

The **tectospinal tract** originates in the deep layers of the **superior colliculus** of the midbrain (▶ Fig. 17.6).
- It terminates in the cervical levels of the spinal cord.
- The function of the tract is not well known. However, due to the fact that the superior colliculus is known to be involved in visual responses, it is likely that this tract facilitates movement of the head in reflex responses to visual stimuli.

17.3 Basal Ganglia

The **basal ganglia** (**BG**) consist of several **subcortical nuclei, subthalamic nucleus,** and the **substantia nigra** (▶ Fig. 17.7a, b).

Damage to these structures or the pathways connecting them with the cortex and spinal cord results in distinct movement disorders. In addition to movement disorders, basal ganglia disease can impact cognitive function and emotions (Clinical Correlation Box 17.1 and 17.2).
- One of the main functions of the basal ganglia is to provide feedback to the cerebral cortex in order to initiate and control movement.
  - Much of the control is inhibitory; thus it modulates output.
  - It is involved in the facilitation of practiced motor activity.
  - It does not initiate voluntary motor movements.
- A significant amount of the output from the basal ganglia is facilitated by the **thalamus** (▶ Fig. 17.8).
- The components of the basal ganglia encompass the telencephalon, diencephalon, and mesencephalon (▶ Fig. 17.9) (▶ Table 17.2).
  - Forebrain structures make up the **corpus striatum**.
    - Putamen
      - Separated from the caudate nucleus by the anterior limb of the internal capsule.
    - **Caudate nucleus**
      - C-shaped
      - Associated with the lateral ventricles

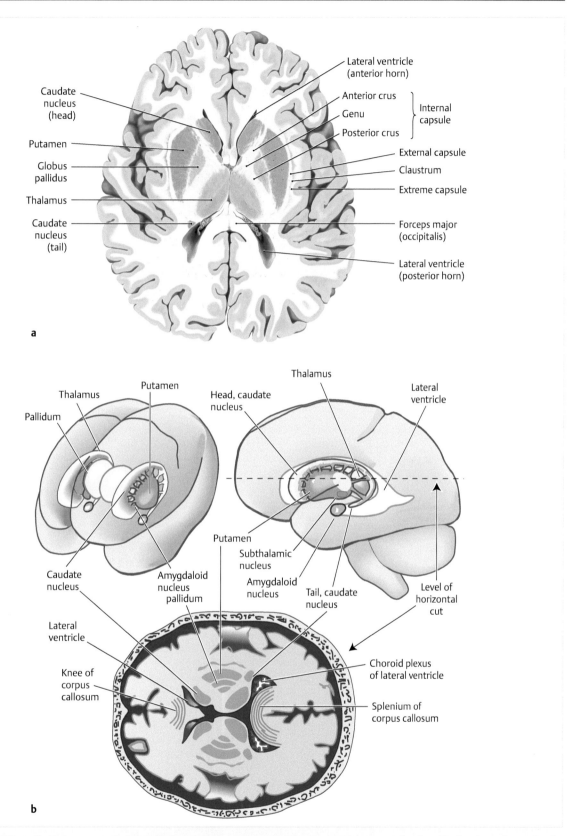

Fig. 17.7 **(a)** Basal ganglia. Transverse section through the cerebrum at the level of the corpus striatum, superior view. The basal ganglia consist of the caudate nucleus, putamen, and globus pallidus and are an essential component of the extrapyramidal motor system, which controls involuntary movement and reflexes and coordinates complex movements. The caudate nucleus and putamen, which are separated from each other by the fibrous white matter of the internal capsule, together constitute the corpus striatum. Deficiency of dopamine in the basal ganglia is responsible for Parkinson's disease. **(b)** Basal ganglia nuclei and their relationship to other cortical structures. (Fig. 17.7a: Reproduced with permission from Schuenke M, Schulte E, Schumacher U. THIEME Atlas of Anatomy Third Edition, Vol 3. © Thieme 2020. Illustrations by Markus Voll and Karl Wesker. Fig. 17.7b: Reproduced with permission from Alberstone CD, Benzel EC, Najm IM, et al. Anatomic Basis of Neurologic Diagnosis. © Thieme 2009.)

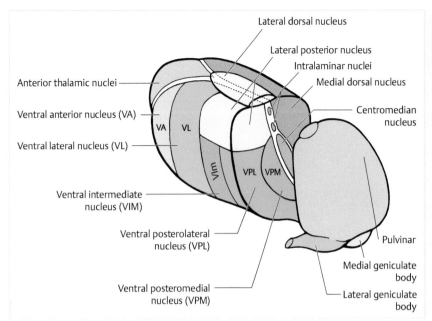

Fig. 17.8 A significant amount of output from the basal ganglia is facilitated from the thalamus. (Reproduced with permission from Baehr M, Frotscher M. Duus' Topical Diagnosis in Neurology. Fourth Edition. © Thieme 2005.)

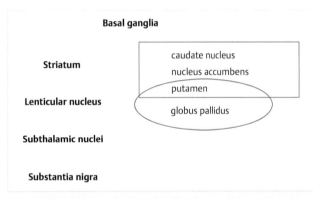

Fig. 17.9 Components of the basal ganglia.

- **Globus pallidus**
- **Nucleus accumbens**
○ **Striatum/neostriatum**
    - Caudate and putamen
○ **Lentiform/lenticular nucleus**
    - Putamen and globus pallidus
○ The subthalamic nucleus is part of the diencephalon.
    - Located inferior to the thalamus.
○ The substantia nigra is found in the midbrain.
    - Plays a significant role in dopaminergic pathways to the striatum.
    - Loss of dopamine secreting neurons in this area results in Parkinson's disease.
- The largest source of afferent fibers to the basal ganglia comes from the cerebral cortex (▶ Fig. 17.10). Afferents from the thalamus also project to the basal ganglia.
○ Cortical input includes motor, sensory, association, and limbic regions.
○ Striatum receives most of the afferents.

Table 17.2 Organization of the basal ganglia

Striatum	Caudate nucleus
	Nucleus accumbens
	Putamen*
Lenticular nucleus	
	Globus pallidus
Subthalamic nucleus	
Substantia nigra	

○ Projections from the cortex are directed toward specific regions of the basal ganglia.
    - The different regions of basal ganglia are arranged somatotopically, much like the motor homunculus found in the primary motor cortex.
- The majority of the output from the basal ganglia is from the globus pallidus and the substantia nigra.
○ The efferents from the basal ganglia and the substantia nigra primarily project to relay nuclei of the thalamus. The thalamic nuclei project to the cerebral cortex (▶ Fig. 17.11).
- There are a several intrinsic connections between the different components of the basal ganglia.
- There are two distinct pathways that are responsible for processing signals through the basal ganglia. These circuits have an opposite effect on the thalamic target structures.
○ **Direct pathway**: Excites thalamic neurons resulting in the excitation of cortical motor neurons (▶ Fig. 17.12a).
○ **Indirect pathway**: Excitations results in inhibition of thalamic neurons resulting in the inability to excite cortical motor neurons (▶ Fig. 17.12b).
○ Normal function of the basal ganglia involves a balance of these two pathways. Disruption of the balance results in motor dysfunction, which is characterized by movement disorders.

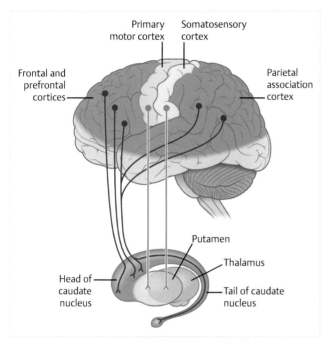

Primary motor cortex Somatosensory cortex

Frontal and prefrontal cortices

Parietal association cortex

Putamen

Thalamus

Head of caudate nucleus

Tail of caudate nucleus

Fig. 17.10 The largest source of afferents to the basal ganglia comes from the cerebral cortex.

- Damage to the basal ganglia typically causes problems with speech, movement, and posture. Collectively, these symptoms are referred to as **parkinsonism.**
  - Symptoms can vary but may include:
    - Movement changes.
    - Increased muscle tone.
    - Muscle spasms and rigidity.
    - Tremors.
    - Difficulty walking.
    - Vocal tics.

Parkinson's disease is the most common condition that causes parkinsonism. Most cases are sporadic although there are cohorts with clearly defined autosomal dominant inheritance patterns. Defining pathological feature is lack of striatal dopamine due to loss of neurons in the substantia nigra. Symptoms include: resting tremors, pill rolling tremor, bradykinesia, rigid muscles, speech changes, and impaired posture and balance. It should be noted that the disease is very heterogeneous with respect to neurochemical and behavioral variations. Treatment includes administration of dopamine or its precursors, stem cell therapy, and transplantation of embryonic dopamine secreting neurons.

Chorea is the term for wild, uncontrolled movements of the distal limbs. **Huntington's chorea** is an inherited autosomal dominant form of the disease. The offspring of patients with Huntington's disease have a 50% chance of inheriting the mutation. Those with the mutated gene will invariably inherit the disease. These patients have degenerative processes occurring in both the striatum and the cerebral cortex. This leads to progressive limb and axial chorea and dementia. In some patients, parkinsonism appears prior to the chorea.

17.4 Cerebellum

The **cerebellum** or "little brain" is a motor structure that plays a key role in movement. It receives information from motor systems and from nonmotor systems such as the **limbic** and **parietal association cortex**. It is also important to note that the cerebellum is involved in much more than movement. Damage to this area can result in language deficiencies and impaired decision-making processes.

- The cerebellum is located at the back of the brain under the occipital and temporal lobes of the cortex.
- It consists of two parts: the **cerebellar deep nuclei** (▶ Fig. 17.13a) and the **cerebellar cortex** (▶ Fig. 17.13b).
  - The deep nuclei are the sole outputs from the cerebellum.
  - The cerebellar cortex encases the deep nuclei. It contains **gyri** and **fissures** much like the cerebral cortex.
- The cerebellum can be divided into transverse and longitudinal subdivisions (▶ Fig. 17.14a, b).
  - Transverse fissures divide the cerebellum into lobes.
    - The posterolateral fissure separates the flocculonodular lobe from the corpus cerebelli (body of the cerebellum).
    - The primary fissure separates the corpus cerebelli into an anterior and a posterior lobe.
  - The cerebellum can also be divided into **longitudinal zones** that run perpendicular to the fissures.
    - The **vermis** is located along the midsagittal plane.
    - Lateral to the vermis is the **intermediate zone**.
    - The **cerebellar hemispheres** are found lateral to the intermediate zone.

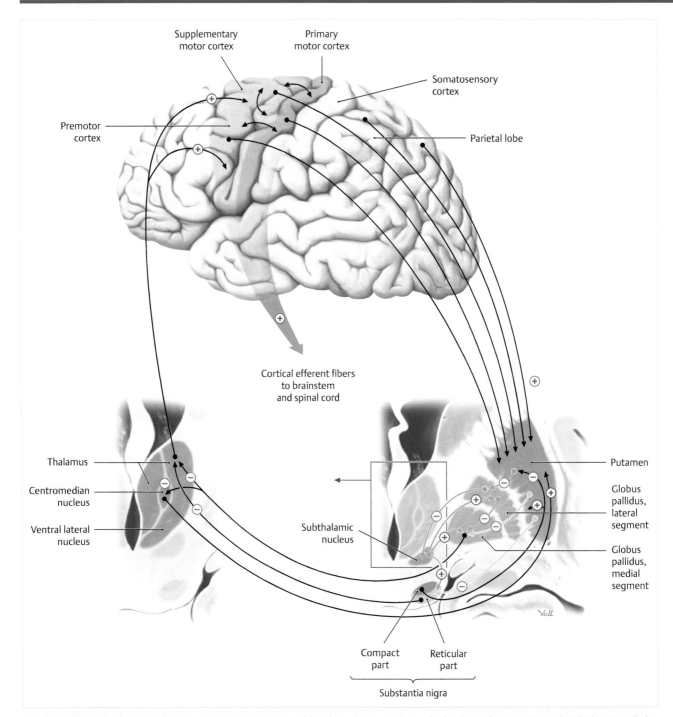

Fig. 17.11 Flow of information between motor cortical areas and basal ganglia: motor loop. The basal ganglia are concerned with the controlled, purposeful execution of fine voluntary movements. They integrate information from the cortex and subcortical regions, which they process in parallel and then return to motor cortical areas via the thalamus (feedback). Neurons from the premotor, primary motor, supplementary motor, and somatosensory cortex and from the parietal lobe send their axons to the putamen. Initially, there is a direct and indirect pathway for relaying the information out of the putamen. Both pathways ultimately lead to the motor cortex by way of the thalamus. In the direct pathway (yellow), the neurons of the putamen project to the medial globus pallidus and to the reticular part of the substantia nigra. Both nuclei then return feedback signals to the motor thalamus, which projects back to motor areas of the cortex. The indirect pathway (green) leads from the putamen through the lateral globus pallidus and subthalamic nucleus to the medial globus pallidus, which then projects to the thalamus. An alternate indirect route leads from the subthalamic nucleus to the reticular part of the substantia nigra, which in turn projects to the thalamus. (Reproduced with permission from Schuenke M, Schulte E, Schumacher U. THIEME Atlas of Anatomy Second Edition, Vol 3. © Thieme 2016. Illustrations by Markus Voll and Karl Wesker.)

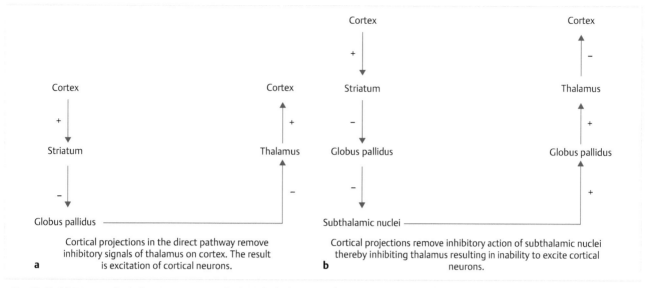

Fig. 17.12 (a) Direct pathway for processing signals through the basal ganglia (excitatory). (b) The indirect pathway of signals to the basal ganglia (inhibitory).

- The cerebellum is attached to the brainstem by three **peduncles** (▶ Fig. 17.15).
  - **Inferior cerebellar peduncle**
    - Composed mainly of afferents to the cerebellum from the spinal cord and brainstem.
  - **Middle cerebellar peduncle**
    - Composed of afferents from the pontine nuclei.
  - **Superior cerebellar peduncle**
    - Composed of efferents from the cerebellum to the red nucleus and the thalamus.
- The functions of the cerebellum include:
  - Maintenance of balance and posture.
  - Coordination of voluntary movements.
  - Motor learning.
  - Cognitive function (Clinical Correlation Box 17.3, 17.4, and 17.5).

Clinical Correlation Box 17.3: Nystagmus

Nystagmus is a condition where the eye makes repetitive, uncontrolled movements. The movement can result in decreased vision and depth perception. The involuntary movements can be up/down or side-to-side or even circular pattern. Nystagmus is typically indicative of a medical condition. Although there are numerous pathologies that can cause this condition, it is commonly associated with cerebellar dysfunction. The characteristics of the nystagmus can indicate the location of the lesion and potential etiology. For example, **upbeat nystagmus**, which is fast beating in an upward direction, is associated with an anterior vermis (cerebellum) lesion. **Horizontal nystagmus** is commonly found in unilateral disease of the cerebral hemispheres. These patients demonstrate a constant drift of the eyes toward the intact cerebellar hemisphere and fast **saccade** (rapid movement) toward the affected hemisphere.

Clinical Correlation Box 17.4: Ataxia

Ataxia is defined as the loss of muscle control or coordination of movement. Ataxia is a symptom of an underlying condition. It can develop over time or come on quite suddenly depending on the etiology. Causes include damage to the cerebellum, trauma, stroke, infections, and autoimmune and hereditary diseases. Drug and alcohol intoxication along with heavy metal poisoning can also induce ataxia. If the ataxia is due to a toxic reaction, it may be reversible. Symptoms include: poor coordination, unsteady walk, difficulty with motor skills, problems with speech, nystagmus, and difficulty swallowing. There is no treatment for the ataxia other than treating the underlying disease that is producing it. If it is due to an infection such as chicken pox or other viruses, it may very likely resolve on its own.

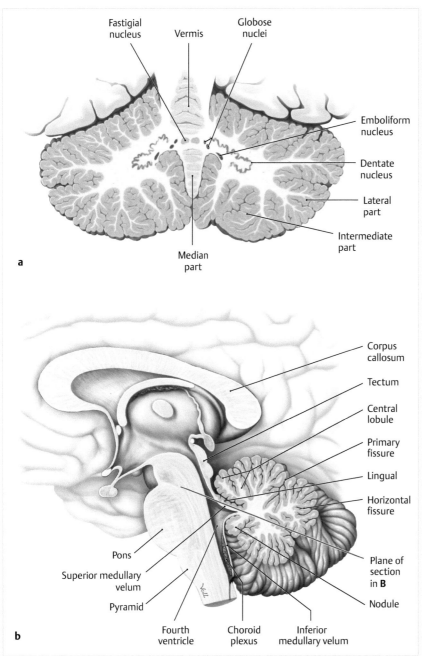

Fig. 17.13 **(a)** Nuclei of the cerebellum. Section through the superior cerebellar peduncles. Deep within the cerebellar white matter are four pairs of nuclei that contain most of the efferent neurons of the cerebellum. **(b)** Cerebellum: Positional relationship and cut surface. Midsagittal section, left lateral view. The cerebellum extends along almost the entire dorsal surface of the brainstem and abuts the tectum of the mesencephalon in the rostral direction and the medulla oblongata in the caudal direction. (Reproduced with permission from Schuenke M, Schulte E, Schumacher U. THIEME Atlas of Anatomy Second Edition, Vol 3. © Thieme 2016. Illustrations by Markus Voll and Karl Wesker.)

Clinical Correlation Box 17.5: Ataxic Dysarthria

Ataxic dysarthria is caused by a lesion in the cerebellum or disruption of its pathways. Phonation is "jerky" and syllables are often separated from one another. Speech tends to be explosive. Although not well understood, it is thought that the problem lies in abnormal speech motor programming in addition to speech execution deficits. Recent research has implicated the speech **feedforward** system of the cerebellum, which uses sensory information prior to planned movement, as at least part of the pathology.

- The cerebellar cortex receives input from multiple sources that are concerned with the regulation of motor function as well as sensory information (▶ Table 17.3). This information is concerned with the status of individual muscles and groups of muscles and sensory information from cutaneous afferents. There are multiple sources of input including:
  - **Dorsal spinocerebellar tract (DSCT)** (▶ Fig. 17.16a, b)
    - Conveys information largely from Golgi tendon organs and muscle spindles regarding the status of individual muscles from the lower limbs.
    - This pathway involves afferent fibers from lower limbs passing into the spinal cord, synapsing on **Clarke's nucleus** and then ascending in the **lateral funiculus** of the spinal cord.

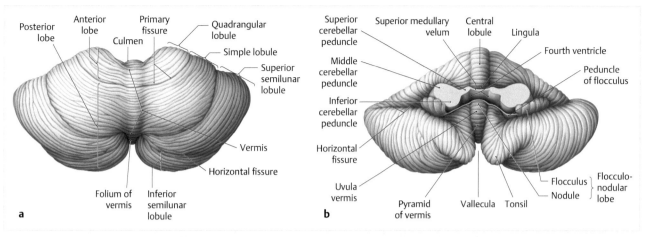

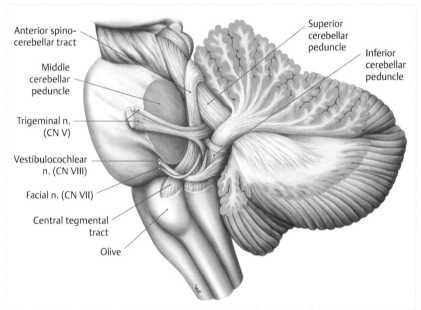

Fig. 17.14 (a) The cerebellum can be divided anatomically into transverse and longitudinal subdivisions. **(b)** Anterior view of the cerebellum. (Reproduced with permission from Schuenke M, Schulte E, Schumacher U. THIEME Atlas of Anatomy Third Edition, Vol 3. © Thieme 2020. Illustrations by Markus Voll and Karl Wesker.)

Fig. 17.15 Cerebellar peduncles. Left lateral view. The substantial mass of the peduncles reflects the extensive neural connections they carry. The cerebellum requires these numerous connections because it is the integrating center for the control of fine movements. It contains and processes vestibular and proprioceptive afferents and modulates motor nuclei in other brain regions and in the spinal cord. (Reproduced with permission from Schuenke M, Schulte E, Schumacher U. THIEME Atlas of Anatomy Third Edition, Vol 3. © Thieme 2020. Illustrations by Markus Voll and Karl Wesker.)

Table 17.3 Sensory input to the cerebellum

Cerebellar Inputs	Information
Dorsal spinocerebellar tract	Golgi tendon organs and muscle spindles from lower extremity
Ventral spinocerebellar tract	Proprioceptive and cutaneous information from leg and trunk
Cuneospinocerebellar tract	Golgi tendon organs and muscle spindles from upper extremity
Brainstem	Motor, sensory, and proprioception
Vestibular system	From inner ear regarding movement and head position

– At the level of medulla, the DSCT travels through the inferior cerebellar peduncle to reach the ipsilateral cerebellum.
  ○ **Ventral spinocerebellar tract (VSCT)** (▶ Fig. 17.16a, b)

– Carries proprioceptive and cutaneous information from the lower body (leg and trunk). This pathway detects whole limb movement.
– The VSCT originates from **spinal border cells** located on the periphery of the ventral horn of the spinal cord. The axons of second order neurons ascend in the **ventral funiculus** to the medulla. From there, the pathway enters the rostral pons and exits the brainstem via the superior cerebellar peduncle. Due to two separate points of decussation, the pathway terminates in the ipsilateral cerebellum.
  ○ **Cuneocerebellar tract** (▶ Fig. 17.17)
– Clarke's nucleus does not exist above C8. Therefore, the dorsal spinocerebellar tract cannot convey information for the upper limb. In its place, the cuneocerebellar tract carries muscle tension and stretch information from the upper limbs.

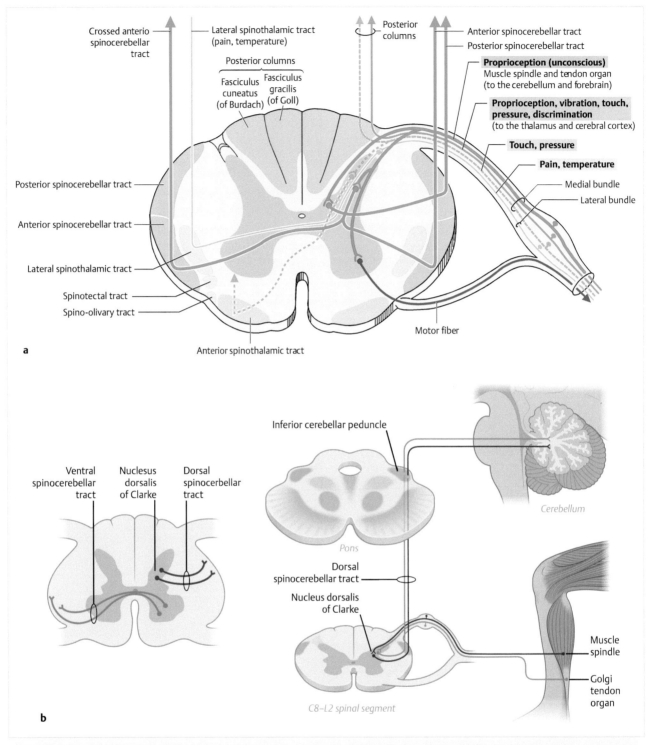

Fig. 17.16 **(a)** Cerebellar input is received from the dorsal spinocerebellar tract and the ventral spinocerebellar tract. **(b)** The dorsal spinocerebellar tract involves afferent fibers from lower limbs passing into the spinal cord. After synapsing on Clarke's nucleus, these fibers ascend in the lateral funiculus. (Fig. 17.16a: Reproduced with permission from Baehr M, Frotscher M. Duus' Topical Diagnosis in Neurology. 4th edition. © Thieme 2005.)

– Afferent fibers from muscle spindles and Golgi tendon organs join the **fasciculus cuneatus** and ascend to the cervical spinal cord, ultimately terminating in the **nucleus cuneatus**. Axons from second order neurons exit the brainstem through the inferior cerebellar peduncle to reach the ipsilateral cerebellum.

○ Brainstem
– In addition to the sensory pathways previously mentioned, a number of brainstem nuclei provide input to the cerebellum (▶ Fig. 17.18).
▪ **Inferior olivary nucleus:** Receives input from both the cortex and the spinal cord.

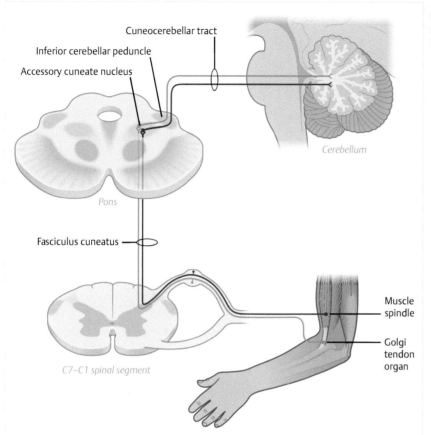

Cuneocerebellar tract

Inferior cerebellar peduncle

Accessory cuneate nucleus

Cerebellum

Pons

Fasciculus cuneatus

C7–C1 spinal segment

Muscle spindle

Golgi tendon organ

Fig. 17.17 The cuneocerebellar tract carries muscle tension and stretch information from the upper limbs.

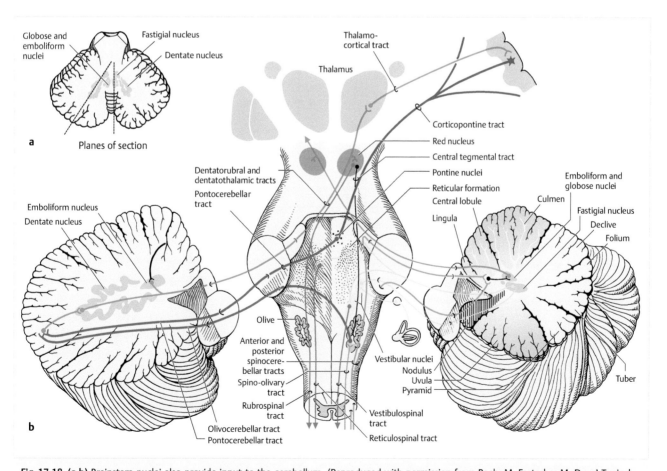

Globose and emboliform nuclei

Fastigial nucleus

Dentate nucleus

Thalamo-cortical tract

Thalamus

a

Planes of section

Dentatorubral and dentatothalamic tracts

Pontocerebellar tract

Emboliform nucleus

Dentate nucleus

Corticopontine tract

Red nucleus

Central tegmental tract

Pontine nuclei

Reticular formation

Central lobule

Lingula

Emboliform and globose nuclei

Culmen

Fastigial nucleus

Declive

Folium

Olive

Anterior and posterior spinocerebellar tracts

Spino-olivary tract

Rubrospinal tract

Olivocerebellar tract

Pontocerebellar tract

Vestibular nuclei

Nodulus

Uvula

Pyramid

Vestibulospinal tract

Reticulospinal tract

Tuber

b

Fig. 17.18 (a,b) Brainstem nuclei also provide input to the cerebellum. (Reproduced with permission from Baehr M, Frotscher M. Duus' Topical Diagnosis in Neurology. Fourth Edition. © Thieme 2005.)

- Inputs from the spinal cord provide information regarding cutaneous and joint afferents as well as stretch from the muscle spindles.
- Input from the cortex includes motor and sensory. Fibers from the inferior olivary nucleus terminate as **climbing fibers** on Purkinje cells.
  - **Vestibular system**

- The vestibular nerve (CN VIII) receives information from the inner ear regarding movement and head position. It relays this information directly to the vestibulocerebellum or flocculolobural lobe or indirectly via the vestibular nuclei (▸ Fig. 17.19).
- CN VIII sends afferents to the cerebellum through the inferior cerebellar peduncle.

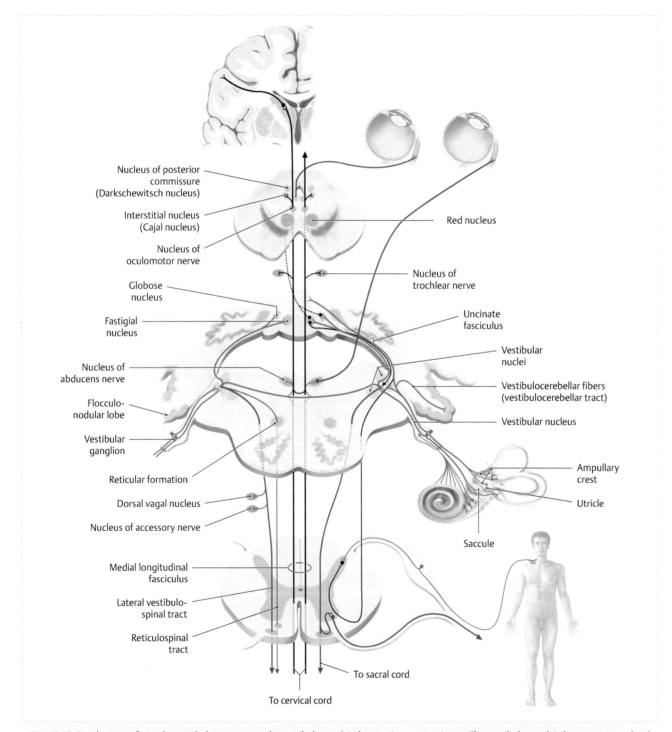

Fig. 17.19 Besides input from the vestibular apparatus, the vestibular nuclei also receive sensory input. The vestibular nuclei show a topographical organization and distribute their efferent fibers to three targets. (1) Motor neurons in the spinal cord via the lateral vestibulospinal tract. These motor neurons help to maintain upright stance, mainly by increasing the tone of extensor muscles. (2) Flocculonodular lobe of the cerebellum (direct sensory input to the cerebellum) via vestibulocerebellar fibers. (3) Ipsilateral and contralateral oculomotor nuclei via the ascending part of the medial longitudinal fasciculus. (Reproduced with permission from Schuenke M, Schulte E, Schumacher U. THIEME Atlas of Anatomy Second Edition, Vol 3. © Thieme 2016. Illustrations by Markus Voll and Karl Wesker.)

□ All afferents from the vestibular nerve terminate as **mossy fibers** on the flocculolobular lobe.
- All outputs from the cerebellum originate from the deep cerebellar nuclei.
  ○ **Fastigial nucleus**
    – Receives input from the vermis and from afferents carrying vestibular, sensory, auditory, and visual information.
  ○ **Interposed nucleus**
    – Receives information from intermediate zone and from afferents carrying spinal, sensory, auditory, and visual information.
  ○ **Dentate nucleus**
    – Receives information from the cerebellar hemispheres and afferents carrying information from the cortex. It projects to the red nucleus and thalamic nuclei.
- Damage to the cerebellum produces movement disorders.
  ○ **Decomposition of movement**
    – Lack of coordinated, smooth movements.
    – Movements broken down into individual component parts.
  ○ **Intention tremors**
    – Involuntary tremor induced by intentional movement toward a target.
  ○ **Dysdiadochokinesia**
    – Difficulty performing rapid, alternating movements.
  ○ **Motor learning problems**
    – Motor learning is the ability to perform movement based on practice or a novel experience. It is necessary for complex movements as well as refining reflex movement. Individuals with deficits have difficulties recalling complex and planned motor activity.

Questions and Answers

1. Which of the following statements is TRUE regarding the reticulospinal tract?
   a) The tract originates in the red nucleus
   b) The tract exits at the spinal cord only at the cervical level
   c) The reticulospinal tracts act as an alternative to the corticospinal tract for motor control.
   d) Pathway is composed of a single tract

Level 1: Easy
Answer C: The reticulospinal tract allows cortical neurons to control motor function via projections from the reticular formation; **(A)** the tract originates in the reticular formation; **(B)** Bothe tracts exit at all spinal levels and **(D)** The pathway is composed of two tracts.
2. A patient with ataxia and resting tremors comes into the ER. Based on these symptoms, what would you suspect might be the issue?
   a) Corticospinal lesion
   b) Basal ganglia lesion
   c) Cerebellar lesion
   d) Flocculonodular lesion

Level 2: Moderate
Answer B: Resting tremors and difficulty walking are hallmark symptoms of BG disease/parkinsonism; **(A)** Corticospinal tract lesion is not associated with tremors or ataxia; **(C)** Cerebellar lesions are associated with ataxia but would display intention tremors and **(D)** Flocculonodular lesion would be the same as a cerebellar lesion.
3. Patient A is experiencing nystagmus, ataxia and intention tremors. Which of the following structures are most likely involved in the patients disorder?
   a) Thalamus
   b) Spinal cord
   c) Basal ganglia
   d) Cerebellum

Level 2: Moderate
Answer D: Cerebellum; **(A)** while thalamic lesions could create cerebellar-like sensory deficits, there would also be sensory issues as well; **(B)** these symptoms are not characteristic of motor tract lesions in spinal cord. **(C)** basal ganglia lesions would not produce nystagmus or intention tremors.
4. Patient B presents with ataxia, uncontrolled movement of the upper limbs and rigidity. During the history & physical, the patient states that his father had similar issues and also suffered from early onset dementia. Patient B also admitted to being a recovering alcoholic. Which of the following diseases do you suspect may be the issue?
   a) Parkinson's disease
   b) Ataxia due to a stroke
   c) Huntington's chorea
   d) Alcoholic induced cerebellar disease

Level 3: Difficult
Answer C: Huntington's chorea is an autosomal dominant disease that presents with symptoms stated in question, especially chorea and family history; **(A)** Individuals with Parkinson's can present with the symptoms stated above; however, the jerky, uncontrolled movements (chorea) are typical of Huntington's and **(D)** Alcohol induced cerebellar disease would have typical cerebellar symptoms which does not include resting tremors or genetic patterns.
5. Which of the following tracts is responsible for coordination of head and eye muscles?
   a) Medial vestibulospinal tract
   b) Lateral vestibulospinal tract
   c) Dorsal spinocerebellar tract
   d) Ventral spinocerebellar tract

Level 1: Medium
Answer A: Medial vestibulospinal tract; **(B)** Lateral vestibulospinal tract travels to cervical, thoracic and lumbar areas; **(C)** Dorsal spinocerebellar tract carries sensory information from the lower limbs **(D)** Ventral spinocerebellar tract carries sensory information from the lower limb and trunk.

18 Integrated Systems

18.1 Autonomic Nervous System (ANS)

18.1.1 Overview

The function of the **autonomic nervous system** (**ANS**) is to maintain homeostasis. It controls several systems such as digestion, respiration, cardiac activity, and exocrine glands among others. The ANS controls are exerted on targeted tissue and cells. The targets of the ANS are: cardiac tissue, smooth muscle, and exocrine glands. This system is made up of visceral motor (general visceral efferent [GVE]) components that operate automatically.

18.1.2 Organization of the ANS

The ANS is divided into three major divisions: the **parasympathetic**, **sympathetic**, and **enteric** nervous system. The enteric system provides the intrinsic innervation for the gastrointestinal tract and mediates reflex peristaltic activity. Due to the unique and specific function of the enteric system, which is independent of the hypothalamus, that particular division will not be included in further discussions in this chapter.

- Both the parasympathetic and sympathetic arms of the ANS involve a two-neuron chain (▶ Fig. 18.1).
  - The first order neuron of the chain is called a **preganglionic** neuron.
    - Its cell body is located within the central nervous system (CNS).
    - Its axon is **myelinated**.
  - The preganglionic axon terminates on the **second-order neuron**.
    - The second order neuron is called a **postganglionic** neuron.
    - Its cell body is located in a peripheral **ganglion**.
    - Its axon is **unmyelinated**.
  - The ANS carries **GVE** fibers that control **visceral motor neurons**.
- Although the divisions are often considered as antagonistic, there are some situations where they work in concert or independently. For example, arrector pili muscles, which are associated with hair follicles in mammals, are solely innervated by sympathetic fibers. Conversely, reproduction requires both sympathetic (ejaculation) and parasympathetic (erection) activity.

18.1.3 Sympathetic Division

- The function of the sympathetic system is to prepare the body for increased activity. It is commonly referred to as the

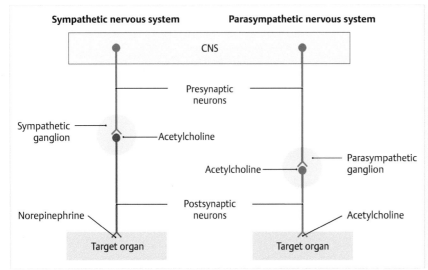

Fig. 18.1 Circuit diagram of the autonomic nervous system. The central first (presynaptic) neuron uses acetylcholine as a transmitter in both the sympathetic and parasympathetic nervous systems neuron. Acetylcholine is also used as a neurotransmitter by the second (postsynaptic) neuron in the parasympathetic nervous system. In the sympathetic nervous system, norepinephrine is used by the noradrenergic neuron. Note: The target cell membrane contains different types of receptors (= transmitter sensors) for acetylcholine and norepinephrine. Each transmitter can produce entirely different effects, depending on the type of receptor. (Reproduced with permission from Schuenke M, Schulte E, Schumacher U. THIEME Atlas of Anatomy. Second Edition, Vol 3. © Thieme 2016. Illustrations by Markus Voll and Karl Wesker.)

Table 18.1 Synopsis of the sympathetic and parasympathetic nervous systems

Organ	Sympathetic Nervous System	Parasympathetic Nervous System
Eye	Pupillary dilation	Pupillary constriction and increased curvature of the lens
Salivary glands	Decreased salivation (scant, viscous)	Increased salivation (copious, watery)
Heart	Increased heart rate	Decreased heart rate
Lungs	Decreased bronchial secretions and bronchodilation	Increased bronchial secretions and bronchodilation
Gastrointestinal tract	Decrease in secretions and motility	Increase in secretions and motility
Pancreas	Decreased exocrine secretions	Increased exocrine secretions
Male sex organs	Ejaculation	Erection
Skin	Vasoconstriction, sweating, piloerection	No effect

(Reproduced with permission from Schuenke. Atlas of Anatomy. Vol. 3, 2nd ed. Thieme; 2017, Table 10.287C.)

Table 18.2 Peripheral sympathetic nervous system

Origin of Preganglionic Fibers*	Ganglion Cells	Course of Postganglionic Fibers	Target
Spinal cord	Sympathetic trunk	Follow intercostal nerves	Blood vessels and glands in chest wall
		Accompany intrathoracic arteries	Visceral targets
		Gather in greater and lesser splanchnic nerves	Abdomen

*The axons of preganglionic neurons exit the spinal cord via the anterior roots and synapse with postganglionic neurons in the sympathetic ganglia.
(Reproduced with permission from Gilroy AM. Atlas of Anatomy. Third Edition. Thieme; 2017, Table 8.4.)

"**fight or flight response.**" Activation of this division will increase heart rate, decrease digestion, and dilate pupils (▶ Table 18.1).

- The sympathetic division of the ANS originates in the **intermediolateral cell column** (**IML**) of the spinal cord (▶ Fig. 18.2a, b).
  - The IML is present in the lateral horn gray matter in vertebral levels T2–L1 (▶ Table 18.2).
    - Due to its range of vertebral levels, the sympathetic arm is also called the **thoracolumbar division** of the ANS (▶ Fig. 18.3a, b).
  - Preganglionic neurons for the head and neck are located in the IML from T1 to T4.
- Sympathetic ganglia house the second order neurons, also known as the postganglionic neuron.
  - The thoracic sympathetic ganglia are described as **paravertebral**. That is, there are two interconnected "**sympathetic chains/trunks**" that run vertically on either side of the vertebral column (▶ Fig. 18.4).
  - In the abdomen and pelvis, sympathetic ganglia lie anterior to the abdominal aorta and are called **prevertebral ganglia**.
- The **superior, middle, and inferior cervical ganglia** (sympathetic ganglia) are located in the head and neck (▶ Fig. 18.5).
  - The superior cervical ganglion is located in the **retrostyloid space** and lies on **longus coli** at approximately C2.
  - The middle cervical ganglion lies medial to the **vertebral artery** at vertebral level C6.
  - The inferior cervical ganglion lies at the level of C7. It often fuses with the first thoracic ganglion in which case it is referred to as the **stellate ganglion**.
  - Preganglionic neurons for the head and neck synapse in the cervical ganglia.

- Sympathetic fibers are widespread in the body.
  - Preganglionic fibers exit the spinal cord via the ventral root of the spinal nerve.
  - The preganglionic fibers enter the sympathetic chain forming **white communicating rami. White rami** are named based on the fact that they contain preganglionic **myelinated** fibers. They are only present from T1 to L2/3 (▶ Fig. 18.6a, b).
  - Some sympathetic preganglionic fibers terminate in the sympathetic chain by synapsing on second order neurons. They can synapse at the vertebral level they entered or they can ascend or descend within the sympathetic chain and synapse at a different level (▶ Fig. 18.7).
  - Postganglionic fibers (unmyelinated) rejoin spinal nerves forming **gray communicating rami**. After joining the spinal nerve, the postganglionic fibers will travel to their target structure (cardiac tissue, smooth muscle, or glands). **Gray rami** are present the entire length of the spinal cord.
  - There are some preganglionic fibers that enter the sympathetic chain via white rami and exit without synapsing such as **splanchnic nerves**. Splanchnic nerves will ultimately synapse on second order neurons that are located in prevertebral ganglia (▶ Fig. 18.8). From there, they will innervate abdominal and pelvic viscera. It should be noted that the term "*splanchnic*" denotes that the nerve innervates viscera. It does not indicate if it is sympathetic or parasympathetic or if it is pre- or postganglionic.
  - There are three groups of thoracic splanchnic nerves that exit the sympathetic chain at different levels (▶ Fig. 18.9):
    - **Greater splanchnics** (T5–T9).
    - **Lesser splanchnics** (T10 and T11).
    - **Least splanchnics** (T12).
  - The greater, lesser, and least splanchnic nerves synapse on prevertebral ganglia in the abdomen. There is significant variability in terms of the specific target ganglia; however, the following relationships are fairly consistent:
    - Greater splanchnics will terminate primarily in the **celiac and superior mesenteric ganglia**. Some fibers will travel directly to the adrenal medulla.
    - The lesser splanchnics will synapse in the **aorticorenal ganglia** or superior mesenteric ganglion.
    - The least splanchnics will terminate in the aorticorenal ganglia.

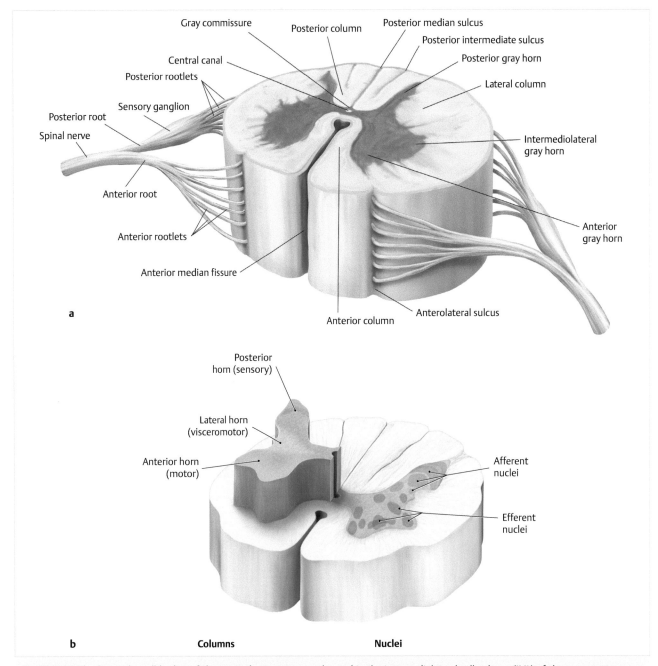

Fig. 18.2 (a) The first order cell bodies of the sympathetic system are located in the intermediolateral cell column (IML) of the gray matter. **(b)** Organization of the gray matter, left oblique anterosuperior view. The gray matter of the spinal cord is divided into three columns (horns): (A) Anterior column (horn): Contains motor neurons (B) Lateral column (horn): Contains sympathetic or parasympathetic (visceromotor) neurons in select regions (C) Posterior column (horn): Contains sensory neurons. Afferent and efferent neurons within these columns are clustered in nuclei according to function. (Reproduced with permission from Schuenke M, Schulte E, Schumacher U. THIEME Atlas of Anatomy Third Edition, Vol 3. © Thieme 2020. Illustrations by Markus Voll and Karl Wesker.)

○ **Lumbar splanchnics** arise from ganglia at vertebral levels L1–L4.
  – Lumbar splanchnics will pass into the **inferior mesenteric ganglia** or a **pelvic plexus** and synapse.
  – The postganglionic lumbar fibers will innervate the **hindgut** and pelvic viscera.

18.1.4 Parasympathetic Division

- The function of the parasympathetic system is to conserve and restore energy. It is often called the "**rest and digest response.**" Activation of this division will slow heart rate, constrict pupils, increase peristalsis, and increase glandular activity (▶ Table 18.1).

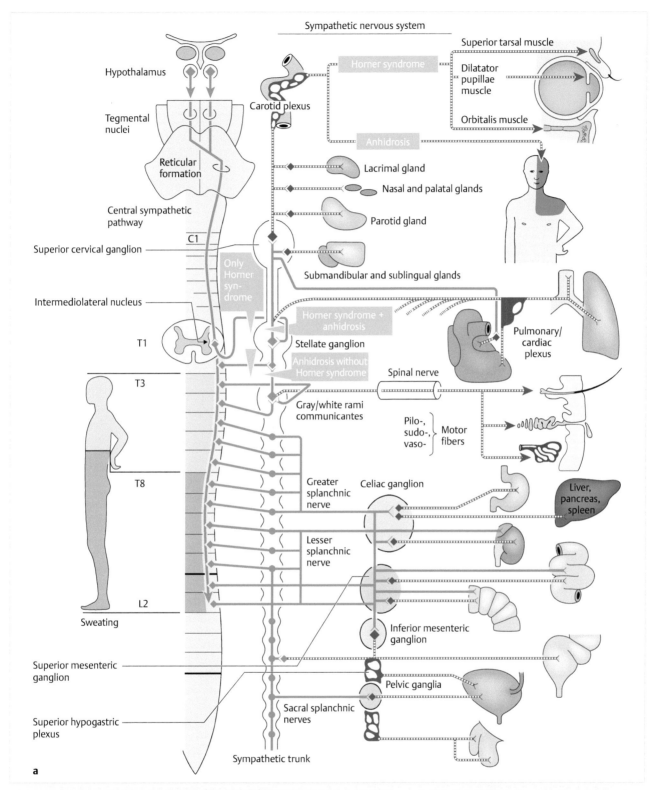

Fig. 18.3 (a) The sympathetic arm of the ANS is also called the thoracolumbar division due to the fact that the first order cell bodies are located in the spinal cord at the thoracic and lumbar levels. ANS, autonomic nervous system. (▶ Fig. 18.3a: Reproduced with permission from Mattle H, Mumenthaler M, Taub E. Fundamentals of Neurology: An Illustrated Guide. Second Edition. © Thieme 2016.

(Continued)

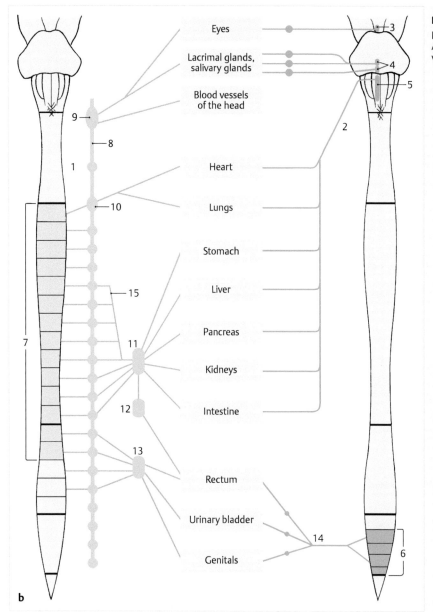

Eyes

Lacrimal glands,
salivary glands

Blood vessels
of the head

Heart

Lungs

Stomach

Liver

Pancreas

Kidneys

Intestine

Rectum

Urinary bladder

Genitals

Fig. 18.3 (*Continued*) **(b)** Reproduced with permission from Kahle W, Frotscher M.Color Atlas of Human Anatomy, Sixth Edition, Vol 3. © Thieme 2011.)

b

- The parasympathetic division originates in the brainstem for most of the body and in the sacral area (IML S2–S4) for the hindgut and pelvic structures. The parasympathetics for the hindgut and pelvic structures are called the **pelvic splanchnics** (▶ Table 18.3).
  - The efferent parasympathetic fibers travel in certain cranial nerves (CNs III, VII, IX, and X) and sacral spinal nerves (S2–S4). Due to its origin, it is sometimes called the **craniosacral division** (▶ Fig. 18.10).
  - First order neurons (preganglionic) of the parasympathetic division are located in brainstem nuclei. The parasympathetic nuclei lie in close proximity to the nuclei of the cranial nerve they travel with. It should be noted that CNs III, VII, IX, and X all have a nucleus of their own motor. The preganglionic fibers from the parasympathetic nuclei travel with cranial nerves to reach their respective ganglia (▶ Fig. 18.11) (▶ Table 18.4). The parasympathetic nuclei:cranial nerves associations are:

  - **Edinger-Westphal nucleus: CN III**
  - **Superior salivatory nucleus: CN VII**
  - **Inferior salivatory nucleus: CN IX**
  - **Dorsal motor nucleus of X: CN X**
  - Second order neurons are located in parasympathetic ganglia in the head or within the walls of the target viscera (▶ Fig. 18.12).
  - Head and neck parasympathetic ganglia are:
    - Ciliary ganglion
      □ Preganglionic fibers travel on CN III to ganglion.
      □ Postganglionic fibers project to the orbit.
      □ Targets are ciliary muscle and sphincter pupillae.
    - Pterygopalatine ganglion
      □ Preganglionic fibers travel with CN VII (greater petrosal followed by nerve of the pterygoid canal).
      □ Postganglionic fibers project to the nasal cavity, palate, paranasal sinuses, and lacrimal gland.
      □ Targets are lacrimal gland and mucous glands.

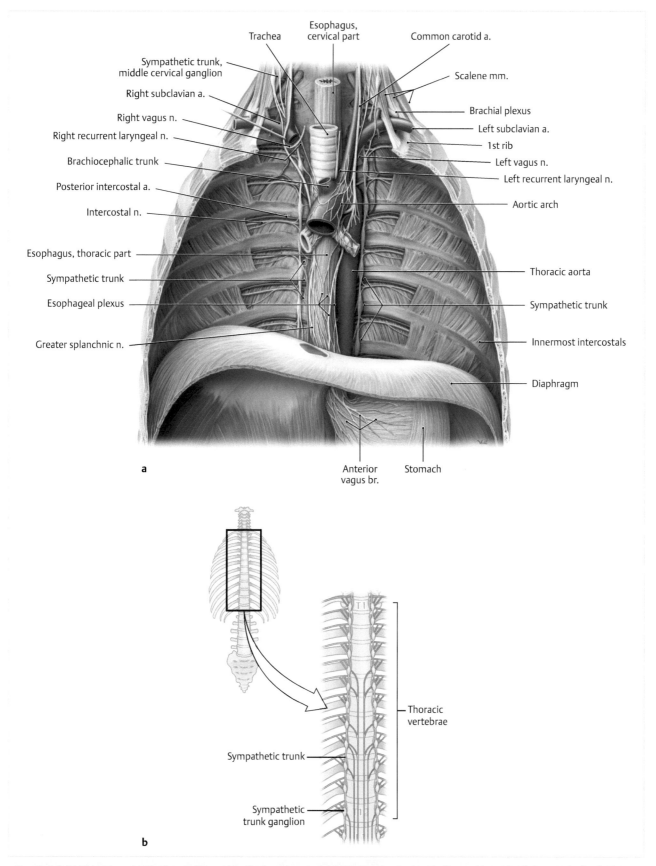

Fig. 18.4 **(a,b)** Thoracic sympathetic ganglia are described as paravertebral because they run vertically on either side of the vertebral column. Reproduced with permission from Gilroy AM, MacPherson BR. Atlas of Anatomy. Third Edition. © Thieme 2016. Illustrations by Markus Voll and Karl Wesker.

- Submandibular ganglion
  - Preganglionic fibers travel in CN VII (chorda tympani and lingual nerves).
  - Postganglionic fibers project to the submandibular and sublingual glands.
  - Target is salivary glands.
- Otic ganglion

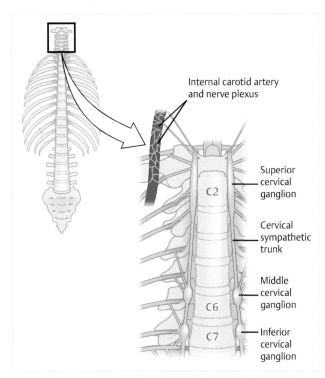

Fig. 18.5 The superior, middle, and inferior sympathetic ganglia are located in the head and neck.

- Preganglionic fibers travel with CN IX (tympanic branch and lesser petrosal).
- Postganglionic fibers project to the parotid gland.
- Target is salivary glands.

18.1.5 Neurotransmitters of the ANS

- Norepinephrine (NE) and acetylcholine (ACh) are the two most common neurotransmitters (NT) of the ANS (▶ Fig. 18.13) (▶ Table 18.5).
  - ACh is secreted by all preganglionic nerve fibers of the ANS (parasympathetic and sympathetic).
  - ACh is secreted by all postganglionic fibers of the parasympathetic division.
  - ACh is secreted by *some* postganglionic sympathetic fibers, specifically, those that innervate sweat glands.
  - NE is secreted by *most* sympathetic postganglionic fibers.
- Receptors of the ANS are classified based on the NT that they bind (cholinergic or adrenergic).
  - ACh binds **cholinergic receptors** (**nicotinic** and **muscarinic**).
    - Nicotinic receptors are found on all postganglionic cell bodies *(parasympathetic and sympathetic)*.
    - Muscarinic receptors are found in the cell membrane of target tissues. ACh, released from *all* postganglionic parasympathetic neurons and *some* sympathetic neurons that innervate sweat glands, binds these receptors.
  - NE binds adrenergic receptors (**alpha** and **beta**).

18.1.6 Autonomic Plexi

- Large collections of sympathetic and parasympathetic efferents, along with **visceral afferents**, form **autonomic nerve plexi**. Branches from these plexi innervate viscera (▶ Fig. 18.14a, b).

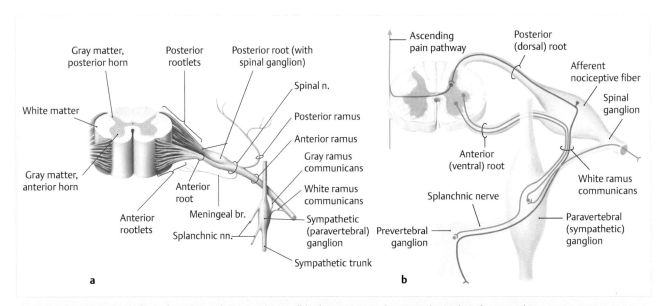

Fig. 18.6 (a) Preganglionic fibers from first order sympathetic cell bodies enter into the sympathetic chain forming white communicating rami. Postganglionic fibers rejoin spinal nerves forming gray communicating rami. (b) White rami are named based on the fact that these axons are preganglionic and therefore myelinated. (Reproduced with permission from Schuenke M, Schulte E, Schumacher U. THIEME Atlas of Anatomy Third Edition, Vol 3. © Thieme 2020. Illustrations by Markus Voll and Karl Wesker.)

- In the thorax, there are **cardiac, pulmonary,** and **esophageal plexi**.
- In the abdomen, the plexi are associated with the aorta and its major branches: **superior mesenteric, inferior mesenteric, renal,** and **superior hypogastric** (▶ Table 18.6).

- Depending on the plexus, the contributing fibers can be preganglionic, postganglionic sympathetic, or parasympathetic.

Summary of parasympathetic and sympathetic divisions of the ANS are provided in ▶ Table 18.7 and ▶ Fig. 18.15.

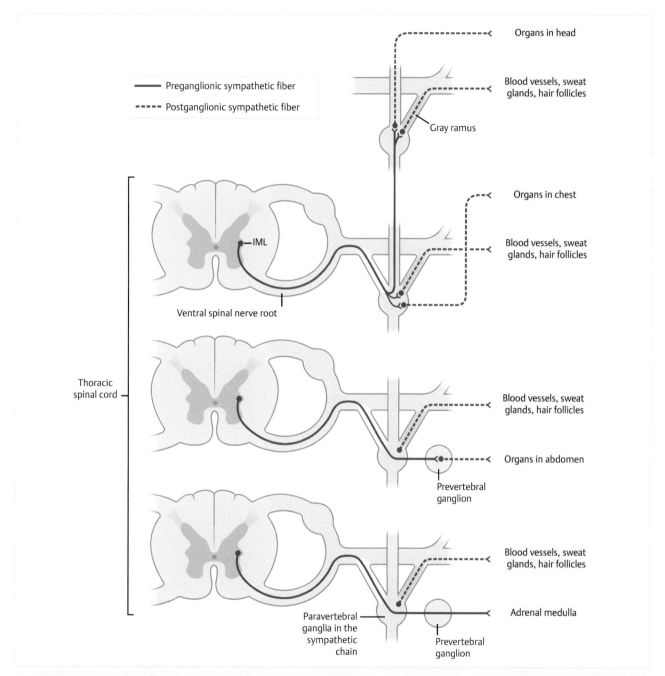

Fig. 18.7 Some preganglionic fibers terminate immediately in the sympathetic chain while others ascend or descend and synapse at a different level.

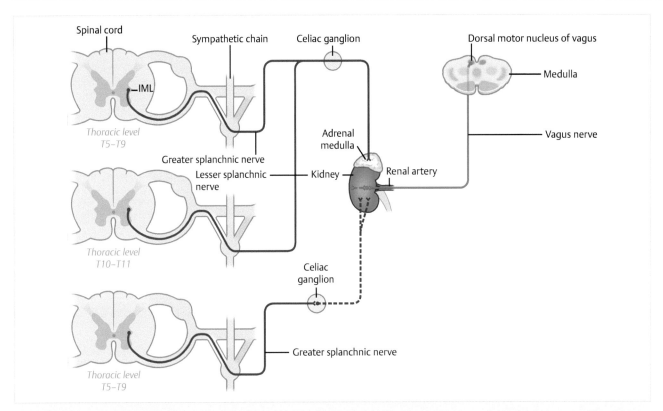

Fig. 18.8 Some preganglionic fibers enter the sympathetic chain via white rami and exit without synapsing such as splanchnic nerves. These nerves innervate abdominal and pelvic viscera.

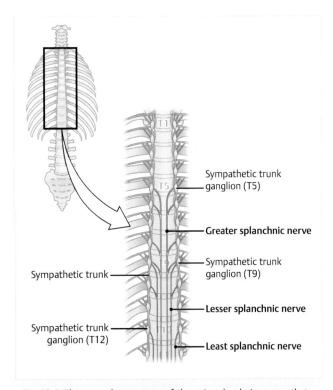

Fig. 18.9 There are three groups of thoracic splanchnic nerves that exit the sympathetic chain at different levels. They are named: greater, lesser, and least splanchnics.

Clinical Correlation Box 18.1: Horner Syndrome

Horner syndrome can be congenital or acquired. The acquired form is caused by an interruption of sympathetic innervation in the head and neck. It can be caused by damage to pre- or postganglionic neurons in the pathway, stroke, tumors, carotid artery disorder, or middle cranial fossa neoplasms. It is fairly uncommon with no gender, racial, or age associations. It is characterized by **ptosis**, pupil constriction (**miosis**), slight elevation of the lower eyelid, and little to no sweating (**anhidrosis**) on the affected side. The ptosis and elevation of the lower eyelid is due to denervation of the superior and inferior tarsal muscles, respectively. The miosis is the result of denervation of the dilator pupillae and anhidrosis is due to the lack of innervation of sweat glands. Vasodilation of the skin arterioles may also occur resulting in flushing of the skin. Treatment is dependent on the underlying cause.

Table 18.3 Peripheral parasympathetic nervous system

Origin of Preganglionic Fibers	Course of Preganglionic Motor Axons*		Target
Brainstem	Vagus nerve (CN X)	Cardiac branches	Cardiac plexus
		Esophageal branches	Esophageal plexus
		Tracheal branches	Trachea
		Bronchial branches	Pulmonary plexus (bronchi, pulmonary vessels)

*The ganglion cells of the parasympathetic nervous system are scattered in microscopic groups in their target organs. The vagus nerve thus carries the preganglionic motor axons to these targets. CN, cranial nerve.
(Reproduced with permission from Gilroy AM. Atlas of Anatomy. Third Edition. Thieme; 2017, Table 8.5.)

Table 18.4 Parasympathetic ganglia in the head

Nucleus	Path of Presynaptic Fibers	Ganglion	Postsynaptic Fibers	Target Organs
Visceral oculomotor (Edinger-Westphal) nucleus	Oculomotor nerve	Ciliary ganglion	Short ciliary nerves	Ciliary muscle (accommodation)
Superior salivatory nucleus	Nervus intermedius (facial nerve root) divides into:		Maxillary nerve → zygomatic nerve → anastomosis → lacrimal nerve	Lacrimal gland
	1. Greater petrosal nerve → nerve of pterygoid canal	Pterygopalatine ganglion	• Orbital branches • Lateral posterior nasal branches • Nasopalatine nerve • Palatine nerves	Glands on: • Posterior ethmoid cells • Nasal conchae • Anterior palate • Hard and soft palate
	2. Chorda tympani →lingual nerve	Submandibular ganglion	Glandular branches	-Submandibular gland -Sublingual gland
Inferior salivatory nucleus	Glossopharyngeal nerve →tympanic nerve →lesser petrosal nerve	Otic ganglion	Auriculotemporal nerve (CN V3)	Parotid gland
Dorsal vagal nucleus	Vagus nerve	Ganglia near organs	Fine fibers in organs, not individually named	Thoracic and abdominal viscera

→ = is continuous with
(Reproduced with permission from Schuenke. Atlas of Anatomy. Second Edition, Vol. 3. Thieme; 2017, Table 10.290B.)

Table 18.5 Summary of neurotransmitters and receptors of the autonomic system

	Parasympathetic	Sympathetic
Preganglionic NT	ACh	ACh
Postganglionic NT	ACh	Mostly NE *Some* ACh (certain blood vessels and sweat glands)
Preganglionic receptor	Nicotinic	Nicotinic
Postganglionic receptor	Muscarinic	Adrenergic (alpha or beta)

Abbreviations: ACh, acetylcholine; NE, norepinephrine; NT, neurotransmitters.

Clinical Correlation Box 18.2: Raynaud's Disease

Raynaud's disease is a disorder that causes extremities (usually fingers and toes) to change color and feel cold and numb. The phenomenon is caused by abnormal constriction of blood vessels and can occur as the primary condition (idiopathic) or secondary to other diseases. The exact etiology is unclear but it is thought to be the result of an exaggerated sympathetic response in the vascular system to triggers such as cold, stress, medications, and other diseases.

Clinical Correlation Box 18.3: Hirschsprung Disease

Hirschsprung disease is a congenital condition characterized by the absence of the **myenteric** and **submucosal plexi** in the distal portion of the colon. The affected bowel has no parasympathetic ganglia present resulting in the inability to relax. As a result, peristalsis is absent and fecal material is not passed. The proximal colon can become massively distended. Complications include perforation, intestinal obstruction, and enterocolitis. Treatment is typically surgery to reroute unaffected large bowel to anus.

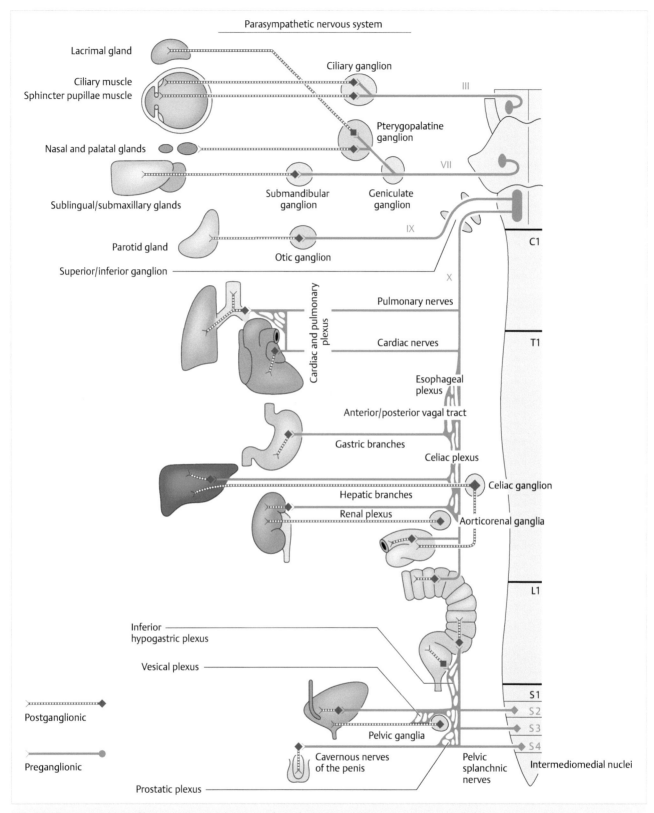

Fig. 18.10 Parasympathetic fibers travel in cranial nerves and sacral spinal nerve. Thus, it is sometimes called the craniosacral division. (Reproduced with permission from Mattle H, Mumenthaler M, Taub E. Fundamentals of Neurology: An Illustrated Guide. Second Edition. © Thieme 2016.

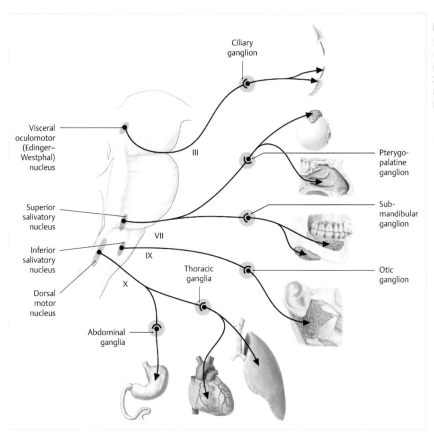

Fig. 18.11 Preganglionic fibers from parasympathetic nuclei travel in cranial nerve to reach their respective ganglia. (Reproduced with permission from Schuenke M, Schulte E, Schumacher U. THIEME Atlas of Anatomy Third Edition, Vol 3. © Thieme 2020. Illustrations by Markus Voll and Karl Wesker.)

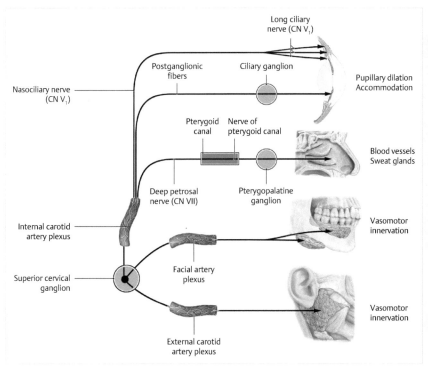

Fig. 18.12 Second-order neurons are located in parasympathetic ganglia of the head or within the walls of the target viscera. (Reproduced with permission from Schuenke M, Schulte E, Schumacher U. THIEME Atlas of Anatomy Third Edition, Vol 3. © Thieme 2020. Illustrations by Markus Voll and Karl Wesker.)

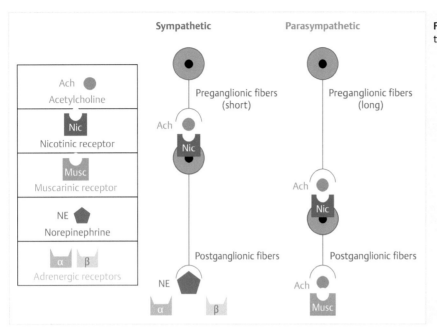

Fig. 18.13 Neurotransmitters and receptors of the ANS. ANS, autonomic nervous system.

18.2 Hypothalamus

18.2.1 Overview

The **hypothalamus** is part of the diencephalon and lies ventral to the thalamus. It mediates endocrine, autonomic, and behavioral activity. It is key in maintaining organ function and producing many of the activities necessary to survival, such as eating, drinking, and reproducing. The hypothalamus facilitates these activities by controlling hormone production as well as the ANS. It is the epicenter for many converging and diverging neural pathways. It is also highly vascularized which is key for hormonal communication.

18.2.2 Anatomy

- The hypothalamus is composed of nuclei. There is significant overlap between the groups (▶ Fig. 18.17a, b).
- These nuclei are organized into zones (▶ Table 18.8).
  - **Periventricular zone**
    - Borders the third ventricle.
    - Important in regulating the release of endocrine hormones from the anterior pituitary gland.
  - **Middle zone**
    - Contains nuclei that regulate the release of **vasopressin** and **oxytocin.**
    - Contains neurons important for regulating the ANS.
    - **Circadian rhythms** are also driven by neurons in this zone.
  - **Lateral zone**
    - Important in emotions.
- The hypothalamus can also be divided in an anterior-posterior orientation.
  - **Anterior region** is the area directly above the optic chiasm.
  - The **tuberal region** is the part that includes the **tuber cinereum.**

- Tuber cinereum is area of the hypothalamus bounded by the **optic chiasm**, **optic tract,** and the posterior edge of the **mammillary bodies**.
- The **posterior region** is the area above and including the mammillary bodies.
- Perforating branches from the **circle of Willis** provide the blood supply to the hypothalamus (▶ Fig. 18.16).
  - The **infundibular stalk** of the pituitary is located approximately in the middle of the circle of Willis.
  - The **arterial circle** surrounds the entire inferior surface of the hypothalamus.

18.2.3 Neural Connections

- Hypothalamic inputs mainly come from the **limbic system** (forebrain), brainstem, and spinal cord.
  - Afferents from the brainstem and spinal cord relay visceral and somatic sensory information.
  - Afferents from the limbic system convey information that the hypothalamus needs to mediate the autonomic and somatic aspects of homeostasis.
  - In addition to **septal nuclei** of the limbic system, major forebrain afferents come from the **hippocampus, amygdala**, **insula**, **orbitofrontal cortex**, other cortical areas, and the **retina**.
- In general, hypothalamic outputs are similar to the inputs. In addition, the hypothalamus controls both the anterior and posterior lobes of the pituitary gland.
  - Other major outputs include descending fibers to the brainstem and spinal cord that influence the ANS and the **mammillothalamic tract**. The function of the mammillothalamic tract is unclear but lesions in this structure are associated with memory and seizure disorders.

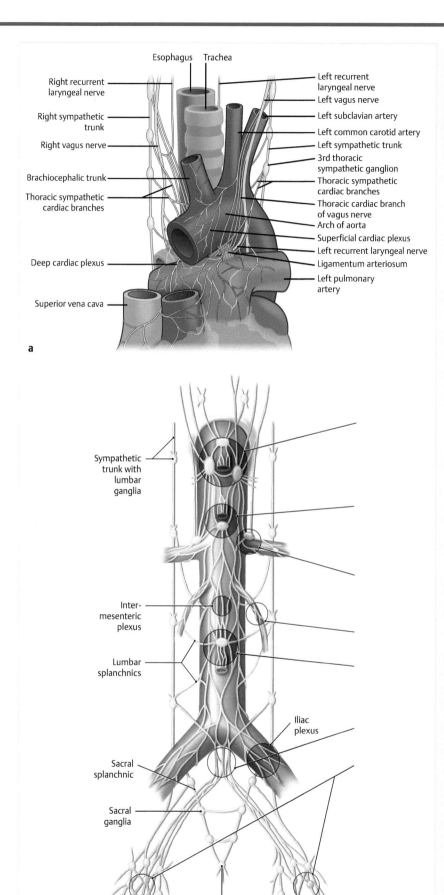

Esophagus
Trachea

Right recurrent laryngeal nerve

Right sympathetic trunk

Right vagus nerve

Brachiocephalic trunk

Thoracic sympathetic cardiac branches

Deep cardiac plexus

Superior vena cava

Left recurrent laryngeal nerve
Left vagus nerve
Left subclavian artery
Left common carotid artery
Left sympathetic trunk
3rd thoracic sympathetic ganglion
Thoracic sympathetic cardiac branches
Thoracic cardiac branch of vagus nerve
Arch of aorta
Superficial cardiac plexus
Left recurrent laryngeal nerve
Ligamentum arteriosum
Left pulmonary artery

a

Sympathetic trunk with lumbar ganglia

Inter-mesenteric plexus

Lumbar splanchnics

Iliac plexus

Sacral splanchnic

Sacral ganglia

Ganglion impar

b

Fig. 18.14 (a) Large collections of autonomic fibers form large plexi. (b) In the abdomen, large autonomic plexi are associated with the aorta.
▶ Fig. 18.14b: Reproduced with permission from Schuenke M, Schulte E, Schumacher U. THIEME Atlas of Anatomy Third Edition, Vol 3. © Thieme 2020. Illustrations by Markus Voll and Karl Wesker.

Table 18.6 Autonomic plexuses in the abdomen and pelvis

Ganglia	Subplexus	Distribution	
Celiac plexus			
Celiac ganglia	Hepatic plexus	Liver, gallbladder	
	Gastric plexus	Stomach	
	Splenic plexus	Spleen	
	Pancreatic plexus	Pancreas	
Superior mesenteric plexus			
Superior mesenteric ganglion	—	• Pancreas (head) • Duodenum • Jejunum • Ileum	• Cecum • Colon (to left colic flexure) • Ovary
Suprarenal and renal plexus			
Aorticorenal ganglion	Ureteral plexus	• Suprarenal gland • Kidney • Proximal ureter	
Ovarian/testicular plexus			
—	—	Ovary/testis	
Inferior mesenteric plexus			
Inferior mesenteric ganglion	Left colic plexus	Left colic flexure	
	Superior rectal plexus	• Descending and sigmoid colon • Upper rectum	
Superior hypogastric plexus			
—	Hypogastric nn.	Pelvic viscera	
Inferior hypogastric plexus			
Pelvic ganglia	Middle and inferior rectal plexus	Middle and lower rectum	
	Prostatic plexus	• Prostate • Seminal vesicle • Bulbourethral gland	• Ejaculatory duct • Penis • Urethra
	Deferential plexus	• Ductus deferens • Epididymis	
	Uterovaginal plexus	• Uterus • Uterine tube	• Vagina • Ovary
	Vesical plexus	Urinary bladder	
	Ureteral plexus	Ureter (ascending from pelvis)	

Note: The two sacral sympathetic trunks converge and terminate in front of the coccyx in a small ganglion, the ganglion impar. (Reproduced with permission from Gilroy AM. Atlas of Anatomy. 3rd ed. Thieme; 2017, Table 16.5.)

Table 18.7 Summary of parasympathetic and sympathetic divisions of the ANS

	Parasympathetic	Sympathetic
Origin	Edinger-Westphal (CN III) Superior salivatory nucleus (CN VII) Inferior salivatory nucleus (CN IX) Dorsal motor nerve of vagus (CN X)	IML T1–L2
Preganglionic outflow	CNs III, VII, IX, and X, and S2–S4	Ventral roots of T1–L2 spinal nerves
Preganglionic neurons	Long, myelinated	Short, myelinated
Postganglionic neurons	Short, unmyelinated	Long, unmyelinated
Ganglia	Present in head and in walls of viscera	Prevertebral and paravertebral

Table 18.8 Functions of the hypothalamus

Region or Nucleus	Function
Anterior preoptic region	Maintains constant body temperature Lesion: Central hypothermia
Posterior region	Responds to temperature changes, e.g., sweating Lesion: Hypothermia
Midanterior and posterior regions	Activate sympathetic nervous system
Paraventricular and anterior regions	Activate parasympathetic nervous system
Supraoptic and paraventricular nuclei	Regulate water balance Lesion: Diabetes insipidus, also lack of thirst response resulting in hyponatremia
Anterior nuclei • Medial part • Lateral part	Regulate appetite and food intake • Lesion: Obesity • Lesion: Anorexia and emaciation

(Reproduced with permission from Schuenke. Atlas of Anatomy. Vol. 3, 2nd ed. Thieme; 2017, Table 14.339D.)

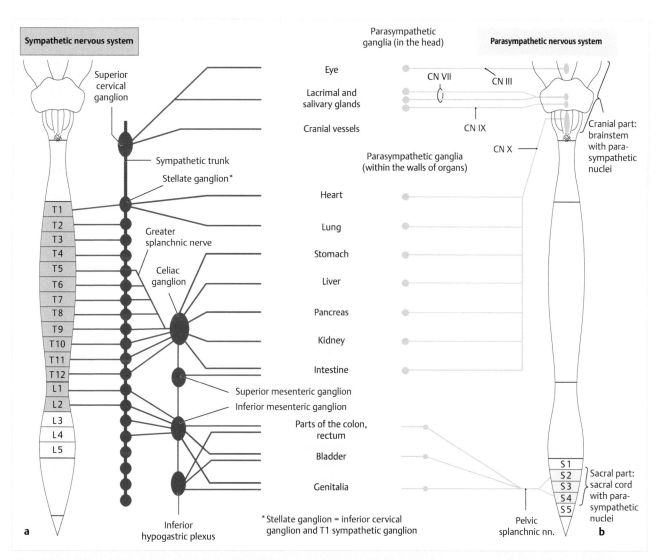

Fig. 18.15 (a,b) Autonomic nervous system—summary. (Reproduced with permission from Schuenke M, Schulte E, Schumacher U. THIEME Atlas of Anatomy Third Edition, Vol 3. © Thieme 2020. Illustrations by Markus Voll and Karl Wesker.)

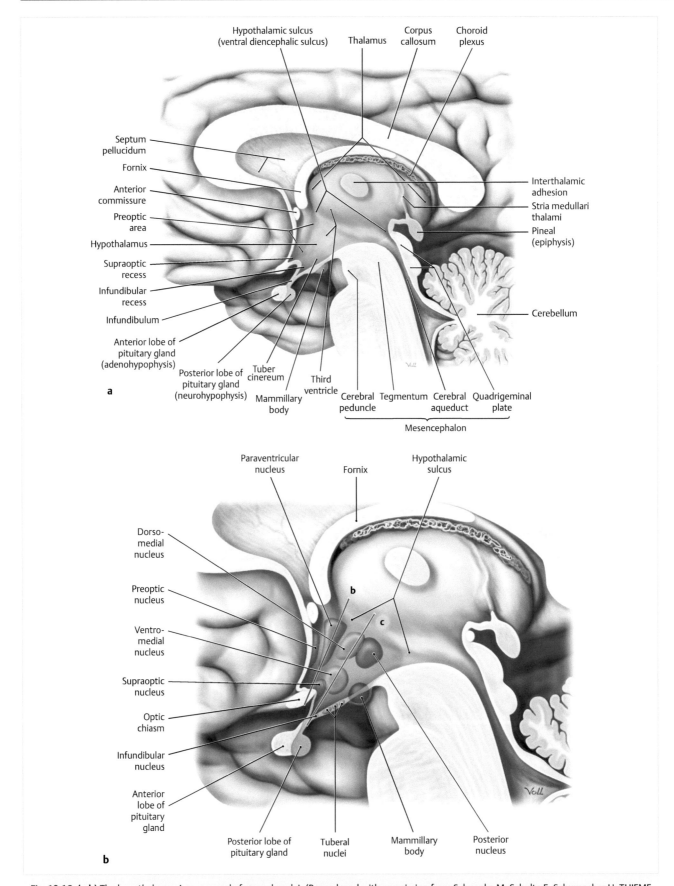

Fig. 18.16 (a,b) The hypothalamus is composed of several nuclei. (Reproduced with permission from Schuenke M, Schulte E, Schumacher U. THIEME Atlas of Anatomy Second Edition, Vol 3. © Thieme 2016. Illustrations by Markus Voll and Karl Wesker.)

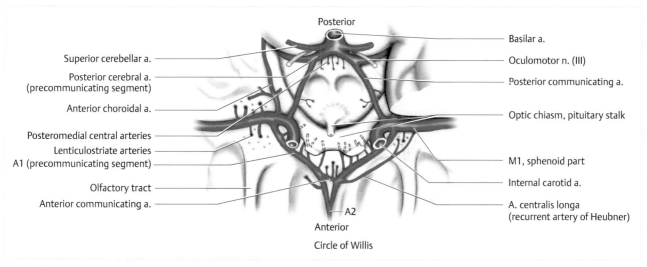

Fig. 18.17 Perforating branches of the circle of Willis provide the blood supply to the hypothalamus. (Modified with permission from Rohkamm R, ed. Color Atlas of Neurology. 2nd Edition. © Thieme 2014.)

- The hypothalamus has a separate neural connection for the **neurohypophysis** (posterior lobe) and a vascular connection to the **adenohypophysis** (anterior lobe) of the **hypophysis** (pituitary gland).

18.3 Limbic System

18.3.1 Overview

The **limbic system** is made up of cortical and subcortical structures that are necessary for normal behavior in humans. Memories, thoughts, personality, and emotions are produced by this system (▶ Fig. 18.18).

18.3.2 Anatomy

- The limbic system was originally named because of its location between the cerebral cortex and the hypothalamus (▶ Fig. 18.19). The term *limbic* means "margin." It is now known that the limbic system includes many other structures outside the border zone. The components of the limbic system include:
  - **Limbic cortex**
    - Cingulate gyrus
    - Parahippocampal gyrus
  - **Hippocampal formation**
    - Dentate gyrus
    - Hippocampus
    - Subicular complex
  - **Amygdala**
  - **Septal area**
- Efferents and afferents to and from the structures of the limbic system form elaborate circuits that allow it to function under normal circumstances. Damage to any of

these areas results in a variety of deficiencies due to their elaborate connections.

18.3.3 Function

- The limbic system works with the hypothalamus and its connection to the ANS and the endocrine system to influence emotional behavior.
  - Fear, anger, and the emotions associated with sexual behavior can trigger an autonomic as well as an endocrine response via the limbic system.
  - Memory.
  - Addiction.
  - Social cognition.
  - Olfaction.
  - Appetite.
  - Sleep patterns and dreaming.

Clinical Correlation Box 18.4: Epilepsy

Temporal lobe epilepsy is the most common form of epilepsy in adults and is often caused by damage to the hippocampus. Involvement can also include the amygdala and the parahippocampal gyrus.

Clinical Correlation Box 18.5: Dementia

Degenerative changes in the limbic system are seen in several neurodegenerative disorders such as Alzheimer. **Plaques** and **tangles**, two classic characteristics of the disease, are seen in both the hippocampus and the amygdala.

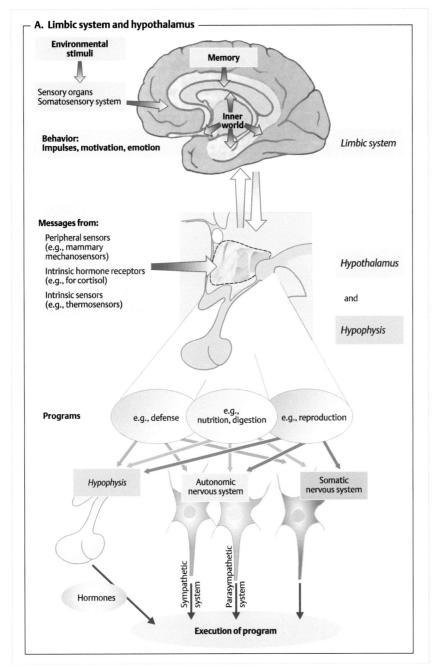

A. Limbic system and hypothalamus

Environmental stimuli

Sensory organs
Somatosensory system

Behavior:
Impulses, motivation, emotion

Memory

Inner world

Limbic system

Messages from:

Peripheral sensors
(e.g., mammary
mechanosensors)

Intrinsic hormone receptors
(e.g., for cortisol)

Intrinsic sensors
(e.g., thermosensors)

Hypothalamus

and

Hypophysis

Programs

e.g., defense

e.g.,
nutrition, digestion

e.g., reproduction

Hypophysis

Autonomic
nervous system

Somatic
nervous system

Hormones

Sympathetic system

Parasympathetic system

Execution of program

Fig. 18.18 Components of the limbic system. (Reproduced with permission from Silbernagl S, Despopoulos A. Color Atlas of Physiology. 6th edition. © Thieme 2009.)

Clinical Correlation Box 18.6: Schizophrenia

Schizophrenics often display symptoms such as disoriented thinking, blunted affect, and emotional withdrawal. In addition, paranoia and hallucinations may be present. Clinical studies have shown that if dopamine receptors in the limbic system are blocked, the severity of the symptoms are lessened.

Clinical Correlation Box 18.7: Kluver-Bucy Syndrome

Kluver-Bucy syndrome is a bilateral temporal lobe disorder. This syndrome is characterized by abnormalities in memory, social function, and idiosyncratic behaviors. Individuals with this disorder display excessive oral tendencies, emotional changes, extreme sexual behavior, and **visual agnosia** (difficulty identifying and processing visual information). Uncontrollable appetite and dementia may be present. This condition is due to temporal lobe damage as a result of trauma or other neurodegenerative disorders. Treatment is supportive along with psychotropic drugs.

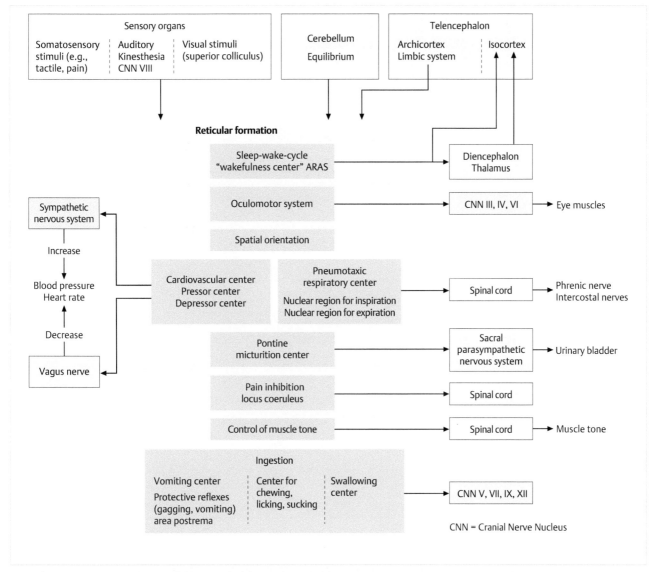

Fig. 18.19 Overview of the reticular system. (Reproduced with permission from Schuenke M, Schulte E, Schumacher U. THIEME Atlas of Anatomy Second Edition, Vol 3. © Thieme 2016. Illustrations by Markus Voll and Karl Wesker.)

18.4 Reticular Formation

18.4.1 Overview

The **reticular formation** is a group of neurons that forms the core of the brainstem. There is significant convergence and divergence of neurons in this structure such that a single neuron can respond to multiple sensory modalities from nearly everywhere on the body. It can influence skeletal muscle, somatic and visceral sensory input, as well as the autonomic and endocrine systems (▸ Fig. 18.20).

Anatomy
- The reticular formation is composed of neurons forming the core of the brainstem (▸ Fig. 18.20).
- It extends from the medulla to the midbrain and is typically divided into three longitudinal zones:
  ○ **Raphe nuclei (median zone)**

- Thin plates of cells located in the sagittal plane of the brainstem.
  ○ **Medial zone**
    - Alongside the midline raphe nuclei.
    - Source of most of the long ascending and descending projections from the reticular formation.
  ○ **Lateral zone**
    - Located lateral to medial zone.
    - Primarily concerned with cranial nerve reflexes and visceral function.

18.4.2 Function

- Neurons in the pontine and medullary reticular formation give rise to the reticulospinal tracts (see Chapter 15) that in general control automatic motor responses such as postural

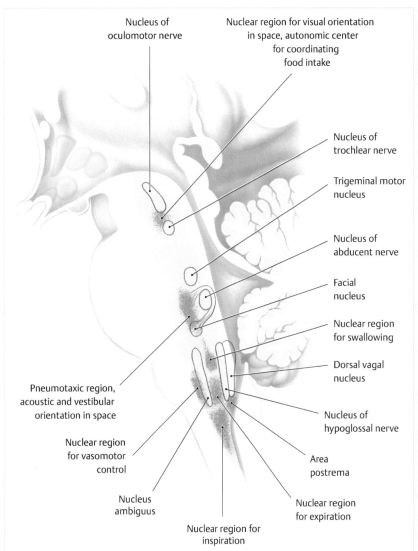

Nucleus of oculomotor nerve

Nuclear region for visual orientation in space, autonomic center for coordinating food intake

Nucleus of trochlear nerve

Trigeminal motor nucleus

Nucleus of abducent nerve

Facial nucleus

Nuclear region for swallowing

Dorsal vagal nucleus

Nucleus of hypoglossal nerve

Area postrema

Nuclear region for expiration

Pneumotaxic region, acoustic and vestibular orientation in space

Nuclear region for vasomotor control

Nucleus ambiguus

Nuclear region for inspiration

Fig. 18.20 The reticular formation forms the core of the brainstem. (Reproduced with permission from Schuenke M, Schulte E, Schumacher U. THIEME Atlas of Anatomy Second Edition, Vol 3. © Thieme 2016. Illustrations by Markus Voll and Karl Wesker.)

adjustments, stepping while walking, and corrections of movement errors.
  ○ The reticular formation connections with the spinal cord and cerebellum facilitate the motor control.
• Participates in pain modulation through transmission of information in descending pathways (see Chapter 14).
• Contains autonomic reflex circuitry.
  ○ Visceral information reaches the reticular formation, which programs appropriate response to environmental changes by projecting to autonomic nuclei in the brainstem and spinal cord.
• Involved in maintaining the normal state of consciousness.

Questions and Answers

1. A 1-year-old boy with a history of constipation and abdominal distension was seen in the ER. The child's mother reported that the constipation had become worse over the last 3 months. Examination showed abdominal distension and a palpable mass in the left lower quadrant. The rectum was empty and not dilated. A barium enema with

radiograph was performed which showed an extremely distended descending colon with a significant change in the lumen diameter at the sigmoid colon. Based on the information provided, which of the following diagnoses is most likely?
a) Hirschsprung's Disease
b) Horner Syndrome
c) Raynaud's Disease
d) Sympathetic injury

Level 3: Difficult
  Answer A: Hirschsprung's Disease; **(B)** Horner's Syndrome results from sympathetic interruption to the head and neck; **(C)** Raynaud's Disease is a sympathetic overreaction of arterioles in the skin, typically the toes and fingers; **(D)** The examination shows lack of peristalsis and gut motility, which indicates a parasympathetic issue.

2. A 23-year-old man with a traumatic brain injury (TBI) was seen by a neurologist upon admission to a rehabilitation facility. The patient displayed aggressive sexual behavior, visual agnosia and excessive oral tendencies (placing objects

in mouth). The neurologist suspects Kluver-Bucy Syndrome. What area of the brain is affected in this disorder?
a) Postcentral gyrus
b) Motor cortex
c) Temporal lobe
d) Prefrontal cortex

Level 3: Difficult

Answer C: Kluver-Bucy is a bilateral temporal lobe disorder; **(A)** Post central gyrus is the sensory strip. Abnormal behaviors presented are not controlled by sensory abnormalities; **(B)** Damage to the motor cortex would cause motor deficiencies; **(D)** prefrontal cortex is responsible for executive function however, the visual agnosia and oral abnormalities do not indicate damage to the prefrontal cortex.

3. Sympathetic preganglionic neurons for the head and neck are located in which of the following structures?
a) Superior cervical ganglia
b) Intermediolateral cell column T1-T4
c) Edinger-Westphal nucleus
d) Ventral horn of the spinal cord T1-T4

Level 2: Easy

Answer B: Preganglionic neurons for the head and neck are located in the IML T1–4; **(A)** Postganglionic neurons for the head and neck are located in the superior (or middle) cervical ganglia; **(C)** Edinger-Westphal nucleus is where preganglionic parasympathetic neurons for the head are located and **(D)**

Motor neurons are located in the ventral horn of the spinal cord. Axons of the sympathetic preganglionic neurons *exit* the spinal cord from the ventral horn however; the cell bodies are not located there.

4. Preganglionic neurons that exit the sympathetic chain without synapsing at T12 are called:
a) Greater splanchnics
b) Lesser splanchnics
c) Least splanchnics
d) Pelvic splanchnics

Level 1: Easy

Answer C: Least splanchnics; **(A)** Greater splanchnics are T5–9; **(B)** Lesser splanchnics are T10–11 and **(D)** Pelvic splanchnics are parasympathetic.

5. Which of the following statements are TRUE regarding the ANS?
a) ACh is secreted by *ALL* preganglionic neurons.
b) NE is secreted by parasympathetic postganglionic fibers.
c) NE binds muscarinic receptors.
d) Sweat glands possess nicotinic receptors.

Level 2: Medium

Answer A: ACh is secreted by ALL preganglionic neurons of the ANS; **(B)** NE is secreted by MOST sympathetic postganglionic fibers; **(C)** NE binds adrenergic receptors and **(D)** Sweat glands possess muscarinic receptors.

Part B

Orofacial Neuroscience

Unit V
Review of Orofacial Structures and Tissues

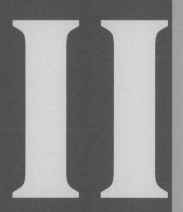

19 Development and Organization of Oropharyngeal Region

19.1 Overview of Oropharyngeal Development

- During the 4th week of development, a portion of the head and neck region, known as the **oropharyngeal region,** begins to differentiate as a functional unit from the **frontonasal process** and **pharyngeal arches**.
  - The frontonasal region corresponds to the midline region of the face and includes the **forehead, nose,** and **philtrum** of the **upper lip.**
  - The pharyngeal arches, which extend from the upper jaw to the level of the cricoid cartilage at vertebral level C6, differentiate to form the oropharyngeal region and includes the **upper** and **lower jaw, palate, oral cavity, pharynx,** and **larynx**.

19.1.1 Pharyngeal Arches (▶ Fig. 19.1)

- The pharyngeal arches (PAs) initially develop as six bilateral tissue swellings that surround the developing pharynx. Early developmental regression of the fifth arch leads to numbering of the arches as PA 1,2,3, 4, and 6. The numbering system reflects the early developmental regression of the fifth arch. The PA derivatives present in the adult are listed in ▶ Table 19.1 and ▶ Fig. 19.1
  - The PAs are covered externally with ectoderm and lined internally with endoderm.
  - Each arch develops in association with an ectodermal lined cleft and an endodermal lined pouch. In the adult, only the

first PA cleft persists and forms the **external auditory meatus** of the **ear**. The pouches give rise to several bilateral structures which are listed in ▶ Table 19.2 (▶ Fig. 19.2).
  - Each arch develops in association with a specific cranial nerve (**CNs V, VII, IX**, and **X**) and gives rise to a central core of tissue consisting of striated muscle, connective tissue, skeletal elements, and a blood vessel (▶ Fig. 19.3).
- The pattern of innervation for adult derivatives reflects their developmental origin from the frontonasal and pharyngeal arch region (▶ Fig. 19.4, ▶ Table 19.3).

19.1.2 Development of Oral Cavity and Face

- During development, the proliferation of tissue in the frontonasal region and the maxillary and mandibular processes of PA 1 gives rise to the primordia of the face and demarcates the boundary of the future oral cavity known as the stomodeum (▶ Table 19.4) (▶ Fig. 19.5) .
- In the adult, the **palatoglossal folds** which form the anterior tonsillar pillars represent the embryonic location of the ectodermal–endodermal boundary and serve as the posterior anatomical boundary of the oral cavity proper. The region posterior to the palatoglossal folds is the oropharynx.

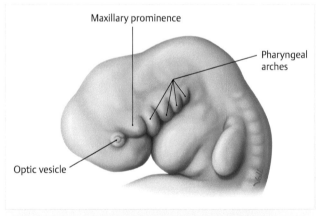

Fig. 19.1 Pharyngeal arch development: Head and neck region of a 5-week-old embryo showing the pharyngeal (branchial) arches and clefts (left lateral view). The pharyngeal arches are instrumental in the development of the face, neck, larynx, and pharynx. Development of the pharyngeal arches begins in the 4th week of embryonic development as cells migrate from the neural crest to the future head and neck region. By the 5th week, a series of four bilateral tissue swellings (first through fourth pharyngeal arches) develop and become visible on the external surface. Each arch is separated externally by four deep grooves (pharyngeal clefts). The pharyngeal arches and clefts are prominent features of the embryo at this stage. (Reproduced with permission from Schuenke M, Schulte E, Schumacher U. THIEME Atlas of Anatomy Third Edition, Vol 1. © Thieme 2020. Illustrations by Markus Voll and Karl Wesker.)

Table 19.1 Development of pharyngeal arches

Pharyngeal Arch	Anatomical Region in the Adult	Muscles*		Skeletal and CT	Cranial Nerve **
		Derivatives of the Pharyngeal Arches			
PA 1	Maxillary and mandibular process of upper and lower jaw	Muscles of mastication • Temporalis • Masseter • Lateral pterygoid • Medial pterygoid • Digastric (anterior) • Tensor tympani • Tensor veli palatini		• Maxilla • Mandible • Zygomatic bone • Palatine bone • Vomer • Squamous part temporal bone • Malleus and incus • Meckel's cartilage • Sphenomandibular ligament • Anterior ligament of malleus	Trigeminal (V)
PA 2	Pharynx	• Muscles of facial expression • Stylohyoid • Digastric (posterior) • Stapedius		• Stapes • Styloid process • Lesser horn hyoid bone • Upper body of hyoid	Facial (VII)
PA 3		Stylopharyngeus		• Greater horn, hyoid • Lower body hyoid bone	Glossopharyngeal (IX)
PA 4 and PA 6	Laryngopharynx Larynx	Pharyngeal and palatal muscles • Levator veli palatini • Uvulae muscles • Palatoglossus • Salpingopharyngeus • Palatopharyngeus • Superior constrictor • Middle constrictor • Inferior constrictor	Laryngeal muscles • Thyroarytenoid • Vocalis • Lateral cricoarytenoid • Cricothyroid • Oblique (inter)arytenoid • Transverse (inter) arytenoid • Posterior cricoarytenoid • Aryepiglottic • Thyroepiglottic	Laryngeal cartilages • Epiglottic • Thyroid cartilage • Cricoid cartilage • Arytenoid cartilage • Corniculate • Cuneiform	Vagus (X)

Notes: *All muscles derived from branchiomeric (pharyngeal) arch mesoderm.
**See Table 19.4 for specific nerve branches derived from each arch.

Table 19.2 Pouch derivatives

Pouch	Germ Layer	Embryonic Structure	Adult Derivative
	Pharyngeal Pouch Derivatives		
1	Endoderm	Tubotympanic recess	Epithelium lining the pharyngotympanic (auditory) (eustachian) tube Middle ear cavity
2		Palatine tonsillar fossa	Epithelium lining tonsillar fossa Epithelium (SSNK) of palatine tonsil
3		Pouch divides dorsal and ventral parts: Dorsal = forms epithelium of inferior parathyroid glands Ventral = forms thymic epithelium	Epithelial (chief/oxyphil) of inferior parathyroid Epithelial reticular cells of thymus
4th and 6th		Pouch divides dorsal and ventral: 4th dorsal pouch = forms epithelium of superior parathyroid glands 4th ventral /6th = forms ultimobranchial body ***Neural crest cells infiltrate ultimobranchial body and differentiate into parafollicular cells; parafollicular cells are incorporated into thyroid gland	Epithelial (chief/oxyphil) cells of superior parathyroid Ultimobranchial = Parafollicular cells incorporated into thyroid

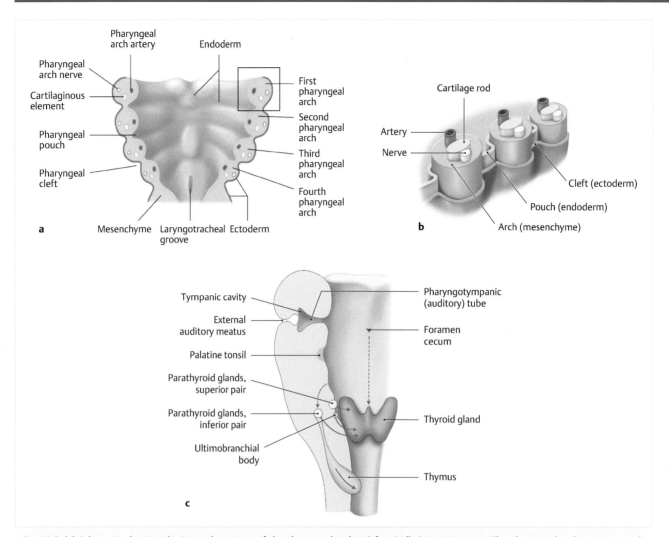

Fig. 19.2 **(a)** Schematic showing the internal structure of the pharyngeal arches (after Sadler). Anterior view. The pharyngeal arches are covered externally by ectoderm and internally by endoderm. Each pharyngeal arch contains an arch artery, an arch nerve, and a cartilaginous element, all of which are surrounded by mesodermal and muscular tissue. The external furrows are called the pharyngeal clefts, and the internal grooves are called the pharyngeal pouches. **(b)** High power view of boxed region shown in **(a)** (after Sadler). Oblique view showing the relationship of pharyngeal arch cartilage, artery, and nerve in the pharyngeal arches. The vessels, nerves, and cartilaginous precursors of each arch are surrounded by mesoderm and developing skeletal muscle tissue. Pharyngeal arches are covered externally by ectoderm (blue) and internally by endoderm (green). **(c)** Migration of the pharyngeal arch tissues (after Sadler). Anterior view. During embryonic development, endoderm of each pharyngeal pouch differentiates bilaterally from the lateral wall of the pharyngeal tube and gives rise to the epithelial cells associated with the auditory tube (PA 1), the palatine tonsils (PA 2), the thymus (PA 3), and the inferior and superior parathyroid glands (PA 3 and PA 4). The epithelium of thyroid gland also develops from endoderm, but it originates from the foramen cecum in the midline of the tongue. Calcitonin-producing C cells, or parafollicular cells, arise from neural crest cells and migrate with the thyroid gland. The thymus, parathyroid glands, and the thyroid gland migrate (arrows) from their sites of developmental origin. The superior and inferior parathyroid glands follow the migratory path of the thyroid glands and come to lie on the posterior surface at the superior and inferior poles of the thyroid. Each lobe of the thymus migrates toward the midline and then descends into the superior mediastinum. (Reproduced with permission from Schuenke M, Schulte E, Schumacher U. THIEME Atlas of Anatomy. Third Edition, Vol 3. © Thieme 2020. Illustrations by Markus Voll and Karl Wesker.)

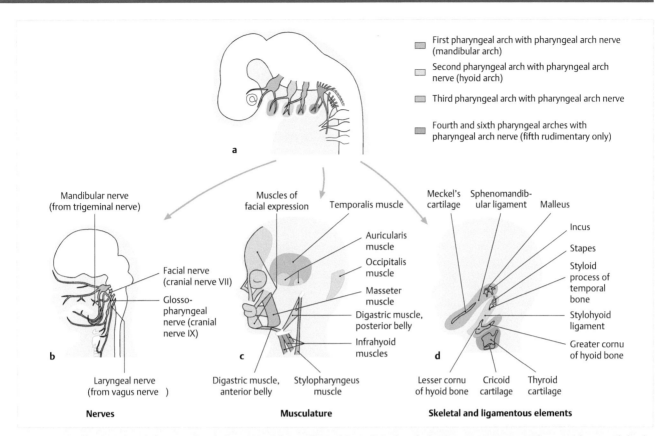

First pharyngeal arch with pharyngeal arch nerve (mandibular arch)

Second pharyngeal arch with pharyngeal arch nerve (hyoid arch)

Third pharyngeal arch with pharyngeal arch nerve

Fourth and sixth pharyngeal arches with pharyngeal arch nerve (fifth rudimentary only)

Mandibular nerve (from trigeminal nerve)

Muscles of facial expression

Temporalis muscle

Meckel's cartilage

Sphenomandib-ular ligament

Malleus

Facial nerve (cranial nerve VII)

Glosso-pharyngeal nerve (cranial nerve IX)

Auricularis muscle

Occipitalis muscle

Masseter muscle

Digastric muscle, posterior belly

Infrahyoid muscles

Incus

Stapes

Styloid process of temporal bone

Stylohyoid ligament

Greater cornu of hyoid bone

b

Laryngeal nerve (from vagus nerve)

c

Digastric muscle, anterior belly

Stylopharyngeus muscle

d

Lesser cornu of hyoid bone

Cricoid cartilage

Thyroid cartilage

Nerves

Musculature

Skeletal and ligamentous elements

Fig. 19.3 (a–d) Schematic of pharyngeal arch derivatives (after Sadler and Drews). Each arch develops in association with a cranial nerve, skeletal muscle derivatives, and connective tissue derivatives. (a) Anlage of the embryonic pharyngeal arches with the associated pharyngeal arch nerves. (b) Definitive arrangement of the future cranial nerves V, VII, IX, and X. (c) Muscular derivatives of the pharyngeal arches. (d) Skeletal derivatives of the pharyngeal arches. (Reproduced with permission from Schuenke M, Schulte E, Schumacher U. THIEME Atlas of Anatomy. Second Edition, Vol 1. © Thieme 2014. Illustrations by Markus Voll and Karl Wesker.)

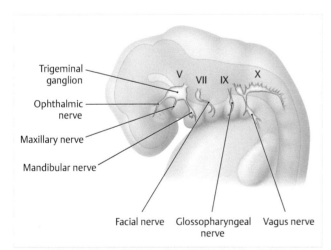

Trigeminal ganglion

Ophthalmic nerve

Maxillary nerve

Mandibular nerve

Facial nerve

Glossopharyngeal nerve

Vagus nerve

Fig. 19.4 Innervation of the pharyngeal arches (left lateral view). Each of the pharyngeal arches is associated with a cranial nerve: First pharyngeal arch is associated with the trigeminal nerve (CNs V2 and V3); second pharyngeal arch, facial nerve (CN VII); third pharyngeal arch, glossopharyngeal nerve (CN IX); fourth and sixth pharyngeal arches, vagus nerve (CN X—superior and recurrent laryngeal nerves). The frontonasal region which contributes to the midline of the face is also associated with the trigeminal nerve, but it is CN V1 division that provides sensory innervation to this part of the face. (Reproduced with permission from Schuenke M, Schulte E, Schumacher U. THIEME Atlas of Anatomy Second Edition, Vol 3. © Thieme 2016. Illustrations by Markus Voll and Karl Wesker.)

19.1.3 Palatal Development (▶ Fig. 19.6)

- Palatal development begins between the 6th and 12th weeks of embryogenesis as a result of differential growth and fusion of external and internal tissues comprising the facial prominences.
- The **primary palate** contains the four maxillary incisors and forms as a small triangular wedge from the **intermaxillary segment** of the frontonasal prominence.
- The **secondary palate** develops as bilateral outgrowths from the **maxillary prominences**. The two palatal shelves fuse together in the midline and fuse anteriorly with the primary palate along the incisive foramen to form the **definitive palate,** which separates the oral and nasal cavities.
- The nasal septum grows inferiorly from the floor of the anterior cranial fossa, fuses with the definitive palate, and divides the nasal cavity into two chambers.

19.1.4 Development of Pharynx

- The pharynx, which develops as a muscular tube from tissue associated with PAs 2 to 6, differentiates into three regions in the adult: the **nasopharynx, oropharynx**, and **laryngopharynx**. Bilateral outpocketings from the

Table 19.3 Pharyngeal arch nerves

Arch		Motor (Voluntary) (SVE)	General Sensory (GSA) (Pain, Temp, Touch)	Special Sensory (SVA) (Taste)	Autonomic (Visceral Motor) Parasympathetic (GVE)
1	Trigeminal CN (V) 3 divisions • Mandibular (V3) • Maxillary (V2) • Ophthalmic (V1)	• Mandibular division (V3) Provides motor function to muscles of PA 1 SVE motor neurons located: Motor nucleus of V	• Mandibular division (V3) • Maxillary division (V2) Carries pain, temp, touch to face, jaw, teeth, oral cavity, TMJ, mucosa ant 2/3 tongue Ganglion = Trigeminal ganglion/semilunar ganglion	none	none
2	Facial N (CN VII)	Facial N—several br. Provides motor function to muscle of PA2 SVE motor neurons located: Motor nucleus of VII	• Facial N— Carries pain, temp, touch to small area behind ear Sensory neurons in ganglion = Geniculate ganglion	• Facial N—chorda tympani br. →via lingual (V3) Carries taste ant 2/3 tongue • Facial N—greater petrosal →via greater and lesser palatine (V2) Carries taste hard and soft palate Special sensory neurons (for taste) in ganglion = Geniculate ganglion	• Facial N—greater petrosal N →n. pterygoid canal • Chorda tympani →lingual Carries parasympathetic fibers to lacrimal, submandibular, sublingual glands, palatal salivary glands Pre-ganglionic neurons • Superior salivatory nucleus Post-ganglionic neurons • Pterygopalatine ganglion • Submandibular ganglion
3	Glossopharyngeal CN (IX)	Glossopharyngeal N—motor Provides motor to one pharyngeal arch muscle of PA 3 Neurons form: nucleus ambiguus	Glossopharyngeal—sensory Carries pain, temp, touch to posterior 1/3 of tongue, oropharynx Somatic general sensory neurons form ganglion = superior glossopharyngeal ganglion	Glossopharyngeal—taste Carries taste to post 1/3 of tongue Special sensory neurons (for taste) form ganglion = inferior (petrosal) glossopharyngeal ganglion	Glossopharyngeal- lesser petrosal N →via auriculotemporal (V3) Carries parasympathetic fibers to parotid gland Preganglionic neurons • inferior salivatory nucleus Postganglionic neurons • otic ganglion
			Pharyngeal arch nerves		
Arch		Motor (voluntary) (SVE)	General sensory (GSA) (pain, temp ,touch)	Special sensory (SVA) (taste)	Autonomic(visceral motor) parasympathetic (GVE)
4	Vagus CN (X)-2 major branches associated with PA 4th Pharyngeal br of (X) Superior laryngeal Br. divides into: • External laryngeal • Internal laryngeal	Vagus— Pharyngeal br of (X) contributes to pharyngeal plexus Provides innervation to Palatoglossus and all palatal, constrictor muscles External laryngeal br of superior laryngeal (X) : Provides motor innervation to cricothyroid muscle SVE motor neurons located : nucleus ambiguus	Vagus— Internal laryngeal br. of vagus Carries pain, temp, touch to root/base of tongue/ epiglottis innervates mucosa in region of larynx above vocal folds Somatic general sensory neurons located in ganglion = Superior vagal (jugular) ganglion	Vagus— Internal laryngeal br. of vagus Carries taste from root/ base of tongue/epiglottis Special sensory (SVA) neurons in ganglion = Inferior vagal (nodose) ganglion	Vagus—pharyngeal and internal laryngeal N carry autonomics Carries parasympathetic fibers to glands of pharynx and larynx Preganglionic neurons • Dorsal motor nucleus of X • Postganglionic neurons located in organ wall
6	Vagus—1 major br associated with PA 6th Recurrent Laryngeal br of X	Recurrent laryngeal br of vagus (X) Provides motor to laryngeal muscles located below the vocal folds SVE motor neurons located: nucleus ambiguus	Recurrent laryngeal branch of vagus (X) : Carries pain, temp, touch to mucosa in region below vocal folds Somatic general sensory neurons in ganglion = inferior vagal (nodose) ganglion	None	Recurrent laryngeal br of X Carries parasympathetic fibers to glands of larynx Preganglionic neurons • Dorsal motor nucleus of X • Postganglionic neurons located in organ wall

Table 19.4 Contributions of the pharyngeal prominences to the face

Pharyngeal Prominence	Adult Facial Structure
Frontonasal prominence * *Single unpaired structure divides into a medial and lateral nasal process* *Medial nasal process further divides into intermaxillary*	Major derivatives: Forehead, part of nose, philtrum of lip, primary palate
• Medial nasal prominence (MNP)	Bridge of nose and tip
o Intermaxillary segment (IM) derived from medial nasal process	Philtrum of upper lip, primary palate
• Lateral nasal prominence (LNP)	Alae of nose; lateral nasal cartilages
Maxillary prominence of PA 1	Upper lip, except philtrum Cheek Maxilla Secondary palate
Mandibular prominence of PA 1	Lower lip Chin Mandible

Notes: *The nose develops in association with the frontonasal process and from the floor of the cartilaginous anterior cranial base.
**The upper lip forms from the union of intermaxillary process and maxillary process.

pharyngeal wall form the pouch derivatives listed in
▶ Table 19.2.

19.1.5 Tongue Development (▶ Fig. 19.7) (▶ Table 19.5)

- As the oral cavity begins to develop, the **pharyngeal arches** begin to proliferate along the inferior boundary of the oral cavity in the region that becomes the floor of the mouth. The tongue and larynx develop as midline structures from the floor of the pharyngeal arch region.
  - PAs 1, 3, and 4 contribute to the **mucosa** of the **tongue**. The pattern of sensory innervation for the tongue reflects the developmental origin of the arches (▶ Table 19.5).
  - **Occipital somites** migrate into the developing tongue along with the **hypoglossal nerve (CN XII)** and differentiate into most of the striated muscle associated with the extrinsic and intrinsic tongue musculature.
    - The extrinsic palatoglossus muscle is the exception to this pattern. Branchiomeric mesoderm (pharyngeal arch mesoderm) of PA 4 gives rise to the palatoglossus muscle. The palatoglossus receives special visceral efferent (SVE) innervation from the pharyngeal plexus (CN X).

19.1.6 Development of the Larynx (▶ Table 19.6)

- The larynx develops during the formation of the tongue and arises from the distal hypobranchial eminence (epiglottic swellings) of PA 4 and the arytenoid swellings of PA 6.
- The true vocal cords serve as the anatomical division between the developmental boundary of the fourth and sixth pharyngeal arches.
- The muscles and mucosa lining the laryngeal region receive innervation from branches of the vagus nerve (CN X). The pattern of innervation reflects the developmental origin of the larynx. The vagal nerve branches which innervate the laryngeal region include the **superior laryngeal, external laryngeal, internal laryngeal (PA 4),** and **recurrent**

(inferior) laryngeal branches of the vagus (PA 6)
(▶ Table 19.6) (▶ Fig. 19.7).

19.2 Overview of Oral Cavity and Oral Mucosa (▶ Fig. 19.8)

19.2.1 Oral Cavity

- The **oral cavity** or **mouth** extends from the lips and cheeks to the palatoglossal folds, which form the anterior tonsillar pillars. Posterior to the tonsillar pillars the oral cavity becomes continuous with the oropharynx.
- The oral cavity consists of two functional regions, the **oral vestibule** and **oral cavity proper,** which are separated by the **dental (alveolar) arches.** The oral vestibule is external to the upper and lower dental arches, and the oral cavity proper lies internal to the dental arches.

19.2.2 Oral Mucosa (▶ Table 19.7)

- The tissue lining the free surfaces of the oral vestibule, oral cavity, and pharynx is a mucous membrane known as **oral mucosa.**
  - The oral mucosa consists of stratified squamous epithelium, which varies with the extent of keratinization, and the amount of underlying connective tissue.
  - The three types of oral mucosa found in the region of the oropharyngeal region include: **lining mucosa, masticatory mucosa,** and **specialized mucosa** (▶ Table 19.7). Regional variations in the type of oral mucosa reflect the functional properties of the specific regions and can be of clinical significance.

Innervation of the Oral Mucosa (▶ Fig. 19.9)

- The oral mucosa contains a high density of sensory receptors that transmit gustatory input, proprioception,

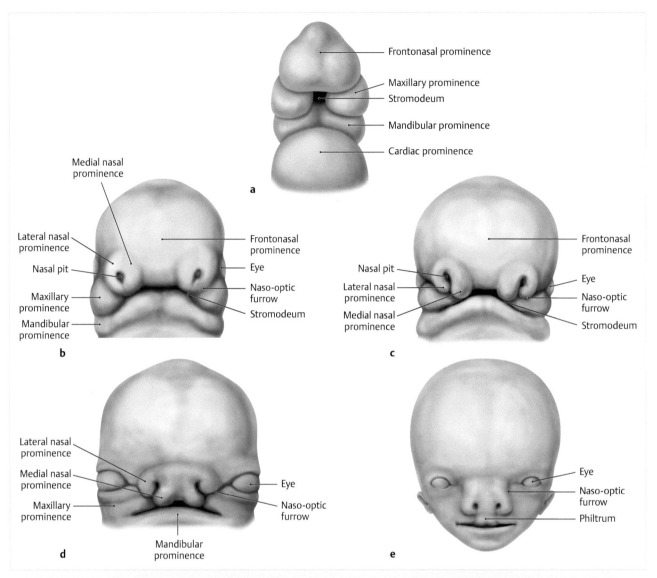

Fig. 19.5 (a–e) Development of the face between 5 and 12 weeks (after Sadler). (a) Anterior view at 24 days. The surface ectoderm of the pharyngeal arch 1 (PA1) invaginates to form the stomodeum, which is a depression between the forebrain and the pericardium in the embryo. It is the precursor of the mouth, oral cavity, and anterior pituitary gland. The stomodeum is surrounded by the frontonasal prominence and bilaterally by the maxillary and mandibular prominence of PA 1. These five prominences contribute to the development of the face. (b, c) Anterior view at 5th and 6th weeks. The nasal placodes, which are ectodermal thickenings, form on each side of the frontonasal prominence and become surrounded by medial and lateral nasal processes. (d, e) Anterior view at 7th to 12th weeks. The medial nasal processes merge to form the intermaxillary segment and the midline of the nose. The lateral nasal processes and maxillary prominences fuse to from side of the nose. The maxillary processes also fuse with the intermaxillary segment to form the upper lip. The mandibular processes and maxillary prominences merge to form the side of the cheek. The frontonasal prominence differentiates to form the nose, philtrum of the upper lip, and region of the forehead. The maxillary process forms the cheek, upper lip, secondary palate, and upper jaw. The mandibular process forms the chin and lower jaw. (Reproduced with permission from Schuenke M, Schulte E, Schumacher U. THIEME Atlas of Anatomy. Third Edition, Vol 3. © Thieme 2020. Illustrations by Markus Voll and Karl Wesker.)

mechanoreception, nociceptive, and thermal stimuli (see Chapter 11 for review).

- Transmission of somatosensory innervation of the oral mucosa covering the oral cavity, pharynx, and laryngeal region occurs through branches of the maxillary (V2) and mandibular (V3) divisions of the trigeminal nerve, the glossopharyngeal (CN IX), and the vagus (CN X) nerves, respectively.
- Gustatory (taste) input and the detection of taste is a discriminative sensation confined to the specific regions of

the oral mucosa which contains taste receptors in **taste buds**.

- Most of the taste buds are associated with the lingual papillae, which comprise the specialized mucosa covering the anterior two-thirds of the tongue. Additional taste buds are scattered on the palate, oropharynx, posterior one-third of the tongue, epiglottis, and laryngeal mucosa (▸ Table 19.7).
- The specific nerve branches that transmit taste from the oropharyngeal region and the central pathways for

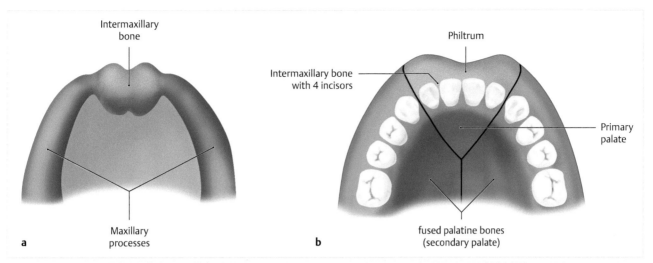

Fig. 19.6 (a, b) Palatal development (after Sadler). Caudal view of palate at 7th weeks. (a) The medial nasal processes fuse together to give rise to the intermaxillary segment. The posterior part of the intermaxillary segment develops into bone tissue and gives rise to the primary palate. In the adult, the primary palate is known as the premaxilla or intermaxillary segment of the maxilla and represents the portion of bone containing the maxillary incisors. (b) Caudal view, adult. The philtrum, an area of soft tissue in the midline of the upper lip, arises from anterior part of intermaxillary segment. The secondary palate develops from the two lateral palatal shelves of the maxillary process. Midline fusion between the lateral shelves forms the secondary palate. Development of the definitive (complete) palate occurs when the tissue of the primary palate fuses with the secondary palate of the maxillary processes. Due to the complexity in palatal development, palatal clefts, which represent defects in the fusion between facial tissue components, can arise. (Reproduced with permission from Schuenke M, Schulte E, Schumacher U. THIEME Atlas of Anatomy. Second Edition, Vol 3. © Thieme 2016. Illustrations by Markus Voll and Karl Wesker.)

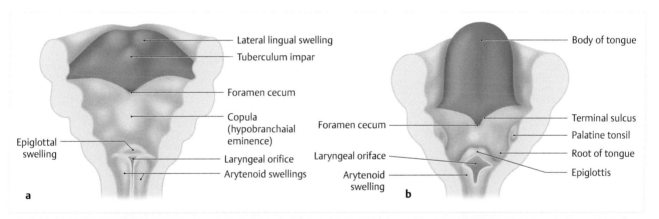

Fig. 19.7 (a, b) Development of the tongue. (a) Early tongue development at 4th week. (b) Late tongue development around week 8. The tongue mucosa develops as swellings from the floor of the pharynx in the region of 1st, 3rd, and 4th pharyngeal arches. The musculature of the tongue is derived from occipital somites. The two lateral lingual swellings from the 1st pharyngeal arch merge together and contribute to the lingual mucosa covering the anterior two-thirds of the tongue. The single midline swelling (the hypobranchial eminence), from the 3rd and 4th pharyngeal arches, contributes to the mucosa covering the posterior one-third of the tongue and epiglottis. A V-shaped terminal depression (sulcus terminalis) separates the anterior two-thirds of the tongue from the posterior one-third. At the apex of the sulcus lies in the foramen cecum which represents the site of origin of the thyroid glands. In the region distal to the hypobranchial eminence, the epiglottic and laryngeal (arytenoid) swellings develop from the 4th and 6th pharyngeal arches and contribute to the epiglottis and laryngeal mucosa. (Reproduced with permission from Schuenke M, Schulte E, Schumacher U. THIEME Atlas of Anatomy Third Edition, Vol 3. © Thieme 2020. Illustrations by Markus Voll and Karl Wesker.)

Table 19.5 Embryonic derivatives of tongue

Developmental Origin	Adult Structure	Innervation Pattern
Pharyngeal arch 1 (PA 1)	Mucosa of anterior two-thirds of tongue	Trigeminal (V3); lingual branch of V3 (GSA) mucosa of anterior two-thirds
Pharyngeal arch 2 (PA 2)	None	Facial VII; chorda tympani branch of facial VII** SVA to taste buds of fungiform papillae on anterior two-thirds of tongue
Pharyngeal arch 3 (PA 3)	Mucosa of posterior one-third of tongue	Glossopharyngeal (IX); lingual and tonsillar branches • GSA to mucosa of posterior one-third • SVA to taste buds circumvallate and foliate papillae
Pharyngeal arch 4 (PA 4)	Mucosa base of tongue and epiglottis	Vagus (X); internal laryngeal (branch of superior laryngeal) • GSA to mucosa base of tongue • SVA to taste buds on epiglottis
Occipital somites	Extrinsic/Intrinsic tongue muscles	Hypoglossal (CN XII); GSE motor
Branchiomeric mesoderm (PA 4)	Palatoglossus muscle	(X) Pharyngeal plexus; SVE motor

The **chorda tympani nerve, a branch of the facial nerve (CN VII), is the nerve associated with region of second arch (PA 2) that is overgrown during tongue development. The chorda tympani nerve, which transmits **taste** from taste buds on the **anterior two-thirds** of the **tongue,** is a remnant of the developmental overgrowth.
Abbreviations: GSA, general somatic afferent; GSE, general somatic efferent; SVA, special visceral afferent; SVE, special visceral efferent.

Table 19.6 Embryonic and adult derivatives of the larynx

Pharyngeal arch	Structures derived from Pharyngeal Arch Lateral plate mesoderm	Cartilaginous	Skeletal muscle	Innervation
Pharyngeal arch	Name of embryonic precursor	Adult derivative	Adult derivative	SVE (motor)
4	Epiglottic /distal hypobranchial swelling	Thyroid and epiglottic cartilage	**External laryngeal muscle** Cricothyroid m	External laryngeal br of X
6	Arytenoid swellings	Cricoid, Arytenoid, Corniculate, Cuneiform cartilage	**Intrinsic laryngeal muscles** (posterior criocoidarytenoid, thyroarytenoid, lateral cricoidarytenoid, transverse and oblique arytenoid, vocalis)	Recurrent laryngeal br of X

Table 19.7 Types of oropharyngeal mucosa

Mucosa Type	Location	Key Characteristics	% Distribution of Oropharyngeal Region
Lining	Labial Buccal Alveolar mucosa Soft palate Ventral tongue Floor of mouth Oropharynx Epiglottis and laryngeal region	• Stratified squamous nonkeratinized (SSNK) epithelium • Loose, flexible attachment submucosa; may require suturing • Faster epithelial turnover than stratified squamous keratinized (SSK) epithelium • Taste buds may be scattered within epithelium of the hard and soft palate (VII), oropharynx (IX), epiglottis, and laryngeal (X) regions	60
Masticatory	Hard palate Gingiva (free and attached)	• Stratified squamous parakeratinized (SSPK) epithelium; some variation of SSK may exist in regions • Firm attachment of submucosa; withstands friction • Slower turnover than SSNK; mucoperiosteum may be present	30
Specialized	Dorsal surface of anterior two-thirds of tongue	• Lingual papillae; surface elevations interspersed with SSK • Lingual papillae are only found on the anterior two-thirds of the tongue • Papillae may contain taste buds • Types of papillae include: ○ Filiform ○ Fungiform** (VII) ○ Circumvallate** (IX) ○ Foliate** (IX)	10

Note: **Contain taste buds.

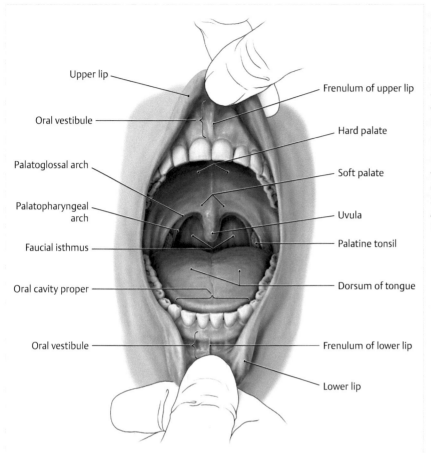

Fig. 19.8 Region of the oral cavity; anterior view. The dental arches (with the alveolar processes of the maxilla and mandible) subdivide the oral cavity into two parts: Oral vestibule: The portion outside the dental arches, bounded on one side by the lips and cheeks and on the other side by the dental arches. Oral cavity proper: The region within the dental arches. The oral cavity proper includes the anterior two-thirds of the tongue and extends from the dental arches to palatoglossal folds (anterior tonsillar pillars). Posterior to folds lies the posterior one-third of the tongue in the region of the oropharynx. (Reproduced with permission from Schuenke M, Schulte E, Schumacher U. THIEME Atlas of Anatomy Third Edition, Vol 3. © Thieme 2020. Illustrations by Markus Voll and Karl Wesker.)

processing and perceiving taste are covered in Chapters 13, 20, and 21.

- Afferent input from low threshold mechanoreceptors and proprioceptors in the oral mucosa plays an integral role in the feedback, perception, and reflexive response concerning the size, texture, and position of objects (**stereognosis)** placed in the oral cavity, including food, liquids, and oral devices.
  - The ability to perceive nociceptive, proprioceptive, and stereognostic inputs is essential for monitoring, adapting, and integrating motor responses involved in occlusion, mastication, swallowing, and speaking, as well as regulating various reflexes (see Chapter 22).
  - Regions of the oral mucosa such as the lips, teeth, periodontal ligaments, anterior and midline regions of the tongue, and palate contain areas of high receptor density with small receptive fields which permits increased sensitivity and greater discrimination of tactile input and oral stereognosis (Clinical Correlation Box 19.2).

Clinical Correlation Box 19.1: Epithelial Turnover

Regional differences in the extent of keratinization influence epithelial turnover rates and can have clinical implications in epithelial homeostasis and wound healing. In the oral mucosa, areas of lining mucosa which contain stratified squamous non-keratinized (**SSNK**) epithelium turnover faster than masticatory mucosa which contains stratified squamous parakeratinized (**SSPK**) epithelium. Furthermore, the proliferative rate of the oral epithelium exceeds that of the epidermis which is a keratinized epithelium (**SSK**), and of oral fibroblasts in the underlying connective tissue. As a result, most oral wounds heal by re-epithelialization rather than scar formation. However, any alteration in normal turnover rates will impact epithelial homeostasis. Radiation and chemotherapy interfere with mitosis and reduce the ability of oral mucosal regeneration. Inhibition of epithelial turnover as an outcome of these treatments leads to an increased susceptibility to form painful ulcers. Cutaneous innervation is also important in maintaining epithelial homeostasis. Inflammatory and immune diseases may lead to changes in cutaneous innervation and alter epithelial turnover and wound healing.

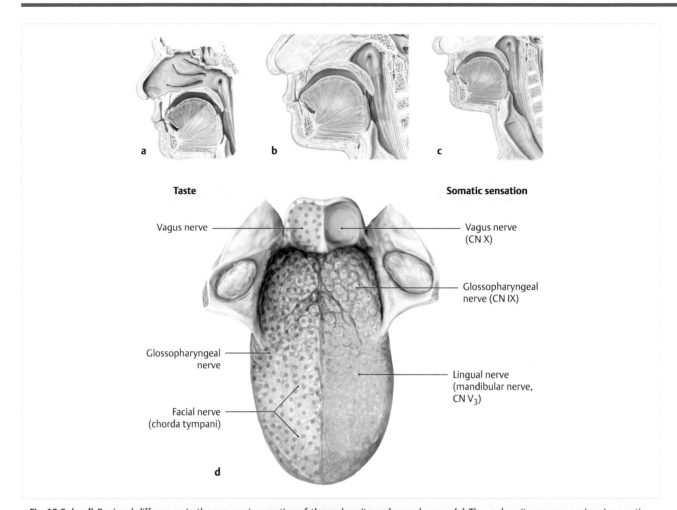

Taste   **Somatic sensation**

Vagus nerve

Vagus nerve
(CN X)

Glossopharyngeal
nerve (CN IX)

Glossopharyngeal
nerve

Lingual nerve
(mandibular nerve,
CN V₃)

Facial nerve
(chorda tympani)

d

Fig. 19.9 (a–d) Regional differences in the sensory innervation of the oral cavity and nasopharynx. **(a)** The oral cavity proper receives innervation from the trigeminal nerve (CN V2 maxillary and CN V3 mandibular). **(b)** Glossopharyngeal (CN IX) carries sensory (GSA/GVA) innervation to the oropharynx. **(c)** The vagus (CN X) transmits sensory input in the region of the laryngopharynx and larynx. **(d)** Anterior view of the somatosensory innervation (left side) and taste innervation (right side) of the tongue. The tongue receives its somatosensory innervation (e.g., touch, pain, thermal sensation) from three cranial nerve branches: Lingual nerve (branch of mandibular nerve, CN V3), glossopharyngeal nerve (CN IX), and vagus nerve (CN X). Three cranial nerves convey the taste fibers: CN VII (facial nerve, chorda tympani), CN IX (glossopharyngeal nerve), and CN X (internal laryngeal of vagus nerve). Thus, a disturbance of taste sensation involving the anterior two-thirds of the tongue indicates the presence of a facial nerve lesion, whereas a disturbance of tactile, pain, or thermal sensation indicates a trigeminal nerve lesion. GSA, general somatic afferent; GVA, general visceral afferent. (Reproduced with permission from Schuenke M, Schulte E, Schumacher U. THIEME Atlas of Anatomy Third Edition, Vol 3. © Thieme 2020. Illustrations by Markus Voll and Karl Wesker.)

- Clinically, changes in the oral mucosa due to systemic or local conditions may modify the sensory perception of pain, tactile input, and taste.
- Changes in tactile perception may occur due to the loss of the periodontal ligament following a tooth extraction, and the placement of dental implants or other oral devices. Alterations in the mechanosensory function of teeth due to malocclusion or disease can impact oral parafunctional behaviors such as bruxism and clenching.
- Medications causing a decrease in salivary flow or vitamin deficiencies lead to atrophy of lingual papillae and may alter the perception of taste.
- Patients following a stroke or individuals with Parkinson's disease often exhibit sensorimotor deficits associated with mastication and swallowing due to a loss in oral stereognosis. The loss in tactile and proprioceptive input may impact the patient's ability to gauge the size of a food bolus before swallowing, to determine the masticatory force and occlusal loads, and to articulate during the process of speaking.

19.3 Structures of Oral Vestibule

- The oral vestibule is a horseshoe-shaped space between the **labial (lip)** and **buccal (cheek)** tissue externally, and the **dental (alveolar) arch** internally. During occlusion, the vestibule connects with the oral cavity proper by the **retromolar space,** which is a gap between the distal edge of the **third molar** and the anterior border of the **ramus** of the **mandible.**
- The structures associated with the oral vestibule include the **lips, cheeks,** and **alveolar arches**. Additionally, the **parotid**

duct, which opens onto the buccal surface opposite the **maxillary second molar,** releases saliva into the vestibule.

19.3.1 Lips and Cheeks (▶ Fig. 19.10)

- The structure of the lips and cheeks are similar. Each contains a core of skeletal muscle, derived from the second pharyngeal arch (PA 2), connective tissue, and several minor salivary glands. The epidermis of the skin covers the external surface of the lips and cheeks and a mucous membrane comprised of **lining mucosa** protects the internal surface facing the vestibule.
  - The skeletal muscle of the lip (**orbicularis oris**) forms a sphincter or circular ring of muscle which functions to close, purse, and protrude the upper and lower lips. The lips also control the degree of protrusion of the maxillary incisors and play an important role in mastication and speech.
  - The **buccinator muscle** of the cheeks aids in mastication by keeping the food bolus between cheek and teeth.
- Motor innervation to the muscles of the lips and cheeks follows the facial nerve (CN VII), while the trigeminal nerve (CN V) innervates the skin and sensory mucosa lining the lips and cheeks (▶ Table 19.8).
  - **SVE** fibers carried by branches of the **facial nerve (CN VII)** provide motor innervation to all **muscles of facial expression,** including the **orbicularis oris** and **buccinator** muscles. The pattern of innervation reflects the embryonic origin of these muscles from the **second pharyngeal arch (PA 2).**
  - **General somatic afferent (GSA) fibers** transmit sensory information from the upper and lower lips and buccal region through terminal branches of maxillary (V2) and mandibular (V3) nerves (▶ Fig. 19.11):
    - The **superior labial branch** from the **infraorbital nerve of V2** supplies the cutaneous and mucosal surfaces of the upper lip. Terminal branches of superior labial also contribute to superior alveolar dental plexus (V2).

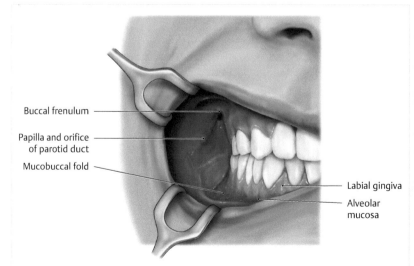

Buccal frenulum

Papilla and orifice of parotid duct

Mucobuccal fold

Labial gingiva

Alveolar mucosa

Fig. 19.10 Oral vestibule with teeth in occlusion. Left lateral view. The maxillary and mandibular dental arches subdivide the oral cavity into two parts: Oral vestibule and oral cavity proper. During occlusion, the oral vestibule, which lies outside the dental arches, bounded by the lips and cheeks, connects with the oral cavity proper by the retromolar space. The retromolar space is the gap between the distal edge of the third molar and the anterior border of the ramus of the mandible. Note the parotid duct papilla is shown on the buccal surface, opposite the maxillary second molar. (Reproduced with permission from Baker EW. Anatomy for Dental Medicine. Second Edition. © Thieme 2015. Illustrations by Markus Voll and Karl Wesker.)

Table 19.8 Summary of innervation to regions of cheek and lip M

	Cutaneous Skin	Lining Mucosa
Cheek (buccal) region	Buccal (long) of V3	Buccal (long) of V3
Upper lip	Superior labial of V2	Superior labial and minor contributions from superior dental plexus (V2)
Lower lip	Mental of V3	Mental of V3 Minor contributions from inferior alveolar of V3

- The **mental nerve**, a terminal branch from the **inferior alveolar (V3)**, supplies the cutaneous and mucosal surface of the lower lip and chin, while the **inferior alveolar nerve** and its **incisive branch** provide innervation to the labial mucosal surface.
    - The **buccal branch** (**long buccal nerve**) of V3 supplies the cutaneous and mucosal surface of the cheek and the alveolar and gingival mucosa along the facial surface of the mandibular molars.

19.3.2 Alveolar Mucosa and Gingiva (▶ Fig. 19.11a, b; ▶ Table 19.9; and ▶ Table 19.10)

- The mandibular and maxillary dental arches demarcate the boundary between the oral vestibule and the oral cavity proper.
    - The outer region of each dental arch faces the oral vestibule and is known as the **facial** or **vestibular surface**. The terms **buccal** and **labial** are also used to demarcate specific regions of the arch.
    - The inner surface of each alveolar arch faces the oral cavity proper. The area of the maxillary arch that meets the hard palate is known as the **palatal surface,** while the part of the mandibular arch which faces the tongue is the **lingual surface** (▶ Fig. 19.12).
- The mucosa covering vestibule forms a mucosal fold, known as the **mucobuccal** (**vestibular**) fold, that reflects from the labial and buccal surfaces onto the alveolar bone of the dental arch to form the **alveolar mucosa**.
- The alveolar mucosa transitions at the **mucogingival junction** to form the **gingiva** surrounding the cervix of the tooth. The transition at the mucogingival junction corresponds to a change from lining mucosa to masticatory mucosa.
    - The gingiva may be further subdivided into the **attached gingiva** and **free gingiva**. The attached gingiva is tightly bound to the periosteum of the alveolar bone while the free gingiva forms an unattached cuff around the cervix (neck) of the tooth (see Chapter 25).
- **GSA** innervation to the alveolar and gingival mucosa covering the maxillary and mandibular arch is carried by terminal branches of maxillary division (V2) and mandibular division (V3) of the trigeminal nerve (see Chapter 20).
- **Maxillary Dental Arch**
    - The alveolar mucosa and gingiva associated with the **facial side** of the maxillary arch transmit sensory input via branches of the **superior (alveolar) dental plexus** of nerves from **V2** (▶ Table 19.9).
    - The superior dental plexus consists of three terminal branches that arise from the infraorbital division and posterior superior alveolar branch of the maxillary nerve (V2) and innervate different regions along the dental arch (▶ Fig. 19.11b).
        - The **anterior superior alveolar** nerve supplies the mucosa, gingiva, and teeth from the maxillary incisors and canines.
        - The **middle superior alveolar nerve,** which is variable in presentation, transmits somatic sensations from the mucosa, gingiva, and maxillary teeth in the region of the premolars and mesiobuccal root of the first molar.
        - The **posterior superior alveolar** nerve innervates the mucosa and teeth in the molar region.
    - On the **palatal surface** of the arch, the **nasopalatine** and **greater palatine nerves** of **V2** transmit GSA input from the gingiva and alveolar mucosa.
- Mandibular Dental Arch (▶ Table 19.10) (see ▶ Fig. 19.11a)
    - In the region of the mandibular arch, the **inferior alveolar nerve**, and its terminal branches, which include the **mental nerve** and **incisive nerve**, carry sensory input received from the facial side of the alveolar mucosa and gingiva in the region of the incisors to the premolars of the mandibular arch.
    - The **buccal branch of V3** supplies the **facial side** of the alveolar mucosa and gingiva in the **mandibular molar region.**
    - The **lingual nerve of V3** transmits sensory input from the **lingual surface** of the mandibular gingiva and alveolar mucosa.
- Specific innervation to the teeth of the dental arches is covered in Chapter 25.

19.4 Structures of the Oral Cavity Proper (▶ Fig. 19.13)

- The oral cavity proper is the region of the mouth that lies internal to the dental arches and is bound by a roof and floor (▶ Fig. 19.13).
    - The oral cavity extends from the anterolateral border of the upper and lower dental arches posteriorly to the **palatoglossal folds (anterior tonsillar pillars).**
    - The **hard** and **soft palates** comprise the **superior boundary** (roof) of the oral cavity.
    - The **mylohyoid muscle** forms the **inferior border** of the oral cavity and provides structural support for the **floor** of the **mouth.**
- The oral cavity communicates posteriorly with the oropharynx through an opening, the **oropharyngeal (faucial) isthmus**. The isthmus to the oropharynx is bound anteriorly by the **palatoglossal fold** and posteriorly by the **palatopharyngeal folds**.
- Structures found within the oral cavity proper include the **maxillary** and **mandibular dental arches**, the **hard** and **soft palates**, and the **anterior two-thirds** of the **tongue.**
- The ducts of the **submandibular** and **sublingual** open into the floor of the oral cavity proper.

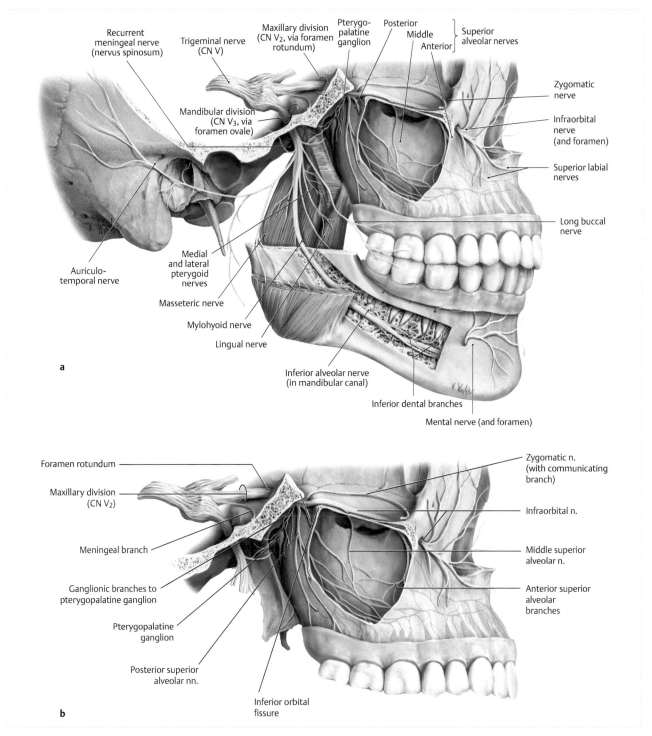

Fig. 19.11 (a, b) Trigeminal nerve distribution of mandibular and maxillary divisions. Right lateral view. The maxillary division of the trigeminal nerve (CN V2) and the mandibular division of the trigeminal nerve (CN V3) innervate the structures of the oral cavity via numerous branches. **(a)** Mandibular division (CN V3). Right lateral view, part of the mandible removed. The mandibular division conveys both motor and sensory information from the region of the lower jaw, tongue, floor of the oral cavity, and TMJ. The long buccal branch (CN V3) transmits somatosensory (GSA) information from the region of the cheek. The mental nerve, a terminal branch of the inferior alveolar nerve (CN V3), conveys GSA information from the lower lip. **(b)** Maxillary division (CN V2). Right lateral view, partially opened right maxillary sinus with the zygomatic arch removed. The infraorbital branch of V2 transmits somatosensory input from the upper lip and alveolar mucosa. From the region of the lip, the infraorbital nerve passes through the infraorbital foramen and then maxillary sinus as the sensory fibers ascend toward the trigeminal ganglion. GSA, general somatic afferent; TMJ, temporomandibular joint. (Reproduced with permission from Schuenke M, Schulte E, Schumacher U. THIEME Atlas of Anatomy Third Edition, Vol 3. © Thieme 2020. Illustrations by Markus Voll and Karl Wesker.)

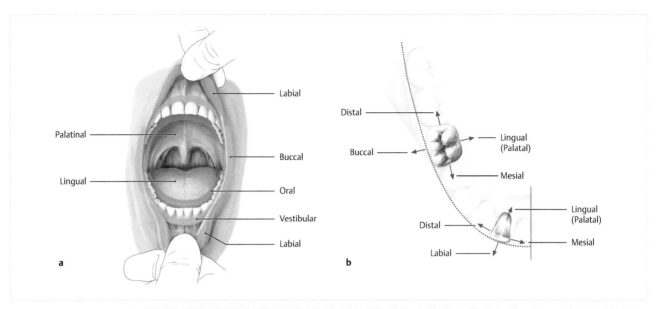

Fig. 19.12 (a) Terms associated with regions of the dental arch, anterior view. Maxillary and mandibular arch demarcate the boundary between the oral vestibule and oral cavity proper. Regions of buccal and labial surface correspond to the outer region of the dental arch, whereas the terms palatal and lingual describe the inner region of the dental arch. (b) Terms used to describe regions of the dental arch and the surfaces of first mandibular molar and lateral mandibular incisor; cranial view of mandibular ramus. Note the terminology changes based on the anatomical region of structure within the arch. (Reproduced with permission from Schuenke M, Schulte E, Schumacher U. THIEME Atlas of Anatomy. Second Edition, Vol 3. © Thieme 2016. Illustrations by Markus Voll and Karl Wesker.)

Table 19.9 Distribution of GSA fibers to maxillary mucosa

Maxillary Arch Region Innervation of Alveolar Mucosa and Gingiva	Anterior Arch (Incisors/Canines)	Middle Arch (Premolar)	Posterior Arch (Molar Regions)
• Facial/Vestibular surface	Anterior superior alveolar nerve of V2 Branch of infraorbital nerve of V2	Middle superior alveolar nerves of V2 Branch of infraorbital nerve of V2	Posterior superior alveolar of V2 Branch of maxillary nerve of V2
• Palatal surface	Nasopalatine nerve of V2	Greater palatine nerve of V2	Greater palatine nerve of V2

Abbreviation: GSA, general somatic afferent.

Table 19.10 Distribution of GSA fibers to mandibular arch mucosa

Mandibular Arch Region Innervation of Alveolar Mucosa and Gingiva	Anterior Arch (Incisors/Canines)	Middle Arch (Premolar)	Posterior Arch (Molar Regions)
• Facial/Vestibular surface	Mental nerve Branch of inferior alveolar of V3	Mental and incisive nerves branch of inferior alveolar of V3	Buccal (long) branch of V3
• Lingual surface	Lingual nerve of V3	Lingual nerve of V3	Lingual nerve of V3

Abbreviation: GSA, general somatic afferent.

19.4.1 Roof of Oral Cavity Proper (▶ Fig. 19.14a–c) (▶ Table 19.11 and ▶ Table 19.12)

- The hard and soft palates form the roof of the oral cavity proper and function to separate the oral cavity from the nasal cavity.

○ The hard palate forms the **anterior two-thirds** of the palatal roof and becomes continuous with the soft palate.

○ Masticatory mucosa covers the two bones comprising the hard palate, the **palatine process of the maxilla,** and **horizontal plate of the palatine bone**. Masticatory mucosa serves to protect the hard palate from masticatory forces during chewing.

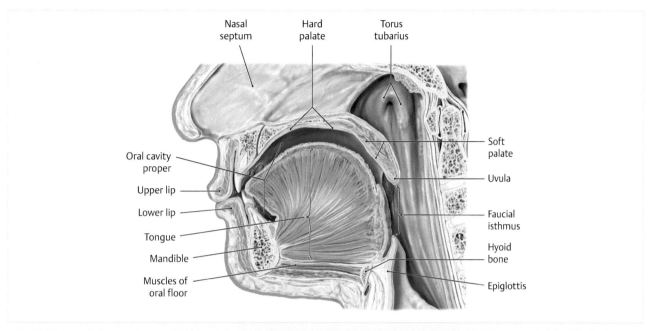

Fig. 19.13 Organization and boundaries of the oral cavity. Midsagittal section; left lateral view. The muscles of the oral floor and the adjacent tongue together constitute the inferior boundary of the oral cavity proper. The roof of the oral cavity is formed by the hard palate in its anterior two-thirds and by the soft palate (velum) in its posterior third. The uvula hangs from the soft palate between the oral cavity and pharynx. The oral cavity, which is located below the nasal cavity and anterior to the oropharynx, communicates posteriorly with oropharynx through an opening, the oropharyngeal isthmus. The oropharynx represents the intersection between the passageway for air and food. (Reproduced with permission from Schuenke M, Schulte E, Schumacher U. THIEME Atlas of Anatomy. Second Edition, Vol 3. © Thieme 2016. Illustrations by Markus Voll and Karl Wesker.)

○ **Somatic sensory** input from the masticatory mucosa covering the hard palate is carried by **GSA** fibers of the **nasopalatine** and **greater palatine** branches of the **maxillary nerve (V2).**
– The **nasopalatine nerve** (V) traverses the nasal cavity and passes through the incisive foramen to transmit sensory input from the anterior one-third of the palate in the region of the four incisors.
– The **greater palatine nerve** (V2) transmits sensory input from most of the palatal mucosa. The greater palatine nerve passes through the **pterygoid fossa** and descends through the **greater palatine canal** before passing through the **greater palatine foramen** to reach the hard palate.
○ **SVE fibers** of the **pharyngeal nerve branch** of **CN X** provide motor innervation via the **pharyngeal nerve plexus** to all skeletal muscles of the soft palate except one, the **tensor veli palatini** muscle. Tensor veli palatini differentiates from the first pharyngeal arch (PA 1) and receives SVE fibers from a terminal motor branch of the **mandibular division of the trigeminal (CN V3)** (▶ Table 19.11).

○ **GSA fibers** of the **lesser palatine nerve** of the **maxillary nerve V2** carry somatic sensory input from the lining mucosa covering the **soft palate, tonsillar fossa,** and **uvulae**. The lesser palatine nerve follows the path of the greater palatine nerve through the pterygopalatine fossa. The lesser palatine nerve passes from the palatal mucosa, enters the **lesser palatine foramen,** and ascends in the **greater palatine canal** with the **greater palatine nerve** to reach the **pterygopalatine fossa** (▶ Fig. 19.15).
○ **Postganglionic parasympathetic (GVE) fibers** arise from the **pterygopalatine ganglion,** a parasympathetic ganglion situated in the **pterygopalatine fossa,** and travel with the **nasopalatine, greater**, and **lesser palatine nerves** of V2 for distribution of GVE fibers to the minor palatal glands of the hard and soft palates.
○ The **greater petrosal nerve (VII)** provides taste **(special visceral afferent [SVA])** for the taste buds associated with the soft and hard palatal mucosa. The taste fibers follow a similar distribution pattern as the GSA and GVE fibers and travel with the lesser palatine and greater palatine nerves of V2.

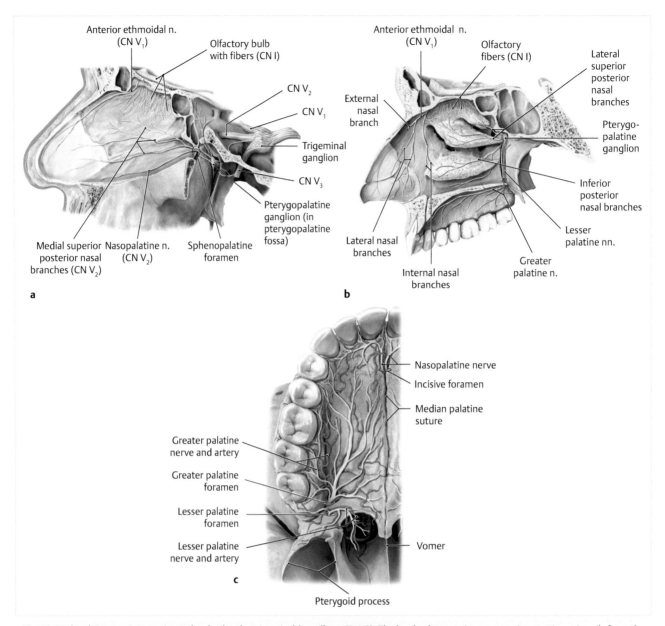

Fig. 19.14 (a–c) Sensory innervation to hard palate by trigeminal (maxillary; CN V2). The hard palate receives sensory innervation primarily from the terminal branches of the maxillary division of the trigeminal nerve (CN V2). **(a)** Left lateral view of branches of maxillary nerve (CN V2) distributed along nasal septum. Demonstrating the nasopalatine nerve passing through the sphenopalatine foramen toward the incisive foramen. The nasopalatine nerve transmits sensory input from the anterior hard palate in the region of the premaxilla. **(b)** Right lateral nasal wall, medial view, showing branches of maxillary nerve demonstrating passage of greater and lesser palatine nerves through the greater palatine canal to exit through the greater and lesser foramen, respectively. **(c)** Inferior view of hard palate. Sensory innervation of palatal mucosa, upper lip, check, and gingiva. Sensory innervation to mucosa of the posterior hard palate and soft palate is mediated by the greater palatine nerve and lesser palatine nerves, respectively. (Reproduced with permission from Schuenke M, Schulte E, Schumacher U. THIEME Atlas of Anatomy Third Edition, Vol 3. © Thieme 2020. Illustrations by Markus Voll and Karl Wesker.)

Table 19.11 Muscles and SVE innervation of soft palate

Muscle	Function	SVE Motor Nerve Supply	Pharyngeal Arch Origin
Levator veli palatini	Elevate soft palate during swallowing	Pharyngeal branch of CN X—motor of pharyngeal plexus	Branchiomeric mesoderm, 4th arch
Palatopharyngeus	Elevates pharynx and larynx Assists in closure of nasopharynx		
Musculus uvulae	Retracts uvulae in posterior superior direction		
Palatoglossus*	Elevates base of tongue Narrow inlet of oropharynx		
Tensor veli palatini	Tense palate; open auditory tube laterally during swallowing/yawning	SVE fibers—motor branch to muscle arises from the main mandibular trunk of V3 (trigeminal nerve)	Branchiomeric mesoderm, 1st arch

Abbreviations: CN, cranial nerve; SVE, special visceral efferent.
Note: *also considered a tongue muscle.

Table 19.12 Summary of palatal innervation

	Hard (anterior)	Hard Palate (posterior)	Soft Palate
Fiber Type	Name of Nerve	Name of Nerve	Name of Nerve
GSA	Nasopalatine nerve (V2) of maxillary	Greater palatine nerve (V2) of maxillary	Lesser palatine nerve (V2) of maxillary
SVA	No innervation	Greater petrosal nerve (VII) via greater palatine nerve (V2) of maxillary	Greater petrosal nerve (VII) via lesser palatine nerve (V2) of maxillary
GVE	Nasopalatine nerve (V2) of maxillary	Greater petrosal nerve (VII) via greater palatine nerve (V2) of maxillary	Greater petrosal nerve (VII) via lesser palatine nerve (V2) of maxillary
SVE	No motor innervation	No motor innervation	• Pharyngeal nerve of CN X via pharyngeal plexus • Muscular branch of V3—tensor veli palatini

Abbreviations: GSA, general somatic afferent; GVE, general visceral efferent, SVA, special visceral afferent; SVE, special visceral efferent.
Note: *SVA and GVE fibers travel with the greater and lesser palatine branches of V2 for distribution to target.

Clinical Correlation Box 19.3: Velopharyngeal Insufficiency

- Proper velopharyngeal closure is essential during swallowing and speech. Structural defects associated with a cleft palate or neurological disorders causing muscle weakness or paralysis due to nerve damage may lead to velopharyngeal insufficiency and result in hypernasal speech and regurgitation while swallowing.

19.4.2 Floor of the Oral Cavity Proper (▶ Fig. 19.16)

- The floor of the oral cavity proper is a small, movable horseshoe-shaped region located medial to the mandible, above the mylohyoid muscle, and below the movable (oral) part of the tongue.
- The contents of the floor of the cavity include a muscular floor comprised of the **mylohyoid** and **geniohyoid muscles**, the **ducts of submandibular** and **sublingual glands**, and the extrinsic muscles which contribute to the **body/root of the tongue** (▶ Fig. 19.16).
  ○ The **tongue** is the largest structure in the floor and rests on the supportive muscles comprising the floor of the oral cavity. The tongue attaches to the mandible and hyoid by the muscles in the root of the tongue.
  ○ The **mylohyoid muscle** forms the **inferior boundary** of the oral cavity proper.
  ○ The **geniohyoid muscle** also contributes to the muscular floor and lies between the mylohyoid muscle and the extrinsic genioglossus muscle of the tongue.
  ○ The region of the muscular floor and the area below constitute a portion of the neck known as the **anterior triangle.** The anterior triangle is further subdivided by the hyoid bone into the **suprahyoid** and **infrahyoid regions**.
    – Three suprahyoid muscles sit below the mylohyoid muscle, the **anterior** and **posterior digastric muscles,** and the **stylohyoid muscles**. The muscles support the floor. The muscles of the suprahyoid and infrahyoid regions play a functional role in swallowing.
- Motor innervation to muscles of the floor and the suprahyoid region is provided by three nerves and reflects the differences in pharyngeal arch development (▶ Table 19.13) (▶ Fig. 19.17)**.**
- A soft, pliable mucous membrane comprised of lining mucosa covers the muscles in the floor of the mouth and reflects onto the ventral (inferior) surface of the tongue. The ventral surface of the tongue remains tethered to the posterior mucosal floor through a midline fold of mucosa known as the **lingual frenulum** (▶ Fig. 19.18).
- The sublingual and submandibular glands lie deep to the mucosa of the floor. The ducts of the glands travel through

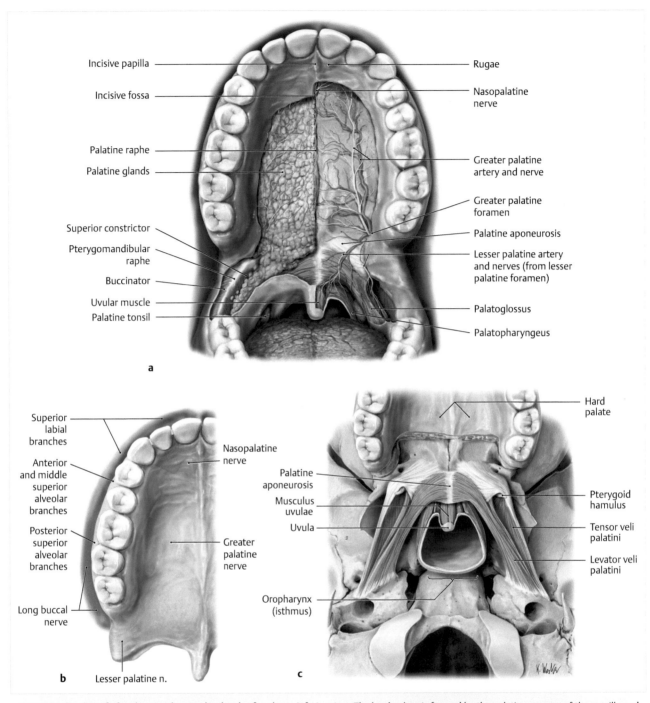

Fig. 19.15 (a–c) Roof of oral cavity showing hard and soft palates, inferior view. The hard palate is formed by the palatine process of the maxilla and the horizontal plate of the palatine bone. It is covered with tough masticatory mucosa, which forms irregular folds anteriorly, known as rugae, which aid in guiding food toward the pharynx. The mucosa is tightly bound to the periosteum of the bones of the hard palate. The palatoglossus, musculus uvulae, and palatopharyngeus are muscles of the soft palate. The two other soft palate muscles, tensor veli palatini and levator veli palatini, are shown in **(c)**. This view also shows the pterygomandibular raphe, which is a ligament formed from the buccopharyngeal fascia. The raphe forms an important landmark for the administration of an inferior alveolar nerve block. The buccinator muscle, a muscle of facial expression, is attached to the pterygomandibular raphe anteriorly. The superior constrictor of the pharynx attaches to pterygomandibular raphe posteriorly. **(b)** Inferior view. The hard palate and soft palate receive sensory innervation primarily from the terminal branches of the maxillary division of the trigeminal nerve (CN V2). Note: The long buccal nerve is a branch of the mandibular division of the trigeminal nerve (CN V3) which transmits sensory information from the lining mucosa of the buccal region. **(c)** Muscles of the soft palate. Inferior view. The soft palate forms the posterior boundary of the oral cavity, separating it from the oropharynx. Muscle of soft palate are all derived from the PA 4 except tensor veli palatini, which is derived from the first pharyngeal arch (PA 1). (Reproduced with permission from Schuenke M, Schulte E, Schumacher U. THIEME Atlas of Anatomy Third Edition, Vol 3. © Thieme 2020. Illustrations by Markus Voll and Karl Wesker.)

Table 19.13 Motor innervation to muscle supporting the floor

Muscle	Pharyngeal Arch (PA) Derivative	Motor Innervation
Geniohyoid (muscular floor)	Not applicable	GSE fibers from C1 carried by the hypoglossal nerve
Mylohyoid (muscular floor)	PA 1	SVE nerve to mylohyoid of mandibular V3
Anterior digastric (suprahyoid)	PA 1	SVE muscular branch of mandibular V3
Posterior digastric (suprahyoid)	PA 2	SVE fibers of facial nerve (CN VII)
Stylohyoid (suprahyoid)	PA 2	SVE fibers of facial nerve (CNVII)

Abbreviations: GSE, general somatic efferent, SVE, special visceral efferent.

the space below the mucous membrane before opening onto the floor of the oral cavity proper.

- ○ The **submandibular duct** (Wharton's duct) opens through two small surface elevations known as the **sublingual papilla (caruncle)**, located along the sides of the lingual frenulum in the midline of the ventral surface of the tongue.
- ○ **Sublingual folds** formed by mucosa on the floor of the mouth contain several small ducts (**ducts of Rivinus**) from the sublingual gland which open onto the floor of the mouth. The largest of these ducts, Bartholin's duct, is the main duct of the sublingual gland, and may also open at the sublingual papilla.
- The **lingual nerve of V3** travels with the **chorda tympani of VII** in the region deep to mucosa lining the floor. The lingual nerve passes between the mylohyoid muscle and hyoglossus muscle, an extrinsic tongue muscle, to provide sensory innervation to the mucosa covering the floor of the mouth, and the anterior two-thirds of the tongue (▶ Fig. 19.19).

19.4.3 Tongue (▶ Fig. 19.20) (▶ Table 19.14)

- The tongue is a large muscular structure important for speech, swallowing, and mastication.
- The oral mucosa covering the tongue varies from specialized to lining mucosa based on function and plays an integral role

in the transmission of sensory input involving taste, temperature, mechanoreception, nociception, and proprioception.

- Anatomically, the tongue consists of three parts: a **movable, oral component**, a **fixed, pharyngeal part**, and **a fixed root.**
- ○ The movable, oral component is in the oral cavity proper. The pharyngeal part forms the anterior wall of the oropharynx. The root of the tongue, which is bound inferiorly by the mylohyoid muscle, and laterally by the sublingual space, is part of the oral cavity situated in the floor of the mouth. The root is anchored by the extrinsic tongue muscles and serves as the point of passage for the neurovascular structures of the tongue.
- The **oral component** (**presulcal**) of the tongue rests on the muscular floor of the oral cavity and comprises the **anterior two-thirds** of the **tongue**. It consists of two parts:
- ○ An **anterior tip**, or apex, which is in contact with the incisors.
- ○ A **body** that extends posteriorly to the **palatoglossal folds** and **sulcus terminalis**.
  - – The **sulcus terminalis** is a shallow v-shaped depression that demarcates the boundary between the oral and pharyngeal parts of the tongue and reflects the embryological origin of each region.
- The oral part of the tongue is movable and possesses a **dorsal** and a **ventral surface**. The dorsal surface of the presulcal tongue faces the palatal roof of the oral cavity, while the ventral surface faces the floor of the mouth.

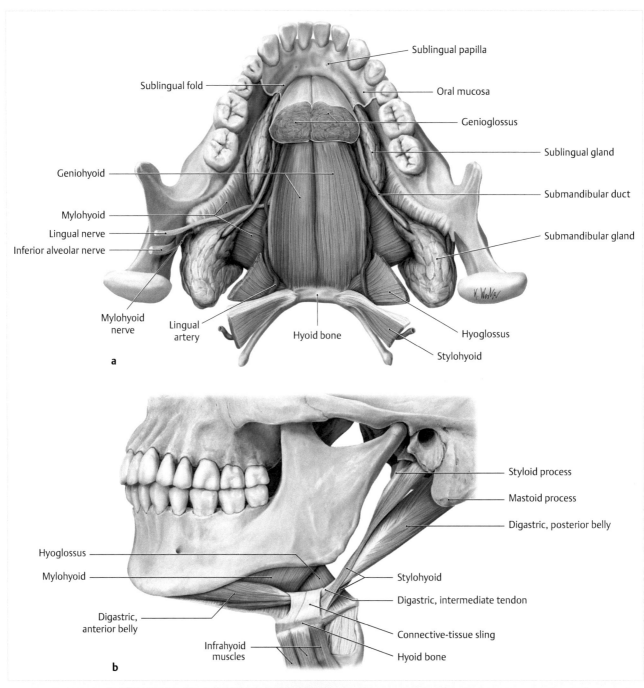

Fig. 19.16 (a, b) Muscles of oral cavity floor. **(a)** Superior view of floor of oral cavity. Genioglossus muscle of the tongue cut. Geniohyoid muscle exposed and covering the mylohyoid. The floor of the oral cavity sits medial to the mandible, below the ventral surface of the tongue, and above the muscular floor that stretches between the mandible. The muscles contributing to the floor reside above the hyoid bone and are known as the suprahyoid muscles. The suprahyoid muscles associated with floor include the mylohyoid, geniohyoid, and anterior digastric. **(b)** Lateral view, suprahyoid muscles. The remaining two suprahyoid muscles are the posterior digastric and stylohyoid. All four muscles function in opening of the jaw and elevating the hyoid bone during swallowing. (▶ Fig. 19.16a: Reproduced with permission from Baker EW. Anatomy for Dental Medicine. Second Edition. © Thieme 2015. Illustrations by Markus Voll and Karl Wesker. ▶ Fig. 19.16b: Reproduced with permission from Schuenke M, Schulte E, Schumacher U. THIEME Atlas of Anatomy Second Edition, Vol 3. © Thieme 2016. Illustrations by Markus Voll and Karl Wesker.)

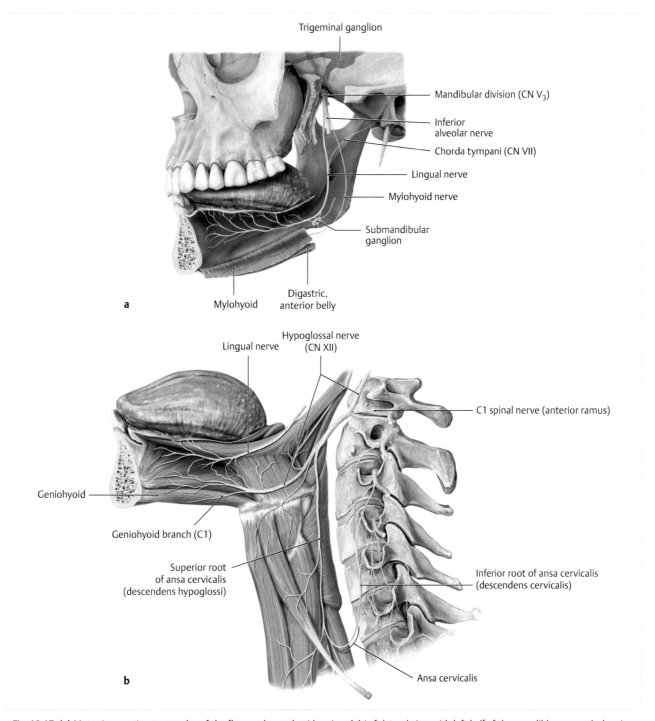

Fig. 19.17 (a) Motor innervation to muscles of the floor and suprahyoid region. **(a)** Left lateral view with left half of the mandible removed, showing the innervation to the tongue and floor of mouth. **(b)** Left lateral view of the muscles of the oral floor. Motor innervation is provided by three cranial nerves and reflects the differences in pharyngeal arch development. The nerve to mylohyoid receives innervation from CN V3; the geniohyoid is innervated by the C1 spinal nerve via the hypoglossal nerve (CN XII). Posterior digastric and stylohyoid muscles receive innervation via the facial nerve (CN VII). (Reproduced with permission from Schuenke M, Schulte E, Schumacher U. THIEME Atlas of Anatomy Third Edition, Vol 3. © Thieme 2020. Illustrations by Markus Voll and Karl Wesker.)

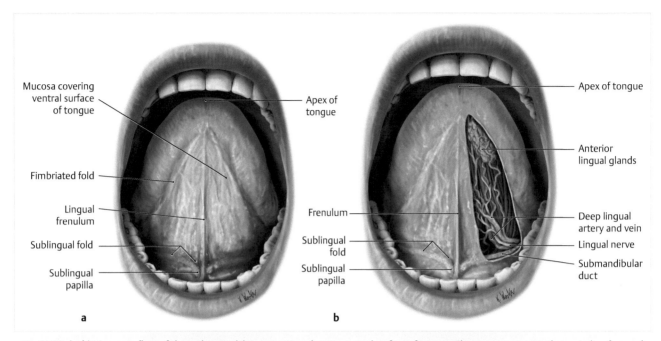

Fig. 19.18 (a, b) Mucosa in floor of the oral cavity. **(a)** Anterior view showing ventral surface of tongue. The mucosa covering the ventral surface and floor of the mouth is a soft pliable mucosa known as lining mucosa. The lingual frenulum is a midline fold of the lingual mucosa which serves to anchor the ventral tongue to the floor of the mouth. Bilaterally, the lining mucosa forms a small fold of tissue located on either side of the lingual frenulum known as the sublingual fold and the sublingual papilla. The sublingual fold covers the sublingual gland, submandibular gland, and submandibular duct that lie on the floor of the oral cavity. **(b)** Anterior view of the ventral tongue. The mucosa is removed on the right side to demonstrate the deep lingual artery, vein, and the lingual nerve (CN V3), which supply the floor of the mouth and ventral tongue. The submandibular duct which sits below the sublingual fold is also visible on the right side. (Reproduced with permission from Schuenke M, Schulte E, Schumacher U. THIEME Atlas of Anatomy Third Edition, Vol 3. © Thieme 2020. Illustrations by Markus Voll and Karl Wesker.)

○ The mucosa covering the dorsal surface of the anterior tongue is **specialized** comprising four types of **lingual papillae: filiform, fungiform, circumvallate (vallate)**, and **foliate papillae.**

○ Lingual papillae are unique to the dorsal surface of the anterior two-thirds of the tongue. Among the four types of the lingual papillae, three of the papillae, **fungiform, foliate,** and **circumvallate (vallate) papillae,** contain **taste buds** which mediate the sensation of taste through **SVA fibers** of **CNs VII** and **IX** (see ▶ Table 19.5 and ▶ Table 19.14).

○ Transmission of somatic sensory innervation from the mucosal surface of the anterior two-thirds of the tongue is through **GSA fibers** of the **lingual branch** of the **mandibular division** of **V3**.

○ The ventral (inferior) surface of the tongue contains the ducts of the minor lingual salivary glands, which open onto the lining mucosa, covering the ventral surface of the tongue.

• The **pharyngeal part** of the **tongue,** also known as the **base** of the **tongue,** lies posterior to the sulcus terminalis, and constitutes the **posterior one-third** or **postsulcal region** of the tongue. The terms pharyngeal or base of the tongue usually refers to the mucosa and tonsillar tissue which are parts of the oropharynx.

○ The posterior tongue forms the floor of the oropharynx and extends posteriorly from the palatoglossal folds to the **glossoepiglottic folds** which connect the pharyngeal part of the tongue with the **epiglottis** of the **larynx** (see ▶ Fig. 19.20).

○ The **base** of the **tongue,** which is immobile and firmly attached by the extrinsic tongue muscles to the mandible and hyoid bone, consists of only a dorsal surface covered with lining mucosa.

○ Lining mucosa of the tongue covers the **lingual tonsils** found on the dorsal surface and reflects laterally onto the **palatine tonsils** in the tonsillar fossa, the pharyngeal walls, and posteriorly onto the epiglottis.

– The oral mucosa, as it reflects from the base of the tongue to the anterior surface of the epiglottis, forms two small mucosal depressions known as the **epiglottic vallecula,** which collect saliva (see ▶ Fig. 19.20).

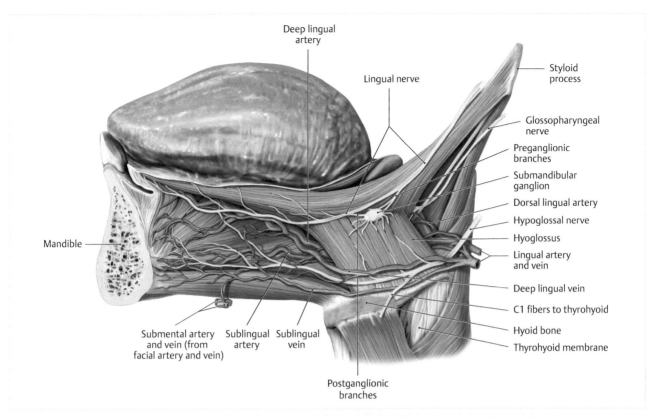

Deep lingual artery

Lingual nerve

Styloid process

Glossopharyngeal nerve

Preganglionic branches

Submandibular ganglion

Dorsal lingual artery

Hypoglossal nerve

Hyoglossus

Lingual artery and vein

Deep lingual vein

C1 fibers to thyrohyoid

Hyoid bone

Thyrohyoid membrane

Mandible

Submental artery and vein (from facial artery and vein)

Sublingual artery

Sublingual vein

Postganglionic branches

Fig. 19.19 Illustration showing the path of the nerves and vessels supplying the tongue; left lateral view; mandible and mylohyoid muscle removed. The nerve supply of tongue reflects to developmental contributions of the pharyngeal arches (PAs 1, 3, and 4). The path of the lingual nerve is shown. GVE and SVA fibers of the chorda tympani travel with the lingual nerve. GVE preganglionic fibers synapse in the submandibular ganglion before supplying submandibular and sublingual glands. SVA fibers transmitting taste from the anterior two-thirds of the tongue travel with lingual nerve. Branches of glossopharyngeal (IX) and vagus (X, not shown) supply the mucosa in the posterior one-third of the tongue and epiglottic regions. GVE, general visceral efferent; SVA, special visceral afferent. (Reproduced with permission from Schuenke M, Schulte E, Schumacher U. THIEME Atlas of Anatomy Third Edition, Vol 3. © Thieme 2020. Illustrations by Markus Voll and Karl Wesker.)

– Lingual papillae are missing from the posterior tongue; however, taste buds are scattered throughout the SSNK epithelial surface and mediate **taste (SVA)** sensation through branches of **CNs IX** and **X** (see ▶ Table 19.14).

- The oral and pharyngeal parts of the tongue exhibit regional differences in mucosal innervation that reflect the pattern of embryonic development.

- Tongue movement occurs through four pairs of **extrinsic** and **intrinsic muscles,** which are separated in the midline by a vertically oriented **fibrous lingual septum**. The lingual septum blends posteriorly with the connective tissue of the hyoglossus muscle to insert onto the hyoid bone and separates the anterior tongue into right and left halves (▶ Fig. 19.21, ▶ Table 19.15).

- The extrinsic and intrinsic muscles work cooperatively to facilitate the complex actions required for mastication, deglutition (swallowing), and phonation (speaking). A description of these neuromuscular functions is covered in Chapter 22.

- **Extrinsic muscles** originate from skeletal elements outside the tongue and function to change the (bodily) position of the tongue (▶ Fig. 19.21a). The extrinsic muscles contribute to the root of the tongue.

- The **intrinsic muscles**, which do not have skeletal attachments, are restricted to the body and root of the tongue, and function to alter the shape of the tongue (▶ Fig. 19.21b).

  ○ Intrinsic muscles fall into three principal groups based on fiber orientation.

- All extrinsic and intrinsic muscles receive motor innervation by **general somatic efferent (GSE) fibers** carried by the **hypoglossal nerve (CN XII)**, except for the **palatoglossus muscle,** which is innervated the **pharyngeal nerve plexus** (▶ Table 19.15).

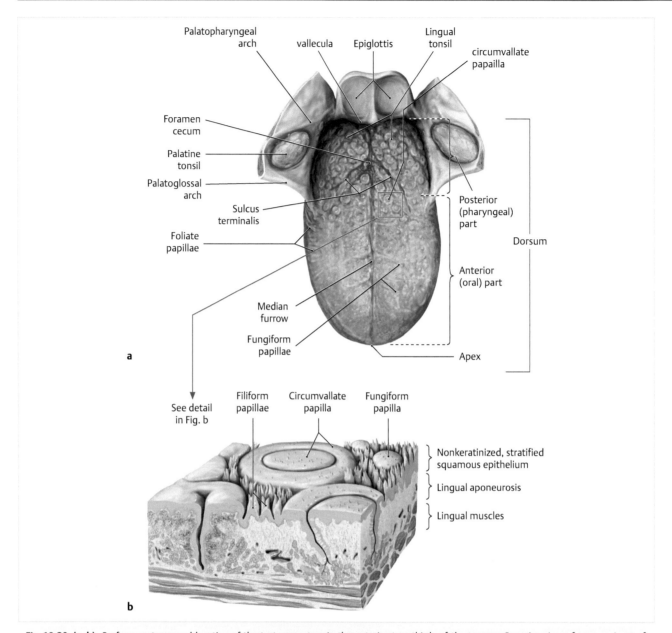

Fig. 19.20 (a–b) Surface anatomy and location of the taste receptors in the anterior two-thirds of the tongue. Superior view of tongue. Inset of papillae shown in Fig. b. **(a)** The parts of the tongue are the root, the ventral (inferior) surface, the apex (tip), and the dorsal (superior) surface. The V-shaped furrow on the dorsum (sulcus terminalis) divides the dorsal surface into an oral portion (comprising the anterior two-thirds) and a pharyngeal portion (comprising the posterior one-third). The mucosa of the anterior dorsum is composed of numerous surface elevations known as lingual papillae. The papillae are divided into four morphologically distinct types: Circumvallate—large dome-shaped structures anterior to the sulcus terminalis, surrounded by a circular depression and minor serous salivary glands; Fungiform—appear as well-vascularized mushroom-shaped structures scattered over the dorsum of anterior two-thirds of tongue; contain mechanical and thermal receptors as well as taste buds; Foliate—located on the lateral margin of the anterior two-thirds of tongue; lie in close association with minor serous salivary glands; Filiform—appear thin and triangular shaped and sensitive to tactile stimuli (the only lingual papillae without taste buds). Lingual papillae are absent from the pharyngeal part of the tongue; however, isolated taste buds are located in the mucous membranes of the soft palate and pharynx (not shown). Humans can perceive five basic taste qualities: sweet, sour, salty, bitter, and umami. (Reproduced with permission from Schuenke M, Schulte E, Schumacher U. THIEME Atlas of Anatomy Third Edition, Vol 3. © Thieme 2020. Illustrations by Markus Voll and Karl Wesker.)

Table 19.14 Summary of GSA and SVA fiber distribution for tongue

Region	Structure Innervated	Fiber Type (Modality)	Name of Nerve	Pharyngeal Arch (PA) Origin
Oral dorsal surface (anterior two-thirds of tongue)	Specialized mucosa (SSK)	GSA (pain, temperature, touch)	Lingual nerve of V3	Lateral lingual swellings of mandibular process (PA 1) overgrows region of second arch (PA 2)
	Lingual papillae* only in anterior 2/3 • Fungiform • Foliate • Circumvallate	SVA (taste)	Chorda tympani (VII) travels with lingual nerve to tongue; innervates the fungiform; glossopharyngeal (IX) supplies circumvallate and foliate	
Oral ventral surface (anterior two-thirds)	Lining mucosa (SSNK) No papilla	GSA	Trigeminal (V); lingual nerve branch of V3	
Pharyngeal (posterior one-third) *dorsal surface only	Lining mucosa (SSNK) No papillae	GSA	Glossopharyngeal (IX); lingual and tonsillar branches	Proximal hypobranchial eminence of third arch (PA 3)
	Taste buds—no papillae	SVA	Glossopharyngeal (IX); lingual and tonsillar branches	
Base of tongue and epiglottis *dorsal surface only	Lining mucosa (SSNK) No lingual papillae	GSA	Vagus (X); internal laryngeal branch of superior laryngeal nerve (X)	Distal hypobranchial eminence of fourth arch (PA 4) Epiglottic swelling of fourth arch (PA 4)
	Taste buds—no papillae	SVA	Vagus (X); internal laryngeal branch of superior laryngeal nerve (X)	

Abbreviations: GSA, general somatic afferent; SSK, stratified squamous keratinized; SSNK, stratified squamous nonkeratinized; SVA, special visceral afferent.

Table 19.15 Extrinsic and intrinsic musculature of tongue

Muscle Group	Muscle	Function	Motor Nerve Supply	Origin of Muscle
Intrinsic group	Superior longitudinal	Shortens and curls apex of tongue upward		
	Inferior longitudinal	Shortens and curls tongue downward		
	Vertical	Widens/compresses tongue		
	Transverse	Narrows and lengthens tongue	GSE fibers Hypoglossal nerve	Mesoderm of occipital somites
Extrinsic group	Genioglossus	Protrusion of tongue		
	Hyoglossus	Depresses tongue		
	Styloglossus	Retrusion of tongue Elevation of tongue		
	Palatoglossus	Elevation of the root of tongue Narrow the entrance of oropharynx isthmus for swallowing	SVE fibers Pharyngeal nerve of X; motor branch of pharyngeal plexus	Branchiomeric (pharyngeal arch [PA]) mesoderm of PA 4

Abbreviations: GSE, general somatic efferent, SVE, special visceral efferent.

19.5 Structures of Pharyngeal Region (▶ Fig. 19.22, ▶ Fig. 19.23, ▶ Fig. 19.24, ▶ Fig. 19.25, ▶ Fig. 19.26, ▶ Fig. 19.27)

- The pharynx which is a muscular tube extending from the base of the skull (basioccipital) to the cricoid cartilage (C6), consists of three functional divisions: **nasopharynx, oropharynx,** and **laryngopharynx** (▶ Fig. 19.22).

- Each division develops in association with the pharyngeal arches and the innervation pattern of the mucosa and muscles reflects the embryonic development of the pharyngeal region.
- Transmission of motor and sensory innervation to the pharyngeal region occurs through the **pharyngeal nerve plexus** (▶ Fig. 19.23).
- The contributions to the pharyngeal nerve plexus include:
  ○ **SVE motor fibers** to the plexus which travel with the **pharyngeal branch** of the **vagus (CN X).**
  ○ **General visceral afferent (GVA) fibers** transmitted by the **pharyngeal branch** of **CN IX** form the predominant

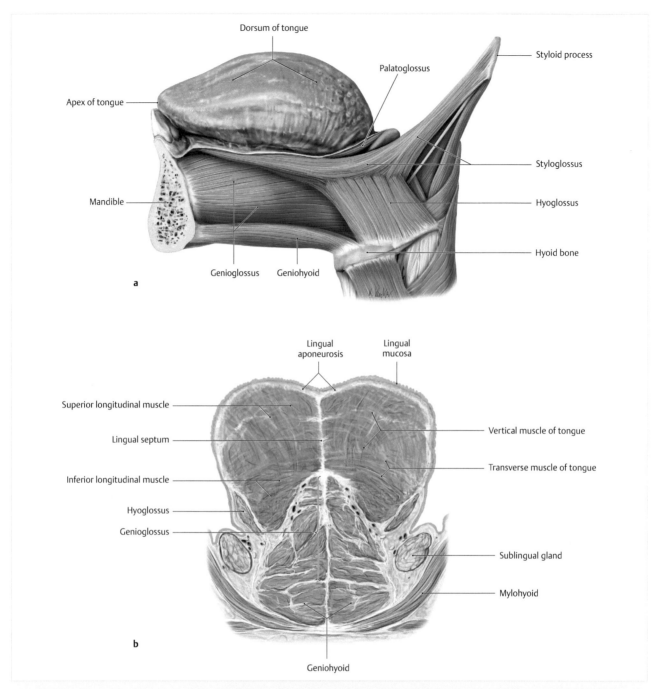

Fig. 19.21 (a, b) Muscles of the tongue. (a) Left lateral view. (b) Anterior view of a coronal section. Tongue movement occurs through four pairs of extrinsic and intrinsic tongue muscles which are separated in the midline by a fibrous lingual septum. The extrinsic and intrinsic muscles work cooperatively to facilitate the complex actions involved in the motor functions of mastication, swallowing, and speaking. The muscles of the tongue arise primarily from occipital somites with the exception of the palatoglossus muscle which is derived from the fourth pharyngeal arch. The hypoglossal nerve (CN XI) provides innervation to all extrinsic and intrinsic glossus muscles except the palatoglossus which is innervated by the pharyngeal plexus. (Reproduced with permission from Schuenke M, Schulte E, Schumacher U. THIEME Atlas of Anatomy. Second Edition, Vol 3. © Thieme 2016. Illustrations by Markus Voll and Karl Wesker.)

Table 19.16 Muscles of pharyngeal regions

Muscle	Function	SVE Motor Nerve Supply	Pharyngeal Arch Origin
Salpingopharyngeus	Elevates the upper and lateral parts of pharyngeal wall	Pharyngeal motor branch of vagus (CN X)	Fourth pharyngeal arch
Palatopharyngeus	Elevates the oropharynx and aids in closing the nasopharynx	Pharyngeal motor branch of vagus (CN X)	Fourth pharyngeal arch
Stylopharyngeus * only muscle innervated by SVE of CN IX	Elevate the pharynx and expand the sides of the pharynx	Glossopharyngeal nerve (CN IX)	Third pharyngeal arch
Superior constrictor	Constricts the upper portion of the pharynx	Pharyngeal motor branch of vagus (CN X)	Fourth pharyngeal arch
Middle constrictor	Constricts the middle portion of the pharynx	Pharyngeal motor branch of vagus (CN X)	Fourth pharyngeal arch
Inferior constrictor • Cricopharyngeus Lower division of inferior constrictor at esophageal boundary	Constricts inferior portion of the pharynx • Upper esophageal sphincter, normally constricted; relaxes as part of swallowing reflex	• Pharyngeal motor branch of vagus (CN X) • Recurrent laryngeal branch of vagus (CN X)	Fourth and sixth pharyngeal arches

Abbreviation: SVE, special visceral efferent.

sensory fiber type associated with **pharyngeal nerve plexus**. The lingual and tonsillar branches of CN IX also provide smaller sensory (GSA/GVA) contributions to the plexus.

○ **Postganglionic sympathetic** (laryngopharyngeal) fibers from the superior cervical ganglion provide vasomotor control to vessels in the region and travel through the plexus.

– *Some authors still describe the cranial root of the accessory nerve (CN IX) as a component of the pharyngeal plexus; however, the literature is controversial and current studies indicate that the motor fibers of the plexus are part of the vagus since the fibers arise from the nucleus ambiguus. The accessory nerve travels with the vagus during its intracranial course and may share the same connective tissue (CT) sheath as it exits the jugular foramen.*

• The pharyngeal muscular wall consists of **three inner longitudinal muscles** and **three outer circular muscles**:

○ The inner longitudinal muscles include the **palatopharyngeus, salpingopharyngeus,** and **stylopharyngeus** which function to elevate the pharynx.

○ The three outer circular muscles are known as the **superior, middle,** and **inferior constrictor muscles** and

function to narrow and constrict the pharynx (▶ Fig. 19.24).

• The muscles comprising the pharyngeal wall originate primarily from branchiomeric (pharyngeal arch) mesoderm of the fourth pharyngeal arch (PA 4) and receive motor innervation from SVE fibers carried by pharyngeal plexus.

○ Two notable exceptions are the **stylopharyngeus** and the **cricopharyngeus** muscle.

○ The stylopharyngeus muscle originates from the third pharyngeal arch (PA 3) and receives SVE fibers from the **glossopharyngeal nerve (CN IX).**

○ The **cricopharyngeus muscle** is a component of the lower division of the inferior constrictor muscle and forms the upper esophageal sphincter (UES). The muscle develops in association with the sixth pharyngeal arch (PA 6) and receives motor (SVE) innervation from the **recurrent (inferior) laryngeal nerve** of **CN X** (▶ Table 19.16). The three constrictor muscles exhibit an overlapping arrangement of muscle fibers with small apertures (openings) created between the adjacent constrictor muscles.

○ The openings allow for the passage of various structures, including nerves and vessels to enter the lumen of the pharyngeal tube (▶ Fig. 19.25) (▶ Table 19.17).

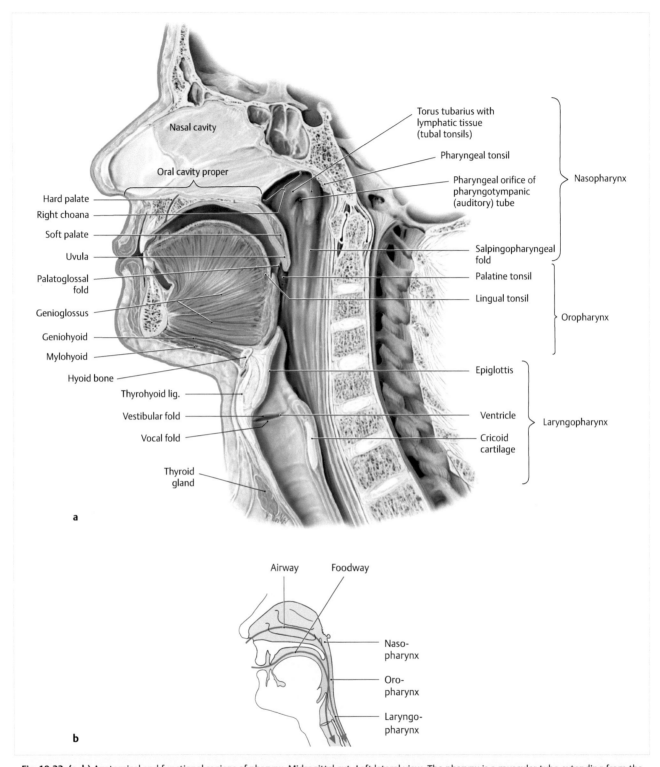

Fig. 19.22 (a, b) Anatomical and functional regions of pharynx. Midsagittal cut. Left lateral view. The pharynx is a muscular tube extending from the base of the skull to the cricoid cartilage (C6) and is anatomically divided into three functional regions: nasopharynx (air passage), oropharynx (food passage), and laryngopharynx/hypopharynx. (Reproduced with permission from Schuenke M, Schulte E, Schumacher U. THIEME Atlas of Anatomy Third Edition, Vol 3. © Thieme 2020. Illustrations by Markus Voll and Karl Wesker.)

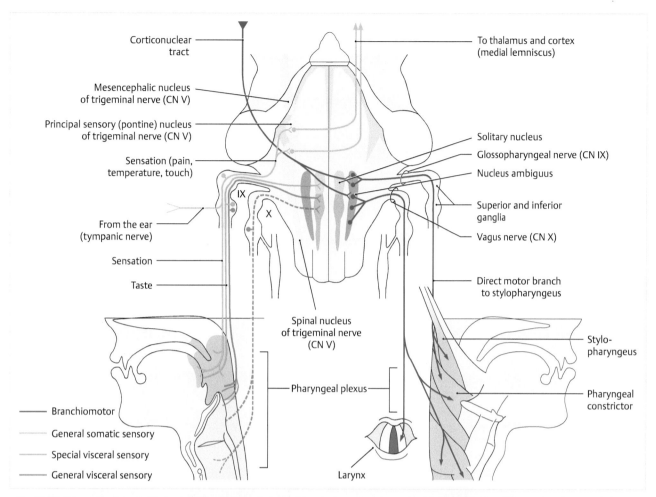

Corticonuclear tract

Mesencephalic nucleus of trigeminal nerve (CN V)

Principal sensory (pontine) nucleus of trigeminal nerve (CN V)

Sensation (pain, temperature, touch)

From the ear (tympanic nerve)

Sensation

Taste

To thalamus and cortex (medial lemniscus)

Solitary nucleus

Glossopharyngeal nerve (CN IX)

Nucleus ambiguus

Superior and inferior ganglia

Vagus nerve (CN X)

Direct motor branch to stylopharyngeus

Spinal nucleus of trigeminal nerve (CN V)

Pharyngeal plexus

Stylopharyngeus

Pharyngeal constrictor

Branchiomotor

General somatic sensory

Special visceral sensory

General visceral sensory

Larynx

Fig. 19.23 Schematic diagram illustrating the pharyngeal plexus. The pharynx receives sensory and motor innervation via the pharyngeal plexus, formed by both the glossopharyngeal (CN IX) and vagus (CN X) nerves, along with postganglionic sympathetic fibers from the superior cervical ganglion. The sensory contributions from the glossopharyngeal nerve (CN IX) include GSA, GVA, and SVA. These sensory fibers contain primary afferent neuron cell bodies in the superior and inferior glossopharyngeal ganglia. The fibers terminate in the spinal trigeminal nucleus (GSA) or the nucleus solitarius. Motor fibers of the vagus which innervate the pharyngeal muscles and contribute to the pharyngeal plexus originate from lower neurons found in the nucleus ambiguus. Note: The vagus predominantly contributes motor fibers to plexus, the stylopharyngeus is supplied directly by CN IX. The pharyngeal motor plexus also provides motor innervation to the palatal muscles with the exception of the tensor veli palatini muscle which is supplied by the mandibular branch of the trigeminal (CN V3) (not shown). GSA, general somatic afferent; GVA, general visceral afferent; SVA, special visceral afferent. (Reproduced with permission from Schuenke M, Schulte E, Schumacher U. THIEME Atlas of Anatomy Third Edition, Vol 3. © Thieme 2020. Illustrations by Markus Voll and Karl Wesker.)

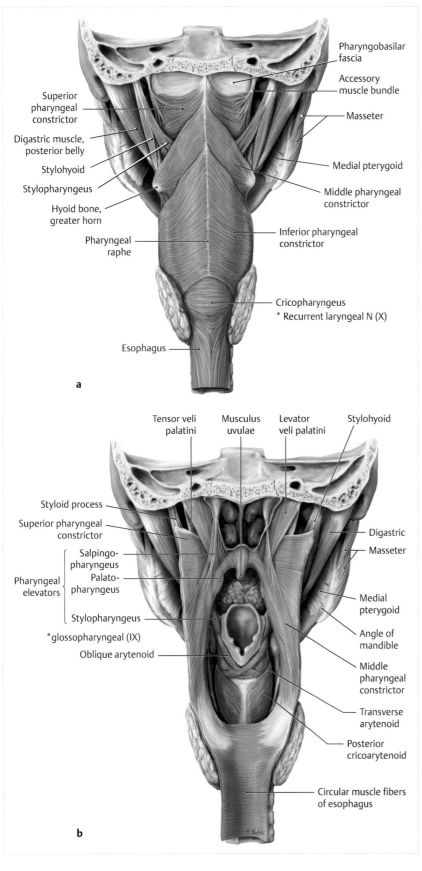

Fig. 19.24 (a, b) Anatomical organization of pharyngeal muscles. Posterior view. **(a)** The muscles of the pharynx consist of three outer circular and three inner longitudinal groups of muscles. The outer circular group consists of the superior, middle, and inferior constrictors. Note how the inferior constrictor fibers blend with circular fibers of esophagus along the inferior border of the constrictor. **(b)** The posterior wall of pharynx open and constrictors retracted back. The inner longitudinal group of pharyngeal muscles consists of three muscles: the salpingopharyngeus, palatopharyngeus, and stylopharyngeus which act as pharyngeal elevators allowing the pharynx to shorten and widen during swallowing. (Reproduced with permission from Schuenke M, Schulte E, Schumacher U. THIEME Atlas of Anatomy Third Edition, Vol 3. © Thieme 2020. Illustrations by Markus Voll and Karl Wesker.)

19.5.1 Nasopharynx (▶ Fig. 19.26 and ▶ Fig. 19.27) (▶ Table 19.18)

- The nasopharynx forms the proximal part of the upper respiratory tract and delivers air from the nasal cavity to the trachea.
- The nasopharynx lies inferior to the base of the skull, attaching to the basioccipital bone, superior to the soft palate and oropharynx, and posterior to the nasal cavity, with which it communicates via the paired nasal choanae.
- The posterolateral wall of the nasopharynx consists of the **superior constrictor muscle** derived from the fourth pharyngeal arch, the **pharyngeal tonsils,** and the openings of the **auditory (pharyngotympanic; eustachian) tubes**.
  - The **auditory tubes** are bilateral cartilaginous structures that connect the nasopharynx to the middle ear cavity and open onto the posterior lateral walls of the nasopharynx.
  - The auditory tube develops from the **first pharyngeal pouch** and functions to equalize air pressure during swallowing.
- A mucous membrane comprised of respiratory mucosa covers the superior region of the nasopharynx and auditory tube before gradually transitioning to lining mucosa toward the soft palate.
- The mucosa of auditory tube and nasopharynx receives GSA fibers from the **tympanic branch of CN IX** via the **tympanic plexus**.
- The nasopharynx also receives GSA innervation from the **pharyngeal branch** of **maxillary (V2) division** of trigeminal nerve and a minor contribution from the sensory component of the **pharyngeal plexus.**

19.5.2 Oropharynx

- The oropharynx, which lies posterior to the oral cavity proper and inferior to the nasopharynx, extends from the soft palate to the level of the hyoid bone and the superior border of the epiglottis.
- The **palatoglossal** and **palatopharyngeal muscles,** which comprise the anterior and posterior tonsillar pillars, form the anterolateral walls of the oropharynx and demarcate the **oropharyngeal inlet (isthmus).**
  - The base (root) of the tongue lies in the midline between the tonsillar pillars and forms the anterior boundary of the oropharynx.
  - The palatine tonsils reside in a small depression located between the tonsillar pillars, known as the tonsillar fossa. The **palatine tonsil** along with **lingual** and **pharyngeal tonsils** found within the pharyngeal wall constitute a ring of nonencapsulated, lymphatic tissue referred to as **Waldeyer's ring** (▶ Fig. 19.27).
  - The oropharynx communicates anteriorly with the oral cavity proper through the oropharyngeal inlet.

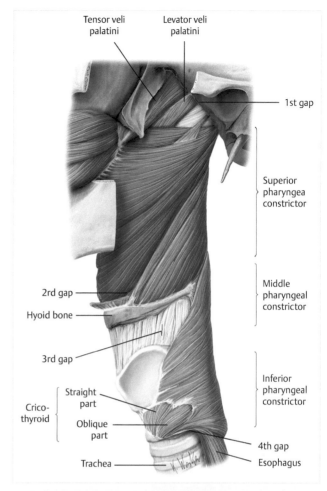

Fig. 19.25 Overlapping arrangement of the pharyngeal constrictors. Left lateral view. The pharyngeal constrictors exhibit an overlapping arrangement of muscle fibers with small apertures created which allow the passage of nerves and vessels to enter the lumen of the pharynx. The gaps are labeled first to fourth and the structures passing through are listed in ▶ Table 19.17. (Reproduced with permission from Schuenke M, Schulte E, Schumacher U. THIEME Atlas of Anatomy Third Edition, Vol 3. © Thieme 2020. Illustrations by Markus Voll and Karl Wesker.)

- The posterolateral wall of the oropharynx consists of superior and middle constrictors, which receive motor innervation from the pharyngeal branch of the **vagus (CN X) through the pharyngeal plexus.**
- Lining mucosa comprised of SSNK epithelium covers the oropharynx. Some areas, such as the base of the tongue, epiglottis, and soft palate, may also contain taste buds.
- **Sensory innervation** to the **oropharynx** is mediated through the pharyngeal, lingual, and tonsillar nerve branches of the glossopharyngeal (CN IX) via the **pharyngeal plexus.**

Glossopharyngeal neuralgia manifests as extreme intermittent unilateral pain which may occur in the pharynx, tonsillar region, base of the tongue, or ear due to mucosal irritation of the pharyngotympanic tube. Attacks, which may last several seconds or minutes, manifest as sharp, stabbing pain radiating from the throat to the ear or vice versa and may be triggered by chewing, swallowing, talking, coughing, or sneezing. Mucosal inflammation and irritation of the glossopharyngeal nerve (CN IX) also serve as the basis for the attack. Due to the involvement of glossopharyngeal nerve, cardiac arrhythmias and syncope (fainting) may also be associated with symptoms. Glossopharyngeal neuralgia is relatively rare and may be indicative of other underlying pathologies such as multiple sclerosis or oropharyngeal cancer. These causative factors may also serve as early warning signs of these diseases.

19.5.3 Laryngopharynx (see ► Fig. 19.27)

- **Laryngopharynx (hypopharynx)** constitutes the inferior division of the pharynx and extends from the level of the epiglottis (C3) to the cricoid cartilage at vertebral level C6, where the muscular wall of the laryngopharynx transitions into the esophagus.
- The laryngopharynx lies posterior to the **larynx** with the **middle** and **inferior constrictor muscles** forming the posterolateral walls. Muscle fibers in the lower part of the inferior constrictor muscle become continuous with the esophagus to form the **cricopharyngeus**, which serves as the upper esophageal sphincter.
  - The **pharyngeal branch of CN X** via the **pharyngeal plexus** supplies motor innervation to the middle and inferior constrictor muscles.
  - The **recurrent laryngeal branch of CN X** provides the majority of **SVE fibers** to the cricopharyngeus muscle before its passage into the infraglottic cavity.
- Lining mucosa covers the walls of the laryngopharynx and reflects onto the aryepiglottic folds of the larynx to form the **piriform recess**, a small cavity (fossa) located on each side of the laryngeal inlet and bound by the lateral wall of laryngopharynx (► Fig. 19.27).
  - During swallowing food is directed around the laryngeal inlet along the piriform recess to enter the esophagus.
- **Sensory (GSA** and **GVA)** fibers from branches of the g**lossopharyngeal nerve (CN IX)** of the pharyngeal plexus transmit afferent input from the mucosal lining of the laryngopharynx.
- The laryngopharynx communicates with the larynx through the laryngeal opening (**laryngeal inlet),** which is a region bound by the **epiglottis, aryepiglottic folds,** and **laryngeal cartilages** (► Fig. 19.27).
  - During swallowing, the muscles of laryngopharynx propel the food bolus toward the esophagus, while the epiglottis inverts to close the laryngeal inlet and protect the airway.

19.6 Structures of the Larynx (► Fig. 19.28, ► Fig. 19.29, ► Fig. 19.30; ► Table 19.19)

- The larynx is a short mucosal lined tube that sits anterior to the laryngopharynx between vertebral levels C3 and C6.
- The larynx functions to protect the airway and deliver air to the lower respiratory tract by connecting the laryngopharynx with the trachea. The larynx is also responsible for producing sound (phonation) through the movement of the vocal (ligaments) cords. The process of phonation is described in Chapter 22.

19.6.1 Cartilage and Muscles of the Larynx

- Nine laryngeal cartilages provide the structural framework for the larynx. The **epiglottic, thyroid** , and **cricoid corniculate** are three large, unpaired cartilages. The **arytenoid, cuneiform**, and **corniculate** are smaller, paired cartilages (► Fig. 19.28a, b).
  - The cartilages, which are held together by several ligaments, connective tissue membranes, and the extrinsic and intrinsic laryngeal muscles, form two flexible joints, the **cricothyroid joint** and **cricoarytenoid joint**. The paired joints permit rotation of the cartilages and aid in the movement of the vocal cords.
  - **Intrinsic laryngeal muscles** alter the length, tension, and position of the **vocal ligaments (cords)**, and affect the diameter of the **rima glottidis.** The rima glottidis is the opening between the vocal cords and is opened or closed by the action of the laryngeal muscles moving the laryngeal cartilage (► Fig. 19.28c).
  - **Extrinsic laryngeal muscles** include the **suprahyoid group** and **infrahyoid group,** which attach to the hyoid bone or thyroid cartilage and function to elevate or depress the larynx during swallowing.
    - Three laryngeal muscles function to **adduct** the **vocal folds**, one functions to **abduct** the **folds** and one alters the **tension** of the **vocal folds** (► Table 19.19).

19.6.2 Regions of the Larynx

- The **laryngeal inlet (aditus)** serves to connect the larynx and laryngopharynx and leads into the lumen of the laryngeal tube. The wall of the laryngeal tube consists of two folds, the **vestibular fold (false vocal cords)** and **vocal fold (true vocal cords)** respectively (► Fig. 19.29a, b).
  - The vestibular folds lie superior to the vocal folds and protect the larynx. The folds consist of a mucous membrane covering the **vestibular ligament**. Closure of the folds occurs reflexively during coughing, micturition, and defecation and causes an increase in intrathoracic and intra-abdominal pressure.

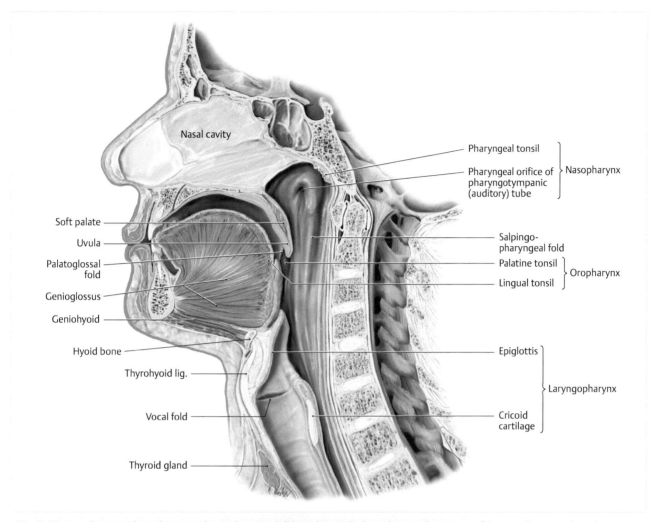

Fig. 19.26 Nasopharynx and oropharynx midsagittal section, left lateral view. The boundaries and structures of the nasopharynx and oropharynx are demarcated. Notable features of the nasopharynx include the two auditory tubes located in the lateral wall (one shown in sagittal view) and the midline position of the pharyngeal tonsil. The oropharynx lies inferior to the nasopharynx. The mucosa of the auditory tube and nasopharynx transmits somatosensory (GSA) input from the tympanic branch of CN IX via tympanic plexus. The region also carries sensory (GSA) information from the pharyngeal branch of the maxillary division of the trigeminal (CN V2), and a small contribution from the pharyngeal plexus (not shown). The posterior boundary of the oropharynx contains the superior and middle constrictor muscles which receive motor innervation from the pharyngeal plexus. The lining mucosa of the oropharynx transmits sensory information via pharyngeal, lingual, and tonsillar branches of the glossopharyngeal nerve (CN IX). GSA, general somatic afferent. (Reproduced with permission from Schuenke M, Schulte E, Schumacher U. THIEME Atlas of Anatomy Third Edition, Vol 3. © Thieme 2020. Illustrations by Markus Voll and Karl Wesker.)

○ The vocal folds, also known as the **vocal cords**, represent a fold of laryngeal mucosa containing the **vocal ligaments (conus elasticus)** and **vocalis muscle.**

– Opening and closing of the vocal folds and the subsequent change in diameter of the rima glottidis occur during breathing and speaking (phonation).

• The vestibular and vocal folds subdivide the laryngeal cavity into three regions, namely, the **supraglottic (vestibule)**, the **ventricle**, and the **subglottic (infraglottic)** regions (▶ Fig. 19.29b) (▶ Table 19.20).

○ The **supraglottic (vestibule)** extends from the inlet to the region above the vestibular fold (false vocal cords). Closure of the inlet occurs during swallowing and protects the respiratory tract from aspiration of foreign material.

○ The **ventricle** is the space between the false and true vocal cords.

○ The **subglottic (infraglottic) cavity** lies below the true vocal cords and leads into the trachea.

19.6.3 Laryngeal Mucosa

• The mucosa covering the laryngeal surface is primarily lining mucosa comprised of pseudostratified ciliated columnar epithelium which continues into the tracheal passageway. The laryngeal mucosa is loosely bound to the underlying submucosa and may become inflamed.

○ One notable exception to the type of mucosa occurs in the region of the **vocal folds (true vocal cords).** The vocal cords which vibrate and modulate airflow during speaking and respiration contain a lining mucosa comprised of SSNK epithelium. The SSNK epithelium is tightly bound to the underlying elastic connective tissue.

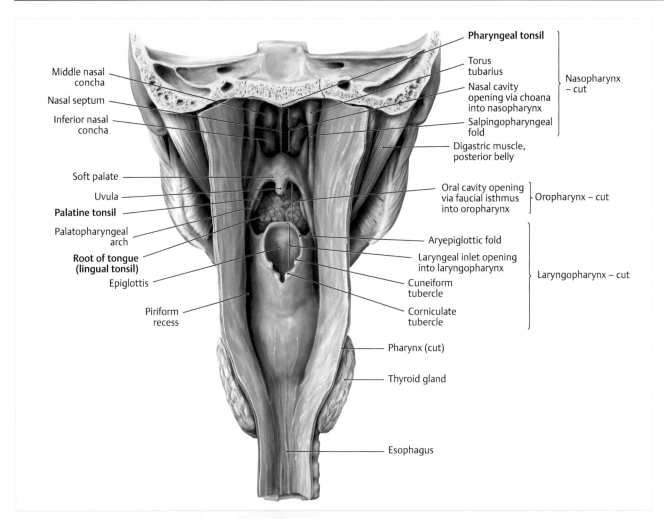

Fig. 19.27 Posterior view of opened pharynx. Schematic demonstrates the relationship and position of the Waldeyer's ring; a tonsillar ring of nonencapsulated lymphatic tissue, comprised of the pharyngeal tonsil, palatine tonsils, and lingual tonsils. Additional smaller groups of lymphatic tissue also contribute but are not shown. (Reproduced with permission from Schuenke M, Schulte E, Schumacher U. THIEME Atlas of Anatomy Third Edition, Vol 3. © Thieme 2020. Illustrations by Markus Voll and Karl Wesker.)

Table 19.17 Structures traversing the apertures in the pharyngeal wall

Region of Aperture (Boundary)	Structures Passing through Aperture	Function of Structure
From base of skull to superior constrictor muscle *aperture above superior constrictor muscle	• Auditory tube • Levator palatini muscle • Ascending pharyngeal artery • Ascending palatine artery	• Auditory tube functions to equalize air pressure between middle ear cavity and nasopharynx • Levator palatini elevates soft palate to close nasopharynx

Between superior and middle constrictor muscles	• Stylopharyngeus muscle
	• Glossopharyngeal nerve branches:
	  ○ Pharyngeal nerve
	  ○ Lingual nerve
	  ○ Tonsillar nerve
	• Tonsillar branch of ascending palatine artery
	• Stylohyoid ligament
		Stylopharyngeus muscle elevates pharynx and expands pharyngeal walls during swallowing and speech
		Glossopharyngeal branches (CN IX) provide
		• GSA and SVA to mucosa of posterior one-third of tongue
		• Contribute GSA and GVA fibers via pharyngeal plexus and innervate mucosa of pharyngeal wall

Between middle and inferior constrictor muscles	• Internal laryngeal nerve branch of vagus (CN X) • Superior laryngeal artery and vein	Vagus nerve branches (CN X) • Carries GSA and SVA fibers to mucosa epiglottis, base of tongue, and laryngeal mucosa above the true vocal cords
Below the inferior constrictor muscle	• Recurrent (inferior) laryngeal nerve of X →continues as inferior laryngeal once it enters through aperture • Inferior laryngeal artery and vein	Vagus nerve branches (CN X) • Carries GSA/GVA fibers to mucosa inferior to true vocal cords • Carries SVE fibers to intrinsic laryngeal muscle

Abbreviations: GSA, general somatic afferent; GVA, general visceral afferent; SVA, special visceral afferent; SVE, special visceral efferent.

Table 19.18 Components of the nasopharynx

Muscular Wall	Function	Motor (SVE) Innervation	Nasopharyngeal Mucosa	Sensory Innervation	PA Derived
Levator palatini	Elevates soft palate posterosuperiorly to close nasopharynx	Pharyngeal plexus Motor fibers from CN X	Transition from **respiratory mucosa** to **lining mucosa** toward inferior boundary of nasopharynx in the region of soft palate Epithelium associated with mucosa: pseudostratified epithelium (PSCC) →stratified squamous nonkeratinized	Tympanic and tubal branches of tympanic plexus of CN IX to auditory tube Pharyngeal branch of V2 mucosa of auditory tube and superior part of nasopharynx	Fourth arch
Superior constrictor	Narrow diameter of nasopharynx	Pharyngeal plexus Motor fibers from CN X		Pharyngeal branch of V2 to superior part of nasopharynx Pharyngeal plexus GSA/GVA fibers from CN IX	Fourth arch
Stylopharyngeus	Elevates pharynx—expansion of lateral walls	Glossopharyngeal (CN IX)		Pharyngeal plexus GSA/GVA fibers from CN IX	Third arch

Abbreviations: GSA, general somatic afferent; GVA, general visceral afferent; PA, pharyngeal arch; SVE, special visceral efferent.

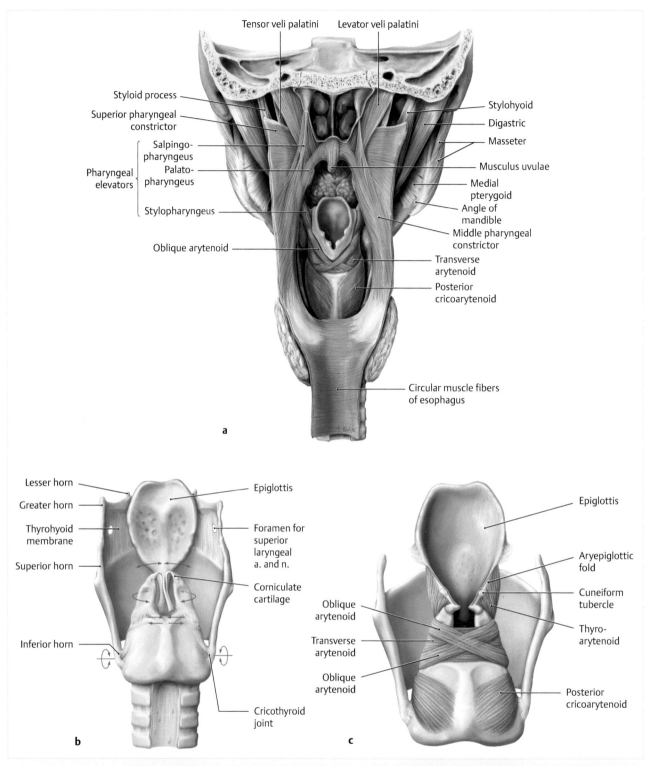

Fig. 19.28 (a–c) Region of the laryngopharynx and structure of the larynx. Posterior view. Constrictor muscle opened and retracted demonstrating the anatomical position of the laryngopharynx and its relationship to the larynx. The laryngopharynx lies posterior to the larynx with the middle and inferior constrictor muscles forming the posterior and inferior boundary of the pharynx. The laryngopharynx represents the region where the muscular wall of the laryngopharynx transitions into esophagus. The region of the larynx is shown in boxed area with a high-power view shown in **(c)**. **(b)** Cartilaginous structures of the larynx. Posterior view. Arrows indicate the direction of movement of the cricothyroid joints. **(c)** Laryngeal muscles. Posterior view. The laryngeal muscles move the laryngeal cartilages relative to one another, affecting the tension and/or position of the vocal folds. (Reproduced with permission from Schuenke M, Schulte E, Schumacher U. THIEME Atlas of Anatomy Third Edition, Vol 3. © Thieme 2020. Illustrations by Markus Voll and Karl Wesker.)

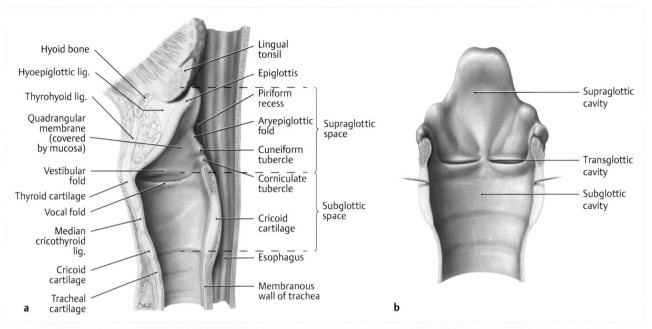

Fig. 19.29 Regions of the larynx. **(a)** Midsagittal section viewed from the left side, demonstrating the anatomical position of the larynx and its relationship to the laryngopharynx. The position of the vocal folds and functional levels are also demarcated. The larynx lies anterior to the laryngopharynx. Air enters through the laryngeal inlet formed by the epiglottis and aryepiglottic folds. Lateral to the aryepiglottic folds are pearshaped mucosal fossae (piriform recesses), which channel food past the larynx and into the laryngopharynx and into the esophagus. The interior of the larynx is lined with mucous membrane that is loosely applied to its underlying tissue (except at the vocal folds). The laryngeal cavity can be further subdivided with respect to the vestibular and vocal folds. The vocal folds (true vocal cords) demarcate the developmental boundary between region of the larynx derived from PA 4 and the area derived from PA 6. **(b)** Posterior view of larynx and esophagus cut along the midline and spread open. Note the functional levels of larynx. (Reproduced with permission from Schuenke M, Schulte E, Schumacher U. THIEME Atlas of Anatomy Third Edition, Vol 3. © Thieme 2020. Illustrations by Markus Voll and Karl Wesker.)

Table 19.19 Intrinsic laryngeal muscles

Muscle	Action on Vocal Cords	Muscle Group	SVE Motor Nerve Supply
Lateral cricoarytenoid	• Adduct vocal cords	Intrinsic group	Recurrent laryngeal nerve
Transverse (inter-) arytenoid	• Close rima glottidis		
Oblique (inter-) arytenoid			
Thyroarytenoid	• Adduction of vocal cords • Close rima glottidis		
Vocalis *inferior fibers thyroarytenoid	• Decrease (shorten) tension vocal cords • No action on rima glottidis		
Posterior cricoarytenoid	• Abduct vocal cords • Open rima glottidis		
Cricothyroid	• Increase tension (lengthen) vocal ligament • No action on rima glottidis	Extrinsic **laryngeal group	External **laryngeal nerve of CN X

Abbreviation: SVE, special visceral efferent.

Notes: *Posterior cricoarytenoid is the only intrinsic muscle to abduct the cords.

**Cricothyroid is the only laryngeal muscle not innervated by recurrent laryngeal nerve; only muscle located outside the larynx that still functions to change vocal cord position.

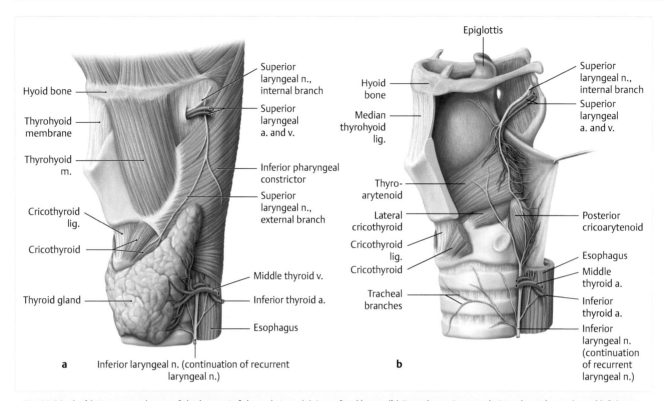

Fig. 19.30 (a, b) Neurovasculature of the larynx. Left lateral view. **(a)** Superficial layer. **(b)** Deep layer. Removed: Cricothyroid muscle and left lamina of thyroid cartilage. Retracted: Pharyngeal mucosa. The superior laryngeal nerve (CN X) divides into the internal laryngeal and external laryngeal nerves. The internal laryngeal nerve passes into the larynx through the thyrohyoid membrane and innervates the mucosa above the vocal folds, including the supraglottic and transglottic regions. The recurrent laryngeal nerve enters the larynx through an opening below the cricopharyngeus muscle to provide motor and sensory innervation to the vocal folds and infraglottic regions. (Reproduced with permission from Schuenke M, Schulte E, Schumacher U. THIEME Atlas of Anatomy Third Edition, Vol 3. © Thieme 2020. Illustrations by Markus Voll and Karl Wesker.)

Clinical Correlation Box 19.5: Lesions of Vocal Folds

- The mucosa covering vocal cords is susceptible to trauma, inflammation, and epithelial dysplasia.
- Depending on the causative factor, the outcome may involve noncancerous (benign) growths known as **nodules** or **polyps** that develop in mucosa covering vocal folds. Nodules and polys may affect voice quality.
- Inflammation of the vocal cords is known as laryngitis and may result from vocal overuse, colds, allergies, smoking, and acid reflux. Laryngitis may lead to a transient or permanent change in the quality of sound produced.
- Widespread inflammation in the mucosal connective tissue due to infection or allergic reaction may result in the accumulation of tissue fluid (edema) and obstruct the laryngeal aperture (rima glottidis), leading to an increased risk of asphyxiation.
- The stratified squamous epithelium which covers the vocal folds is susceptible to dysplasia and is a frequent site of laryngeal squamous cell carcinoma in smokers. Squamous cell carcinoma in the larynx often manifests as a sore throat and ear pain.

19.6.4 Innervation to Larynx

- Innervation to the region of the larynx is mediated through several branches of the vagus nerve (▶ Fig. 19.30).
  - Specifically, the **superior laryngeal nerve** of **CN X,** which carries motor and sensory fibers, divides into two terminal branches, the **external laryngeal nerve of CN X** and **internal laryngeal branches of CN X.**
    - The **external laryngeal nerve** supplies one muscle, the cricothyroid muscle, derived from PA 4 mesoderm. This muscle functions to lengthen the vocal cords and increase cord tension which alters voice pitch.
    - The **internal laryngeal nerve of CN X,** which pierces the thyrohyoid membrane to gain access to the laryngeal cavity, carries GSA and GVA fibers from the laryngeal mucosa in the region of the epiglottis and to the mucosa covering the supraglottic region *above* the vocal folds. The internal laryngeal nerve also carries SVA from the epiglottic region. This region is developmentally associated with PA 4.
  - The region of mucosa which covers the vocal folds and the subglottic (infraglottic) area transmits sensory information via the **recurrent laryngeal branch of the vagus (CN X).**

Table 19.20 Divisions of laryngeal cavity

Laryngeal Region	Mucosal Boundaries	Innervation of Mucosa
Supraglottic cavity (laryngeal vestibule)	Laryngeal inlet to vestibular folds (supraglottic mucosa)	GSA/GVA—internal laryngeal branch of CN X
Ventricle/Transglottic space (intermediate laryngeal cavity)	Region between vestibular fold and superior border of vocal folds (anterior subglottic mucosa)	GSA/GVA—internal laryngeal branch of CN X
Subglottic cavity (Infraglottic space)	Vocal folds to the inferior border of cricoid cartilage (subglottic mucosa)	GSA/GVA—recurrent laryngeal branch of CN X **also carry proprioceptive fibers from muscle spindles

Abbreviations: GSA, general somatic afferent; GVA, general visceral afferent.

– The recurrent laryngeal nerves on the right and left sides follow slightly different courses; however, on both sides of the neck, the recurrent laryngeal nerve enters the laryngeal cavity by passing through the aperture below the lower border of the inferior constrictor (see ▶ Table 19.20).
• The specific pathway and functional role of the superior laryngeal nerve (CN X) in mediating laryngeal function are covered in Chapters 20 to 22.

Questions and Answers

1. The cranial nerve branch that provides both motor (SVE) and general somatic sensation (GSA) innervation to skeletal muscles and mucosa derived from the region of the sixth pharyngeal is the _____ nerve.
   a) Superior laryngeal
   b) External laryngeal
   c) Pharyngeal plexus
   d) Internal laryngeal
   e) Recurrent laryngeal

Level 2: Moderate

Answer E: The recurrent laryngeal nerve is a terminal branch of the vagus (CN X) and supplies the mucosa in the region of the vocal folds and below. It also innervates all of the intrinsic muscles of the larynx. The recurrent laryngeal does not innervate the external laryngeal muscle, known as the cricothyroid muscle. The recurrent laryngeal nerve is the nerve associated with the derivatives of PA 6. The superior laryngeal (A) carries motor and sensory fibers and divides into two terminal branches, the (B) external laryngeal and (D) internal laryngeal nerves of CN X. The external laryngeal supplies motor innervation to the cricothyroid muscle. The cricothyroid muscle is derived from PA 4. The internal laryngeal branch carries sensory fibers to the mucosa above the vocal folds. This region also develops in association with PA 4. The pharyngeal plexus (C) contains both motor fibers from the vagus and sensory fibers primarily from the glossopharyngeal. The pharyngeal plexus provides innervation to the oropharynx and not the region of the larynx. The motor and sensory fibers of the plexus are associated with PA 4 (vagus) and PA 3 (glossopharyngeal).

2. Which of the following is an extrinsic tongue muscle derived from paraxial mesoderm of the fourth pharyngeal arch (PA 4) and innervated by a branch of the vagus (CN X)?
   a) Hyoglossus
   b) Styloglossus
   c) Palatopharyngeus
   d) Genioglossus
   e) Palatoglossus

Level: Moderate

Answer E: The palatoglossus muscle is an extrinsic tongue muscle derived from PA 4 mesoderm and is innervated by the vagus (pharyngeal plexus). The palatopharyngeus (C) is also derived from PA 4 and innervated by the pharyngeal plexus (CN X); however, the palatopharyngeus contributes to the posterior wall of the pharynx and not the tongue. The other muscles listed, hyoglossus (A), styloglossus (B), and genioglossus (D), are extrinsic muscles of the tongue, which develop from occipital somites. These muscles are not considered pharyngeal arch derivatives. They are innervated by GSE fibers of hypoglossal nerve (CN XII).

3. The name of the embryological precursor that gives rise to the lining mucosa covering the pharyngeal portion of the tongue is the _____.
   a) Copula
   b) Lateral lingual swellings
   c) Tuberculum impar
   d) Hypobranchial eminence
   e) Arytenoid swellings

Level 1: Easy

Answer D: The hypobranchial eminence may be divided into proximal and distal components. The proximal component gives rise to lining mucosa covering the posterior one-third (pharyngeal part) of the tongue. The distal segment of the hypobranchial eminence and the epiglottic swelling give rise to the base of the tongue, while the arytenoid swelling (E) contributes to the larynx. The lateral lingual swellings (B) overgrow the tuberculum impar (C) and form the mucosa of the anterior two-thirds of the tongue. The copula (A) is also overgrown and doesn't contribute to the mucosa of the tongue.

4. Each of the following palatal muscles receives SVE innervation from a branch of the vagus nerve **EXCEPT** one. Which one is the exception?
   a) Palatoglossus
   b) Palatopharyngeus
   c) Musculus uvulae
   d) Tensor veli palatini
   e) Levator veli palatini

Leve 2: Moderate

Answer D: The exception is the tensor veli palatini muscle. All the muscles listed are palatal; however, the tensor veli palatini muscle is derived from the first pharyngeal arch (PA) and receives SVE motor innervation from the mandibular division of the trigeminal nerve (V3). All other palatal muscles, the palatoglossus (**A**), the palatopharyngeus (**B**), musculus uvulae (**C**), and the levator veli palatini (**E**) are muscles derived from branchiomeric mesoderm of PA 4. Each muscle is innervated by the pharyngeal nerve branch of CN X, which contributes SVE motor fibers to the pharyngeal plexus.

5. Which nerve lesion would lead to a loss of taste on the left side of the anterior two-thirds of tongue?
   a) The left lingual nerve in the floor of the oral cavity
   b) The right chorda tympani as it passes through pterygopalatine fossa
   c) The left inferior alveolar nerve in the infratemporal fossa
   d) The left hypoglossal nerve in the floor of mouth
   e) The right superior salivatory nucleus

Level 2: Moderate

Answer A: The chorda tympani of VII travels (hitch-hikes) with the lingual nerve in the floor of the oral cavity; therefore, an injury to the lingual nerve will also damage the accompanying chorda tympani. This will cause a deficit of both SVA and GSA input on the same side (ipsilateral) of the lesion. In this case, the left lingual nerve traveling with the chorda tympani of VII (SVA) to the left side of the anterior two-thirds of the tongue is damaged, leading to the loss of taste. The right chorda tympani (**B**), if damaged, would cause a loss of taste on the right side.

The left inferior alveolar nerve of V3 (**C**) and its terminal branches carry GSA fibers to the mandibular arch and provide sensory input to the teeth, gingiva, lower lip, and chin. The hypoglossal nerve (**D**), which is susceptible to damage in the floor of the mouth, carry only GSE (motor) fibers to the tongue. Damage to the left hypoglossal nerve at that point would cause the tongue to deviate to the left (side of the lesion) when protruded. The right superior salivatory nucleus (**E**) contains the preganglionic cell bodies for the GVE neurons of VII. The damage would affect lacrimation and salivation but not taste directly.

20 Overview of Orofacial Pathways Part I—Trigeminal and Facial Nerves

20.1 Introduction

The trigeminal (CN V), facial (CN VII), glossopharyngeal (CN IX), vagus (CN X), and hypoglossal (CN XII) nerves develop con-comitantly with the pharyngeal arches during orofacial development and innervate defined regions of the head and neck. Among the cranial nerves supplying the head and neck region, CNs V, VII, IX, X, and XII play an integral role in transmitting afferent and efferent responses necessary for proper sensori-motor function of the orofacial region. Most oropharyngeal functions, including swallowing, chewing, and speech, depend on sensory input or feedback to coordinate and modulate the bilateral motor activity of the orofacial muscles. The planning, execution, and control of motor behaviors is a complex neural process that requires input from multiple peripheral sensory modalities. The absence of correct input or difficulty in processing sensory information may result in abnormal or inaccurate motor output. In the region of the face and oral cavity, the trigeminal and facial nerves provide critical sensory feedback which aid in the execution of mastication, swallowing, and speech articulation. The lower cranial nerves work cooperatively in the region of the oropharynx to coordinate these oromotor activities. The present chapter is designed to serve as a detailed reference describing the path of the trigeminal (CN V) and facial (CN VII) nerves to provide a foundation for understanding the oromotor activities involved in mastication, swallowing, and articulation. Chapter 21 covers the lower CNs IX, X, and XII.

20.2 Trigeminal Nerve: Overview of Functional Components

- The trigeminal nerve is the largest of cranial nerves and provides the primary source of **somatic afferent** (general somatic afferent [GSA]) input from the face, oral and nasal cavities, orbit, jaw, teeth, temporomandibular joint (TMJ), and anterior tongue.
- The trigeminal nerve, which develops in association with the first pharyngeal arch and frontonasal regions, consists of a **large sensory root** formed by the convergence of the **ophthalmic (V1)**, **maxillary (V2)**, and **mandibular (V3)** divisions of the trigeminal nerve.
  - In the periphery, the terminal branches of the **ophthalmic, maxillary,** and **mandibular divisions** exhibit a defined distribution pattern that correlates with distinct regions of the head (▶ Fig. 20.1a–c).
- A small motor root associated with mandibular (V3) division transmits **efferent (special visceral efferent [SVE])** fibers and innervates the skeletal muscles derived from the first pharyngeal arch.
- An overview of the functional modalities carried by each of the three divisions of the trigeminal nerve is provided in ▶ Table 20.1 and ▶ Table 20.2.
- The distribution of the sensory and motor divisions and the course of each peripheral branch are outlined in the following section and summarized in ▶ Table 20.4, ▶ Table 20.5, ▶ Table 20.6, ▶ Table 20.7, ▶ Table 20.8, ▶ Table 20.9.

20.2.1 Overview of Peripheral Distribution of Trigeminal GSA Fibers

Afferent Sensory Receptors

- The general sensory afferent (GSA) fibers receive input from two classes of receptors: **exteroreceptors** and **proprioceptors** (▶ Table 20.3; also see Chapter 11).
  - Exteroreceptors convey two types of sensations classified as **protopathic** and **epicritic**.
  - Proprioceptors provide kinesthetic feedback concerning the position and movement of joints.
- Two additional functions associated with GSA fibers include:
  - GSA fibers function in reflexive activity and comprise the afferent limb of several protective reflexes. GSA input also provides feedback to motor neurons for sensorimotor control involved in mastication, swallowing, and articulation (see Chapter 22).
  - Postganglionic parasympathetic fibers arising from autonomic ganglia of CNs III, VII, and IX accompany

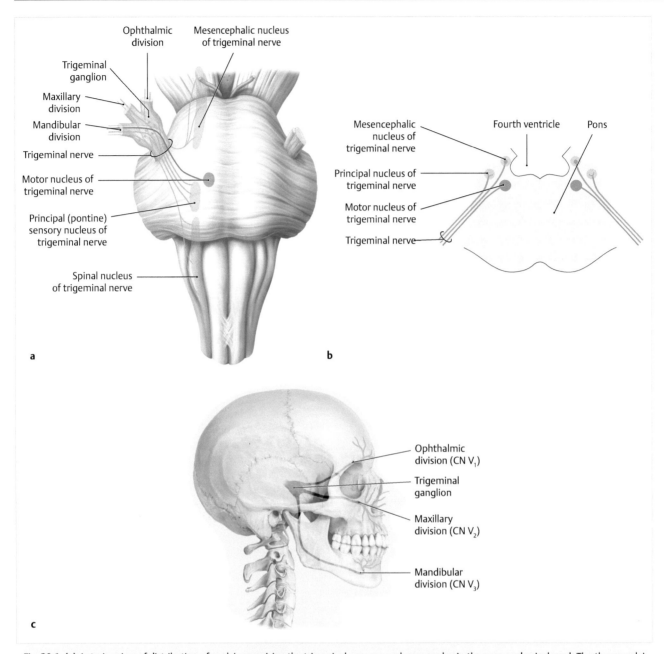

Fig. 20.1 **(a)** Anterior view of distribution of nuclei comprising the trigeminal sensory nuclear complex in the pons and spinal cord. The three nuclei which comprise the trigeminal sensory complex include the mesencephalic, chief (principal), and spinal trigeminal nucleus. A small motor root arises from the motor nucleus of the trigeminal nerve and provides motor innervation to the muscles of mastication. **(b)** Schematic cross section through the pons at the level of trigeminal nerve. **(c)** Right lateral view of distribution pattern of the terminal divisions of the trigeminal nerve. (Reproduced with permission from Schuenke M, Schulte E, Schumacher U. THIEME Atlas of Anatomy Third Edition, Vol 3. © Thieme 2020. Illustrations by Markus Voll and Karl Wesker.)

Table 20.1 Overview of trigeminal motor components

Overview of Trigeminal Motor Component							
Functional Component	Trigeminal Division	Associated Ganglia	Associated Nuclei	Trigeminal (V3) Major Motor Branches	Distribution /Functional Role	Key Features of General Path	Clinical Signs of Peripheral Damage
SVE	Voluntary motor to the skeletal muscles derived from PA 1	**Mandibular (V3)**	Not applicable	SVE neurons **Trigeminal motor nucleus** in pons	**Main trunk** • Medial pterygoid **Anterior division** • Masseteric* • Deep temporal* • Lateral pterygoid **Posterior division** • Nerve to mylohyoid • Nerve to anterior digastric	Mediates chewing, bolus formation, and articulation Innervates masticatory jaw opening and jaw closing muscles: Masseter, temporalis, pterygoids; mylohyoid, digastric (anterior), tensor tympani, tensor veli palatini	Motor branch emerges from pons and passes inferior to sensory ganglia of CN V (trigeminal ganglia). SVE fibers travel with mandibular (V3) sensory division; divide to form anterior and posterior divisions of V3 in the infratemporal fossa	Weakness and atrophy of jaw; ipsilateral deviation of jaw during opening

Abbreviation: SVE, special visceral efferent.
Note: *Mixed, carry motor and sensory fibers.

Table 20.2 Overview of trigeminal sensory components

Functional Component	Trigeminal Division	Associated Ganglia	Associated Nuclei	Trigeminal (V) Major Sensory Branches of Division	Region Innervated/ Functional Role	Key Features of General Path
GSA	Types of receptors for each division Extero-receptors: • Epicritic (tactile) • Protopathic (pain, temperature, crude touch) Proprioceptor (positional information)	Ophthalmic CN V1	**Trigeminal (semilunar) sensory ganglion** Contains primary afferent cell bodies for epicritic and protopathic	**Trigeminal sensory nuclear complex** • Trigeminal spinal nucleus • Chief (principal) sensory nucleus • Mesencephalic nucleus * (contains primary afferent neurons of proprioceptive fibers)	• Lacrimal • Frontal • Nasociliary • Meningeal	Upper one-third of face, orbit, sinuses Afferent input from forehead, upper eyelid, cornea, conjunctiva, orbit, nasal cavity, dorsum of the nose, frontal, ethmoid, and sphenoid paranasal sinuses, and dura of some of the anterior cranial fossa	• V1 enters the cranium from the orbit via the **superior orbital fissure** • V1 passes through lateral wall of **cavernous sinus**
		Maxillary CN V2	**Trigeminal (semilunar) sensory ganglion** Contains primary afferent cell bodies for epicritic and protopathic	**Trigeminal sensory nuclear complex** • Trigeminal spinal nucleus • Chief (principal) sensory nucleus • Mesencephalic nucleus * (contains primary afferent neurons of proprioceptive fibers)	• Meningeal • Zygomatic • Infraorbital • Posterior superior alveolar • Ganglionic (pterygopalatine) branches	Middle one-third of face; nose, maxillary arch/palate Afferent input from upper lip, lateral and posterior portions of nose, upper cheek, anterior temple, mucosa of nasal cavity, maxillary sinus, maxillary dental arch, palatal region of oral cavity, nasopharynx, and part of dura in middle cranial fossa	• V2 enters the cranium from pterygopalatine fossa via the **foramen rotundum** • V2 passes through inferolateral wall of **cavernous sinus**

(Continued)

345

Table 20.2 (*Continued*) Overview of trigeminal sensory components

Functional Component	Trigeminal Division	Associated Ganglia	Associated Nuclei	Trigeminal (V) Major Sensory Branches of Division	Region Innervated/ Functional Role	Key Features of General Path
	Mandibular CN V3	Trigeminal (semilunar) sensory ganglion Contains primary afferent cell bodies for epicritic and protopathic	Trigeminal sensory nuclear complex • Trigeminal spinal nucleus • Chief (principal) sensory nucleus • Mesencephalic nucleus * (contains primary afferent neurons of proprioceptive fibers)	• Meningeal • Buccal (long) • Deep temporal* • Masseteric* • Auriculotemporal • Lingual • Inferior alveolar *mixed nerves (motor and sensory)	Lower one-third of face; jaw/TMJ Afferent input from lower lip, chin, posterior cheek, temple, mucosa of lower jaw, anterior two-thirds of the tongue, and portions of the dura of anterior and middle cranial fossae	• V3 enters the cranium from the **infratemporal fossa** via the foramen **ovale** • Fibers pass **outside cavernous sinus** as they pass to ganglion

• Clinical signs of peripheral damage: Hemifacial anesthesia; loss of sensation to ipsilateral side of face if sensory root damaged; specific pattern of loss isolated to specific division indicates extracranial injury.
Abbreviations: GSA, general somatic afferent; TMJ, temporomandibular joint.

Table 20.3 Overview of somatosensory receptors for orofacial region

Sensory Modality Transmitted	Receptor Location	Primary Afferent Fiber Type
Exteroceptors **Protopathic sensations** (pain, temperature, crude touch, itch)	Each division transmits **protopathic** sensations from specific locations based on dermatome pattern V1: Orbit, upper one-third of face, sinuses V2: Middle one-third of face; nasal cavity; teeth (pulp) upper jaw; palate V3: Lower one-third of face; oral cavity; anterior tongue; teeth (pulp); lower jaw	Nonencapsulated free nerve endings: Thinly myelinated Aδ fibers Unmyelinated C fibers Includes polymodal nociceptors that respond to noxious and nonnoxious stimuli (temperature; mechanical distortion, chemicals)
Exteroceptors **Epicritic sensations** (tactile; fine discrimination, pressure, vibration, stretch; conscious proprioception, stereognostic input)	Each division transmits **epicritic** sensations from specific locations based on dermatome pattern V1: Orbit, upper one-third of face, sinuses V2: Middle one-third of face; nasal cavity; teeth (pulp); upper jaw; palate V3: Lower one-third of face; oral cavity; anterior tongue; teeth (pulp) lower jaw	Encapsulated and nonencapsulated mechanosensory receptors Large diameter, myelinated Aβ fibers Low threshold mechanoreceptors Include: Meissner's and Ruffini's corpuscles, Merkel's cells
Proprioceptors (detect the static position and movement of joints and muscles' stereognostic input) Unconscious proprioception	Each division transmits unconscious proprioceptive sensations from the specific location based on dermatome pattern V1: Extraocular eye muscles V2: PDL, gingiva V3: PDL, gingiva, TMJ; Muscle spindles in jaw closing muscles; tongue; * Mechanoreceptors play a critical role in managing bite force during mastication	Encapsulated proprioceptors Myelinated large diameter Aα (Ia) and type II Muscle spindles Mechanoreceptors (myelinated Aβ fibers); Ruffini's corpuscles

Abbreviations: PDL, periodontal ligament; TMJ, temporomandibular joint.

Table 20.4 Ophthalmic division (V1): Peripheral distribution of (GSA) sensory branches

Peripheral Sensory Distribution of Ophthalmic VI			
Major Branches of V1	Associated Postganglionic Autonomic Fibers (GVE) and Ganglion	Terminal Branches	Sensory Region Innervated
Lacrimal nerve Course: Afferent fibers pass from lacrimal gland along the superior border of lateral rectus below roof of orbit to enter the cranium through **superior orbital fissure**	**Pterygopalatine ganglion** Located in pterygopalatine fossa **Preganglionic parasympathetic** fibers from **greater petrosal of facial (CN VII)** synapse in ganglion **Postganglionic parasympathetic** originates from ganglion and travels with **zygomatic branch of V2** and then travels with **lacrimal branch (V1)** to supply secretomotor fibers to lacrimal gland	Does not divide further	**Lacrimal nerve** receives somatic sensations from the lacrimal gland and conjunctiva distributes postganglionic parasympathetic fibers (GVE) to lacrimal gland
Frontal nerve Divides into two terminal nerve branches Course: Passes between the roof of orbit and levator palpebrae toward the superior orbital fissure	Not associated	• Supratrochlear nerve • Supraorbital nerve	**Supratrochlear nerve** receives input from medial upper eyelid **Supraorbital nerve** receives input from bridge of nose, forehead, frontal sinus

Nasociliary nerve
Divides into five terminal branches
Course:
Passes between the medial rectus and superior oblique
Crosses superior to the optic nerve (CN II) to enter the superior orbital foramen
	Ciliary ganglion
	Located in orbit
	Preganglionic parasympathetic fibers of oculomotor nerve (CN III) synapse in the ganglion
	Postganglionic parasympathetic originating from the ganglion travels with the **short ciliary nerve of nasociliary branch (V1)**
	Postganglionic sympathetic fibers follow the internal carotid plexus and then travel with the long ciliary to the dilator pupillae muscle
		• Anterior ethmoidal nerve
		  ○ Internal nasal branch
		  ○ External nasal branch
			Anterior ethmoidal transmits sensory information from anterior and middle ethmoid sinuses
			Internal nasal nerve supplies lateral nasal cavity and anterior nasal septum
			External nasal nerve transmits sensory input from the skin of ala and apex of nose

		• Infratrochlear nerve	**Infratrochlear nerve** transmits sensory input from the lacrimal sac and caruncula, conjunctiva, skin of medial eyelid, skin of side of nose
		• Long ciliary nerve	**Long ciliary nerve** transmits sensory information from iris, sclera, cornea Postganglionic sympathetic fibers travel with the long ciliary to the dilator pupillae muscle
		• Sensory ciliary ○ Short ciliary	• **Short ciliary** fibers transmit somatic sensations (GSA) from the sclera; pass through ciliary ganglion—no synapse • Serve as sensory afferent limb of corneal reflex—projects to spinal trigeminal nucleus (STN) • Postganglionic parasympathetic (GVE) travels with short ciliary nerves; distribute to sphincter pupillae and ciliary muscle
		• Posterior ethmoidal nerve	**Posterior ethmoidal** receives input from ethmoid and sphenoid sinus

Abbreviations: GSA, general somatic afferent; GVE, general visceral efferent.

individual sensory branches from each of the three divisions of the trigeminal nerve. The branches serve to distribute general visceral efferent (GVE) fibers to their target organs and are listed in each table covering the peripheral distribution of the fibers.

20.2.2 GSA Peripheral Distribution of Trigeminal Divisions

GSA V1: Peripheral Sensory Distribution

- Ophthalmic division (V1) transmits only **somatic afferent (GSA)** input from peripheral receptors found in the upper one-third of the face, and mucous membranes of the orbit and sinuses (▶ Fig. 20.2).
- The ophthalmic (V1) division also carries GSA (type Ia) fibers from muscle spindles of the extraocular muscles which provide information about the position and movement of the eye within the orbit and maintain binocular vision.
- GSA input follows the three terminal branches of the ophthalmic division (V1), the **lacrimal, frontal,** and **nasociliary nerves** (▶ Table 20.4).
- The three peripherally distributed branches pass through the orbit via the **superior orbital fissure** to join to form the ophthalmic division of the trigeminal (V1) in the middle cranial fossa.

GSA V2: Peripheral Sensory Distribution

- The maxillary division (V2) of the trigeminal nerve consists of five principal branches, **the meningeal (middle meningeal), zygomatic, posterior superior alveolar, infraorbital** (▶ Table 20.5), and the **ganglionic (pterygopalatine) nerve branches** (▶ Table 20.6) (▶ Fig. 20.3a–c).
- Each branch transmits GSA input from several terminal branches associated with peripheral afferent receptors found in the skin of the middle third of the face, and the mucous membranes lining the maxillary sinus, nose, palate, and maxillary dental arch.
- The terminal branches converge in the pterygopalatine fossa to form the maxillary division (V2) before entering the cranium via the foramen rotundum.

GSA V3: Peripheral Sensory Distribution

- In comparison to terminal branches of the ophthalmic and maxillary divisions, the terminal branches of the **mandibular division (V3) of the trigeminal nerve** may be mixed nerves and carry both **special visceral motor (SVE) fibers** and **GSA fibers** (▶ Fig. 20.4a–c).
- The sensory component of V3 consists of seven main peripheral branches: the **meningeal, buccal, masseteric, posterior deep temporal, auriculotemporal, inferior alveolar,** and **lingual nerve** branches.
- Each branch transmits GSA input from terminal branches associated with peripheral afferent receptors found in the skin of the lower third of the face, TMJ, lower dental arch jaw, anterior tongue, and floor of the oral cavity.

- The meningeal branch (recurrent meningeal or nervus spinosum) transmits GSA input from the dura of the middle and anterior cranial fossa (▶ Table 20.7). The sensory fibers contribute directly to the main mandibular trunk.
- The remaining six primary branches enter the infratemporal fossa and contribute to the formation of the **anterior** and **posterior divisions of V3** (▶ Table 20.8 and ▶ Table 20.9).
- The anterior and posterior divisions unite to form a **common (main) mandibular trunk,** which enters the cranium through foramen ovale.

20.2.3 GSA: Intracranial and Central Path of Trigeminal Sensory Divisions

(See ▶ Table 20.10 **for summary paths)**
- The three divisions of the trigeminal (CNs V1, V2, and V3) converge at the **trigeminal sensory (semilunar) ganglion**, which contains the cell bodies for the primary afferent neurons carrying protopathic and epicritic sensations (see ▶ Fig. 20.1a). The cell bodies of the primary afferent neurons that mediate unconscious proprioception reside in the **mesencephalic nucleus** of the trigeminal sensory nuclear complex.
- The central processes for the primary afferent neurons found in the trigeminal ganglion and mesencephalic nucleus synapse on specific nuclei within the **trigeminal sensory nuclear complex,** or form synaptic connections involved in reflex activities. The primary ascending sensory pathways originating from the trigeminal sensory nucleus are summarized in ▶ Table 20.10 (see Chapter 13 for specific details).
  ○ Additional ascending pathways to the cerebellum (trigeminocerebellar path) and reticular formation (trigeminoreticular path), as well as projections from the Ventral posteromedial (VPM) of the thalamus to intralaminar thalamic nuclei, are not included below. These pathways that provide proprioceptive feedback and are important for processing pain are covered in Chapter 13.

20.2.4 Special Visceral Efferent Component

SVE Fibers: Origin, Central Connections, and Course

- **SVE fibers** originate from **α** and **γ lower motor neurons (LMNs)** located in the **trigeminal motor nucleus,** a small nucleus situated medial to the trigeminal sensory nuclear complex in the pontine tegmentum.

The **trigeminal motor nucleus** receives central input from several sources, including **direct bilateral input** from upper motor neurons (UMNs) in the orofacial cortex, the masticatory central pattern generator, and the mesencephalic nucleus. There is additional indirect input from the cerebellum and the sensorimotor cortex. Central input is outlined in ▶ Table 20.11.

Table 20.5 Maxillary division (V2): Peripheral distribution of main (GSA) sensory branches

Maxillary Branches Associated with Face and Maxillary Dental Arch			
Major Branches of V2	Associated Autonomic Fibers (GVE) and Ganglion	Terminal Branches	Sensory Region Innervated
Meningeal branch **Course:** Branches from maxillary nerve in middle cranial fossa	None	No named terminal branches	Dura mater of middle cranial fossa

Four principal branches, the **zygomatic, infraorbital nerve branches, posterior superior alveolar,** and **ganglionic (pterygopalatine)**, receive GSA input from several terminal branches. The four branches enter the **pterygopalatine fossa** and converge to form the maxillary division (V2) of the trigeminal nerve.
• The **zygomatic branch** of V2 and the six terminal branches associated with the **ganglionic (pterygopalatine)** nerve of V2 also distribute autonomic (GVE) fibers to target tissue.

Major Branches of V2	Associated Autonomic Fibers (GVE) and Ganglion	Terminal Branches	Sensory Region Innervated
Zygomatic branch Divides into two terminal branches **Course:** Terminal branches of zygomatic nerve pass through the lateral wall of the orbit, join as the zygomatic nerve, and travel along the orbit floor and pass through **inferior orbital fissure** to the pterygopalatine fossa	**Pterygopalatine ganglion** **Preganglionic parasympathetic** fibers from **greater petrosal of facial (CN VII)** synapse in ganglion **Postganglionic parasympathetic fibers** of greater petrosal of facial (CN VII) originate from pterygopalatine ganglion and travel with **zygomaticotemporal of V2**; GVE fibers then travel with **lacrimal branch (CN V1)** to supply secretomotor fibers to lacrimal gland	• Zygomaticofacial • Zygomaticotemporal	**Zygomaticofacial** Transmits GSA input from the prominence of the cheek **Zygomaticotemporal** Transmits GSA input from the lateral scalp above the zygomatic arch Distributes GVE fibers to lacrimal nerve (CN V1) to lacrimal gland
Infraorbital branch Divides into two terminal branches within the infraorbital canal Divides into three terminal branches on the face **Course:** Afferent fibers of terminal branches of infraorbital nerve pass through infraorbital foramen, and travel through the infraorbital canal in the floor of the orbit. The fibers join to form the infraorbital nerve. The infraorbital nerve passes through the **inferior orbital fissure** to the pterygopalatine fossa.	None associated	Terminal branch associated with infraorbital canal pass through maxillary sinus: • Middle superior alveolar • Anterior superior alveolar Terminal branches on face pass through **infraorbital foramen:** • Superior labial branch • External nasal branch • Inferior palpebrae branch	Middle and anterior superior alveolar branches join the posterior superior alveolar branch of V2 in the maxillary sinus to form the **superior dental plexus** **Middle** and **anterior superior alveolar branches** transmit GSA input from the periodontal ligament, labial gingiva, and pulp of the maxillary incisors, canines, premolars, and the mesiobuccal root of the first maxillary molar Carry sensory input from mucosa of maxillary sinus as they pass through sinus Cutaneous branches to skin of face carry GSA sensation from region of the **superior labial branch** of skin and labial mucosa of upper lip; **external nasal branch** of lateral side (ala) of external nose; **inferior palpebrae branch** of skin of lower eyelid respectively
Posterior superior alveolar branch **Course:** Afferent fibers from the maxillary sinus, posterior dental arch from the infratemporal fossa through pterygomaxillary fissure to enter the pterygopalatine fossa Posterior superior alveolar nerve joins with other terminal branch to form the maxillary division	None	No named terminal branches	Contributes to innervation of the maxillary sinus Innervates the periodontal ligament, buccal gingiva, and pulp of the **maxillary molars** **possible exception mesiobuccal root of first maxillary molar Contributes to superior dental plexus** formed by anterior and middle alveolar nerves

(Continued)

Table 20.5 (*Continued*) Maxillary division (V2): Peripheral distribution of main (GSA) sensory branches

Maxillary Branches Associated with Face and Maxillary Dental Arch			
Major Branches of V2	Associated Autonomic Fibers (GVE) and Ganglion	Terminal Branches	Sensory Region Innervated
Ganglionic branch of V2 **Course:** • One to two ganglionic nerve branches connect the ganglion to maxillary division (V2) • Ganglionic branch contributes to the maxillary division • Ganglionic branch receives GSA input from six terminal branches arising from six terminal branches which pass through the ganglion	**Pterygopalatine** (sphenopalatine) **ganglion** Located in pterygopalatine fossa GSA fibers from periphery pass through ganglion without synapsing	Terminal branches of ganglionic/pterygopalatine nerve branch pass from periphery to pterygopalatine fossa (terminal ganglionic branches and distribution listed in ▶ Table 20.6)	

Abbreviations: GSA, general somatic afferent; GVE, general visceral efferent.

Table 20.6 Maxillary division (V2): Peripheral distribution of terminal ganglionic branches

Sensory (GSA) Branches of V2 Associated with Pterygopalatine Ganglion in Pterygopalatine Fossa			
Major Branches of V2	Associated Autonomic Fibers (GVE) and Ganglion	Terminal Branches	Sensory Region Innervated

Terminal branches of ganglionic (pterygopalatine) nerve branch of V2
Course:
• Six terminal ganglionic nerve branches convey somatic sensations from peripheral targets
• Terminal ganglionic nerve branches of V2 enter pterygopalatine fossa and pass through the pterygopalatine ganglion without synapsing
	Pterygopalatine (sphenopalatine) **ganglion**
	Located in pterygopalatine fossa
	Nerve of pterygoid canal (vidian nerve)
	Connects to ganglion
	Formed by:
	• Preganglionic parasympathetic fibers of **greater petrosal** (CN VII)
	• Postganglionic sympathetic fibers of **deep petrosal nerve**
	• Preganglionic parasympathetic fibers of CN VII **synapse** in ganglion
	• Postganglionic sympathetic fibers pass through **without synapsing**
		Six terminal sensory branches:
		• Greater palatine
		• Lesser palatine
		• Pharyngeal
		• Posterior superior nasal
		  ○ Lateral nasal
		  ○ Medial nasal
		• Nasopalatine
		• Orbital
		Each branch carries:
		• **GSA** from mucosa to CNS
		• Postganglionic parasympathetic (**GVE**) to glands
		• Postganglionic sympathetic (**GVE**) to glands
			Greater palatine nerve innervate the hard palate, palatal gingiva in the premolar and molar region
			Lesser palatine nerve innervates the soft palate
			• **Greater** and **lesser palatine** nerves pass from the palatal region to the ganglion in the pterygopalatine fossa via greater and lesser palatal foramen, respectively, and greater palatine canal. These nerves distribute GVE to palatal glands and transmit GSA from the palatal mucosa. SVA from palatal taste buds also follows the GSA fibers to ganglion and then joins the greater petrosal (CN VII) fibers
			Pharyngeal branch innervates the nasopharynx fibers, pass to pterygopalatine fossa via the pharyngeal canal
			Posterior superior nasal branch, and its two divisions, **lateral and medial nasal branches**, innervate the mucosa of lateral wall and nasal septum walls. Posterior superior nasal branches pass from the nasal cavity to the pterygopalatine fossa via the sphenopalatine foramen.
			Nasopalatine branch transmits GSA input from the palatal gingiva associated with maxillary incisors and canines. Passes from palatal roof through the incisive canal to the nasal cavity. Passes through the nasal cavity along the nasal septum to ganglion in the pterygopalatine fossa via sphenopalatine foramen.
			Orbital branch transmits GSA input from orbital periosteum and posterior ethmoid and sphenoid sinuses to ganglion in pterygopalatine fossa via inferior orbital fissure.

Abbreviations: CNS, central nervous system; GSA, general somatic afferent; GVE, general visceral efferent; SVA, special visceral afferent.

Table 20.7 Mandibular division (V3): Peripheral sensory (GSA) distribution of mandibular trunk

Sensory Branches of V3 from the Main Mandibular Trunk			
Major Branches of V3	Associated Autonomic Fibers (GVE) and Ganglion	Terminal Branches	Sensory Region Innervated
Meningeal branch Course: Afferent fibers pass from dura through the foramen spinosum to join the main mandibular trunk of V3 as it passes through the foramen ovale	None associated	Does not divide further	**Meningeal branch** receives somatic sensations from the dura of middle cranial fossa

Abbreviations: GSA, general somatic afferent; GVE, general visceral efferent.

Table 20.8 Mandibular division (V3): Peripheral sensory (GSA) distribution of anterior division

Sensory (GSA) Branches of V3 from the Anterior Division			
Major Branches of V3	Associated Autonomic Fibers (GVE) and Ganglion	Terminal Branches	Sensory Region Innervated
Buccal nerve (long buccal) Course: Cutaneous afferent buccal fibers pierce the buccinator muscle, enter the oral cavity, and travel posteriorly in the cheek, deep to masseter muscle. Buccal nerve passes between the two heads of lateral pterygoid to join the anterior division of V3.	None associated	Does not divide further	**Buccal branch** receives somatic sensations from the oral mucosa lining the vestibule of oral cavity and innervates the gingiva and alveolar mucosa on the buccal side in the mandibular molar region of the dental arch Transmits somatic sensations from skin over the buccinator
Masseteric nerve * *mixed nerve* Course: Sensory fibers lie anterior to TMJ capsule and deep to the temporalis tendon Fibers pass from TMJ through the mandibular notch to join the anterior division	None associated	No named branches	**Masseteric nerve (articular branch)** transmits sensory information from CT capsule surrounding the **TMJ**
Posterior deep temporal branch * *mixed nerve* Course: Contributes a few sensory fibers that lie anterior to TMJ capsule and deep to the temporalis muscle. Fibers pass from TMJ joint to join the anterior division.	None associated	No named branches	**Posterior deep temporal branch** transmits some sensory information from CT capsule surrounding the **TMJ**

Abbreviations: CT, connective tissue; GSA, general somatic afferent; GVE, general visceral efferent; TMJ, temporomandibular joint.

Table 20.9 GSA mandibular division (V3): Peripheral sensory (GSA) distribution: Posterior division

Sensory (GSA) Branches of V3 from the Posterior Division			
Major Branches of V3	Associated Autonomic Fibers (GVE) and Ganglion	Terminal Branches	Sensory Region Innervated
Auriculotemporal branch Course: Sensory nerve branches pass deep to lateral pterygoid and the neck of the mandible; splits into two roots to encircle the middle meningeal artery; fibers join the posterior division of V3	**Otic ganglion** Located in infratemporal fossa inferior to foramen ovale **Preganglionic parasympathetic fibers of lesser petrosal (CN IX)** synapse in **otic ganglion** **Postganglionic parasympathetic** originates from ganglion and accompanies the **deep auriculotemporal nerve** to mediate secretomotor activity for parotid **Postganglionic sympathetic** vasomotor fibers from the external carotid plexus follow branch of maxillary artery and pass through otic ganglion without synapsing to parotid gland *Damage to postganglionic GVE fibers can lead to inappropriate regeneration of parasympathetic and sympathetic innervation to parotid glands (see Chapter 24, Frey's syndrome)	• Superficial auriculotemporal branch ○ Anterior auricular ○ Superficial temporal • Deep auriculotemporal branch ○ Parotid • Articular branch of auriculotemporal	**Auriculotemporal branch** Superficial branches transmit somatic sensations from the skin over the temporal region, tragus of ear, external auditory meatus, and external tympanic membrane. Deep branches which lie deep to parotid convey somatic sensations from region of parotid gland. Distribute postganglionic parasympathetic secretomotor fibers (GVE) to parotid gland Distribute postganglionic sympathetic vasomotor fibers to parotid **Articular branch** transmits sensory information from CT capsule surrounding the temporomandibular joint (**TMJ**) *Auriculotemporal nerve at risk of damage during temporomandibular joint surgery and parotidectomy

(Continued)

Table 20.9 (*Continued*) GSA mandibular division (V3): Peripheral sensory (GSA) distribution: Posterior division

Sensory (GSA) Branches of V3 from the Posterior Division			
Major Branches of V3	Associated Autonomic Fibers (GVE) and Ganglion	Terminal Branches	Sensory Region Innervated
Lingual nerve **Course:** Sensory fibers from mucosa of the tongue and oral cavity pass posteriorly, crossing the submandibular duct and the lateral surface of hyoglossus. Lingual nerve continues between the medial pterygoid and ramus of mandible to enter the infratemporal fossa and join the posterior division of V3. The **chorda tympani branch of facial (CN VII)** joins the posterior border of lingual nerve in the infratemporal fossa. Chorda tympani nerve conveys SVA fibers from the anterior tongue. Accompanies the lingual nerve from the oral cavity to the infratemporal fossa.	**Submandibular ganglion** Ganglion is suspended from the lingual nerve at the posterior border of mylohyoid muscle. **Preganglionic parasympathetic fibers of CN VII** synapse in **submandibular ganglion**. **Postganglionic parasympathetic** fibers originate from the ganglion and **accompany lingual nerve** to submandibular and sublingual glands and minor salivary glands to mediate secretomotor activity. **Postganglionic sympathetic** fibers from the external carotid plexus follow branch of maxillary artery to parotid gland.		**Lingual nerve** Conveys somatic sensations from the mucosa lining the dorsal and ventral surfaces of anterior two-thirds of the tongue and floor of mouth Transmits sensory input from gingiva and alveolar mucosa on the lingual surface of mandibular dental arch Distributes postganglionic parasympathetic fibers (GVE) to submandibular and sublingual glands, minor labial, and lingual salivary glands Conveys taste fibers from anterior tongue
Inferior alveolar nerve* *mixed nerve* Divides into two terminal sensory branches **Course:** The mental and incisive branches join to form the inferior alveolar nerve at the level of second premolar near the mental foramen. Inferior alveolar nerve passes posteriorly through the **mandibular canal** in the body of the mandible. Passes through mandibular foramen between the sphenomandibular ligament and the ramus of mandible and enters to the infratemporal fossa. Joins the posterior division in the infratemporal fossa.		Terminal branch travels within the mandible • **Incisive branch** Terminal branch passes through the **mental foramen** from face • **Mental nerve**	**Inferior alveolar** and **incisive branch** form an inferior dental plexus Transmits sensory information from the periodontal ligament (PDL) and all teeth in the mandibular dental arch **Mental branch** conveys sensory input from skin of the chin, lower lip, and the mucosa of the oral vestibule and facial gingiva from the premolar region anteriorly to the incisors in the midline.

Abbreviations: CT, connective tissue; GSA, general somatic afferent; GVE, general visceral efferent; SVA, special visceral afferent.

Intracranial Course of SVE Fibers

- SVE fibers emerge from the motor nucleus of CN V, pass between the motor and main sensory nucleus to exit the pons, and then travel inferior to the trigeminal ganglion.
- SVE fibers traverse the **foramen ovale** along with the sensory root of the mandibular (V3) division as the **main mandibular trunk** to enter the infratemporal fossa.

SVE V3 Fibers: Peripheral Motor Distribution

- In the **infratemporal fossa,** the following motor branches arise from the main trunk and anterior and posterior divisions:

  - **Medial pterygoid nerve** arises from the **main mandibular trunk**.
  - **Anterior and posterior deep temporal branches,** the **lateral pterygoid nerve, and masseteric branches** arise from the **anterior division.**
  - The **nerve to mylohyoid** arises from the **posterior division.**
- Terminal branches carrying SVE fibers innervate the muscles derived from the first pharyngeal arch (▶ Table 20.12, ▶ Table 20.13, ▶ Table 20.14) (▶ Fig. 20.5).

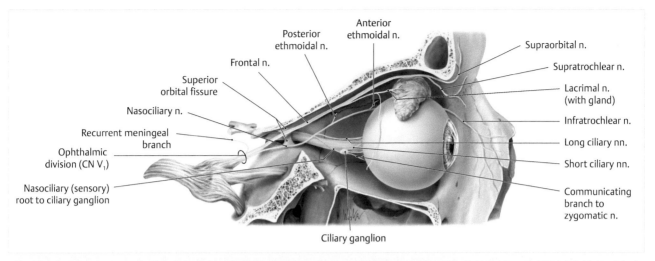

Fig. 20.2 Peripheral course of ophthalmic division (CN V1) of trigeminal nerve. Ophthalmic division (V1), partially opened right orbit. (Reproduced with permission from Schuenke M, Schulte E, Schumacher U. THIEME Atlas of Anatomy Third Edition, Vol 3. © Thieme 2020. Illustrations by Markus Voll and Karl Wesker.)

Clinical Correlation Box 20.1: Lesions to Trigeminal Nerve

Bilateral or unilateral damage to the trigeminal sensory and motor system may result from peripheral or central lesions. Symptoms will vary based on the location and extent of the injury.

- **Central lesions** may result from damage to higher cortical neurons, injury to ascending sensory or descending motor tracts, or to lesions in the brainstem.
- **Peripheral lesions** involving one of the divisions or specific terminal branches of the trigeminal nerve will be ipsilateral. Depending on the site of the lesion, it may be associated with anesthesia in the sensory distribution area, an absent corneal reflex, or trigeminal neuralgia (see Chapter 13). Unilateral atrophy or weakness of the masticatory muscles may result from motor damage to the mandibular division and usually involves sensory loss. Paralysis of only the mandibular motor branches without sensory disturbances is rare.

Central (supranuclear) lesions: Upper motor lesions involving the trigeminal

- Muscles of mastication receive bilateral innervation from UMNs. Due to bilateral corticobulbar input to LMNs situated in the trigeminal motor nucleus in the mid-pons, any unilateral lesion to UMNs, or the region above the level of the trigeminal motor nucleus, does not cause obvious deficits in jaw function.
- Large bilateral lesions to regions above the trigeminal motor nucleus may cause weakness and limited jaw opening. However, the chewing process, which involves rhythmic movements elicited through brainstem mediated reflexes, will still function if the lesion occurs above these interneurons. The action of chewing may become hyperactive and uncoordinated due to loss of cortical feedback to central pattern generators which control the rhythmic chew cycle.

Additionally, articulation is significantly affected by supranuclear lesions, and the patient exhibits an exaggerated jaw jerk reflex (hyperreflexia) (see Chapter 13).

Central brainstem lesions: Damage to the trigeminal motor nucleus

- Brainstem lesions of the LMNs found within the trigeminal motor nucleus result in ipsilateral atrophy to muscles of the first pharyngeal arch. Typically, the jaw deviates to the affected (weak) side upon opening due to the unopposed action of the opposite lateral pterygoid. Injury to LMNs or peripheral nerve branches carrying SVE may lead to atrophy and weakness (flaccid paralysis) of affected muscles. Damage to the trigeminal motor nucleus will also result in the loss of the monosynaptic jaw jerk reflex. The reflex, which is elicited by lightly tapping the relaxed open jaw in a downward direction, involves proprioceptive afferent input from the mesencephalic nucleus and efferent motor output from jaw-closing neurons found in the trigeminal motor nucleus.

Central brainstem lesions: Ascending somatosensory tracts

- Central lesions involving the brainstem may impact the trigeminal sensory nuclear complex or damage to the ascending trigeminothalamic (trigeminal lemniscus) tracts. The extent of sensory loss will depend on the site of injury.

Given the proximity of the ascending trigeminal sensory tracts with the somatosensory tracts of the body, lesions that affect the trigeminothalamic tract may also affect the lateral spinothalamic tract or the medial lemniscus to cause associated sensory deficits in the body (see Chapters 12 and 13) (▶ Fig. 20.6).

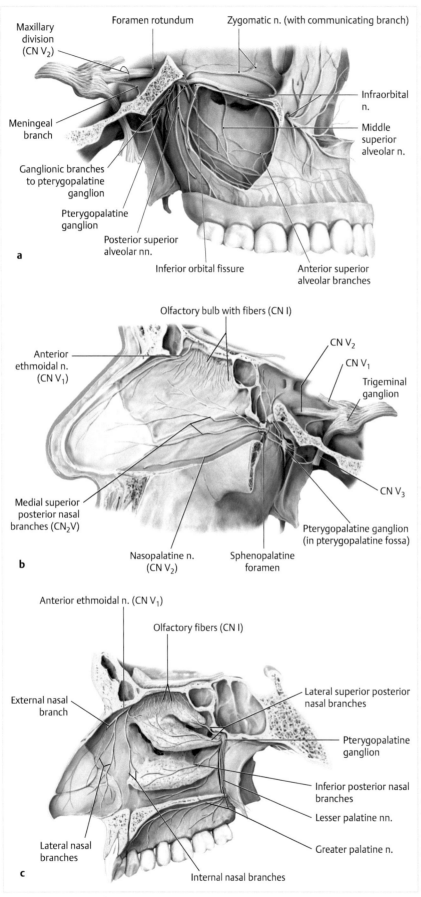

a

Maxillary division (CN V₂)

Foramen rotundum

Zygomatic n. (with communicating branch)

Meningeal branch

Ganglionic branches to pterygopalatine ganglion

Pterygopalatine ganglion

Posterior superior alveolar nn.

Inferior orbital fissure

Infraorbital n.

Middle superior alveolar n.

Anterior superior alveolar branches

b

Olfactory bulb with fibers (CN I)

Anterior ethmoidal n. (CN V₁)

CN V₂

CN V₁

Trigeminal ganglion

Medial superior posterior nasal branches (CN₂V)

CN V₃

Nasopalatine n. (CN V₂)

Sphenopalatine foramen

Pterygopalatine ganglion (in pterygopalatine fossa)

c

Anterior ethmoidal n. (CN V₁)

Olfactory fibers (CN I)

External nasal branch

Lateral superior posterior nasal branches

Pterygopalatine ganglion

Inferior posterior nasal branches

Lesser palatine nn.

Greater palatine n.

Lateral nasal branches

Internal nasal branches

Fig. 20.3 **(a)** Peripheral course of maxillary division (V2). A partially opened right maxillary sinus with zygomatic arch removed. **(b)** Peripheral course of maxillary division—branches to nasal septum, left lateral view. **(c)** Peripheral course of maxillary division—branches to right lateral nasal wall, medial view. (Reproduced with permission from Schuenke M, Schulte E, Schumacher U. THIEME Atlas of Anatomy Third Edition, Vol 3. © Thieme 2020. Illustrations by Markus Voll and Karl Wesker.)

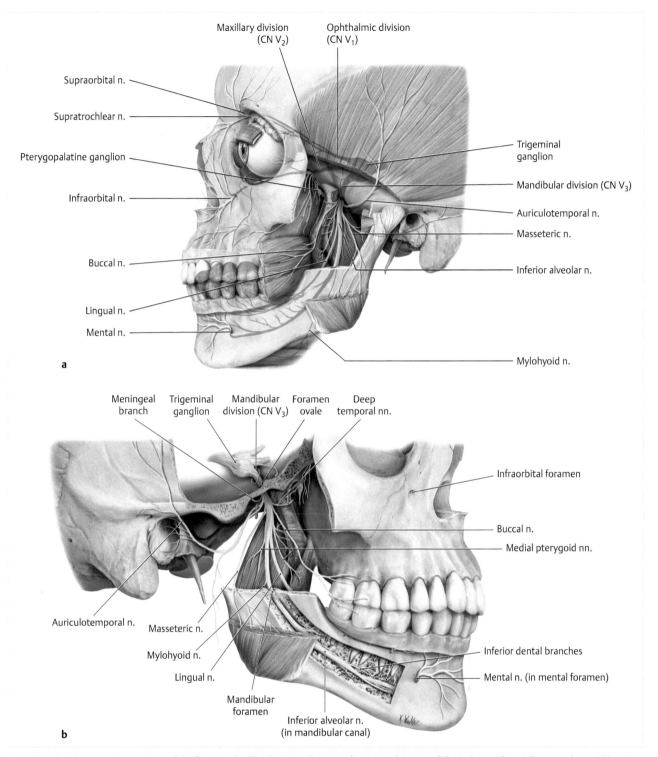

Supraorbital n.

Supratrochlear n.

Pterygopalatine ganglion

Infraorbital n.

Buccal n.

Lingual n.

Mental n.

Maxillary division (CN V₂)

Ophthalmic division (CN V₁)

Trigeminal ganglion

Mandibular division (CN V₃)

Auriculotemporal n.

Masseteric n.

Inferior alveolar n.

Mylohyoid n.

a

Meningeal branch

Trigeminal ganglion

Mandibular division (CN V₃)

Foramen ovale

Deep temporal nn.

Infraorbital foramen

Buccal n.

Medial pterygoid nn.

Auriculotemporal n.

Masseteric n.

Mylohyoid n.

Lingual n.

Mandibular foramen

Inferior alveolar n. (in mandibular canal)

Inferior dental branches

Mental n. (in mental foramen)

b

Fig. 20.4 (a) Cutaneous innervation of the face supplied by the three divisions of trigeminal nerve. Left lateral view of partially opened mandible with zygomatic arch removed. (b) Peripheral course of mandibular division (V3). Partially opened mandible showing middle cranial fossa windowed. The main mandibular trunk located in the middle cranial fossa gives off two branches, the meningeal (recurrent, nervus spinosus) branch (GSA) and nerve to medial pterygoid (SVE), before dividing into an anterior and posterior divisions which pass through the foramen ovale.

(Continued)

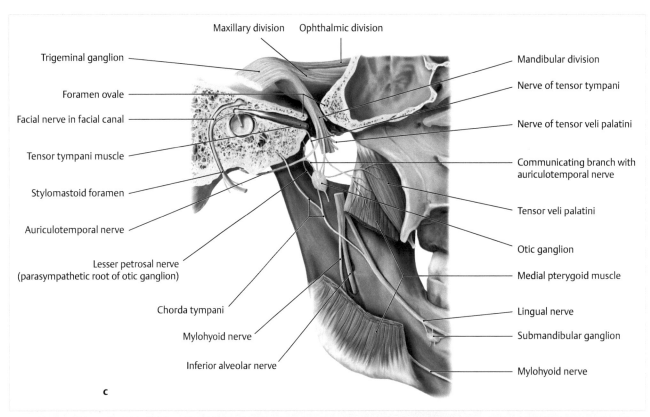

Fig. 20.4 (*Continued*) (**c**) Peripheral course of mandibular division (V3), right lateral view, opened oral cavity with right half of mandible removed. The otic and submandibular parasympathetic ganglia illustrated. The otic ganglion contains parasympathetic fibers of the glossopharyngeal (CN IX). Postganglionic (GVE) fibers arising from the ganglia accompany the auriculotemporal branch (V3) to the parotid and buccal minor salivary glands. The submandibular ganglion contains postganglionic (GVE) fibers of the chorda tympani branch of CN VII which accompany the lingual nerve (V3) to the submandibular and sublingual glands. Taste (SVA) sensations carried from the anterior two-thirds of the tongue by the chorda tympani of CN VII also accompany the lingual nerve (V3). GSA, general somatic afferent; GVE, general visceral efferent; SVE, special visceral efferent. (Reproduced with permission from Schuenke M, Schulte E, Schumacher U. THIEME Atlas of Anatomy Third Edition, Vol 3. © Thieme 2020. Illustrations by Markus Voll and Karl Wesker.)

Table 20.10 Overview of ascending pathways and trigeminal sensory nuclear complex

Trigeminal Sensory Nuclear Complex			
Trigeminal Nuclei	**Spinal Trigeminal Nucleus** (aka spinal nucleus of CN V (second-order neurons) • Pars oralis • Pars interpolaris • Pars caudalis	**Chief Sensory Nucleus of CN V** (second order) *(aka main sensory, pontine trigeminal, principal nucleus)	**Mesencephalic Nucleus of CN V** (unique nucleus—only nucleus containing first-order neurons in the CNS)
Functional component and pathway	Protopathic sensations of orofacial skin, oral mucosa Pathway for pain, temperature, crude touch	Epicritic sensation of orofacial skin and oral mucosa Pathway for fine tactile discrimination and conscious proprioception (pressure, vibration)	Proprioceptive input from muscle spindles in jaw closing muscles, tongue and extraocular eye muscles, and mechanoreceptors of PDL and TMJ Pathway for unconscious proprioception:
Territory of trigeminal	All three divisions transmit GSA input from: Skin, mucosa, gingiva, PDL, TMJ, and region of eye GSA fibers of CN VII, CN IX< and CN X also terminate in spinal trigeminal nucleus and follow same ascending pathway as CN V (see Chapter 13)	All three divisions transmit from: skin, mucosa, teeth, gingiva, PDL, and region of eye	Received primarily from V2 and V3: V1 carries some proprioceptive from extraocular eye muscles
Principal ascending tract	Ventral trigeminothalamic tract (VTT) (contralateral path to somatosensory cortex) **Key summary:**	**1. Dorsal trigeminothalamic tract (DTT)** (ipsilateral path to somatosensory cortex) **2. Ventral trigeminothalamic tract**	Monosynaptic reflex to **trigeminal motor nucleus** **some proprioceptive fibers follow VTT and DTT to cortex for conscious

(Continued)

Table 20.10 (*Continued*) Overview of ascending pathways and trigeminal sensory nuclear complex

Trigeminal Sensory Nuclear Complex		
Protopathic fibers decussate for VTT →contralateral VPM of thalamus →somatosensory cortex	(VTT) (contralateral path to cortex) **Key summary:** Epicritic fibers of chief sensory nucleus may either remain ipsilateral in DTT or cross and join protopathic fibers in VTT.	processing**

Abbreviations: CNS, central nervous system; GSA, general somatic afferent; PDL, periodontal ligament; TMJ, temporomandibular joint; VPM, ventral posteromedial.

Notes: *Epicritic fibers join protopathic fibers in ventral trigeminothalamic tract at the level of pons. Collectively, fibers ascend as the trigeminal lemniscus which is near medial lemniscus and lateral to spinothalamic tracts.

**Additional connections of each pathway not included above (see Chapter 13).

Table 20.11 Trigeminal motor nuclei and central input for SVE fiber

Functional Component	Central Input	CN V Motor Nucleus	Territory and Terminal Branches	Functional Outcome

SVE fibers of V3	Trigeminal motor nucleus receives input from following sources:
	• Receives **bilateral** input via **corticobulbar tract** from the supranuclear (**UMN**) neurons in both motor cortices to provide voluntary control of mastication
	• Receives indirect input from the cerebellum and basal ganglia via **extrapyramidal tracts**
	• Receives input from the **masticatory central pattern generator** in the pontomedullary reticular formation to coordinate masticatory activity and unconscious rhythm of chewing
	• Receives sensory input indirectly from the **trigeminal sensory nuclear complex** via the **sensorimotor cortex** and other **cranial nerves** to modulate efferent motor responses through sensorimotor feedback
	• Receive direct input from **mesencephalic nucleus** for reflexive control of jaw opening
		Trigeminal motor nucleus (contains LMN) SVE fibers originate from nucleus, pass ventral to sensory root, and exit with sensory division of CN V3 Exit skull via **foramen ovale**	Terminal branches of motor root of V3 arise in **infratemporal fossa** SVE fibers innervate first pharyngeal arch muscles
			• **Main mandibular trunk:**
			  ○ Medial pterygoid nerve
			• **Anterior division:**
			  ○ Anterior deep temporal
			  ○ Lateral pterygoid nerve
			• **Posterior division**
			  ○ Masseteric branch
			  ○ Posterior deep temporal branch
				Masticatory muscles primarily control mandibular movement
				• **Depression** is produced by the lateral pterygoid and digastric muscles and by gravity.
				• **Elevation** is due to the temporalis, masseter, and medial pterygoid muscle.
				• **Protrusion** is caused by the pterygoid muscles and the masseter.
				• **Retraction** results from the posterior fibers of the temporalis.
				• **Lateral side-to-**side movements depend on an interaction between all the muscles of mastication.

Abbreviations: LMN, lower motor neuron; SVE, special visceral efferent; UMN, upper motor neuron.

Notes: *Regions of motor cortex include the cortical masticatory area of primary motor cortex (M1); the premotor cortex (PMC), and supplementary motor area (SMA).

**See Chapters 16 and 17 for the complete motor path involving the corticobulbar (pyramidal tract) and extrapyramidal tract.

20.3 Facial Nerve

- The facial nerve (CN VII) develops in association with the second pharyngeal arch and carries both motor and sensory modalities. The modalities carried include two motor components, SVE and GVE, and three sensory modalities, GSA, general visceral afferent (GVA), and special visceral afferent (SVA) fibers.
- The largest component of the facial nerve, the **facial nerve proper,** provides the primary source of voluntary motor innervation to the face and transmits **special visceral motor** (SVE) fibers to the skeletal muscles derived from second pharyngeal arch.
- A smaller division, the **nervus intermedius** (**intermediate nerve**), serves as the sensory and visceral motor division of CN VII. The nerve transmits **taste (SVA), somatic sensory (GSA) fibers, visceral sensory (GVA) fibers**, and **visceral motor (GVE)** fibers of the parasympathetic division (see ▶ Table 20.15 for summary of functional modalities).
- The facial nerve proper and the nervus intermedius follow a similar path through the temporal bone (▶ Fig. 20.7a–c).

Table 20.12 SVE peripheral fiber distribution: Main trunk of V3

Motor (SVE) Branches from Main Trunk of V3			
Major Branches of V3	Terminal Branches	Motor Target Innervated	Action of Muscle
Nerve to medial pterygoid Course: Fibers arise from the main trunk and innervate deep and superficial heads of medial pterygoid muscle. Some fibers from medial pterygoid nerve pass through otic ganglion without synapsing to innervate both tensor muscles.	**Nerve to medial pterygoid** gives rise to two muscular branch: • **Nerve to tensor tympani** • **Nerve to tensor veli palatini**	**Nerve to medial pterygoid** provides special visceral motor function to medial pterygoid muscle **Nerve to tensor tympani** penetrates the auditory tube to innervate the tensor tympani muscle **Nerve to tensor veli palatini** innervates tensor veli palatini muscle *Note tensor veli is the only palatal muscle to receive innervation from trigeminal nerve.	**Medial pterygoid muscle** Bilateral actions: Elevates mandible Assists to protrude mandible Side-to-side excursion (lateral excursion) Unilateral contraction acts to deviate mandible to contralateral side *Muscle most often involved in trismus (lockjaw) following inferior alveolar nerve block **Tensor tympani muscle** Tenses tympanic membrane and dampens sound produced by pulling malleus (ear ossicle) medially **Tensor veli palatini muscle** Tenses soft palate prior to palatal elevation

Abbreviation: SVE, special visceral efferent.

Table 20.13 SVE peripheral fiber distribution: Anterior division of V3

Motor (SVE) Branches of V3 from Anterior Division			
Major Branches of V3	Terminal Branches	Motor Target Innervated	Action of Muscle
Deep temporal nerve Divides into two terminal motor branches **Course:** Fibers arise from anterior division of V3 in the infratemporal fossa. Terminal branches of deep temporal nerve ascend and pass superior to lateral pterygoid muscle between the skull and temporalis muscle and innervate the deep surface of temporalis.	• Anterior deep temporal nerve • Posterior deep temporal nerve	**Deep temporal nerve and terminal branch** innervate the temporalis muscle	**Temporalis muscle** Vertical (anterior) fibers: Elevate mandible Horizontal (posterior) fibers: Retract mandible Aids in side-to-side movement (lateral excursion) of mandible
Masseteric nerve *mixed nerve **Course:** Fibers from anterior division pass laterally from infratemporal fossa and above the lateral pterygoid muscle to pass though the mandibular notch which sits anterior to the TMJ to provide motor fibers to the medial side of muscle.	No additional named branches	**Masseteric nerve** Innervates the masseter	**Masseter muscle** Bilateral action: Elevates mandible Protrudes the mandible Aids in side-to-side movements (lateral excursion)
Nerve to lateral pterygoid **Course:** Fibers arise from anterior division and immediately enter the deep surface of both heads of the lateral pterygoid; may run with buccal of V3 or originate from buccal branch as it passes between two heads of lateral pterygoid.	No named terminal branches	**Nerve to lateral pterygoid** Innervates both heads of the lateral pterygoid muscle	**Lateral pterygoid muscle** Bilateral action: Protrudes mandible Superior head elevates mandible during chew cycle power stoke Inferior head depresses mandible *Aided by gravity and digastric muscles Side-to-side movement (lateral excursion) during chewing Unilateral movement causes mandible to deviate to the contralateral side *Muscle most commonly involved in myofascial pain syndrome due to masticatory muscle spasm; often associated with chronic pain or TMJ disorders

Abbreviations: SVE, special visceral efferent; TMJ, temporomandibular joint.

Table 20.14 SVE peripheral fibers distribution: Posterior division of V3

Motor (SVE) Branch of V3 from the Posterior Division			
Major Branches of V3	Terminal Branches	Sensory Region Innervated	Action of Muscle
Mylohyoid nerve Divides and gives rise to one terminal motor branch **Course:** The mylohyoid nerve splits from the inferior alveolar branch of V3 at the level of mandibular canal. Mylohyoid nerve travels anteriorly in a groove located on the medial surface of ramus of the mandible. The nerve divides at the inferior border of mylohyoid to give rise to the nerve to anterior belly of digastric.	• **Nerve to anterior belly of digastric** Divides from mylohyoid nerve at the inferior border of mylohyoid muscle	**Mylohyoid nerve** Provides motor innervation to mylohyoid muscle **Nerve to anterior belly of digastric** Provides motor innervation to anterior belly of digastric muscle *Note: The posterior belly of digastric is derived from the second pharyngeal arch and receives SVE fibers by the facial nerve	• **Mylohyoid muscle** Elevates the floor of the oral cavity Assists in elevating the hyoid bone Aid in depressing mandible (jaw opener) • **Anterior belly digastric muscle** Elevates hyoid bone Depresses the mandible (jaw opener) Aids in swallowing

Abbreviation: SVE, special visceral efferent.

20.3.1 Facial SVE Fibers: Origin, Central Connections, and Course

CN VII SVE Fibers: Central Course

- The SVE fibers of the **facial nerve proper** originate from cell bodies of LMNs located in the **facial motor nucleus** of the pontine tegmentum and form the **motor root of CN VII** (▸ Fig. 20.7b).
- The neuronal cell bodies within the facial motor nucleus comprise two distinct groups: a **dorsal** and a **ventral motor group**.
  - The dorsal motor group innervates muscles of the forehead and eye (**upper facial muscles of expression**), which function in bilateral facial movements such as blinking, squeezing the eyes shut, and wrinkling the forehead.
  - The ventral motor group innervates the facial muscles below the eye (**lower facial muscles of expression**). Lower facial muscles contribute to unilateral movements associated with expressive functions of the mouth.

Central Control of LMNs in the Facial Motor Nucleus

- The **facial motor nucleus** receives input from several sources which allow for voluntary and involuntary control of facial muscles of expression. The specific connections are described in ▸ Table 20.16 and include descending input from the pyramidal (direct activation) and extrapyramidal (indirect activation) tracts, the limbic system, the brainstem

central pattern generators (CPG) in the reticular formation, and sensory feedback from peripheral receptors.
- **Cortical input** provides voluntary control of the upper and lower facial muscles through bilateral and contralateral input to LMNs in the dorsal and ventral facial motor nucleus, respectively.
  - **UMNs** in the **motor cortices** descend via the corticobulbar tract to innervate the LMNs in the dorsal and ventral motor groups of the facial nerve.
    - The dorsal part of the facial motor nucleus receives bilateral innervation from both the left and right cerebral hemispheres, while the ventral part receives contralateral innervation. The variation in cortical innervation patterns to the LMNs innervating the upper and lower facial muscles is of clinical significance and is important in diagnosis (see Clinical Correlation Box 20.2 and 20.3) (▸ Fig. 20.8a–c).
- **The limbic system** functionally elicits involuntary emotive control of facial expression.
  - The limbic system, which receives and processes visceral and emotional inputs, provides indirect input to the facial motor nucleus. Input from the limbic system influences the activity of cortical supranuclear (UMNs) neurons and functionally couples emotional signals to facial expression.
- **Masticatory CPGs** and sensorimotor feedback coordinate oromotor behaviors such as chewing, bolus formation, and articulation with appropriate facial movements.
- **Extrapyramidal system** coordinates motor movements and corrects for motor errors.

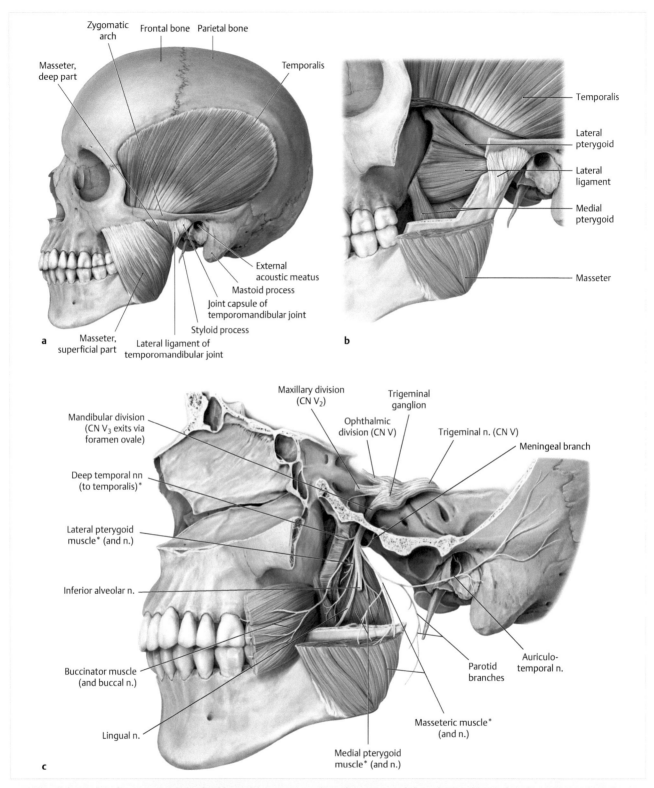

Fig. 20.5 **(a)** Muscles of mastication. Superficial layer showing temporalis and masseter. Left lateral view. **(b)** Muscles of mastication. Deep layer. Lower temporalis and coronoid process of mandible removed. Masseter, temporalis, and medial pterygoid elevate the mandible. The lateral pterygoid depresses the mandible. **(c)** Motor innervation of jaw muscles. Left lateral view. The mandibular division of trigeminal nerve (CN V3) supplies motor innervation to the muscles of mastication. Some sensory branches of ophthalmic (CN V1) and maxillary division (CN V2) are also shown. (Reproduced with permission from Schuenke M, Schulte E, Schumacher U. THIEME Atlas of Anatomy Third Edition, Vol 3. © Thieme 2020. Illustrations by Markus Voll and Karl Wesker.)

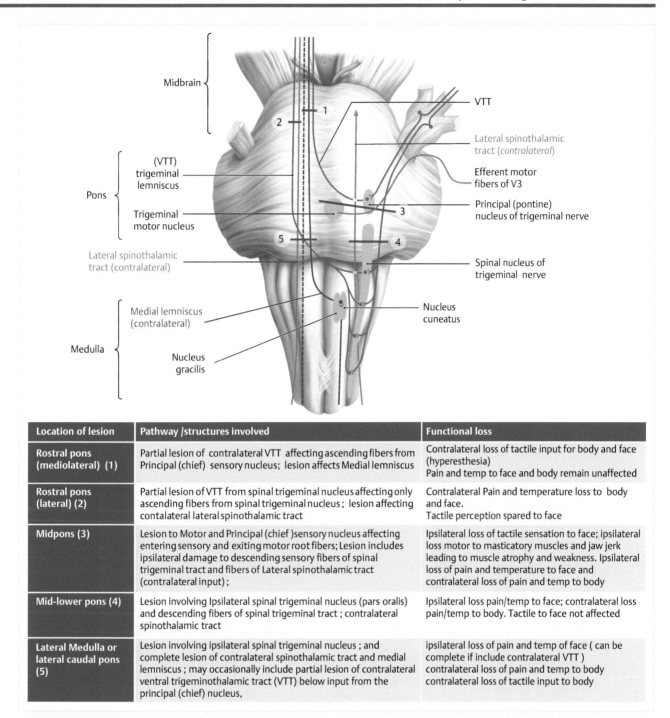

Location of lesion	Pathway /structures involved	Functional loss
Rostral pons (mediolateral) (1)	Partial lesion of contralateral VTT affecting ascending fibers from Principal (chief) sensory nucleus; lesion affects Medial lemniscus	Contralateral loss of tactile input for body and face (hyperesthesia) Pain and temp to face and body remain unaffected
Rostral pons (lateral) (2)	Partial lesion of VTT from spinal trigeminal nucleus affecting only ascending fibers from spinal trigeminal nucleus ; lesion affecting contalateral lateral spinothalamic tract	Contralateral Pain and temperature loss to body and face. Tactile perception spared to face
Midpons (3)	Lesion to Motor and Principal (chief)sensory nucleus affecting entering sensory and exiting motor root fibers; Lesion includes ipsilateral damage to descending sensory fibers of spinal trigeminal tract and fibers of Lateral spinothalamic tract (contralateral input) ;	Ipsilateral loss of tactile sensation to face; ipsilateral loss motor to masticatory muscles and jaw jerk leading to muscle atrophy and weakness. Ipsilateral loss of pain and temperature to face and contralateral loss of pain and temp to body
Mid-lower pons (4)	Lesion involving Ipsilateral spinal trigeminal nucleus (pars oralis) and descending fibers of spinal trigeminal tract ; contralateral spinothalamic tract	Ipsilateral loss pain/temp to face; contralateral loss pain/temp to body. Tactile to face not affected
Lateral Medulla or lateral caudal pons (5)	Lesion involving ipsilateral spinal trigeminal nucleus ; and complete lesion of contralateral spinothalamic tract and medial lemniscus ; may occasionally include partial lesion of contralateral ventral trigeminothalamic tract (VTT) below input from the principal (chief) nucleus,	ipsilateral loss of pain and temp of face (can be complete if include contralateral VTT) contralateral loss of pain and temp to body contralateral loss of tactile input to body

Fig. 20.6 Location of central brainstem lesions involving the trigeminal and somatosensory system. (Reproduced with permission from Schuenke M, Schulte E, Schumacher U. THIEME Atlas of Anatomy Second Edition, Vol 3. © Thieme 2016. Illustrations by Markus Voll and Karl Wesker.)

Table 20.15 Functional modalities of transmission by the facial nerve: Facial nerve proper and nervus intermedius

Facial Nerve Proper					
Functional Component	Associated Nuclei	Associated Ganglia	Facial Nerve Branch	Region Innervated	Clinical Signs of Peripheral Damage
SVE	Voluntary motor to skeletal muscles of PA 2. Aid in bolus formation, swallowing, and convey emotion	Facial motor nucleus	Not applicable	Stapedius Posterior digastric Posterior auricular Stylohyoid Temporal Zygomatic Buccal Mandibular Cervical	Stapedius, digastric (posterior belly), stylohyoid, muscles of facial expression	Ipsilateral **facial palsy** (paralysis) Loss of corneal (blink) reflex (efferent limb VII)

Nervus intermedius					
Functional component	Associated nuclei	Associated ganglia	Facial nerve branch	Region innervated/Functional role	Clinical signs of peripheral damage
GVE	Parasympathetic (secretomotor) activity to glands	Superior salivatory nucleus	Pterygopalatine parasympathetic ganglion Submandibular parasympathetic ganglion	Greater petrosal Chorda tympani	Lacrimal gland, nasal glands, minor salivary glands of hard and soft palate and pharynx, submandibular and sublingual labial salivary glands Secretomotor function	Dry mouth (xerostomia) Decreased lacrimation—dry eye
GSA	Protopathic and epicritic sensations from exteroreceptors	Spinal trigeminal nucleus of CN V	Geniculate sensory ganglion	Sensory auricular Travels with posterior auricular nerve of CN VII	Skin behind the ear, auricle	Minor
SVA	Taste from chemoreceptors of taste buds	Nucleus of tract of solitarius (rostral)	Geniculate sensory ganglion	Greater petrosal Chorda tympani	Hard and soft palates; scattered taste buds in mucosa Anterior two-thirds of tongue; taste buds associated with lingual fungiform papilla Mediate taste	Loss of taste in ipsilateral tongue
GVA	Mucosal irritation	Nucleus of tract of solitarius (rostral)	Geniculate sensory ganglion	No named branches	Mucous membranes of posterior soft palate and nasopharynx	Minor

Abbreviations: GSA, general somatic afferent; GVA, general visceral afferent; GVE, general visceral efferent; SVA, special visceral afferent; SVE, special visceral efferent.

Table 20.16 Central input and intracranial course of facial nerve SVE fibers

Functional Component	CN VII Motor Nucleus	Central Input to Facial Motor Nucleus	Central Course	Intracranial Path and Skull Exit	Distribution of SVE Fibers
SVE fibers of facial nerve proper	**Facial motor nucleus** (contains LMNs) Located lower to pontomedullary junction SVE fibers originate from the dorsal group and ventral group of facial motor nuclei	LMNs in facial motor nucleus comprised dorsal and ventral groups, receive input from following sources **Volitional control of facial muscles:** Provided by supranuclear (UMNs) in motor cortex Project via **corticobulbar** tract to: • Upper facial muscle: Dorsal motor group of CN VII receives **bilateral** input • Lower facial muscles: Ventral motor group of CN VII receives unilateral input from UMNs in **contralateral** motor cortex **Involuntary (emotive) control** • **Limbic system** provides indirect input via motor cortex to LMNs for	SVE originates in facial nucleus, loops around abducens nerve, forms internal genu→ Exits brainstem at cerebellopontine angle with trigeminal (CN V) and vestibulocochlear nerves (CN VIII)→ CN VII SVE fibers travel with nervus intermedius (CN VII) and CN VIII to enter the **internal auditory canal**	SVE fibers of facial nerve exit **internal auditory meatus**→ ear→enters **facial canal**→pass by **tympanic cavity** of middle ear→exits facial canal via **stylomastoid foramen**	Facial nerve gives rise to one motor branch in facial canal: • Stapedius Facial nerve emerges from stylomastoid foramen, give rise to three branches: • Posterior belly digastric • Stylohyoid • Posterior auricular *Mixed nerve Enters parotid glands to form parotid plexus Five named branches of parotid plexus: • Temporal • Zygomatic • Buccal

(Continued)

Table 20.16 (*Continued*) Central input and intracranial course of facial nerve SVE fibers

Functional Component	CN VII Motor Nucleus	Central Input to Facial Motor Nucleus	Central Course	Intracranial Path and Skull Exit	Distribution of SVE Fibers
		involuntary facial movements associated with emotions **Feedback control** • LMN receives sensory input from the **sensorimotor cortex** and **CPGs** to modulate efferent motor output from LMNs • Receives indirect input from the cerebellum and basal ganglia via **extrapyramidal tracts** (see Chapter 17); serves to correct motor errors and coordinate movements			• Marginal mandibular • Cervical Regionally distributed with extensive cross branching Terminates on muscles of facial expression

Abbreviations: CPG, central pattern generator; LMN, lower motor neuron; SVE, special visceral efferent; UMN, upper motor neuron.
Notes: *Regions of motor cortex include the cortical masticatory area of primary motor cortex (M1), premotor cortex (PMC), and supplementary motor area (SMA).
**Regions of limbic system and subcortex include the anterior cingulate gyrus, amygdala, hippocampus, and basal ganglia.

Clinical Correlation Box 20.2: Central (Supranuclear) Lesions Causing Facial Paralysis (▶ Fig. 20.8a, b)

• The variation in cortical innervation to the upper and lower facial muscles leads to differential effects in the voluntary control of movements following unilateral damage to UMNs in the primary motor cortex, the internal capsule, or the descending corticobulbar tract. These injuries are known as **supranuclear lesions** that occur in regions above the facial motor nucleus.
  ○ A unilateral upper motor lesion to the primary motor cortex leads to the contralateral loss of lower facial muscles. Upper facial muscles retain voluntary control and are generally not affected due to bilateral innervation patterns.
  ○ However, the facial muscle located below the eyes receive only contralateral cortical projections and exhibit unilateral weakness in the voluntary control of lower facial muscles on the opposite side of the cortical lesion.
• A common cause of a supranuclear lesion involving the facial nerve is a stroke occurring at or above the internal capsule of the thalamus. Strokes occurring in this area disrupt descending motor pathways carrying corticobulbar fibers and lead to contralateral facial weakness of the lower facial muscle. Strokes in this region may also interrupt the passage of corticospinal fibers and lead to contralateral motor weakness of the limbs.
• Given the sensorimotor connections between the somatosensory cortex, limbic system, and premotor cortex, a patient experiencing unilateral damage to the primary motor cortex can still respond spontaneously to emotional stimuli without apparent weakness or loss of facial symmetry due to premotor and limbic connections remaining intact.

CN VII SVE Fibers: Intracranial Course

• The facial nucleus lies in the caudal part of the pons, just inferior and lateral to the nucleus of the abducens nerve. The SVE fibers which comprise the motor root of CN VII exit from the **facial motor nucleus**, loop around the abducens nerve as the **internal genu** of the facial nerve, and form a small elevation known as the **facial colliculus** in the floor of the fourth ventricle.
• The SVE motor fibers of the **facial nerve proper** travel with the **nervus intermedius** and emerge together from the caudal pons at the **pontomedullary (cerebellopontine) junction** (see ▶ Fig. 20.7a).
• Both divisions of the facial nerve travel with vestibulocochlear nerve (CN VIII) through the **internal acoustic meatus** in the petrous portion of the **temporal bone**.
• The fibers of the facial nerve pass along the roof of the vestibular labyrinth of the inner ear and enter the **facial canal** of the **temporal bone**.
• Within the **facial canal**, at the level of the **geniculate sensory ganglion**, the nervus intermedius and the motor root of CN VII gives rise to three branches (see ▶ Fig. 20.7c)
  ○ **Greater petrosal nerve** (GVE)
  ○ **Chorda tympani nerve** (GVE; SVA)
  ○ **Stapedial nerve** (SVE)
    – The stapedial nerve, the only motor branch to arise from the facial nerve proper in the facial canal, supplies the stapedius, a middle ear muscle.
    – The stapedius attaches to the stapes and functions to attenuate sound and dampen loud noises. Damage to the nerve may lead to increased sensitivity to noise and certain frequencies (**hyperacusis**).
    – It forms the efferent component of the stapedial reflex.
• **SVE fibers** of the motor root pass through geniculate ganglion without synapsing, bend 90 degrees to form the **external genu (geniculum)**, and then pass inferior and medial to the middle ear (tympanic) cavity before exiting the skull via the **stylomastoid foramen**.
• Damage to the facial nerve during its peripheral course may be caused by temporal bone fractures, inflammation

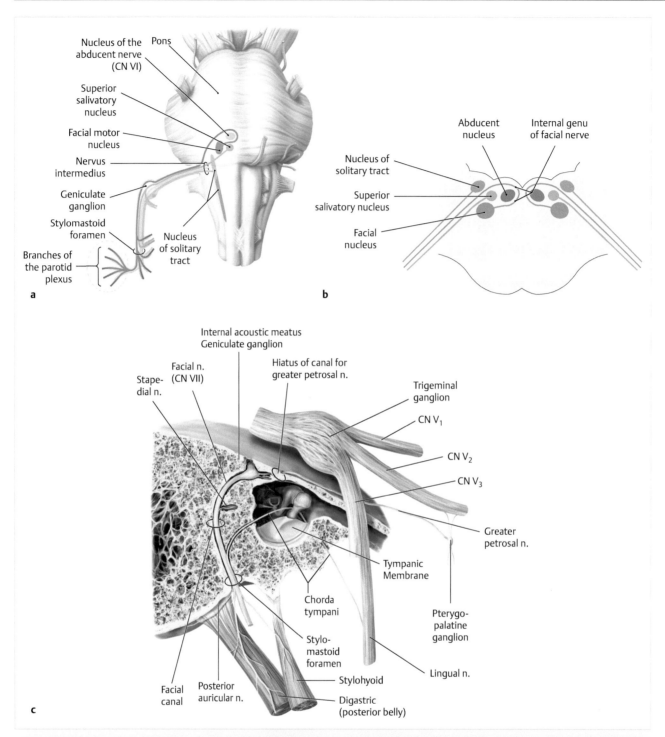

Fig. 20.7 **(a)** Anterior view of brainstem. Associated nuclei and principal branches of the facial nerve. CN VII originates in four nuclei in the pons and medulla. These nuclei all combine to travel, via the internal auditory meatus, to the geniculate ganglion. The branchiomotor component (SVE), which innervates the muscles of facial expression and the stapedius muscle of the ear, originates in the pons at the facial nucleus. It circles around CN VI. The visceral motor component, which innervates the lacrimal, submaxillary, and submandibular glands, originates in the medulla at the superior salivatory nucleus. The visceral sensory (SVA) component, which conveys taste for the anterior two-thirds of the tongue, contains neuron cell bodies in the geniculate ganglion and projects to the solitary tract nucleus in the medulla. The somatic sensory component (GSA) of CN VII contains cells bodies in the geniculate ganglion, and transmits external ear sensation to the medulla and to the spinal nucleus of CN V. **(b)** Cross section through pons at the level of the internal genu of facial nerve and floor of fourth ventricle. **(c)** Intracranial course of facial nerve. Right lateral view. Branches of facial nerve pass through the internal acoustic meatus and the facial canal in the temporal bone. Three nerves branch from the facial nerve during its course through the facial canal. The greater petrosal nerve (SVA and GVE), the nerve to the stapedius (SVE), and the chorda tympani (SVA and GVE) exit the facial canal. The remaining branches of the facial nerve (SVE) arise after exiting the stylomastoid foramen and supply to muscles of facial expression. GSA, general somatic afferent; GVE, general visceral efferent; SVA, special visceral afferent; SVE, special visceral efferent. (Reproduced with permission from Schuenke M, Schulte E, Schumacher U. THIEME Atlas of Anatomy Third Edition, Vol 3. © Thieme 2020. Illustrations by Markus Voll and Karl Wesker.)

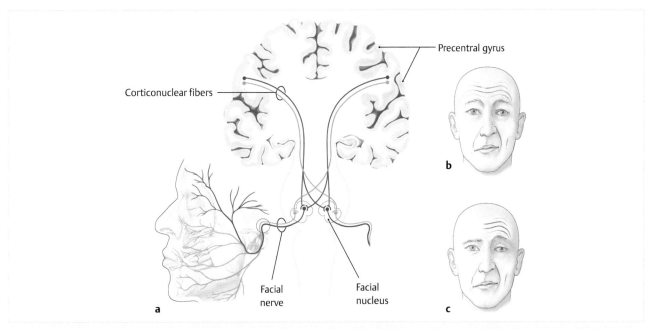

Fig. 20.8 (a) Central and peripheral facial paralysis. Demonstrating location and connections between upper motor neurons (supranuclear) and lower motor neurons of the facial motor nucleus. Dorsal part of facial motor nucleus receives bilateral input from both cortices, while the ventral part of the nucleus receives only contralateral input. Corticonuclear fibers shown from left hemisphere partially control the upper left and right side facial muscles and completely control the lower facial muscles on the right side. **(b)** Central (supranulclear) lesions. Lesion of upper motor neurons (UMNs) shown on left side leads to facial paralysis of the contralateral muscles in the lower half of face. The nasolabial fold flattens and the corner of the mouth sags on the right (contralateral) side due to weakness of orofacial muscles. Speech articulation may be impaired. Due to bilateral input from UMN the patient can wrinkle forehead and close both eyes. **(c)** Brainstem and peripheral lesions of CN VII. Brainstem lesions of lower motor neurons (LMNs) of the facial motor nucleus, or damage to SVE fibers in their peripheral course, leads to unilateral facial muscle paralysis of ipsilateral upper and lower facial muscles. Patient shown with right-side lesion exhibits drooping on right side of mouth, and inability to wrinkle forehead and close right eye. Additional deficits may also be present (see ▶ Table 20.17). (Modified with permission from Schuenke M, Schulte E, Schumacher U. THIEME Atlas of Anatomy. Second Edition, Vol 3. © Thieme 2016. Illustrations by Markus Voll and Karl Wesker.)

Table 20.17 Comparison of UMN and LMN lesions of facial nerve

	UMN	LMN
Voluntary motor movements • Upper facial group • Lower facial group	Present for upper facial muscle Lost lower facial group—contralateral side	Lost upper and lower groups—ipsilateral side
Involuntary facial movements associated with emotion	Present	Lost
Corneal (blink) reflex	Present	Lost
Lacrimation, salivation, taste, hearing,	Present	Lost or diminished taste, salivation, lacrimation, hyperacusis—minor defect *Loss depends on location
Drooling	Uncommon	Common
Ability to wrinkle forehead	Present	Lost on affected side

Abbreviations: LMN, lower motor neuron; UMN, upper motor neuron.

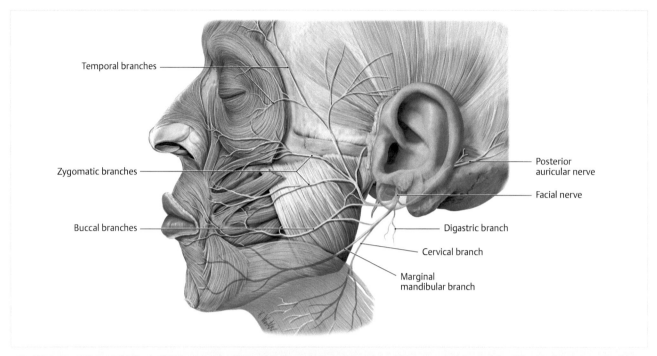

Fig. 20.9 Special visceral efferent (SVE) motor distribution and branching pattern of the facial nerve proper. Left lateral view showing point of exit from stylomastoid foramen and terminal branching of parotid plexus to supply the muscles of facial expression. Signs and symptoms of facial nerve damage depend on the exact anatomical site of the lesion during its course. The more peripheral the site of the injury, the signs and symptoms become less diverse. (Reproduced with permission from Schuenke M, Schulte E, Schumacher U. THIEME Atlas of Anatomy Second Edition, Vol 3. © Thieme 2016. Illustrations by Markus Voll and Karl Wesker.)

resulting from infection, or trauma. Signs and symptoms vary based on the exact site of the lesion (see Clinical Correlation Box 20.3 and ▶ Fig. 20.10).

20.3.2 CN VII SVE Fibers: Peripheral Course

- As the facial nerve exits the stylomastoid foramen it gives rise to three muscular branches: the **posterior auricular nerve** that supplies the posterior auricular muscle and the **occiptiofronatalis muscle**, the nerve to the **posterior belly of the diagastric**, and the **nerve to the stylohyoid muscle**.
- The facial nerve enters the posterior boundary of the parotid gland and divides into **temporofacial** and **cervicofacial** divisions to form the **parotid nerve plexus**.

The facial nerve does not innervate the parotid gland but can be at surgical risk during parotid surgery.

- The five terminal branches arising from the parotid plexus of the facial nerve include the **temporal, zygomatic, buccal, marginal mandibular,** and **cervical** branches. The terminal branches provide a regional pattern of innervation to the upper and lower muscles of facial expression (▶ Fig. 20.9).

Clinical Correlation Box 20.3: Brainstem and Infranucluear Lesions to Facial Motor Nucleus (LMN) (see ▶ Fig. 20.8c)

- Damage to LMNs in the facial motor nucleus, or to SVE fibers during their peripheral course, leads to a loss of voluntary motor control to both upper and lower facial muscle groups and results in unilateral facial muscle paralysis of the entire ipsilateral face.

Depending on the site of the lesion, patients may be at risk of corneal ulcerations on the affected side due to decreased lacrimation. Additional deficits may manifest food pocketing in cheek, difficulty in bolus formation, drooling, diminished taste, and difficulty in speech articulation. A comparison between UMN and LMN lesions of the facial nerve is provided in ▶ Table 20.17.

- Cerebrovascular accident (stroke) causing a nuclear lesion of the facial motor nucleus often involves the abducens (CN VI) motor nucleus due to its anatomical proximity to the facial nucleus in the pons. Vascular lesions occurring in this region will cause ipsilateral loss of innervation to the lateral rectus muscle and may also impact the corticospinal tract leading to limb weakness on the contralateral side (see ▶ Fig. 20.7b).

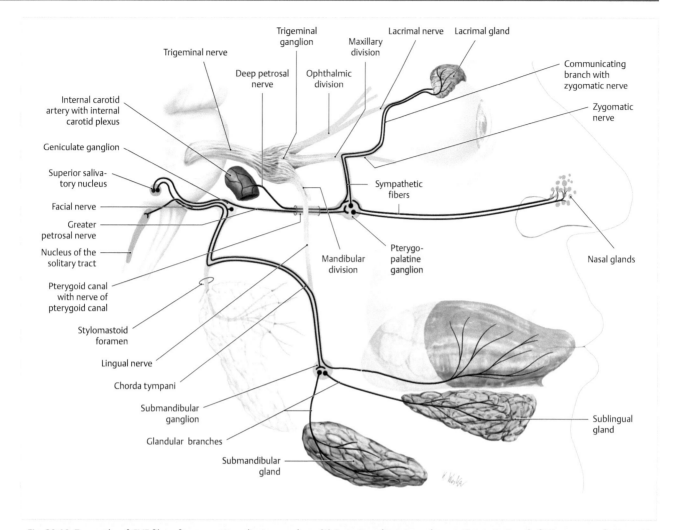

Fig. 20.10 Two paths of GVE fibers from superior salivatory nucleus: (1) Superior salivatory nucleus –> Greater petrosal of VII –> nerve of pterygoid canal –> synapse in pterygopalatine ganglion in the pterygopalatine fossa –>target glands (nasal, palatal and glossopalatine glands) via greater and lesser palatine N of V2. (2) Superior salivatory nucleus of VII –> chorda tympani of VII –> synapse in submandibular ganglion in floor of oral cavity –> target glands (submandibular, sublingual, labial, and anterior lingual glands) via lingual N of V3. (Reproduced with permission from Schuenke M, Schulte E, Schumacher U. THIEME Atlas of Anatomy Second Edition, Vol 3. © Thieme 2016. Illustrations by Markus Voll and Karl Wesker.)

Clinical Correlation Box 20.4: Bell's Palsy (▶ Fig. 20.10)

Bell's palsy or facial palsy is the most common acute cause of LMN paralysis of the face and is hallmarked by rapid onset with a lack of trauma. It is often associated with viral infections, such as herpes simplex, leading to inflammation and compression of the facial nerve during its peripheral course through the facial canal. Symptoms vary depending on the location of the lesion within the facial canal; however, motor paralysis is complete on the ipsilateral side of the face, with some dysfunction of the nervus intermedius. In addition to complete unilateral facial paralysis, there may be concomitant loss of glandular and sensory function due to compression of the nervus intermedius. Prognosis depends on the extent of peripheral nerve damage to the axon and whether the injury leads to Wallerian degeneration (see Chapter 3 clinical correlation).

20.3.3 CN VII GVE Fibers

GVE CN VII: Origin, Central Connections, and Course (see ▶ Fig. 20.7c and ▶ Fig. 20.10)

- **Preganglionic parasympathetic fibers** originate from GVE neurons in the **superior salivatory nucleus** in the **caudal pons** and travel in the **nervus intermedius**. The nervus intermedius which does not loop around the abducens nerve exits the caudal pons just lateral to the SVE fibers carried in the facial nerve proper.
- Preganglionic parasympathetic neurons in the superior salivatory nucleus receive modulatory input and reflexive stimuli from several sources that function to control the efferent outflow of salivary gland secretion (see Chapter 24 for detail).
  - Preautonomic neurons in the **hypothalamus** and **amygdala** provide reflexive input to salivatory neurons via

dorsal longitudinal fasciculus in response to visceral input such as odors, nausea, and emotional states including fear, joy, and sadness.

○ Reflexive afferent input associated with **gustatory (taste) input, oral tactile stimulation, pain,** or **irritation** may project to superior salivatory nucleus directly from the **nucleus solitarius,** the **chief sensory nucleus,** and the **spinal trigeminal nucleus,** respectively.

CN VII GVE Fibers: Intracranial Course

- GVE fibers of the nervus intermedius follow the same intracranial course as SVE fibers to enter the facial canal. Within the facial canal the **preganglionic parasympathetic (GVE) fibers** branch from the facial nerve at the level of the geniculate sensory ganglion and divide into the **chorda tympani nerve** and **greater petrosal nerve**.
- Preganglionic GVE fibers of both the **chorda tympani nerve** and **greater petrosal nerve** pass through the geniculate sensory ganglion without synapsing and then follow either a submandibular route or a lacrimal route to exit the skull and synapse in their designated parasympathetic ganglia (see ▸ Fig. 20.11).
- A description of each route, along with the path of the chorda tympani and greater petrosal nerve branches, is summarized in ▸ Table 20.18 and ▸ Table 20.19.

20.3.4 Sensory Component of the Facial Nerve: SVA, GSA, and GVA

- The sensory modalities carried by the nervus intermedius of CN VII include **SVA, GVA,** and **GSA** fibers. Taste (SVA) conveyed from taste buds in the anterior two-thirds of the tongue and palatal mucosa represents the most significant sensory component of the facial nerve. Taste fibers from the tongue and palate follow the chorda tympani and greater petrosal branches of CN VII, respectively. The SVA fibers follow a similar path as the secretomotor fibers (GVE) carried by these nerves (see ▸ Fig. 20.11). GSA and GVA provide only a minor contribution of sensory input from the orofacial region. GSA fibers provide innervation behind the external ear and travel with the posterior auricular branch of CN VII as it emerges from the stylomastoid foramen.
- The **primary afferent neuronal cell bodies** of each sensory modality reside in the **geniculate sensory ganglion** and the fibers pass through the ganglion without synapsing.
- Central axons of primary afferent fibers join the nervus intermedius and enter the brainstem at the cerebellopontine angle with the facial nerve proper. The central axons synapse on the following target nuclei before ascending to higher brain centers.
  ○ Central axons of **SVA** and **GVA neurons** project to the **nucleus solitarius.**
  ○ Central **GSA fibers** synapse in the **spinal trigeminal nucleus.**
- A description of the specific path for each modality is outlined in ▸ Table 20.20, ▸ Table 20.21, ▸ Table 20.22.

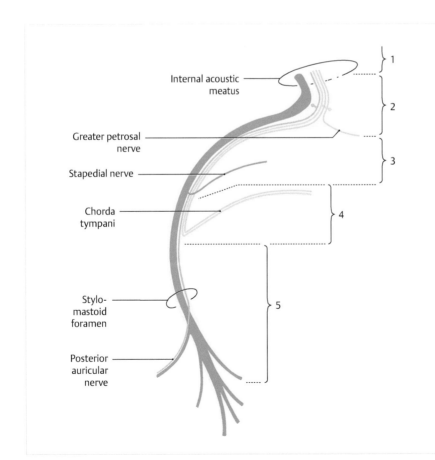

Internal acoustic meatus

Greater petrosal nerve

Stapedial nerve

Chorda tympani

Stylo-mastoid foramen

Posterior auricular nerve

1
2
3
4
5

Fig. 20.11 Path of parasympathetic general visceral efferents (GVEs) and gustatory special visceral afferent (SVA) of the facial nerve. Preganglionic parasympathetic neurons reside in superior salivatory ganglion. The two distribution paths of secretomotor (GVE) fibers to the lacrimal, nasal, and salivary glands are shown. Taste (SVA) fibers, which arise from the anterior two-thirds of tongue, travel with the lingual nerve (CN V3) and chorda tympani nerve of CN VII. During their course, SVA fibers accompany some GVE fibers, but pass through the submandibular ganglion without synapsing (shown). SVA fibers from palatal taste buds travel with the greater petrosal nerve of CN VII. SVA taste fibers originate from pseudounipolar neurons in the geniculate ganglion and ascend to nucleus tract of solitarius. 1: Complete ipsilateral motor paralysis of all upper and lower facial muscles; vestibulocochlear dysfunction including deafness, vertigo, loss of taste, lacrimation, salivation. 2: Complete Ipsilateral motor paralysis, loss of taste, lacrimation, salivation. 3: Complete ipsilateral motor paralysis, loss of taste, decreased salivation. 4: Loss of upper and lower muscles; stapedial function spared, loss of taste, and decreased salivation. 5: Ipsilateral loss of upper and lower facial muscle only. (Reproduced with permission from Schuenke M, Schulte E, Schumacher U. THIEME Atlas of Anatomy. Second Edition, Vol 3. © Thieme 2016. Illustrations by Markus Voll and Karl Wesker.)

Table 20.18 GVE fiber distribution: Submandibular route: Chorda tympani of CN VII

Parasympathetic Innervation: Submandibular Route via Chorda Tympani Nerve of CN VII						
Functional Component	Cranial Nerve Branch	Cranial Nerve Motor Nuclei	Intracranial Path and Skull Exit	Parasympathetic Ganglion	Peripheral Course	Effector Target
GVE Secretomotor to salivary and nasal glands	Chorda tympani	Superior salivatory nucleus (location of preganglionic parasympathetic neurons)	GVE fibers of facial nerve enter **internal auditory meatus**→ ear→enters **facial canal**→ pass medial to tympanic membrane through middle ear (**tympanic**) cavity →exits skull through **petrotympanic fissure** → enters infratemporal fossa → travels with lingual nerve to submandibular ganglion	Submandibular ganglion	Postganglionic fibers travel with the **lingual nerve** V3 through floor of oral cavity for distribution of GVE fibers to glands	• Submandibular • Sublingual • Lower labial* • Anterior lingual*

Abbreviation: GVE, general visceral efferent.
Note: *Minor salivary glands.

Table 20.19 GVE fiber distribution: Lacrimal route: Greater petrosal nerve of CN VII

Parasympathetic Innervation: Lacrimal Route via Greater Petrosal Nerve of CN VII						
Functional Component	Cranial Nerve Branch	Cranial Nerve Motor Nuclei	Intracranial Path and Skull Exit	Parasympathetic Ganglion	Peripheral Course	Effector Target
GVE Secretomotor to salivary and nasal glands	Greater petrosal	Superior salivatory nucleus (location of preganglionic parasympathetic neurons)	GVE fibers of facial nerve enter **internal auditory meatus**→ ear→enters **facial canal**→ exit facial canal through facial hiatus →enters pterygoid canal and joins the **deep petrosal nerve** which carries postganglionic sympathetic fibers. Both nerves travel as the **nerve of pterygoid canal (vidian nerve)**. → enters pterygopalatine fossa Preganglionic parasympathetic synapse in ganglion	Pterygopalatine ganglion	Postganglionic fibers distributed by branches of **ophthalmic (V1)** and **maxillary (V2)** • Fibers follow **zygomaticotemporal** (V2) →enters **inferior orbital fissure** → travels with lacrimal nerve (V1) • Fibers follow named terminal branch of V2 from ganglion in pterygopalatine fossa	Distribution via V1 • **Lacrimal gland** Distribution via V2 • **Nasal and paranasal glands via** • **Posterior superior lateral and medial nasal branch** • Nasopalatine branch • Posterior superior alveolar nerve branch • **Palatal and pharyngeal glands** via greater and lesser palatine nerve

Abbreviation: GVE, general visceral efferent.

Clinical Correlation Box 2.5: Loss of Taste

Diminished or loss of taste known as **dysgeusia** or **ageusia**, respectively, may occur to the anterior two-thirds of the tongue due to injury to the facial nerve. Associated deficits in addition to the loss of taste correlate to the site of injury (see ▶ Fig. 20.10).

• Injury to the lingual nerve just distal to the point of junction with the chorda tympani will cause a loss of ipsilateral taste, loss of general sensation, and decreased salivation of the submandibular and sublingual glands.

• Injury to the chorda tympani distal to its branching from the facial nerve leads to a loss of taste to anterior two-thirds of tongue and secretomotor activity.

• Injury to the facial nerve proximal to branching within the facial canal results in loss of taste, general sensation to posterior ear, lacrimation, and salivation from the sublingual and submandibular glands, and paralysis of all ipsilateral facial muscles.

Table 20.20 Course of SVA fibers for facial nerve (CN VII)

Special Visceral Afferent (SVA) Course					
Cranial Nerve Branch Names	Peripheral Afferent Input and Location	Cranial Ganglia Location of primary afferent neurons	Sensory Nuclei Location of secondary afferent neurons	Central Target *	Central Termination *
SVA (taste) **Chorda tympani branch of CN VII**	Chemoreceptors on neuroepithelial cells Taste for anterior two-thirds of tongue Afferent fibers travel with lingual nerve (V3) from floor of mouth SVA fibers join the chorda tympani in infratemporal fossa and enters skull via petrotympanic fissure. Fibers pass through ganglion.	**Geniculate—primary afferent neurons** Central processes travel via nervus intermedius. Descend in tract of solitarius to medulla and synapse on second-order neurons in nucleus tractus solitarius (NTS).	**Nucleus tractus solitarius** (rostral part)	Secondary afferents ascend bilaterally in **central tegmental tract** Target: VPM nuclei of thalamus Target: Hypothalamus	Project to primary taste area (gustatory cortex) of somatosensory cortex and insula for conscious perception of taste Termination in limbic system • Hippocampus (memory) • Amygdala • Hypothalamus For emotional processing of eating and reflexive input to salivatory centers in response to taste
SVA **Greater petrosal branch of CN VII**	Chemoreceptors on neuroepithelial cells of taste buds in palatal mucosa SVA fibers travel with greater and lesser palatine (V2) from palatal mucosa →ascend through palatine canal to enter the pterygopalatine fossa. SVA fibers pass through pterygopalatine ganglion without synapsing and join the greater petrosal nerve → SVA fibers project toward geniculate ganglion	**Geniculate—primary afferent neurons** Central processes travel via nervus intermedius	**Nucleus solitarius** (rostral part)	Same central target as above	Same central terminations as above

Abbreviation: SVA, special visceral afferent; VPM, ventral posteromedial.
Note: *The central taste pathway which ascends from the nucleus solitarius to higher brain centers for processing is a common pathway shared by CNs VII, IX, and X.

Table 20.21 Course of GSA fibers for facial nerve (CN VII)

General Somatic Afferent (GSA) Branches of Facial Nerve					
Cranial Nerve Branch Names	Peripheral Afferent Input	Cranial Ganglia Location of primary afferent neurons	Sensory Nuclei Location of secondary afferent neurons	Central Target	Central Termination
Sensory auricular branch Travels with posterior auricular branch Fibers to skin behind external ear, auricle * Communicates with auricular branch of vagus	Cutaneous nociceptors, mechanoreceptors in the skin behind the ear and auricle of ear Short peripheral course: Fibers from posterior region of ear enter skull through **stylomastoid foramen,** pass through **facial canal** → GSA fibers pass through geniculate ganglion without synapsing	**Geniculate ganglion** Central processes travel via nervus intermedius to enter pons → GSA fibers descend in spinal trigeminal tract to synapse on second-order neurons in spinal trigeminal nucleus	**Spinal trigeminal nucleus**	Secondary afferents ascend in ventral trigeminal tract Project to the contralateral VPM of thalamus	Facial region of primary somatosensory cortex in postcentral gyrus of parietal lobe

Abbreviations: GSA, general somatic afferent; VPM, ventral posteromedial.

Table 20.22 Course of GVA fibers for facial nerve (CN VII)

General Visceral Afferent (GVA) Fibers of Facial Nerve					
Facial (CN VII)	Peripheral Afferent Input	Cranial Ganglia Location of primary afferent neurons	Sensory Nuclei	Central Target	Central Termination
GVA No named branches Very small contribution to mucous membranes in nasopharynx	Polymodal nociceptive give rise to GVA fibers. GVA fibers travel along path of GVE fibers from greater petrosal. GVA pass from the nasopharynx and soft palate to pterygopalatine fossa →via the **lesser palatine foramen** → enters the skull through the pterygoid canal and greater petrosal hiatus → travel with greater petrosal toward geniculate ganglion. GVA fibers pass through without synapsing.	Geniculate ganglion Central processes travel via nervus intermedius to enter brainstem	Nucleus solitaries (caudal part)	• VPM of thalamus • Subcortical neurons, amygdala, hypothalamus input may modulate activity in premotor cortex facial expression in response to emotional interpretation of sensory input	Primary somatosensory cortex in postcentral gyrus of parietal lobe Premotor cortex in frontal lobe via input from cortical and subcortical structures

Abbreviations: GVA, general visceral afferent; VPM, ventral posteromedial.

Questions and Answers

1. A lesion destroying the spinal trigeminal tract in the caudal pons results in the loss of the _____.
   a) Contralateral pinprick sensation to the forehead
   b) Ipsilateral corneal reflex
   c) Pressure sense to the skin covering the thyroid gland
   d) Jaw jerk reflex
   e) Two-point discrimination in the ipsilateral cheek

Level 2: Moderate

Answer B: The GSA afferent fibers that carry crude touch, pain, and temperature sensations are the Aδ and C fibers of the trigeminal nerve (CN V). These fibers provide the afferent limb of the corneal reflex. The SVE fibers of facial nerve form the efferent limb. Afferent fibers arising from the cornea travel with a branch of the ophthalmic nerve, pass through the trigeminal ganglion, and then enter the spinal trigeminal tract to synapse on second-order neurons in the spinal trigeminal nucleus. A loss of two-point discrimination (**E**) and pinprick (**A**) sensations are considered tactile input and do not travel in the spinal trigeminal tract. The nerve fibers transmitting this type of GSA input are myelinated Aβ fibers that synapse on second-order neurons of the chief sensory nucleus. The chief sensory nucleus lies lateral to the trigeminal motor nucleus in the midpons. These structures lie rostral to the spinal trigeminal tract and nucleus. The tactile pressure sensations to the skin of the neck near the thyroid gland (**C**) is provided by branches of the superficial cervical plexus and does not project to the spinal trigeminal tract. The tactile input from mechanoreceptors will follow the fasciculus cuneatus of the dorsal column medial lemniscus (DCML) pathway. Pain and thermal sensations from the neck usually follow the spinothalamic tract; however, it is possible to have overlap/convergence of sensory input between the cervical and trigeminal system from the cervical region due to the position of the pars caudalis nucleus extending to the level of C2. The loss of the jaw jerk reflex (**D**) occurs in

lesions of the mesencephalic nucleus (afferent limb) found in the rostral pons, or due to damage to the trigeminal motor nucleus (efferent limb).

2. The nerve branches that arise from the facial nerve during its course through the facial canal include each of the following EXCEPT one. Which one is the exception?
   a) Nerve to the stapedius
   b) Posterior auricular nerve
   c) Chorda tympani nerve
   d) Greater petrosal nerve

Level 1: Easy

Answer B: The posterior auricular nerve branch arises from the facial nerve upon exiting the facial canal at the stylomastoid foramen. The nerve to the posterior belly and stylohyoid muscle also arises from the facial nerve at this point. The facial canal may be divided into three segments: the labyrinthine, the tympanic, and the mastoid regions. (**A**) The nerve to the stapedius muscle (SVE) exits from tympanic section of the canal to provide motor fibers to the stapedius muscle. Damage to this nerve causes hyperacusis. (**C**) The chorda tympani, which transmits both GVE and SVA fibers, exits the facial canal through the tympanic canaliculus. The nerve provides secretomotor innervation to the sublingual and submandibular glands and conveys taste from anterior two-thirds of the tongue. (**D**) The greater petrosal nerve carries preganglionic parasympathetic (GVE) fibers that control the secretion of the lacrimal, nasal, and palatal glands. It exits the facial canal through the facial hiatus at the level of the geniculate ganglion.

Use the following scenario to answer questions 3 and 4

A patient with a history of hypertension and type 2 diabetes presents with sudden onset of slurred speech, facial droop, medial deviation of the right eye (estropia, a form of strabismus), double vision (horizontal diplopia), and contralateral limb weakness (hemiplegia). The magnetic resonance imaging

(MRI) shows signs of an ischemic stroke in the region of the right caudal pons.

3. The initial presentation of symptoms suggests involvement of each of the following structures EXCEPT one. Which one is the exception?
   a) Right facial motor nucleus
   b) Right abducens nucleus
   c) Right trochlear nucleus
   d) Right corticospinal tract

Level 2: Moderate

Answer C: The right trochlear nerve (CN IV) is found in the midline of the midbrain, just caudal to the inferior colliculus. It is too far rostral to be affected by an infarct in the caudal pons. The trochlear nerve innervates the superior oblique muscle and functions to turn the eye inward and down. (**A**) The facial nucleus lies in caudal pons just inferior and lateral to the abducens motor nucleus. A lesion of the lower motor neurons in the facial nucleus results in slurring of words and right-side facial droop due to paralysis of facial muscles of expression. (**B**) The abducens nerve lies medial to the facial motor nucleus. The motor fibers of the facial nerve loop around the abducens nerve, forming an elevation known as the facial colliculus. A stroke involving the facial nerve may also involve the abducens due to the proximity of the two nuclei. (**D**) The corticospinal tracts pass from the cortex through the brainstem to reach the spinal cord. It carries motor fibers for the trunk and extremities and will decussate at the level of the pyramids in the medulla to supply the contralateral side of the body. Corticobulbar fibers, the inferior salivatory nucleus of CN VII, and the nervus intermedius of CN VII, along with other structures not listed, may also be involved depending on the extent of the stroke.

4. In the scenario above, which of the following findings may be seen upon clinical examination of the patient's facial movements?
   a) Right-side weakness of the lower facial muscles, with sparing of frontalis
   b) Left-side weakness of the frontalis muscle
   c) Right-side weakness of all muscles of facial expression
   d) Left-side weakness of all muscles of facial expression

Level 2: Moderate

Answer C: The symptoms described and the location of the lesion are consistent with damage to the lower motor neurons in the right facial motor nucleus in the pons. Unilateral lesions of the facial motor nucleus result in ipsilateral facial nerve palsy. Facial palsy (Bell's palsy) results in motor loss to ALL of the muscles of facial expression on the side of the lesion.

Choice (**D**) would not be the result because the lesion occurs in the right facial motor nucleus. LMNs provide ipsilateral innervation to the skeletal muscles. (**A**) In comparison, unilateral cortical lesions of UMNs result in contralateral loss of ONLY the lower facial muscles. Lower facial muscles receive innervation from the contralateral primary motor cortex. These cortical fibers terminate in the ventral part of the facial motor nucleus. Upper facial muscles receive bilateral input from the cortex, and the cortical fibers terminate in the dorsal part of the nucleus. (**B**) The bilateral input to upper facial muscles spares the forehead (frontalis) and eye (orbicularis oculi) muscles from paralysis due to unilateral UMN lesions, so paralysis or weakness of the forehead would not occur.

5. An infranuclear (peripheral) lesion of the left facial nerve that occurs just distal to the geniculate ganglion will result in each of the following clinical signs EXCEPT one. Which one is the exception?
   a) Loss of taste in left anterior two-thirds of tongue
   b) Decreased salivation of the sublingual and submandibular glands
   c) Decreased lacrimation
   d) Complete facial paralysis
   e) Hyperacusis

Level 2: Moderate

Answer C: The greater petrosal nerve of CN VII carries parasympathetic (GVE) fibers to the lacrimal gland to control lacrimation. The greater petrosal arises from the facial nerve at the level of the geniculate ganglion in the facial canal and lies proximal to the lesion, so it is not affected. The other nerve branches of the facial nerve, each branch distal to the lesion, will be affected. (**A**) The chorda tympani branches from the facial nerve distal to the lesion in the tympanic part of the canal and carries taste (SVA) from taste buds found in the papillae in the anterior two-thirds of the tongue. (**B**) The chorda tympani nerve also transmits parasympathetic (GVE) to the sublingual and submandibular glands to control salivation. (**D**) Complete ipsilateral facial paralysis will result due to the compression of all motor (SVE) branches of CN VII during its course through the facial canal. (**E**) Hyperacusis result from damage to the nerve of the stapedius. This motor branch causes contraction of the stapedial muscle which helps to attenuate loud noises. Overall, hyperacusis causes minimal clinical impact; however, patients may complain of sensitivity to certain frequencies, with a decreased tolerance to loud noises, or may perceive sounds louder than produced.

21 Overview of Orofacial Pathways Part II— Glossopharyngeal, Vagus, and Hypoglossal Nerves

Learning Objectives

1. Describe the location of lower cranial nerve motor nuclei and sensory nuclei.
2. Describe the functional modalities carried by the glossopharyngeal, vagus, and hypoglossal nerves.
3. Explain the significance and clinical signs associated with a lower motor lesion affecting the nucleus ambiguus.
4. Describe the sensory distribution of taste fibers to posterior one-third of tongue and ascending path to cerebral cortex.
5. What is the pathway by which protopathic sensation from the larynx reaches the somatosensory cortex?
6. Explain the cortical input to the lower motor neurons in cranial motor nuclei of CNs IX, X, and XII.
7. Compare the differences between an upper motor neuron (central) and lower motor neuron lesion to the tongue.
8. Explain the pathway for the GVE fibers carried by the glossopharyngeal nerve.

21.1 Introduction

The lower cranial nerves IX, X, and XII are important in executing several oromotor functions including phonation and swallowing. The cranial nerves work cooperatively with the trigeminal and facial nerves to mediate mastication, swallowing, and speech articulation. The close proximity of the lower cranial motor nuclei within the medulla, along with their overlapping peripheral course as they descend in the neck, puts the lower cranial nerves at risk for injury. Lesions affecting lower cranial nerves may result from numerous causes and should be suspected in cases of disturbed speech, difficulty in swallowing, pharyngeal pain, or sensory loss. Examples of nerve lesions involving the lower cranial nerves are presented throughout the chapter as four Clinical Correlation Boxes 21.1–21.4. The last clinical box, 21.4, discusses the possible outcome if a lesion affects several of the lower cranial nerves. This chapter describes the specific path for each of the lower cranial nerves to provide a baseline for understanding oromotor function and sensorimotor reflexes. Oromotor function is covered in Chapter 22.

21.2 Glossopharyngeal

- The glossopharyngeal nerve (CN IX) develops in association with the third pharyngeal arch and carries both motor and sensory modalities. The modalities carried include two motor components, namely, special visceral efferent (SVE) and general visceral efferent (GVE) fibers, and three sensory modalities, namely, general somatic afferent (GSA), general visceral afferent (GVA), and special visceral afferent (SVA) fibers (▶ Fig. 21.1). The functional modalities associated with the glosspharyngeal nerve are outlined in Table 21.1.

21.2.1 Special Visceral Efferent Component of Glossopharyngeal

CN IX SVE Fibers: Origin, Central Connections, and Course

- Motor fibers arising from corticonuclear (upper motor neurons [UMNs]) neurons in the orofacial area of the primary motor cortex and premotor areas descend in the **corticobulbar (pyramidal) tract,** through the posterior internal capsule, to synapse **bilaterally** on lower motor neurons (LMNs) in the **nucleus ambiguus.**

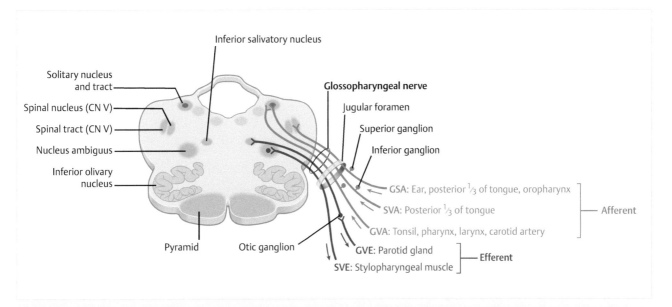

Fig. 21.1 Motor and sensory modalities carried by the glossopharyngeal nerve (CN IX). SVE and GVE motor fibers originate from the nucleus ambiguus and inferior salivatory nucleus, respectively. GSA afferent sensations project to the spinal trigeminal nucleus, whereas GVA and SVA fibers terminate in the nucleus tractus solitarius. GSA, general somatic afferent; GVA, general visceral afferent; GVE, general visceral efferent; SVE, special visceral efferent.

- **SVE fibers** of **CN IX** arise from LMNs found in the **rostral part** of the **nucleus ambiguus.**
  - The caudal portion of nucleus ambiguus contains the LMNs for the SVE component of the vagus nerve (CN X). Nuclear lesions affecting LMNs in the nucleus ambiguus will potentially impact both CNs IX and X; however, the motor deficit of the vagus (CN X) will be more significant due to its motor contribution to the pharyngeal plexus.
  - Comparable to other orofacial cranial nerve nuclei, the LMNs in the nucleus ambiguus receive input from central pattern generators (CPGs) involved in generating rhythmic patterned movements and reflexive activity.
  - The extrapyramidal system also provides indirect feedback to the nucleus ambiguus to coordinate motor activities and correct for motor error.
- The remaining functional components of CN IX join with the SVE fibers to form the **main trunk** of the glossopharyngeal nerve. The glossopharyngeal nerve exits the medulla from the postolivary sulcus located between the olive and inferior cerebellar peduncle, just superior to the vagus nerve and accessory nerve (CN IX).
- Glossopharyngeal nerve passes through the posterior cranial fossa to exit the skull via the **jugular foramen.** The vagus (CN X), the accessory (CN IX), and the internal jugular vein accompany the glossopharyngeal nerve as it exits the skull.

SVE Fibers: Peripheral Course (▶ Fig. 21.2)

- SVE fibers of CN IX descend in the neck between the internal carotid and internal jugular vein, deep to the stylohyoid process, to innervate the **stylopharyngeus muscle** derived from the **third pharyngeal arch branchiomeric mesoderm.** The stylopharyngeus muscle elevates the pharynx during swallowing and speech (see Chapter 22).

21.2.2 GVE of CN IX

GVE Fibers: Central and Intracranial Course

- **GVE fibers** arise from **preganglionic parasympathetic cell bodies** found within the **inferior salivatory nucleus.**
- The inferior salivatory nucleus receives modulatory input and reflexive stimuli from several sources that function to control the efferent outflow of salivary gland secretion (see Chapter 24 for detail).

- Preautonomic neurons in the **olfactory, hypothalamus,** and **amygdala** provide reflexive input to salivatory neurons via **dorsal longitudinal fasciculus** in response to visceral input such as odors, nausea, and emotional states including fear, joy, and sadness.
- Reflexive afferent input associated with **gustatory (taste) input, oral tactile stimulation, pain,** or **irritation** may project to the **inferior salivatory nucleus** from the **nucleus solitarius,** the **chief sensory nucleus,** and from the **spinal trigeminal nucleus** (see Chapter 24).
- Preganglionic parasympathetic (GVE) fibers follow the other functional fiber components of CN IX to exit the skull through the **jugular foramen.** GVE fibers join the **tympanic branch** of CN IX as it branches from the main trunk of the glossopharyngeal nerve.
- The tympanic nerve carrying GSA fibers along with GVE fibers passes through a small opening, the **tympanic canaliculus,** to enter the middle (tympanic) ear cavity, and forms the tympanic nerve plexus. GVE fibers pass through the plexus to form the **lesser petrosal nerve** (▶ Fig. 21.3).

GVE Peripheral Course

- The **lesser petrosal nerve** exits the middle ear cavity, re-enters the middle cranial fossa, and then travels with mandibular branch V3 through the **foramen ovale** to enter infratemporal fossa.
- The **lesser petrosal** synapses on the **otic ganglion** that lies immediately inferior to the foramen ovale.
- **Postganglionic fibers** emerging from the otic ganglion accompany the **auriculotemporal nerve (CN V3)** of the **mandibular division** for distribution of secretomotor fibers to the **parotid gland** and minor **buccal salivary glands.** The pathway for GVE fibers associated with the glossopharyngeal nerve are outlined in Table 21.2.

21.2.3 GSA of CN IX

GSA Fibers: Peripheral Course

- **Nociceptors, mechanoreceptors,** and **thermoreceptors** give rise to primary somatic afferent fibers which transmit general sensory input from three areas along the following nerve branches:
  - GSA information from the mucosa of **the auditory tube (pharyngotympanic tube)** and **the inner surface of the tympanic membrane** travel via the **tympanic plexus** and **tympanic nerve.**

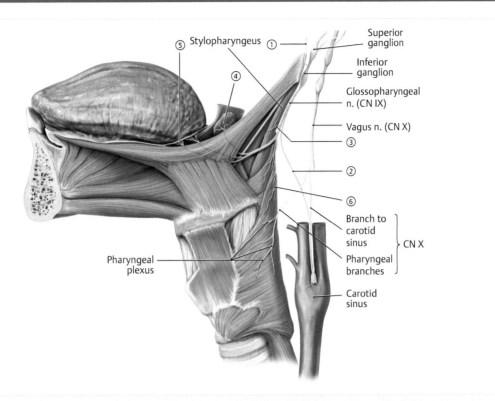

Fig. 21.2 Peripheral distribution and course of motor and sensory fibers of the glossopharyngeal nerve. The glossopharyngeal nerve carries predominantly sensory fibers except for the SVE motor fibers innervating the stylopharyngeus muscle. The lower motor neurons for the stylopharyngeus reside in the rostral part of the nucleus ambiguus. The pharyngeal nerve branch of CN IX, along with minor contributions from the tonsillar and lingual branches of CN IX, provides sensory (GVA/GSA) innervation to the pharynx and combines with the vagus (CN X) to form pharyngeal plexus. The nerve to carotid sinus communicates with the vagus nerve to carry visceral afferent signals from the baroreceptors in the carotid sinus and chemoreceptors in the carotid body toward the nucleus tractus solitarius (NTS) in the medulla. The NTS is important for the integration of cardiorespiratory reflexes and vasomotor control. The nucleus ambiguus and the nucleus tract solitarius mediate functions associated with both the glossopharyngeal and vagus. CNs IX and X are often tested together when assessing brainstem lesion and cranial nerve function. GSA, general somatic afferent; GVA, general visceral afferent; SVE, special visceral efferent. (Reproduced with permission from Schuenke M, Schulte E, Schumacher U. THIEME Atlas of Anatomy Third Edition, Vol 3. © Thieme 2020. Illustrations by Markus Voll and Karl Wesker.)

○ GSA input from the mucosa of **posterior one-third of tongue, upper pharynx, and tonsillar fossa** travel via the **lingual** and **tonsillar** branches of the glossopharyngeal nerve. The peripheral nerve processes arising from the oropharynx pass through the aperture between the superior and middle constrictors to ascend toward the superior ganglion.

○ GSA fibers from the **skin covering the external ear** initially travel with the **auricular branch** of **CN X.**

• Primary afferent fibers ascend toward the GSA afferent neurons located in the **superior ganglion** of **CN IX** which resides in the jugular foramen. GSA fibers pass through the ganglion without synapsing.

The specific pathways for each peripheral branch are outlined in ▶ Table 21.3.

CN IX GSA: Intracranial and Central Course

• Central processes of afferent fibers emerge from superior ganglion of CN IX and pass through the **jugular foramen** to enter the **brainstem at the medulla.**

• GSA fibers for each branch of CN IX follow the same central path as the protopathic fibers of CNs V, VII, and X. Secondary afferents ascend to the cortex via the **trigeminothalamic tract** (trigeminal lemniscus—a summary of the path is provided in ▶ Table 21.3 and a detailed description of the trigeminothalamic tract may be found in Chapter 13).

21.2.4 GVA of CN IX

GVA Fibers: Peripheral Course

• **GVA fibers** of the glossopharyngeal nerve travel primarily through **carotid (sinus) nerve** and **pharyngeal nerve of CN IX.**

• The GVA fibers of the **carotid sinus nerve** arise from specialized baroreceptors and chemoreceptors located in the wall of the internal carotid and common carotid artery at the point of bifurcation. These receptors provide afferent input for vasomotor reflexes mediated through cardiovascular and respiratory centers in the medulla and the activation of the autonomic system.

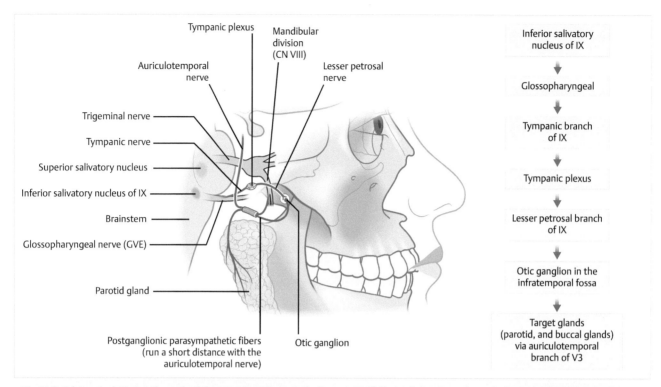

Fig. 21.3 Schematic depicting the path of the parasympathetic visceral motor (GVE) fibers of the glossopharyngeal nerve to the parotid and buccal salivary glands. Right, lateral view. GVE, general visceral efferent.

○ **Baroreceptor reflex**: Baroreceptors detect changes in systolic blood pressure and reside in the **carotid sinus** and **aortic sinus**.

– GVA fibers follow the carotid sinus nerve of CN IX to the **nucleus tractus solitarius (NTS)** to synapse on second-order neurons. Secondary afferents project to cardiac vagal parasympathetic neurons in the nucleus ambiguus and the dorsal motor nucleus of CN X. Secondary afferents also project to the neurons in the reticular formation of the medulla for sympathetic control of the heart.

– The vagus serves as the efferent limb of the baroreceptor reflex. Vagal parasympathetic (GVE) fibers terminate on the SA node of the heart and causes a decrease in heart rate (**bradycardia**) in response to elevated blood pressure and baroreceptor stimulation.

○ **Chemoreceptor reflex**: Chemoreceptors, which respond to decreased levels of oxygen (**hypoxia**), increased level of carbon dioxide (**hypercapnia**), or decreased levels in pH (**acidosis**), are found in the **carotid body** and **aortic body**.

– The aortic branch of the vagus nerve, which conveys GVA input from the aortic sinus and aortic body, travels with the GVA fibers of the carotid sinus nerve branch of the glossopharyngeal nerve to the nucleus tract of solitarius in the central nervous system (CNS).

– The central afferent GVA fibers synapse in the **NTS** before projecting to vasomotor and respiratory reflex centers in the medullary reticular formation and hypothalamus to control parasympathetic and sympathetic activity. The outcome of chemoreceptor stimulation is to increase respiratory activity and may also increase cardiac output.

• GVA fibers also arise from **polymodal nociceptors** from the **mucosa** lining the **oropharynx, tonsillar fossa, parotid gland,** and **soft palate.** These provide the principal afferent input for the sensory component of the pharyngeal plexuses and serve as the afferent limb of the gag reflex (**see Chapter 22**).

• The peripheral processes of GVA fibers pass through the inferior ganglion of CN IX without synapsing and then ascend to the NTS (solitary nucleus) to synapse on second-order neurons.

• The central pathway for the branches carrying GVA fibers is described in ▶ Table 21.4.

21.2.5 SVA of CN IX

SVA Fibers: Peripheral Course

• **SVA fibers** receive gustatory input through specialized taste (chemoreceptors) receptors in the neuroepithelial cells comprising the taste buds in the posterior one-third of the tongue, circumvallate papillae, and posterior foliate papillae.

Vagus nerve branches in the neck	
1	Pharyngeal branches
2	Superior laryngeal n.
3R	Right recurrent laryngeal n.
3L	Left recurrent laryngeal n.
4	Cervical cardiac branches

Table 21.1 Functional modalities transmitted by the glossopharyngeal nerve

Functional Component		Associated Nuclei	Associated Ganglia	Glossopharyngeal Branch	Region Innervated	Clinical Signs of Peripheral Damage
SVE	Voluntary motor to the skeletal muscle of third pharyngeal arch *Aids in elevating pharynx during swallowing	SVE fibers originate from **nucleus ambiguus**	Not applicable	**Stylopharyngeus nerve**	Stylopharyngeus muscle	**Dysphagia** (difficulty swallowing)
GVE	Parasympathetic (secretomotor) activity to glands Salivary reflex (efferent limb)	GVE fibers originate from **inferior salivatory nucleus**	**Otic ganglion** (postganglionic parasympathetic neurons)	**Tympanic nerve → lesser petrosal branch*** *Name changes with continuation of tympanic branch from plexus	Parotid gland Minor buccal glands	**Xerostomia** (dry mouth)
GSA	Protopathic and epicritic sensations from nociceptors and mechanoreceptors found in mucosa of oropharynx	Primary afferent fibers terminate in (pars caudalis) **spinal nucleus of V**	**Superior ganglion of CN IX** (primary afferent neuron cell bodies)	**Tympanic branch*** *Contributes to tympanic plexus **Lingual branch Tonsillar branch Auricular branch**	Internal tympanic membrane, auditory tube, and mastoid air cells Posterior one-third of tongue (postsulcal region), oropharynx, tonsillar fauces Skin behind the ear	**Anesthesia** of posterior tongue, oropharynx Weak or absent gag reflex Difficulty initiating swallowing due to sensory loss Glossopharyngeal neuralgia (stabbing pain)
SVA	Taste from chemoreceptors of taste buds Salivary reflex (afferent limb)	Primary afferent fibers terminate in rostral part of **nucleus tractus solitarius**	**Inferior (petrous) ganglion of CN IX** (primary afferent neuron cell bodies)	**Lingual branch Tonsillar branch**	Posterior one-third of tongue Circumvallate papillae Foliate papillae	**Dysgeusia** (loss of taste in posterior tongue)
GVA	Mucosal irritation Baroreceptors /Chemoreceptors* *Reflexive control of blood pressure Gag reflex (afferent limb) Swallow reflex (afferent limb)	Primary afferent fibers terminate in caudal part of **nucleus tractus solitarius (nucleus solitarius)**	**Inferior (petrous) ganglion of CN IX** (primary afferent neuron cell bodies)	**Carotid (sinus) branch Pharyngeal branch*** *Main sensory component of pharyngeal nerve plexus *Lingual /Tonsillar branch—minor contribution to sensory pharyngeal plexus	• Carotid sinus • Carotid body • Mucous membranes covering the pharyngeal walls, nasopharynx, oropharynx, tonsillar fossa, middle ear cavity	Loss of carotid sinus baroreflex *If bilateral, associated with chronic hypertension

*Tympanic plexus receives contributions from GSA of tympanic nerve, GVE postganglionic sympathetic fibers, and GVE preganglionic parasympathetic fibers.
*Pharyngeal plexus contains a sensory component primarily from GVA pharyngeal nerve of CN IX, minor contributions of GSA from lingual and tonsillar branch, SVE motor of plexus arising primarily from vagus, and GVE postganglionic sympathetic.

*Peripheral lesion will manifest ipsilaterally on the side of the injury.

Abbreviations: GSA, general somatic afferent; GVA, general visceral afferent; GVE, general visceral efferent; SVA, special visceral afferent; SVE, special visceral efferent.

- The SVA fibers project from the receptors and travel via the **small lingual** and **tonsillar branches** of **CN IX** and ascend toward the **primary SVA neurons** found within the **inferior (petrosal) ganglion** of **CN IX**. The SVA fibers pass through the ganglion without synapsing.
- The peripheral and central path for the branches carrying SVA fibers of the glossopharyngeal nerve is described in ▸ Table 21.5. The ascending gustatory pathway for processing taste is part of a shared taste pathway that is followed by the secondry afferent fibers of CNs VII, IX, and X (see Chapter 15).

21.3 Vagus

- The **vagus nerve (CN X)** develops in association with the **fourth** and **sixth pharyngeal arches** and carries two motor components, **SVE** and **GVE**, and three sensory modalities, **GSA, GVA,** and **SVA** (▸ **Table 21.6.**). The vagus provides motor and sensory innervation to the head, pharynx, and larynx, and serves as the principal source for parasympathetic innervation to the heart, lungs, and abdominal viscera (▸ Fig. 21.4). The functional modalities of the vagus nerve are outlined in ▸ Table 21.6.

Table 21.2 GVE fiber distribution: Parotid and buccal glands

Functional Component	Cranial Nerve Branch	Cranial Nerve Motor Nuclei	Central Course	Intracranial Path and Skull Exit	Parasympathetic Ganglion	Peripheral Course	Effector Target
GVE	Lesser petrosal	**Inferior salivatory nucleus** Contains preganglionic parasympathetic neuron cell bodies	GVE fibers arise from inferior salivatory nucleus in the medulla GVE fibers travel with main trunk of CN IX and exit skull via **jugular foramen**	GVE fibers join tympanic branch → enters the middle ear (tympanic) cavity via tympanic canaliculus → contributes to the **tympanic plexus** → branches from plexus as lesser petrosal nerve → exits skull via **foramen ovale** → lesser petrosal nerve synapses on otic ganglion	Otic ganglion Postganglionic fibers originate from ganglion→ travel with V3	Postganglionic fibers travel with **auriculotemporal branch** (V3)	• Parotid gland • Minor buccal glands

Abbreviation: GVE, general visceral efferent.

Table 21.3 GSA distribution for glossopharyngeal nerve

Functional Component/ Region Innervated/ Branch Names	Peripheral Course	Sensory Ganglion	Sensory Nuclei	Central Target	Central Termination
GSA **Receptors** Nociceptors Mechanoreceptors Thermoreceptors **Regions:** Posterior one-third of tongue Tonsillar fossa Oropharynx **Lingual branch** **Tonsillar branch** **Pharyngeal branch** *Contributes to pharyngeal plexus	**Path** GSA fibers pass from posterior one-third, tonsillar fossa, and oropharynx → pass between aperture in superior and middle constrictor to exit pharynx → ascends in the neck between the internal and external carotid → passes through superior ganglion of CN IX	**Superior ganglion of CN IX** Central process of GSA fibers passes from ganglia, enters skull via jugular foramen to enter the medulla Fibers descend in spinal trigeminal tract and synapse in **pars caudalis of spinal trigeminal nucleus**	Spinal trigeminal nucleus (second-order neurons) Secondary afferents form ascending tracts	Secondary afferents ascend to **ventral trigeminothalamic tract (VTT)** Third-order neurons in VPM of thalamus → posterior internal capsule → cortex GSA fibers of CNs V, VII, and X travel same path—secondary afferents ascend in VTT	Primary somatosensory cortex (orofacial region) for conscious perception of pain, temperature, and crude touch Afferent contributions to CGPs to alter CPG output to cranial motor nuclei V, VII, IX, and X for sensorimotor feedback for swallowing
GSA **Receptors** Nociceptors Mechanoreceptors Thermoreceptors **Regions:** Mucosa covering internal surface of tympanic membrane, auditory (pharyngotympanic) tube, middle ear cavity, mastoid air cells **Branch** **Tympanic branch of CN IX**	GSA fibers pass from the tympanic plexus from tympanic membrane and auditory tube in middle ear cavity → enters skull via tympanic canaliculus to join main trunk of glossopharyngeal				

Abbreviations: CPG, central pattern generator; GSA, general somatic afferent; VPM, ventral posteromedial.

• Several regional branches arise from the vagus throughout its descending course, including cervical, thoracic, and abdominal segments (▶ Fig. 21.5).

21.3.1 SVE of Vagus

CN X SVE Fibers: Origin, Central Connections, and Course

• LMNs in the nucleus ambiguus receive bilateral innervation from UMN in the primary motor cortex and premotor cortical areas. Motor fibers descend via the **corticobulbar tract** and pass through the posterior limb of the internal capsule to the **nucleus ambiguus**.

• LMNs in the nucleus ambiguus also receive input from the extrapyramidal tract and CPGs in the reticular formation of the brainstem, which serves to coordinate oromotor movements and modulate motor activity in response to sensory feedback.

• SVE fibers originate from LMN in the **nucleus ambiguus** and exit along with other modalities of the vagus as a series of 8 to 10 rootlets from the dorsolateral (postolivary sulcus) of the medulla. The rootlets converge to form the main trunk of the vagus and exit the skull through the jugular foramen,

Table 21.4 Pathway of GVA fibers of glossopharyngeal nerve

Functional Component/ Region Innervated/ Branch Names	Peripheral Course	Sensory Ganglion	Sensory Nuclei	Central Target	Central Termination
GVA receptors: • Baroreceptors in carotid sinus (arterial blood (systolic) pressure) • Chemoreceptors in carotid body (maintain arterial blood levels of CO_2, O_2, and pH) **Region:** Wall of internal carotid **Branch:** • **Carotid sinus branch of CN IX**	**Path:** Fibers from baroreceptors (carotid sinus) and chemoreceptors (carotid body) → join the main trunk of CN IX in the neck and pass between the internal and external carotid artery Fibers ascend along the surface of internal carotid artery to the inferior ganglion housed within jugular foramen Afferent fibers do not synapse in the ganglion.	**Inferior (petrous) ganglion of CN IX** Central processes from baroreceptors → enter medulla → GVA fibers synapse ipsilaterally in nucleus tractus solitarius **(NTS)** Central processes from chemoreceptors synapse on neurons of the dorsal respiratory group (DRG) located in NTS	**Nucleus tractus solitarius (NTS)** (caudal) (second-order neurons)	• Secondary afferents from NTS project to the following location: 1. Secondary afferents carrying input from baroreceptors project to **dorsal motor nucleus** and **nucleus ambiguus** and synapse on cardiac preganglionic parasympathetic vagal neurons 2. Secondary afferents carrying chemoreceptive input from DRG in NTS project to **respiratory CPGs in ventral respiratory nucleus of medulla**	• Fibers project to cardiac, vasomotor, and respiratory reflex centers in the medullary reticular formation and hypothalamus **Carotid sinus baroreflex** In response to parasympathetic input from vagal parasympathetic fibers, the pacemaker cells of heart slow contraction **Carotid body chemoreflex** In response to input from the ventral respiratory nucleus→ motor neurons in phrenic nucleus of spinal cord are stimulated and pulmonary ventilation increases
Receptors: Polymodal nociceptor gives rise to GVA **Branches** • **Pharyngeal branch of CN IX** • **Lingual and tonsillar** **Region:** *Pharyngeal branch principal contributor to **sensory component of pharyngeal plexus**. Plexus also receives GSA input from pharyngeal, lingual, and tonsillar branches.	**Path:** GVA fibers from mainly oropharynx → contribute sensory component of pharyngeal plexus → Fibers pass through aperture of the superior and middle constrictor to join the main trunk of glossopharyngeal in the neck with main branch → Fibers ascend toward inferior ganglion	**Inferior (petrous) ganglion of CN IX** Central processes of GVA fibers synapse in nucleus tractus solitarius **(NTS)**	**Nucleus tractus solitarius (NTS)** (caudal) (second order neurons)	• Swallowing CPGs in **medullary reticular formation** (Chapter 22) • project to **salivatory nuclei** (Chapter 24) • project to **nucleus ambiguus** for afferent limb of **gag reflex**	• Mediate salivatory reflex • Elicit swallowing reflex • Elicit gag afferent limb of reflex

Abbreviations: GSA, general somatic afferent; GVA, general visceral afferent.

along with glossopharyngeal (CN IX) and accessory nerve (CN XI).

• The main vagal trunk descends in the neck between the internal jugular and the internal carotid artery within the carotid sheath.

SVE of CN X: Peripheral Course of the Vagus

• Inferior to the jugular foramen the vagus nerve exhibits two sensory ganglia, the **superior (jugular) ganglion** and **inferior (nodose) ganglion**. The SVE fibers travel past the ganglion and join the other modalities to form a common vagal trunk.

• Vagus descends vertically in the neck within the carotid sheath between the internal jugular vein and internal carotid artery. Four branches arise from the cervical segment of the

vagus nerve in the neck. Among these, the **pharyngeal, external laryngeal,** and **recurrent laryngeal nerves** carry **SVE fibers.**

• Lesions affecting the LMN or peripheral motor branches are discussed in Clinical Correlation Box 21.1.

• The remaining branches which arise from the vagus in the neck, thorax, and abdomen carry visceral (GVA) and autonomic (GVE) fibers are covered in Chapter 18.

Peripheral Distribution of SVE Fibers of Cervical Branches of CN X

Pharyngeal Nerve: Peripheral Course

• The pharyngeal nerve of CN X, which serves as the principal (SVE) motor nerve for the skeletal muscles of the pharynx, passes between the internal and external carotid arteries to

Table 21.5 SVA fiber distribution for glossopharyngeal (CN IX)

Functional Component/ Region Innervated/ Nerve Branches	Peripheral Course	Sensory Ganglion	Sensory Nuclei	Central Target	Central Termination
SVA Taste **Receptors** Chemoreceptors in taste buds **Region:** Posterior one-third of tongue, circumvallate papillae, foliate papillae **Branches:** Lingual branch Tonsillar branch	**Path:** SVA fibers pass from taste buds in posterior one-third of tongue → pass between aperture in superior and middle constrictor → exit pharynx → ascend between the internal and external carotid → and pass the inferior ganglion of CN IX	**Inferior (petrosal) ganglion** Central process of SVA fibers enter the medulla, ascend in the tract of solitarius, and synapse on second-order neurons in nucleus tractus solitarius (NTS)	**Nucleus tractus solitarius (NTS) (rostral)**	Secondary afferents ascend via **central tegmental tract** Target VPM of thalamus Target **hypothalamus**	Primary taste area (gustatory cortex) of **somatosensory cortex** and insula for conscious perception of taste Termination in **limbic system** • Hippocampus (memory) • Amygdala • Hypothalamus For emotional processing of eating

Abbreviations: SVA, special visceral afferent; VPM, ventral posteromedial.
Note: The central taste pathway which ascends from the nucleus solitarius to higher brain centers for processing is a common pathway shared by CNs VII, IX, and X.

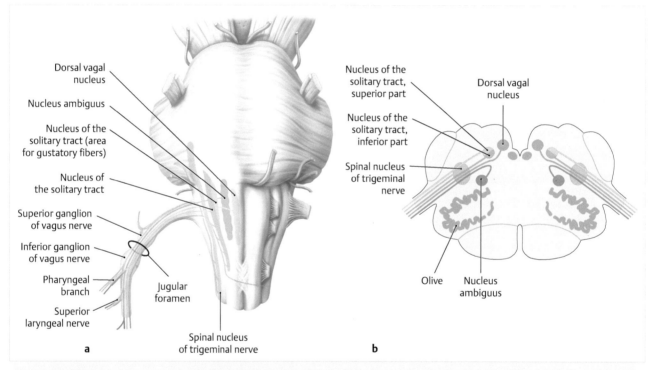

Fig. 21.4 (a, b) Nuclei of the vagus nerve (CN X). **(a)** Anterior view of the medulla showing the site of emergence of the vagus nerve and passage through the jugular foramen. **(b)** Cross section of medulla at the level of superior olive, depicting the motor and sensory nuclei of the vagus nerve. The vagus exits the skull through the jugular foramen along with glossopharyngeal nerve (CN IX) and accessory nerve (CN XI). Compression of these nerves within the jugular foramen may occur due to tumors, vascular lesions, or trauma, and lead to unilateral loss of sensory input and paralysis of motor fibers. (Reproduced with permission from Schuenke M, Schulte E, Schumacher U. THIEME Atlas of Anatomy. Second Edition, Vol 3. © Thieme 2016. Illustrations by Markus Voll and Karl Wesker.)

pierce the middle constrictor and then forms the motor component of the pharyngeal plexus.

- Pharyngeal branch of CN X innervates all skeletal muscles of the pharynx and soft palate except the **stylopharyngeus (CN IX)** and **tensor veli palatini (CN V3)**. The pharyngeal muscles innervated by the vagus originate from the fourth pharyngeal arch and include the superior, middle, inferior constrictors, the levator palatini, palatoglossus,

palatopharyngeus, and salpingopharyngeus (see Chapter 19, Table 19.16 for details).

Superior Laryngeal Nerve: Peripheral Course

- **The superior laryngeal nerve** branches from the vagus just distal to the pharyngeal nerve, descends bilaterally adjacent to the pharynx, between the external and internal carotid

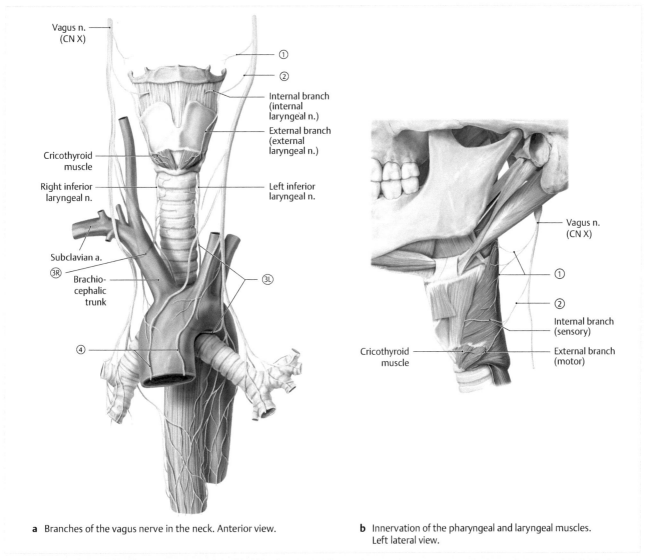

a Branches of the vagus nerve in the neck. Anterior view.

b Innervation of the pharyngeal and laryngeal muscles. Left lateral view.

Fig. 21.5 Peripheral distribution and course of motor and sensory fibers of the vagus nerve in the neck. **(a)** Anterior view of the neck. The vagus nerve travels within the carotid sheath where it is located posterior and lateral to internal and common carotid arteries and medial to the internal jugular vein. Both the right and left vagus nerves pass anterior to the subclavian artery, and then each sends a terminal branch, known as the recurrent laryngeal nerve, to ascend from the mediastinum to enter the larynx. Note the right recurrent laryngeal branch of the vagus loops around the right subclavian artery, and the left recurrent nerve branch hooks around the arch of the aorta. During its descent in the neck, four branches arise from the vagus nerve: pharyngeal branches, superior laryngeal nerve, recurrent laryngeal branches, and cervical (superior) cardiac branches. **(b)** Left lateral view of the neck. The superior laryngeal nerve of CN X divides into the internal laryngeal branch and the external laryngeal branch. (Reproduced with permission from Schuenke M, Schulte E, Schumacher U. THIEME Atlas of Anatomy Third Edition, Vol 3. © Thieme 2020. Illustrations by Markus Voll and Karl Wesker.)

arteries, and then divides into the **external laryngeal nerve** and **internal laryngeal nerve** branches (▶ Fig. 21.6).

○ The **external laryngeal branch** passes deep to the inferior constrictor to innervate the **cricothyroid muscle.** It also provides a small motor contribution to the cricopharyngeus muscle of the inferior constrictor.

○ The **internal laryngeal nerve,** which carries **sensory (GSA, SVA) fibers,** pierces the thyrohyoid membrane to enter the lumen of the pharynx and provides sensory innervation to the region of the epiglottis,

laryngopharynx, and the laryngeal mucosa above the true vocal folds.

Recurrent Laryngeal Nerve: Peripheral Course (▶ Fig. 21.6)

• Recurrent laryngeal nerves, which carry SVE, GVE, GSA, and GVA fibers, branch from the vagus as it descends into the thorax. Each recurrent nerve follows a different path on the left and right sides.

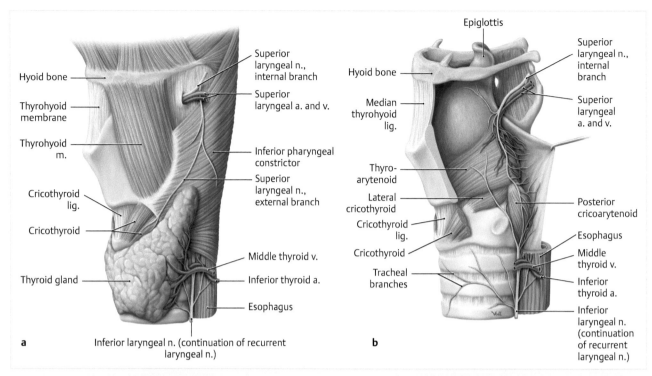

Fig. 21.6 Path of superior laryngeal and recurrent laryngeal nerve of the vagus (CN X). **(a)** Left lateral view of the larynx. Superficial dissection depicting the branching of the superior laryngeal nerve into the internal laryngeal nerve, which pierces the thyrohyoid membrane to provide sensation to the epiglottis and laryngeal mucosa, and the external laryngeal nerve, which provides motor innervation to the cricothyroid muscle. **(b)** Deep dissection showing the internal laryngeal nerve supplying the region above the vocal folds and the inferior laryngeal nerve, which is a continuation of the recurrent laryngeal nerve as it enters the larynx. (Reproduced with permission from Schuenke M, Schulte E, Schumacher U. THIEME Atlas of Anatomy Third Edition, Vol 3. © Thieme 2020. Illustrations by Markus Voll and Karl Wesker.)

○ The **left recurrent nerve** branches from the vagus at the level of the aortic arch and hooks around the **aortic arch.**
○ The **right recurrent laryngeal nerve** separates from the vagus nerve at the level of the thoracic inlet and loops around the **right subclavian artery.**
• Both the right and left recurrent laryngeal nerves ascend in the neck, and pass through a small aperture below the inferior margin of inferior constrictor to enter the **infraglottic (subglottic) cavity** of the larynx.
• The **recurrent (inferior) laryngeal nerves** provide SVE fibers to all the intrinsic muscles of the larynx except the cricothyroid muscle, which receives motor innervation from the external laryngeal nerve of CN X (see Chapter 19, Table 19.20).
• The striated muscles comprising the upper esophageal sphincter (UES) and upper one-third of the esophagus also receive motor innervation from the recurrent laryngeal nerve. The pattern of innervation to laryngeal and esophageal muscles by the recurrent laryngeal nerve is functionally important for swallowing reflexes.

- Collectively, LMN lesions and damage to cervical vagal branches of the vagus will vary in severity based on whether the damage is unilateral or bilateral. Damage to LMN associated with SVE fibers or damage to the pharyngeal, laryngeal, or recurrent laryngeal nerves during their peripheral course may manifest as difficulties in speaking, swallowing, and respiratory distress.
  - Unilateral lesions in LMNs in the nucleus ambiguus may affect the laryngeal muscles which act on the vocal cords as well as the pharyngeal and soft palatal muscles involved in swallowing. Unilateral lesions may result in muscle paralysis, atrophy, or weakness and manifest as hoarseness, problems with phonation or sound production (dysphonia), speech production (dysarthria), and difficulties in swallowing (dysphasia).
- Peripheral nerve lesions in specific branches during their course in the anterolateral neck may also occur. The point of injury will determine the extent of damage and symptoms (▶ Fig. 21.7).
  - Unilateral lesions of **pharyngeal nerve fibers** supplying the soft palate cause difficulty in swallowing due to flaccid paralysis of the soft palate and failure to elevate on the affected side. Upon visual inspection, the uvula deviates away from the paralyzed side to the unaffected (normal) side due to the unopposed action of the levator palatini. Patients may exhibit hypernasality in speech due to palatal weakness (▶ Fig. 21.8).
  - The **recurrent laryngeal nerve** is susceptible to injury given its course through the neck and superior mediastinum. Compression of the recurrent laryngeal nerve resulting from metastatic lung cancer or damage to the recurrent laryngeal nerve during surgical procedures involving removal of the thyroid or parathyroid glands can result in paralysis of all intrinsic muscles of the larynx on the affected side. Unilateral damage to the recurrent laryngeal nerve causes hoarseness and **dysphonia** (difficulty in sound production). Bilateral damage causes **aphonia** (inability to speak) and significant respiratory distress (**dyspnea**) due to loss in the ability to abduct the vocal cords. The cough reflex, which is mediated by afferent and efferent contributions from the vagus, is also compromised. The most significant risk to a patient with a unilateral lesion of the recurrent laryngeal nerve is the loss of protective laryngeal reflexes leading to possible aspiration or choking (see Chapter 22).

21.3.2 GVE of CN X

GVE Fibers: Origin of Central Connections and Intracranial

- Preganglionic parasympathetic (GVE) fibers originate from the **dorsal nucleus of CN X** on the floor of the fourth ventricle and travel with SVE fibers to exit jugular foramen as a part of the main vagal trunk. Most of the preganglionic parasympathetic fibers travel with the thoracic and abdominal divisions of the vagus nerve.
- Central input from preautonomic neurons in the hypothalamus and reticular formation provides regulation of autonomic function and projects to preganglionic parasympathetic nuclei.
  - The dorsal vagal nucleus receives central input from the preautonomic neurons in the **hypothalamic nuclei** and the visceral reflex centers of the **reticular formation.**
  - Sensory input from the olfactory and visuals systems, along with gustatory and visceral afferent sensations from the **nucleus of the tract of solitarius,** also projects to the dorsal vagal nucleus and mediates cephalic reflexes and sensorimotor responses involved in feeding.
- Preganglionic parasympathetic (GVE) fibers originating from the dorsal vagal nucleus travel with nerve branches arising from the cervical, thoracic, and abdominal divisions of the vagus. Preganglionic fibers synapse on postganglionic parasympathetic neurons located in intramural ganglia.
- Clinical outcomes resulting from damage to GVE fibers of X are highlighted in Clinical Correlation Box 21.2.

GVE of CN X: Peripheral Course

Cervical GVE Fiber Distribution of CN X

- Cervical branches of the **pharyngeal** and **internal laryngeal** nerves distribute secretomotor fibers to **pharyngeal mucosal glands** and the **laryngeal glands** located above the level of the vocal folds.
- The **recurrent laryngeal nerve,** once it enters the infraglottic cavity, distributes secretomotor fibers to laryngeal glands below the vocal folds.

Thoracic and Abdominal GVE Fibers of CN X

- The majority of the **vagal GVE fibers** descend as the **right** and **left vagal trunks** into the thorax and form the **cardiac, pulmonary,** and **esophageal plexuses.** The preganglionic parasympathetic fibers of the vagus (CN X) synapse in intramural ganglia associated with each organ and short postganglionic fibers travel to effector cells. The path for the thoracic and esophageal plexuses are covered in Chapter 18.

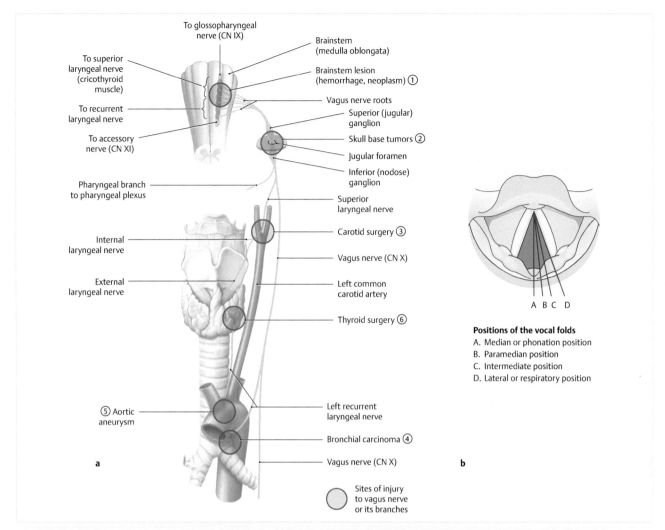

Fig. 21.7 Lesions of the vagus nerve. **(a)** Anterior view depicting sites of lesions. Lesions in the vagus nerve may cause motor paralysis or sensory loss. Symptoms and the extent of damage will vary based on the site of the lesion, and whether the damage is unilateral or bilateral. Central lesions occurring unilaterally in the brainstem or higher may disrupt input from UMNs of the corticobulbar tract. Due to predominantly bilateral input to the nucleus ambiguus, a unilateral lesion results in limited paralysis and motor weakness (not shown). **(1)** Unilateral damage to LMNs in the nucleus ambiguus or the SVE motor fibers of CN X during their peripheral course may be associated with flaccid paralysis. **(2)** Tumors occurring at the skull base or within the jugular foramen will cause multiple motor and sensory symptoms due to the compromised function of CNs IX, X, and XI, which exit the base of the skull through the jugular foramen. The most notable feature will be unilateral paralysis of all intrinsic and extrinsic laryngeal muscles, as well as the pharyngeal and most palatal muscles on the affected side. Dysfunction in soft palate elevation and vocal cord movements cause difficulties in speaking, sound production, and swallowing. The gag reflex mediated by the glossopharyngeal (afferent limb) and vagus (efferent limb) may also be lost. There may be diminished taste and sensation from the posterior third of the tongue and epiglottis. **(3)** Peripheral nerve lesions of the vagus may occur due to tumors, trauma, or surgery. The superior laryngeal and recurrent laryngeal **(4, 5, 6)** are most susceptible due to their anatomical pathway. Damage to the superior laryngeal nerve manifests as mild hoarseness (dysphonia) with a possible change in pitch and voice projection due to unilateral paralysis of the external laryngeal nerve and the cricothyroid muscle. The recurrent laryngeal nerve results in unilateral paralysis of all intrinsic laryngeal muscles, including the vocalis muscle on the affected side. **(b)** Unilateral vocal fold (cord) paralysis results in reduced mobility and incomplete closure of the vocal folds causing hoarseness, difficulties in speaking, and breathing (B and C represent possible vocal fold positions during paralysis.). LMNs, lower motor neurons; SVE, special visceral efferent; UMNs, upper motor neurons. (Reproduced with permission from Schuenke M, Schulte E, Schumacher U. THIEME Atlas of Anatomy Third Edition, Vol 3. © Thieme 2020. Illustrations by Markus Voll and Karl Wesker.)

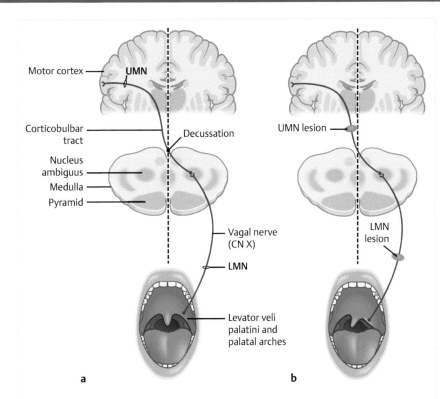

Fig. 21.8 Innervation of the palatal arches and uvula. Branches of the glossopharyngeal nerve transmit sensory innervation to the palatal mucosa through the afferent fibers of the pharyngeal plexus. Motor innervation to the palatal muscles and uvulae is mediated by contributions of the vagus nerve via the pharyngeal plexus. The nucleus ambiguus receives predominantly bilateral input from UMNs; therefore, a unilateral UMN lesion may only demonstrate mild contralateral weakness. Motor fibers carried by the vagus project unilaterally from LMNs in the nucleus ambiguus to the ipsilateral side of the palate. A unilateral LMN lesion results in the complete paralysis of the palatal muscles on the side of the lesion. The integrity of palatal innervation and assessment of palatal function may be tested by asking the patient to say "ah" and observing the position of the palate. (a) Normal position. The palate elevates equally as shown on both sides. (b) A contralateral UMN lesion (right) or a unilateral LMN lesion (left) both exhibit similar outcomes. The palate arch sags on the ipsilateral side (affected, left side), and the uvula deviates contralaterally to the intact side (normal, right side) due to the unopposed action of the levator veli palatini muscle. LMN, lower motor neuron; UMN, upper motor neuron.

Labels on figure:
Motor cortex — UMN
Corticobulbar tract — Decussation
Nucleus ambiguus
Medulla
Pyramid
Vagal nerve (CN X)
LMN
Levator veli palatini and palatal arches
a

UMN lesion
LMN lesion
b

21.3.3 GSA of CN X

CN X GSA: Peripheral (Extracranial) Course

- **Nociceptors, mechanoreceptors,** and **thermoreceptors** give rise to primary somatic afferent fibers which transmit general sensory input from several regions along the following nerve branches:
  ○ A small **meningeal branch** conveys GSA input from the meningeal dura mater in the posterior cranial fossa.
  ○ GSA information is also transmitted by the auricular branch, the internal laryngeal branch, and recurrent laryngeal nerves.
- The peripheral pathway and distribution of the branches are listed in ► Table 21.7.

CN X GSA: Intracranial and Central Course

- Central processes of somatic afferent fibers emerge from the **superior vagal ganglion of CN X** and join the main vagal trunk as it passes through the jugular foramen to enter the **brainstem at the medulla.** GSA fibers of vagus follow the same path as protopathic sensations for CNs V, VII, and IX.
- The fibers travel in the **spinal trigeminal tract** before synapsing on second-order neurons in the pars caudalis of the **spinal nucleus of V.**
- Secondary afferent fibers ascend via the **ventral trigeminothalamic tract** to **contralateral** third-order relay neurons in the ventral posteromedial **(VPM)** of the **thalamus.**
- Thalamic fibers project via the **posterior limb of the internal capsule** to terminate in the **primary somatosensory cortex** for conscious perception of pain, crude touch, and temperature.

21.3.4 GVA of CN X

GVA Fibers of CN X: Peripheral Course

- The visceral sensory component of the vagus provides unconscious sensory input from baroreceptors and chemoreceptors found within the aorta, as well as sensations arising from visceral polymodal nociceptors in the pharynx, larynx, heart, bronchi, lungs, esophagus, and abdominal viscera.

Table 21.6 Functional modalities of vagus

Functional Component		Associated Nuclei	Associated Ganglia	Vagus Nerve Branch	Region Innervated	Clinical Signs of Peripheral Damage
SVE	Voluntary motor to the skeletal muscles derived from fourth and sixth PA	SVE fibers originate in **nucleus ambiguus** Receive predominantly bilateral input from cortical UMNs Receive input from cerebellum and basal ganglia and CPGs	Not applicable	**Pharyngeal nerve**	Principal motor contribution to pharyngeal plexus—all palatal and pharyngeal muscles except stylopharyngeus (CN IX) and tensor veli palatini (CN X)	Dysphasia (difficulty swallowing—dysfunction in palatal elevation and peristalsis) Gag reflex weak or lost; palatal deviation to contralateral (unaffected) side
				Superior laryngeal of CN X* → **External laryngeal nerve**	Cricothyroid muscle	**Dysphonia** (hoarseness; decreased sound production if unilateral)
				Recurrent laryngeal nerve	All intrinsic laryngeal muscles EXCEPT cricothyroid	Dyspnea (difficulty breathing if bilateral) Nonproductive cough (bovine cough) due to failure adduct vocal folds
GVE	Parasympathetic (secretomotor) activity to glands, smooth muscle, and cardiac muscle	GVE fibers originate from **dorsal nucleus of CN X**	**Intramural ganglion** in walls of heart, trachea, bronchi, esophagus, gut, viscera	Distributed with pharyngeal, internal laryngeal, and recurrent laryngeal branch	Mucosal glands in the lower pharynx and larynx	Digestive issues may be associated with changes in peristalsis Cardiac arrhythmias (tachycardia) may be present
				Cardiac plexus	Cardiac and nodal fibers of heart (inhibitory)	
				Pulmonary plexus	Mucosal glands and smooth muscle in trachea, bronchial tree	
				Esophageal plexus → anterior and posterior gastric branches → abdominal plexuses	Esophagus, stomach, liver, pancreas, gallbladder, and intestines as far as the splenic flexure	
GSA	Protopathic and epicritic sensations from exteroceptors	Primary afferent fibers terminate in **spinal nucleus of V**	**Superior vagal (jugular) ganglion** (locus: primary afferent neuron cell bodies)	**Auricular branch**	Skin behind the ear, external tympanic membrane, external auditory meatus	Sensory disturbances and partial anesthesia to external auditory meatus and laryngeal region Sensory input facilitates swallowing and protective reflexes
				Meningeal branch	Dura mater in posterior cranial fossa	
			Inferior vagal (nodose) ganglion (locus: primary afferent neuron cell bodies)	Superior laryngeal of CN X* → **Internal laryngeal branch** → upper and lower branches	Mucosa base of tongue, epiglottis, vallecula, laryngeal vestibule piriform fossa, mucosa above false vocal cords	
				Recurrent laryngeal nerve	Mucosa of vocal cords and infraglottic region	
GVA	Interoceptors: Baroreceptors and chemoreceptors Polymodal nociceptors found in viscera and blood vessel walls that monitor the body's internal state and function in unconscious visceral reflexes	Primary afferent fibers terminate in **nucleus tract of solitarius (NTS)**	**Inferior vagal (nodose) ganglion** (locus: primary afferent neuron cell bodies)	**Aortic branch of CN X**	Baroreceptors of aortic sinus Chemoreceptors of aortic body in wall of aorta	Changes in arterial pressure, heart rate, and respiratory rate—minor; more significant if carotid receptors are damaged Partial anesthesia to mucosa Dysphasia—initiating reflexive swallowing Susceptible to choking
				Superior laryngeal of CN X* → **Internal laryngeal branch** → upper and lower branches	Base of tongue, epiglottis, vallecula, laryngeal vestibule piriform fossa, mucosa above false vocal cords	

(Continued)

Table 21.6 (*Continued*) Functional modalities of vagus

Functional Component		Associated Nuclei	Associated Ganglia	Vagus Nerve Branch	Region Innervated	Clinical Signs of Peripheral Damage
				Recurrent laryngeal nerve	Mucosa of vocal cords and infraglottic region	and aspiration during swallowing due to loss of sensory feedback Loss/diminished cough reflex (afferent limb)
SVA	Chemoreceptors (taste), receptors of neuroepithelial cells	Primary afferent fibers terminate in **NTS**	**Inferior vagal (nodose) ganglion** (locus: primary afferent neuron cell bodies)	Superior laryngeal branch of CN X* → Internal laryngeal branch → upper and lower branches	Mucosa of base of tongue, epiglottis, vallecula	Insignificant

Abbreviations: CPGs, central pattern generators; GSA, general somatic afferent; GVA, general visceral afferent; GVE, general visceral efferent; PA, pharyngeal arch; SVA, special visceral afferent; SVE, special visceral efferent; UMNs, upper motor neurons.
Note: *Superior laryngeal branch of CN X divides into two terminal branches in the neck: external laryngeal (SVE) and internal laryngeal branches (GSA/SVA/GVA).

Table 21.7 Peripheral distribution of GSA fiber

Branch Name and Function	Receptors and Location	Peripheral Path
Auricular branch Ganglion: Superior vagal ganglion	**Receptors** Nociceptors Mechanoreceptors Thermoreceptors **Regions:** External surface of tympanic membrane; external auditory meatus	• GSA fibers travel from the skin of the ear, pass posterior to the internal jugular vein → and then traverse the tympanomastoid fissure to the jugular fossa • A small communicating branch from the glossopharyngeal (CN IX) joins the auricular branch of CN X in the jugular fossa before the peripheral afferent fibers of the auricular nerve enter the **superior (jugular) ganglion of CN X**
Internal laryngeal nerve Ganglion: Inferior vagal ganglion	**Receptors** Nociceptors Mechanoreceptors Thermoreceptors **Regions:** **Pharyngeal mucosa** near base of tongue, epiglottis, and laryngeal mucosa region of **false vocal folds**	• GSA fibers travel with GVA of the internal laryngeal nerve • Exits the laryngopharynx by piecing the **thyrohyoid membrane** → in the neck it merges with the **external laryngeal nerve** → forms the **superior laryngeal nerve** • The superior laryngeal nerve joins the main vagal trunk and ascends in the neck within the carotid sheath toward the inferior and superior sensory ganglia of CN X
Recurrent laryngeal nerve Ganglion: Inferior vagal ganglion	Mechanoreceptors and polymodal nociceptors in laryngeal mucosa covering the **true vocal folds** and **area below folds** (subglottic region)	GSA fibers travel with GVA of the recurrent laryngeal nerve → exit the larynx through an aperture below the inferior margin of inferior constrictor → fibers then join the main vagal trunk and ascend in the carotid sheath toward the inferior sensory ganglion of CN X

Abbreviations: GSA, general somatic afferent; GVA, general visceral afferent.

- The cell bodies of the **GVA neurons** reside within the **inferior (nodose) ganglion of CN X.** The GVA fibers pass through the inferior (nodose) ganglion without synapsing.
- The specific branches and pathways are listed in
  ▸ Table 21.8.

GVA of CN X: Intracranial Course and Central Course

- Central processes of GVA neurons of CN X pass through the jugular foramen, enter the medulla of the brainstem, and then descend ipsilaterally in the **tract of solitarius** to synapse on the second-order neurons found in the **caudal part** of **NTS**. The GVA fibers from the vagus follow a similar pathway as CN IX to visceral reflex centers.
- Secondary afferent fibers project bilaterally from the nucleus solitarius via the **dorsal longitudinal fasciculus** to neurons in the cardiac, vasomotor, respiratory, and reflex centers of the nucleus ambiguus, the dorsal motor nucleus of CN X, the **hypothalamus,** and **medullary reticular formation** for reflexive responses to changes in cardiac output, respiration, and blood pressure.

Table 21.8 Peripheral distribution of GVA fibers

Branch Name and Function	Receptors and Location	Peripheral Path
Aortic branch of CN X Principal role: Mediating vasomotor reflexes	**Baroreceptors** of the **aortic sinus** and **chemoreceptors** of the **aortic body** reside in the wall of the aortic arch and detect changes in pressure and oxygen saturation levels, respectively	The aortic branch ascends in the neck, passing between internal carotid and external carotid to join the vagal trunk, and travels toward the inferior (nodose) ganglion Primary afferents of central processes target caudal nucleus tractus solitarius (NTS) → secondary afferents follow path similar to GVA of CN IX for vasomotor reflexes *see GVA fibers of CN IX for details
Internal laryngeal nerve Principal role: • Initiate swallow reflex due to afferent input • Protective reflexes in glottic closure for airway protection • Cough reflex	Mechanoreceptors and polymodal nociceptors in **pharyngeal mucosa** near base of tongue, epiglottis, and **laryngeal mucosa above vocal folds**	GVA fibers travel with GSA fibers, then join the main vagal trunk and ascend in the carotid sheath toward the inferior sensory, the inferior (nodose) ganglion
Recurrent laryngeal nerve Principal role • Protective reflexes in glottic closure for airway protection • Cough reflex	Mechanoreceptors and polymodal nociceptors in laryngeal mucosa covering the **vocal folds** and **area below folds** (subglottic region)	GVA fibers travel with GSA fibers, then join the main vagal trunk and ascend in the carotid sheath toward the inferior (nodose) ganglion
Vagal branches of the pulmonary plexuses Principal role: Mediate protective reflexes • Cough reflex • Respiratory reflex, i.e., Hering-Breuer inflation reflex	Mechanoreceptors and polymodal nociceptors in **walls of viscera**	GVA fibers follow GVE fibers from viscera, then join the right and left vagal branches to ascend toward inferior (nodose) ganglion
Right and left vagal branches from abdominal and esophageal plexuses Principal role: Visceral feedback about distention, nausea	Mechanoreceptors and polymodal nociceptors in walls of viscera	GVA fibers follow GVE fibers from viscera, then join the right and left vagal branches to ascend toward the inferior (nodose) ganglion

Abbreviations: GSA, general somatic afferent; GVA, general visceral afferent; GVE, general visceral efferent.

21.3.5 SVA of CN X

SVA Fibers: Peripheral Course

- **SVA fibers** receive gustatory input through specialized taste (chemoreceptors) receptors in the neuroepithelial cells comprising the taste buds in the epiglottis, vallecula, and supraglottic region of the laryngopharynx.
- The SVA fibers project from the receptors and travel via the **internal laryngeal nerve** and ascend toward the **primary SVA neurons** found within the **inferior (nodose) ganglion of CN X.** The SVA fibers pass through the ganglion without synapsing.

SVA of CN IX: Intracranial and Central Course

- SVA fibers join the vagus and pass into the skull through the jugular foramen and enter the medulla to synapse on second-order neurons found in the **rostral part of the nucleus solitarius (gustatory).**
- Secondary afferent fibers of the vagus follow the same taste pathway as the facial and glossopharyngeal nerves. Fibers ascend **bilaterally** in the **central tegmental tract** to the ipsilateral and contralateral tertiary relay neurons in the **VPM of the thalamus**.
- Tertiary neurons project bilaterally through the **posterior limb of the internal capsule** to the **primary cortical**

gustatory area of the **somatosensory cortex** and **insular cortex** for conscious taste perceptions.
- Fibers traveling in the **central tegmental tract** also project to the **hippocampus, hypothalamus,** and **amygdala** of the **limbic system** and mediate reflex activities involving memory creation and emotional aspects of taste.

21.4 Hypoglossal

- The musculature of the tongue plays a critical role in a variety of critical human oral functions, including articulation, swallowing, mastication, and respiration.
- The hypoglossal nerve (CN XII) is a motor nerve that mediates tongue movement by controlling the shape and position of the tongue.
- The hypoglossal nerve (CN XII) only carries somatic efferent (GSE) fibers and innervates all intrinsic and extrinsic muscles of the tongue except for the palatoglossus muscle, which receives innervation from the pharyngeal plexus (CN X). The skeletal tongue muscles develop from the occipital somites which migrate into the pharyngeal arch region during development.
- A functional overview of GSE fibers carried by the hypoglossal nerve are outlined in (▶ Table 21.9)

Table 21.9 Functional overview of hypoglossal nerve (CN XII)

Functional Component		Associated Nuclei	Associated Ganglia	Hypoglossal Nerve Branch	Region Innervated	Clinical Signs of Peripheral Damage
GSE	Voluntary motor to the skeletal muscles derived from occipital somites	GSE fibers originate from **hypoglossal nucleus**	Not applicable	Muscular branches not specifically named ****C1 fibers travel with hypoglossal nerve for distribution to geniohyoid and thyrohyoid muscle.** **C1 not part of hypoglossal nerve.*	All extrinsic and intrinsic tongue muscle EXCEPT palatoglossus supplied by CN X of pharyngeal plexus Functional role: Mediates all tongue movements by changing shape and position of tongue	Slurred speech due to difficulty in articulating; problems with bolus formation and swallowing; atrophy of muscles and fasciculations (small spontaneous muscle contractions) may be present Damage to one motor nucleus or unilateral peripheral nerve damage causes: Unilateral atrophy and ipsilateral deviation of tongue to affected side upon protrusion If bilateral damage occurs, such as in bulbar palsy, the tongue is immobile and can't protrude

Abbreviation: GSE, general somatic efferent.

Table 21.10 Central input and course for hypoglossal nerve (CN XII)

Functional Component	CN XII Motor Nucleus	Central Input to Hypoglossal Motor Nucleus	Central Course Intracranial Path and Skull Exit	Peripheral Course
GSE fibers of hypoglossal nerve	**Hypoglossal motor nucleus** (contains LMNs) Located in lower pontomedullary junction SVE fibers originate from dorsal group and ventral group of facial motor nucleus	LMNs receive input for voluntary and **involuntary (reflexive) movements** **Volitional control of tongue muscles** Contralateral cortical input from UMNs in primary, premotor cortices Travel via corticobulbar tract to LMNs in hypoglossal motor nucleus **Involuntary (reflexive) control** **Feedback control** • LMNs receive indirect sensory input from NTS and spinal trigeminal nuclear complex for protective reflexes • Receive input from masticatory and swallowing CPGs to coordinate and modulate oromotor movements • Receives indirect input from the cerebellum and basal ganglia via extrapyramidal tracts (see Chapter 16); serves to correct motor errors and coordinate movements	• GSE fibers from hypoglossal motor neurons exit from lower medulla as small rootlets • Rootlets merge to form the hypoglossal nerve and then exit the skull via the **hypoglossal (condylar) canal** • Hypoglossal nerve lies in close proximity with CNs IX, X, and XI at point of exit from cranial base	• Hypoglossal nerve descends lateral to vagus, external to carotid sheath • Enters root of tongue above hyoid bone to distribute lingual branches to extrinsic and intrinsic muscles **See text for details.*

Abbreviations: CPGs, central pattern generators; GSE, general somatic efferent; LMNs, lower motor neurons; NTS, nucleus tractus solitarius; SVE, special visceral efferent; UMNs, upper motor neurons.

21.4.1 GSE of CN XII

GSE of CN XII: Origin, Central Connections, and Intracranial Course

• The **GSE** fibers of the **hypoglossal nerve** originate from the cell bodies of the LMNs located in the **hypoglossal motor nucleus** of the caudal medulla.

Central Control of LMNs in the Hypoglossal Motor Nucleus

• The **hypoglossal motor nucleus** receives input from the following sources, which allows for voluntary and involuntary (reflexive) control of movement. The specific connections, which are described in ▶ Table 21.10, include descending input from the pyramidal and extrapyramidal

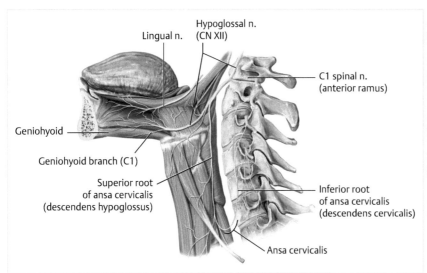

Lingual n.
Hypoglossal n. (CN XII)
Geniohyoid
Geniohyoid branch (C1)
Superior root of ansa cervicalis (descendens hypoglossus)
C1 spinal n. (anterior ramus)
Inferior root of ansa cervicalis (descendens cervicalis)
Ansa cervicalis

Fig. 21.9 Peripheral path of the hypoglossal nerve. Left lateral view. As the hypoglossal nerve passes forward to innervate the tongue muscles, it travels with fibers from C1 cervical branches. The C1 branch innervates the geniohyoid and thyrohyoid muscles and contributes to the superior root of the ansa cervicalis loop. The inferior (descending) root of ansa cervicalis arises from C2–C3 spinal nerves. (Reproduced with permission from Schuenke M, Schulte E, Schumacher U. THIEME Atlas of Anatomy Third Edition, Vol 3. © Thieme 2020. Illustrations by Markus Voll and Karl Wesker.)

tracts, the brainstem CPGs in the reticular formation, and sensory feedback from peripheral receptors.

- **Cortical input** provides voluntary control of the extrinsic and intrinsic tongue musculature. **UMNs** originating primarily from the **contralateral** primary motor cortex and premotor cortical areas descend via the **corticobulbar tract.** Corticobulbar fibers pass through the posterior limb of the internal capsule to terminate on LMN in the **contralateral hypoglossal nucleus**.
- **Masticatory** and **swallowing CPGs** in the brainstem reticular formation, along with sensorimotor feedback, coordinate oromotor behaviors such as chewing, bolus formation, and articulation with appropriate lingual movements (see Chapter 22).
  - Sensory feedback originating from cervical proprioceptors that supply lingual muscle spindles, along with taste receptors, nociceptors, and mechanoreceptors, mediates the lingual reflexes involved in protecting the tongue during mastication and airway protection during swallowing (see Chapter 22).
  - The hypoglossal nucleus indirectly receives input in response to proprioceptive, taste, and tactile stimulation from the **trigeminal sensory nuclear complex** and the **NTS**. Secondary afferent fibers arising from sensory nuclei project to CPGs or to the hypoglossal motor nuclei to modulate and coordinate lingual movements.

Intracranial Course of CN XII

- General somatic efferent fibers from **LMNs** found in the **hypoglossal nucleus** exit from the preolivary sulcus in the lower medulla as small rootlets. The rootlets merge to form the **hypoglossal nerve** and then exit the skull via the **hypoglossal (condylar) canal** in the posterior cranial fossa.

GSE of CN XII: Peripheral Distribution (▶ Fig. 21.9)

- The hypoglossal nerve descends from the base of the skull, emerging between the internal carotid artery and internal

Table 21.11 Summary of GSE innervation to tongue musculature

Muscle Group	Muscle	Motor Nerve Supply
Intrinsic group	Superior longitudinal	GSE fibers Hypoglossal nerve
	Inferior longitudinal	
	Vertical	
	Transverse	
	Genioglossus	
Extrinsic group	Hyoglossus	
	Styloglossus	
	Palatoglossus	SVE fibers Pharyngeal nerve of CN X; motor branch of pharyngeal plexus

Abbreviations: GSE, general somatic efferent; SVE, special visceral efferent.

jugular vein. It descends external to the carotid sheath and lateral to the vagus nerve.

- **C1 cervical branches** emerge from the spinal cord in close proximity to the hypoglossal nerve. **C1 cervical fibers** accompany the hypoglossal nerve to supply the **geniohyoid** and **thyrohyoid** muscles.
- Fibers of **C1** then contribute to the **superior root** of **ansa cervicalis**, while the **inferior root** of the **ansa cervicalis** arises from **C2–C3**. The ansa cervicalis innervates the infrahyoid (strap) muscles, which are important in swallowing.
- The nerve enters the root of the tongue above the level of the hyoid bone. The nerve courses toward the submandibular region, passing deep to the posterior belly of the digastric muscle and stylohyoid muscle.
- The nerve passes superficial to the hyoglossus muscle, inferior to lingual nerve and submandibular duct, and then passes deep to the mylohyoid muscle to innervate the hyoglossus, genioglossus, styloglossus, and intrinsic tongue muscles (▶ Table 21.11).
- Clinical outcomes associated with UMN and LMN lesions of the hypoglossal nerve are discussed in Clinical Correlation Box 21.3.

Nuclear and infranuclear: LMN lesions of the hypoglossal nerve

Unilateral damage to LMNs in the hypoglossal nucleus, or to the hypoglossal nerve during its peripheral course through the condylar (hypoglossal canal), or as a result of an injury to the neck, may cause **hypoglossal nerve palsy** or **paralysis** to the hypoglossal nerve which supplies motor innervation to the tongue muscles. In each case, damage causes muscle weakness, and the tongue deviates upon protrusion toward the side of the lesion due to the unopposed action of the genioglossus muscle on the intact side. Prolonged damage may lead to unilateral **atrophy** (decrease in muscle size) of the tongue muscles on the affected side. **Fasciculations,** which are spontaneous small muscle twitches, may also occur while the tongue is at rest. **Flaccid paralysis,** atrophy, and tongue weakness often lead to difficulty in articulation due to the loss of coordinated tongue movement. Motor disorders affecting speech articulation are known as **dysarthria** and often manifest as slurred speech and difficulty in consonant pronunciation. Additional problems with bolus formation and swallowing may also occur due to motor weakness. Sensory loss to the mucosa of the tongue is not a feature of isolated hypoglossal nerve lesions.

Supranuclear: UMN lesions of the hypoglossal nerve

Strokes, tumors, and UMN diseases result in very limited tongue atrophy due to loss of neural input. In comparison to LMN lesions, damage to UMNs results in contralateral muscle weakness of the tongue and causes the tongue to deviate to the opposite side of the UMN lesion due to the predominant contralateral input of the corticobulbar fibers. Muscle atrophy is typically not associated with cortical lesions; however, UMN lesions may cause **spastic paralysis,** which may manifest as uncoordinated tongue movements and spastic dysarthria. Spastic dysarthria is often characterized by monotonous, slow, strangled speech.

Brainstem lesions involving the lower cranial nerves IX, X, and XII are common following a stroke due to the proximity of the cranial motor nuclei. Additionally, the four lower cranial nerves which travel close together are also at risk of injury during their peripheral descending course in the neck. Injuries to the posterior cranial base, infections in the retromandibular or post-styloid parapharyngeal spaces, or a tumor compressing structures as they emerge from the jugular foramen will most likely compromise CNs IX, X, and XI. The hypoglossal nerve (CN XII), which emerges from the hypoglossal canal medial to CNs IX, X, and XI, along with the sympathetic fibers that accompany the internal carotid artery may also be compressed if the mass involves the parapharyngeal space. Possible clinical outcomes include the following:

- Flaccid paralysis, atrophy, weakness of tongue. Motor involvement of the hypoglossal nerve may lead to difficulty in speech articulation due to the loss of coordinated tongue movement. Motor disorders affecting speech articulation are known as dysarthria. Additional problems with bolus formation and swallowing may occur due to tongue weakness.
- Unilateral involvement of the vagus will cause an inability to adduct the vocal cords, leading to hoarseness, and difficulty in sound production (dysphonia). Damage to the vagus will cause pharyngeal muscle weakness and may comprise swallowing due vagal contributions to the pharyngeal plexus. The uvula will deviate to the opposite side of the lesion due to the unopposed action of the levator veli palatini.
- Unilateral anesthesia to the oropharyngeal area on the affected side may also occur due to the loss of the glossopharyngeal nerve. Patients may exhibit diminished taste in the posterior one-third of the tongue. Individuals may be at risk for choking and aspiration of liquids into the trachea due to compromised glottic closure reflexes (see Chapter 22).
- The involvement of sympathetic fibers may result in clinical signs of ptosis of the upper eyelid, and pupillary constriction (miosis) due to interruption of sympathetic innervation to the dilator pupillae muscle.

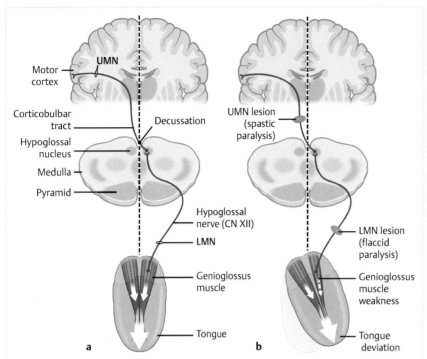

Fig. 21.10 Motor innervation to the tongue. **(a)** Normal innervation to the genioglossus muscle by the CN XII. **(b)** Tongue with UMN or LMN lesions resulting in paralysis of the genioglossus muscle. UMN projects predominantly via corticobulbar tract to the contralateral hypoglossal motor nucleus. A UMN lesion (shown right) causes deviation of the protruded tongue to the contralateral side (left) due to paralysis of the left genioglossus muscle. LMN provides unilateral motor innervation to the muscle on the ipsilateral side of the tongue. LMN lesion (left side shown) will cause flaccid paralysis and atrophy of the tongue muscles and cause ipsilateral paralysis of the genioglossus muscle. The protruded tongue will deviate to the affected weak side (left side) due to genioglossus paralysis and the unopposed action of the opposite genioglossus muscle. LMN, lower motor neuron; UMN, upper motor neuron.

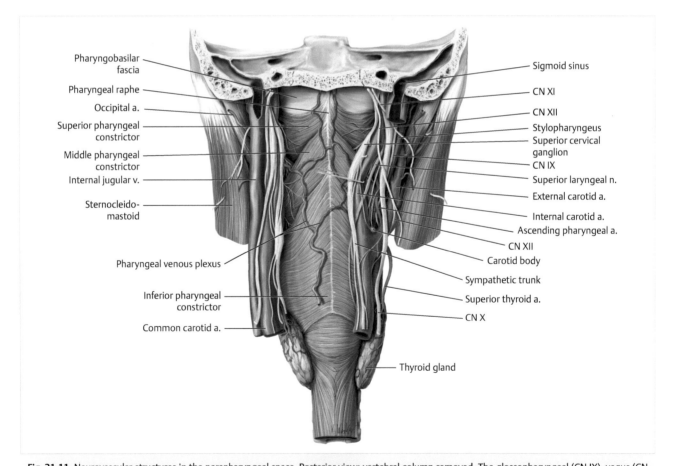

Fig. 21.11 Neurovascular structures in the parapharyngeal space. Posterior view; vertebral column removed. The glossopharyngeal (CN IX), vagus (CN X), and spinal accessory (CN XI) nerves exit the jugular foramen with the internal jugular at the cranial base and enter the parapharyngeal space. The hypoglossal nerve (CN XII), exiting from the hypoglossal canal, is also found in the parapharyngeal space, along with the superior cervical ganglion of the sympathetic trunk. The proximity of these structures places the nerves at risk from compression injuries resulting from tumors, or fractures involving the posterior skull. The structures are also at risk from infections spreading from the oral cavity, salivary glands, palatine tonsils, adenoids, or retropharyngeal space into the posterior (post-styloid) compartment of the parapharyngeal space. Compression of CNs IX, X, XI, and XII and vascular structures will lead to significant motor and sensory deficits. Clinical signs may include difficulties in phonation, bolus formation, swallowing, and speech articulation, which may be accompanied by ptosis and miosis due to sympathetic involvement. (Reproduced with permission from Schuenke M, Schulte E, Schumacher U. THIEME Atlas of Anatomy Third Edition, Vol 3. © Thieme 2020. Illustrations by Markus Voll and Karl Wesker.)

Questions and Answers

1. An isolated ipsilateral lesion to the rostral portion of the nucleus ambiguus will result in mild dysphagia due to paralysis of which of the following muscles?
   a) Palatopharyngeus
   b) Salpingopharyngeus
   c) Middle pharyngeal constrictor
   d) Stylopharyngeus
   e) Levator veli palatini

Level 2: Moderate

Answer D: Stylopharyngeus is the only muscle to receive innervation from the glossopharyngeal nerve (CN IX). The muscle aids in widening and elevating the pharynx during swallowing. The LMNs of the stylopharyngeus are found in the rostral part of the nucleus ambiguus and damage to these neurons or the motor (SVE) nerve fibers of CN IX to the stylopharyngeus will result in mild dysphasia. The caudal part of the nucleus ambiguus contains LMNs of the vagus nerve. The vagus innervates **(A)** palatopharyngeus, **(B)** salpingopharyngeus muscle, **(C)** the middle constrictor, and **(E)** the levator veli palatini via motor branches from the pharyngeal plexus. LMNs of the vagus also provide innervation to the laryngeal muscles, the superior and inferior pharyngeal constrictors, and the palatoglossus and musculus uvulae which are not listed as choices. The palatal, pharyngeal, and laryngeal muscles innervated by the vagus contribute significantly to swallowing mechanism and also phonation (sound production).

Use the clinical scenario below to answer questions 2 and 3

A 23-year-old man presents with fever and painful swelling of the left side of the neck due to a bacterial infection in the parotid that has spread to the posterior (post-styloid) compartment of the parapharyngeal (lateral pharyngeal) space. Neurologic examination shows left-sided ptosis, miosis, paresis of the sternocleidomastoid and trapezius muscles, difficulty swallowing, hoarseness, and left tongue deviation. Laryngoscopy shows left vocal cord paralysis.

2. Each of the following clinical findings EXCEPT one may also be present due to the location of the injury. Which one is the exception?
   a) Left palatal sagging, deviation of uvula to right
   b) Weakness turning head to right
   c) Hyperactive jaw reflex
   d) Decreased sensitivity to taste on the left posterior third of tongue
   e) Loss of sensation of the pharyngeal mucosa on left

Level 3: Difficult

Answer C: A hyperactive jaw reflex is the exception and would not be seen in association with this infection. Infections in the posterior parapharyngeal space will compress the contents of the space. The jaw reflex is mediated by proprioceptive input to the mesencephalic nucleus of V and motor nucleus of V. A loss of the jaw reflex occurs with unilateral damage to cranial nerve nuclei, whereas bilateral supranuclear (central) lesion to UMNs or the corticobulbar tract will cause spastic paralysis and a hyperactive jaw reflex.

Trismus (lockjaw) is often associated with infections spreading anteriorly within the parapharyngeal space. Structures found in the posterior parapharyngeal space include the content of the carotid sheath (internal jugular vein, internal carotid artery, and vagus, CN X), along with sympathetic chain, the glossopharyngeal nerve (CN IX), hypoglossal nerve (CN XII), and the accessory nerve (CN XI). The trigeminal nerve lies anterior to this space and the motor division is not affected. The jaw reflex is mediated by proprioceptive input to the mesencephalic nucleus of V and motor nucleus of V. A loss of the jaw reflex occurs with unilateral damage to cranial nerve nuclei, whereas bilateral supranuclear (central) lesion to UMNs or the corticobulbar tract will cause spastic paralysis and a hyperactive jaw reflex.

Trismus (lockjaw) is often associated with infections spreading anteriorly within the parapharyngeal space. Choice **(A)** is correct; left palatal sagging and uvula deviation to the unaffected right side will occur due to injury to CN IX and CN X on the left side. CN IX innervates the pharyngeal mucosa and CN X innervates the palatal muscles. The gag reflex, if tested, would be absent on the affected left side due to damage of CNs IX and X. Evaluation of palatal elevation by asking the patient to say "ah" would show deviation of the uvula to right due to the damage of the left vagus (CN X), and the unopposed action of the levator veli palatini muscles on the right. **(B)** Weakness in turning head away from the side of the infection is correct. CN XI lies in the post-styloid parapharyngeal space and innervates the sternocleidomastoid and trapezius muscles. The sternocleidomastoid functions to turn the head to the contralateral (opposite) side, so a loss in innervation will produce weakness in the movement. Choices **(D)** and **(E)** are also correct. CN IX carries sensory input from pharyngeal mucosa and taste from the posterior third of the tongue. Both modalities will be absent due to compression of CN IX on the left side.

3. The clinical findings support the compression of each of the following nerves EXCEPT one. Which one is the exception?
   a) Accessory nerve
   b) Hypoglossal
   c) Vagus
   d) Sympathetic chain
   e) Trigeminal

Level 2: Moderate

Answer E: The trigeminal nerve is the exception. The trigeminal nerve is not in the region of the posterior (post-styloid) compartment of the parapharyngeal space. The trigeminal nerve exits the middle cranial fossa and lies anterior to the infection. The anterior parapharyngeal space does contain branches of V3, including the inferior alveolar, lingual, and auriculotemporal nerves, along with the internal maxillary artery. The symptoms listed are not associated with these nerves. Choice **(A)** accessory nerve and vagus **(C)** exit the jugular foramen, along with the internal jugular vein, and the glossopharyngeal nerve. These structures along with the internal carotid artery and sympathetic chain **(D)**, and hypoglossal nerve **(B)**, lie in the posterior parapharyngeal space. Damage to the vagus **(C)** leads to ipsilateral weakness of the palatal and pharyngeal muscles that are important in swallowing and the laryngeal muscles necessary for phonation. The ipsilateral weakness of the laryngeal muscles is noted by the vocal cord paralysis and hoarse voice. The accessory nerve (**A**) innervates the sternocleidomastoid and trapezius, and damage leads to weakness in contralateral head rotation and shoulder drop. Compression of the sympathetic nerve (**D**) causes pupillary constriction (miosis) and eyelid droop (ptosis). Damage to the hypoglossal (**B**) leads to ipsilateral weakness of the genioglossus muscle causing the tongue to deviate to the weak side. Although not noted in the clinical description, the patient would most likely exhibit dysarthria, which is a disturbance in speech articulation due to the weakness of the laryngeal, pharyngeal, palatal, and tongue muscles. These muscle groups need to work bilaterally to produce a coordinated response and proper articulation.

Use the following clinical scenario to answer questions 4 and 5

A 68-year-old patient presents with bilateral carotid stenosis due to atherosclerotic plaque formation. Given the patient's increased risk of stroke, a carotid endarterectomy is performed in the left carotid artery, causing surgical damage to the ipsilateral carotid sinus. This leads to a partial loss of the baroreceptor reflex and subsequent postoperative hypertension.

4. Which cranial nerve carries the afferent fibers that mediate the baroreflex of the carotid sinus?
   a) Vagus
   b) Accessory nerve
   c) Hypoglossal
   d) Glossopharyngeal

Level 1: Easy

Answer D: The carotid sinus nerve of the glossopharyngeal nerve innervates the baroreceptors of the carotid sinus and the chemoreceptors in the carotid body. These peripheral receptors monitor changes in blood pressure and the chemical composition of the blood, respectively. Stimulation of the peripheral receptors leads to the activation of cardiovascular and respiratory centers in the medulla and activation of the autonomic nervous system. Carotid endarterectomy (CAE) and carotid artery stenting (CAS) are two procedures used to reduce the risk of stroke caused by clots associated with carotid atherosclerotic stenosis. Both types of procedures can surgically damage the baroreceptors of the carotid sinus and lead to disruption of baroreflex activity and subsequent hypertension. (**A**) The aortic branch of the vagus transmits GVA input from the baroreceptors in the aortic sinus and chemoreceptors in the aortic body, not the carotid sinus. The aortic nerve of CN X follows a similar route as CN IX and has a similar reflex response;

however, the aortic sinus and body contribute less to the baroreflex and chemoreflex than that of CN IX. (**B**) The accessory nerve (CN XI) and (**C**) hypoglossal nerve (CN XII) do not contribute to this reflex. During a carotid endarterectomy the vagus, glossopharyngeal, and hypoglossal nerve are possibly at risk given their proximity to the carotid artery. The accessory nerve runs posterolateral to these structures and should not be an issue.

5. During the patient's carotid endarterectomy, the hypoglossal nerve and ansa cervicalis are both injured. Each of the following clinical findings EXCEPT one may be associated with damage to the hypoglossal nerve. Which one is the exception?
   a) Anesthesia of anterior two-thirds of tongue
   b) Atrophy and fasciculations on left side
   c) Dysarthria
   d) Deviation of the tongue to the left

Level 2: Moderate

Answer A: Anesthesia of the anterior two-thirds of tongue is the exception. The transmission of general somatic sensations from the anterior two-thirds of the tongue occurs by the lingual branch of V3. The hypoglossal nerve provides (GSE) ipsilateral motor innervation from the hypoglossal motor nucleus to all intrinsic muscles and the styloglossus, hyoglossus, and genioglossus muscles. The palatoglossus muscle is supplied by the vagus. (**D**) Deviation of the tongue to left is correct. The genioglossus muscle is responsible for protrusion of the tongue, and ipsilateral damage to the nerve during its course leads to paralysis of the genioglossus and deviation of the tongue to the damaged side. (**B**) Left-side atrophy and fasciculations are correct. LMN lesions to the hypoglossal nucleus or damage to the hypoglossal nerve during its peripheral course will be associated with fasciculations, flaccid paralysis, and muscle atrophy due to loss of neural input to the muscle. (**C**) Dysarthria is also correct. Dysarthria is characterized as a disturbance in speech articulation due to weakness of the laryngeal, pharyngeal, palatal, and tongue musculature. Difficulties with tongue movement and placement during articulation will most likely manifest as problems with consonant and vowel pronunciation. The hypoglossal motor nuclei predominantly receive contralateral innervation from the primary motor cortices. As a result, UMN lesions affecting the hypoglossal nerve will lead to the contralateral deviation of the tongue. UMN lesions will also show signs of increased muscle tone and spastic paralysis, which in the tongue is manifested as slow movements. This leads to speech that sounds stilted and strangled.

22 Neuromuscular Control of Mastication, Swallowing, and Speech

22.1 Overview of Oropharyngeal Region

The present chapter summarizes the processes of chewing, swallowing, and speech and outlines the neural pathways involved in coordinating these oromotor activities. Each of the oromotor activities involves both volitional control and involuntary reflexive patterns that are essential to its function. The chapter begins with a brief overview of motor and sensory input to the orofacial region and highlights the areas of functional overlap between oromotor activities. The chapter then describes the functional processes of mastication, swallowing, and speech and the neural pathways which control these oromotor activities.

22.1.1 Functional Overlap of Oromotor Activities

- **Mastication** (chewing), **deglutition** (swallowing), **phonation** (sound production), and **articulation** (formation of speech sounds) represent complex motor functions unique to the head and neck region.
- Each oromotor process utilizes similar anatomical structures and shares a common functional passageway with the respiratory system. Due to the level of functional overlap, these oromotor activities require a high degree of sensory input, neuromuscular control, and precise coordination to permit respiration and prevent aspiration (▶ Table 22.1).
- The execution of oromotor activities occurs through a unique set of striated muscle groups derived primarily from pharyngeal arch (branchiomeric) mesoderm.
  - The muscle groups include the **perioral** muscles of facial expression, the **muscles of mastication**, the **suprahyoid** and **infrahyoid muscles**, the **tongue**, and the **palatal, pharyngeal**, and **laryngeal musculature (Reference Chart A)** (▶ Fig. 22.1). These muscle groups are discussed in Chapter 19.
- Each oropharyngeal muscle group plays an integral role in mediating and coordinating the complex movements involved in chewing, swallowing, and speech.
- These oromotor tasks differ from those performed by trunk and limb muscles and these functional differences are reflected in structural variations in the skeletal muscle groups comprising the oromotor system (▶ Table 22.2).

22.1.2 Overview of Oropharyngeal Motor and Sensory Activity

- Oromotor functions, such as chewing, swallowing, and speech, involve bilateral activation of several different muscle groups in the oropharyngeal region to ensure proper integration and sequencing of function.
- The ability to perform complex oromotor movements involves the integration of several intricate neural circuits linked together by numerous neurons.

Table 22.1 Common anatomical passageways for oromotor functions

Anatomical Passageway	Description of Region	Functional Process				
		Mastication	Deglutition	Speech—Phonation	Speech—Articulation	Respiration
Oral cavity	Cavity bound by lips, cheeks, teeth, tongue, and palate Connected posteriorly to oropharynx Considered part of vocal tract	Site of chewing and food reduction via coordinated jaw movements occurring through masticatory apparatus	Bolus preparation Oral transport via activity of masticatory apparatus	Oral cavity functions as resonator to modulate filter and amplify sounds	Changes in shape, size, and position of oral articulatory structures along with jaw movement produces oral sounds of vowels and consonants	Mouth breathing when nasal cavity closed or blocked
Nasal cavity	Cavity superior to palate and connected posteriorly to nasopharynx	Not directly involved Facilitates breathing during chewing	Sealed off during swallowing by soft palate	Resonance chamber for production of vocal sounds	Produces nasal sounds when soft palate (velum) depressed toward tongue	Nasal breathing when mouth closed or blocked
Pharynx Three parts: • Nasopharynx • Oropharynx • Laryngopharynx (hypopharynx)	Common passage for swallowing and breathing, phonation Muscular tube that connects the oral and nasal cavities to the larynx (anteriorly) and esophagus (posteriorly) Considered part of vocal tract	Minor role; oropharynx receives food; aids in bolus formation; nasopharynx serves airway	Directs food (bolus) transport to esophagus Produce phasic contractions and relaxations of constrictors during swallowing	Act as resonance chamber to modulate filter and amplify sounds Changes in diameter and length alter frequency of vibrational pitch (low vs. high)	Assists in articulation through cooperative action of pharyngeal constrictors and soft palate to close nasopharynx—prevents nasality in speaking	Directs airflow Pharynx dilates for airway patency
Larynx	Connects pharynx to trachea; part of vocal tract Position of rima glottidis (opening between vocal fold), rima vestibule (opening between the vestibular false folds), and the vestibule (opening to larynx) changes based on functions of swallowing, phonation, respiration	Not directly involved	Protects airway from aspiration during swallowing Rima glottidis, rima vestibule, and vestibule closed; vocal cords and false vocal folds adducted (closed); epiglottis inverts; arytenoid cartilages adduct and pull forward to close inlet	Production of sound due to vocal cord vibration during expiratory phase of air passage Rima glottidis closed; vocal cords adducted; rima vestibule open	Resonance chamber—limited activity Changes in length alter frequency of vibrational pitch (low vs. high)	Directs airflow; produces phasic contractions and relaxation during expiration and inspiration Rima glottidis, rima vestibule, and vestibule open; vocal cords abducted during inspiration→ vocal cords close → then forced open in expiration
Trachea	Part of conducting portion of upper respiratory system Extends inferiorly from larynx to bronchial tree Considered part of vocal tract	Not involved	Not involved	Air passage during phonation Aids in vocal cord vibration	Not involved	Passage for air during expiration and inspiration
Esophagus	Communicates with pharynx superiorly; pharynx connects oral cavity and esophagus	Not directly involved	Receives bolus; transports bolus via peristaltic actions to stomach	Not involved	Not involved	Not involved

Note: *The term **vocal tract** includes the region of the trachea, larynx, pharynx, and oral cavity.

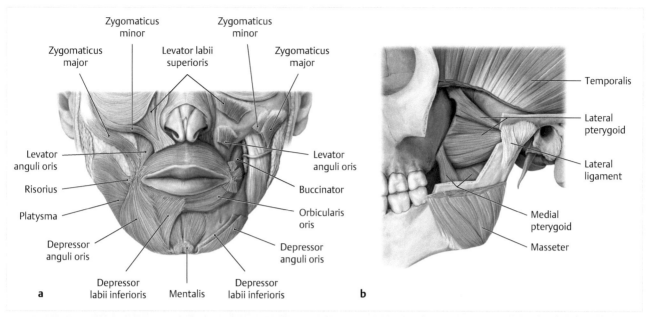

Fig. 22.1 Muscles of facial expression: Perioral groups. Anterior view. **(a)** The muscles of facial expression that surround the mouth are known as the perioral group or buccolabial muscle groups. The muscles in this group include the circumferentially arranged orbicularis oris muscles, several muscles that are radially arranged from the orbicularis oris, along with the buccinator of the cheek, and the risorius that extends from the corners of the mouth. The facial modiolus (not labeled) is an area of fibromuscular tissue that lies 10 to 12 mm lateral to the angle of the mouth and represents the point of intersection for the perioral musculature. The modiolus functions to maintain constriction during mastication, aid in bolus positioning, prevent spillage during chewing, and facilitate the oral phase of swallowing. The perioral muscles also serve a functional role in the articulation of vowels and consonants by mediating positional and shape changes of the lips. **(b)** Muscles of mastication. Left lateral view; deep layer. A portion of the mandible, including the coronoid process, and fibers of the lower temporalis are removed. The primary muscles of mastication include the masseter, medial and lateral pterygoids, and the temporalis. The muscles collectively work together to stabilize the temporomandibular joint (TMJ) and move mandible relative to maxilla via elevation, depression, protrusive, retrusive, and lateral excursive movements. The actions of the muscles mediate chewing, swallowing, and speaking behaviors. (Reproduced with permission from Schuenke M, Schulte E, Schumacher U. THIEME Atlas of Anatomy Third Edition, Vol 3. © Thieme 2020. Illustrations by Markus Voll and Karl Wesker.)

- As described in Chapter 16, skeletal muscle is under voluntary control, and while some actions can occur as simple protective reflexes, the execution of most **volitional** movements involves complex neural circuits, which integrate both voluntary and involuntary neural pathways (▶ Fig. 22.2).
- In the oropharyngeal region, the striated muscles controlling oromotor activities receive direct innervation from lower motor neurons (LMNs) that reside bilaterally within the brainstem or the laminae (IX) of the spinal cord ventral horn (▶ Table 22.3).
- The oromotor activities of mastication, swallowing, and speech exhibit functional overlap, and use the same LMNs to perform these different tasks. To coordinate these motor responses, the LMNs, which control oropharyngeal movements, receive descending input from several cortical and subcortical regions, along with input from specific groups of interneurons in the brainstem reticular formation.
- In addition to these descending pathways, several ascending pathways transmit sensory information from proprioceptors, mechanoreceptors, and nociceptors, which modulate motor activity and initiate protective reflexes.

22.2 Summary of Neural Control Mechanisms

22.2.1 Cortical Input

- Cortical input that provides volitional control for oromotor tasks originates from the prefrontal association cortex and the cortical motor areas of the frontal lobe. The motor commands for planning and selecting the sequence of complex voluntary movements originate from premotor neurons in the prefrontal cortex (PFC) based on sensory input from cortical association areas and project to **upper motor neurons (UMNs)** in the cortical motor regions (▶ Fig. 22.3).
- As discussed in Chapter 16, the cortical motor areas which contain UMNs involved in the sequencing and execution of movements consist of three regions: the **primary motor cortex (M1),** the **premotor cortex (PMC),** and the **supplementary motor area (SMA).**
  - These three motor regions (M1, PMC, and SMA) receive sensory input from the **thalamus** and the **primary somatosensory cortex** of the parietal lobe.

Table 22.2 Oropharyngeal head musculature

Characteristic	Head and Neck
Developmental origin	Pharyngeal head (branchiomeric) mesoderm
Location of primary afferent neurons	Cranial sensory ganglia of CNs V, VII, IX, and X *Mesencephalic nucleus (proprioception)
Location of upper motor neurons and cortical input • Somatotopic arrangement in motor cortex for limb trunk and face	Primary motor cortex (oromotor area) Cortical input is primarily bilateral causing bilateral contraction—exception is LMNs of facial motor nucleus (CN VII) and hypoglossal nerve (CN XII)
Location of lower motor neurons (LMNs)	Cranial nerve motor nuclei of brainstem CNs V, VII, IX, X, and XII
Motor (LMN) innervation muscle	SVE fiber of cranial nerves *Except CN XII and cervical plexus C1–C3 (GSE)

Types of motor units
• **Type I**
(slow-twitch; fatigue resistant)
• **Type IIa**
(fast-twitch; fatigue resistant)
• **Type IIb**
(fast-twitch; fatigable)
  ○ Motor unit is the α-motor neuron (LMN) and innervates all muscle fibers (see Chapter 16)
  ○ A motor unit is comprised of one fiber type which confers functional properties
  ○ Type of fiber is based on the contractile properties of myosin protein
  ○ Contraction strength is determined by number of motor units recruited (activated)
	• Different muscles contain different ratios of motor unit types based on function
	• Oropharyngeal muscles also contain unique fiber types and hybrid muscle fiber types, which presumably provides differences in contractile forces and speed of contraction

Size of motor unit (innervation ratio) • The size of the motor unit corresponds to the innervation ratio which represents the total number of muscle fibers innervated by single motor unit • The innervation ratio contributes to the level of precision and control created by the muscle	Oropharyngeal muscles typically exhibit smaller innervation ratios, which allows for precise, graded movements, and fine control
Types of proprioceptors • **Muscle spindles (Ia fibers)** (detect changes in muscle length; provide resistance to stretch) • **Golgi tendon organs (Ib fiber)** (detect changes in muscle tension) • **Joint receptors (Aβ)** (detect positional changes and movement of joint)	• Differential distribution of muscle spindles ○ Muscle spindles present only in jaw-closing muscles, some laryngeal muscles, tongue, and extraocular eye muscles • Golgi tendon, few or absent • Joint receptor distribution in temporomandibular joint (TMJ) comparable to body
Types of other sensory receptors • Mechanoreceptors • Nociceptors • Thermoreceptors	General distribution: Overall higher receptor density and smaller receptive fields throughout face and oropharyngeal areas as compared to body Regional variations within oral cavity
Receptor density/receptive field High receptor density and small receptive field, more discriminative input	Include areas of teeth, lips, tip, and midline of tongue; oropharyngeal isthmus; pharyngeal wall, vocal folds

Abbreviations: GSE, general somatic efferent; SVE, special visceral efferent.

○ Based on the functional and physiological coupling of the motor cortex with cortical sensory association areas, the two cortices are collectively known as the **sensorimotor cortex.**

– Reciprocal connections between the motor and sensory cortex facilitate sensorimotor integration that is necessary for the acquisition and performance of motor skills. In the orofacial region, these reciprocal connections play an important role in adaptive behavior associated with changes to the oral environment following the placement of a dental prosthesis or tooth extractions.

○ UMNs that are essential in executing oromotor functions reside near the lateral sulcus of the primary motor strip (M1), and include the **masticatory motor area (CMA),** the **cortical swallowing area (CSA),** and the **laryngeal (speech) motor cortex (LMC).** Functional overlap exists between these orofacial areas to aid in synchronizing bilateral orofacial movements (▶ Fig. 22.4).

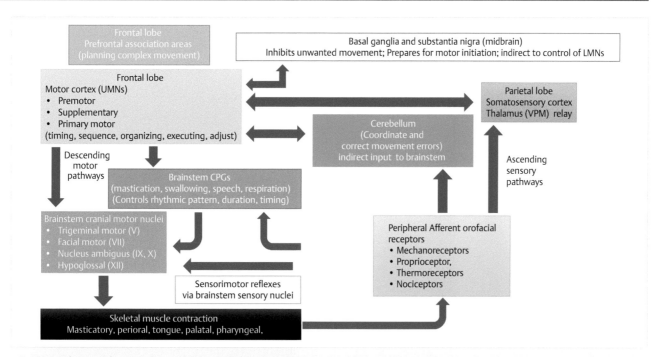

Fig. 22.2 Schematic diagram of sensorimotor pathways involved in the control of movement. The execution of complex voluntary movements involves the integration of several voluntary and involuntary motor pathways. Motor responses depend on sensory input provided from the somatosensory and association cortices and from cerebellum and basal ganglia. Collectively, the cortical and subcortical regions function to coordinate movements, correct for error, and modulate rhythmic patterns of movement generated by central pattern generators. The sensorimotor regions work cooperatively together as components of feedback loops through which the cortex and subcortical areas influence each other.

Table 22.3 Summary of LMN location for oropharyngeal muscles

	Trigeminal (CN V3)	Facial (CN VII)	Glossopharyngeal and Vagus (CNs IX and X*)	Hypoglossal (CN XII)	Cervical Spinal
Motor nuclei	Trigeminal motor nucleus	Facial motor nucleus	Nucleus ambiguus	Hypoglossal motor nucleus	Cervical spinal group
Location	Mid-pons	Caudal pons	Rostral medulla	Caudal Medulla	Level C1–C3 spinal cord ventral horn
Modality*	SVE	SVE	SVE	GSE	GSE
Cranial nerve branch	Mandibular (CN V3)	Facial nerve	Glossopharyngeal (CN IX) Pharyngeal plexus via pharyngeal branch of CN X Superior laryngeal; external laryngeal branch (CN X) Recurrent laryngeal (CN X)	Hypoglossal	C1 nerve to thyrohyoid and geniohyoid Ansa cervicalis (C1–C3)
Muscle group	Muscles of mastication Tensor veli palatini Mylohyoid Anterior digastric	Facial expression Perioral muscles (buccinator, orbicularis oris) Posterior digastric Stylohyoid	Palatal except tensor veli palatini* V3 Pharyngeal muscles Laryngeal muscles Upper esophagus	Tongue Extrinsic and intrinsic musculature	Infrahyoid and suprahyoid muscles
Functional role and overlap	• Mastication • Swallowing (oral phase) • Speaking—jaw movement	• Mastication bolus formation • Swallowing (oral phase) • Speaking/ articulation of vowels and consonants	• Swallowing (pharyngeal phase) (esophageal) • Speech/phonation (vocal cord movement)	• Mastication (bolus placement) • Swallowing (oral phase) • Speech/ articulation of vowels and consonants	• Mastication—assist in opening (depression) jaw via infrahyoid group • Swallowing (pharyngeal phase) stabilize, raise, and lower hyoid bone via infrahyoid and suprahyoid group

Abbreviations: GSE, general somatic efferent; LMN, lower motor neuron; SVE, special visceral efferent.
Note: *Oropharyngeal muscles develop from pharyngeal arch (branchiomeric) mesoderm and somatic mesoderm and receive SVE and GSE fibers respectively.

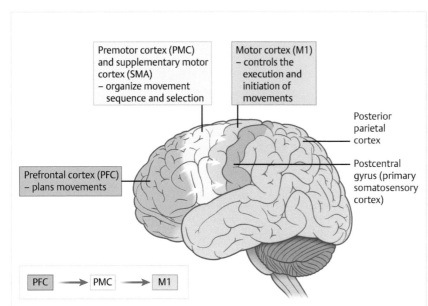

Fig. 22.3 Cortical areas involved with motor function. Lateral view of the left hemisphere. The motor regions reside in the prefrontal gyrus of the frontal cortex and sensory regions reside in the postcentral gyrus of the parietal cortex. The planning and execution of complex voluntary movements involve interaction between several cortical areas. The prefrontal cortex (PFC) plans and directs complex movements and motor behaviors based on goals and knowledge gained from previous experience. The region of the premotor cortex (PMC) and supplementary motor area interpret the plan and determine the sequence of movements. The premotor neurons in the PMC and supplementary motor area (SMA) project to primary motor cortex (M1) which serves to execute the response and produce specific movements. The primary somatosensory and sensory association cortices, as well as input from the basal ganglia and cerebellum, serve to modulate the motor response and correct for error.

- The sensorimotor cortices, which exhibit a somatotopic arrangement, comprise a large component of the motor and sensory representation within the M1 and S1 territories. The large areas of cortical representation reflect the functional complexity of movements performed by the orofacial muscles and the high degree of sensory acuity required for feedback and sensorimotor integration.
- UMNs arising from these orofacial regions provide excitatory and inhibitory cortical input via corticobulbar pathways to LMNs in the brainstem motor nuclei of the trigeminal (CN V), facial (CN VII), glossopharyngeal (CN IX), vagus (CN X), and hypoglossal (CN XII) cranial nerves (see Chapter 16).
  - Cortical input to these cranial nerve nuclei is direct and bilateral with the exception of the hypoglossal motor neurons and the motor neurons innervating the lower facial muscles. These LMNs receive only contralateral input (see Chapters 20 and 21).
  - UMNs from the orofacial areas of the motor cortex also project to groups of interneurons within the brainstem that are involved in controlling the timing, duration, and rhythm of orofacial movements. These interneurons act as **central pattern generators** (**CPGs**).
- Other cortical areas necessary in controlling oromotor activities include the **anterior cingulate gyrus (limbic), insular cortex,** and **gustatory cortex**. These areas mediate emotional behavior and influence the spontaneous rhythmic activity of chewing, swallowing, and forms of nonverbal communication such as crying and laughing.

22.2.2 Cerebellar and Subcortical Input

- The sensorimotor cortex also exhibits reciprocal connections with the cerebellum and several subcortical structures including the basal ganglia, thalamus, and limbic system. Based on sensorimotor feedback, these subcortical areas provide indirect input to the cranial motor nuclei via the extrapyramidal pathways and function to modulate movement and correct for motor errors (see Chapter 17).
  - Cerebellar and basal ganglia dysfunction results in impaired initiation, execution, and coordination of motor function. In the orofacial region, these areas play an important role in modulating jaw position and coordinating muscular movements. Damage to these areas may manifest as unintentional movements, jaw tremors, and difficulty in chewing and swallowing, or appear as slurred speech due to difficulty in coordinating oromotor movements.

22.2.3 Brainstem Input

Several areas of the brainstem reticular formation contain groups of excitatory and inhibitory interneurons that act as CPGs.
- CPGs integrate reflexive responses and create the rhythmic activity involved in chewing, swallowing, speech, and respiration through direct projections to the LMNs in the cranial motor nuclei of CNs V, VII, IX, X, and XII.
- CPGs may generate rhythmic movement independently; however, sensory feedback from orofacial receptors and

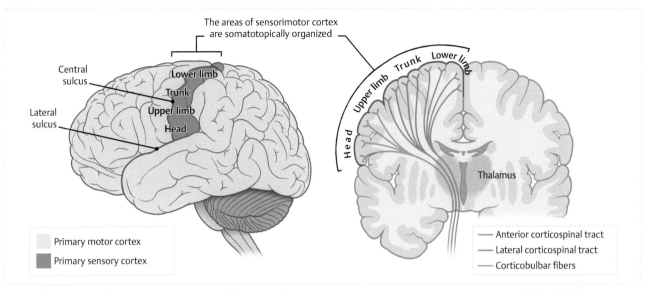

Fig. 22.4 Areas of cortical representation corresponding to orofacial function. **(a)** Lateral view of left hemisphere demonstrating the location of primary motor and somatosensory cortices. **(b)** Anterior view of the precentral gyrus showing the somatotopic map. The primary motor (M1) region resides in the precentral gyrus of the frontal cortex, and the primary somatosensory (S1) region resides in the postcentral gyrus of the parietal cortex. The two regions, which work cooperatively together, are functionally known as the sensorimotor cortex. Both cortical regions exhibit a somatotopic arrangement, such that each body area maps, point for point, to specific territories within the M1 and S1 cortices. The amount of area represented correlates with the functional importance of that area of the body. As depicted in the diagram, the neurons responsible for motor execution and sensory processing of information from the orofacial region in the head reside in the M1 and S1 cortex near the lateral sulcus (fissure). Both regions represent disproportionately large cortical areas when compared with the corresponding body area. The discrepancy in the size of cortical representation reflects the functional complexity of movements performed by the orofacial muscles and the high degree of sensory acuity required for feedback and sensorimotor integration.

descending cortical and subcortical inputs may modulate CPG output to the cranial motor nuclei and alter the timing and duration of the activities.

- Individual CPGs exist for distinct oromotor activities and reside in separate regions of the brainstem (▶ Table 22.4).
- Many oromotor tasks exhibit functional overlap and require the same LMNs to mediate mastication, swallowing, and speech. Given the degree of functional overlap, it is predicted that individual CPGs that modulate these tasks interact with each other to ensure that the oromotor responses are synchronized and executed in a coordinated manner (▶ Fig. 22.5).

22.2.4 Sensory Input

- An important aspect of motor control is the role of proprioceptors, mechanoreceptors, and nociceptors in providing sensorimotor feedback (see Chapters 11 and 13).
- The oropharyngeal region exhibits a high number of sensory receptors throughout the facial skin, oral mucosa, periodontal ligament (PDL), muscles, and temporomandibular joint (TMJ). The high receptor density, small receptive field, and pattern of distribution throughout the orofacial region confer a high level of discrimination, proprioception, and stereognostic input which is critical for modulating oromotor output (▶ Table 22.5).

- Afferent fibers project to the brainstem sensory nuclei, the CPGs, subcortical areas, and higher cortical regions to provide feedback. Sensory input modulates oromotor activities, initiates protective reflex responses, and adapts the motor response to changes in the oral environment.

22.3 Neural Reflexes of Oromotor System

- In the oropharyngeal region, feedback from oral sensory receptors contributes to several orofacial reflex pathways. Orofacial reflexes serve to protect and modulate various neuromuscular activities by altering motor neuron activity (▶ Table 22.6, ▶ Table 22.7, ▶ Table 22.8, ▶ Table 22.9, ▶ Table 22.10, ▶ Table 22.11, ▶ Table 22.12, ▶ Table 22.13, ▶ Table 22.14).
- The reflexes involving the jaw play a role in protecting the masticatory apparatus from damage and provide feedback to CPGs to adjust the chewing cycle and accommodate changes in bolus consistency.
- Pharyngeal and laryngeal reflexes play a critical role in airway protection and function in the coordination of swallowing and respiratory motor activities.

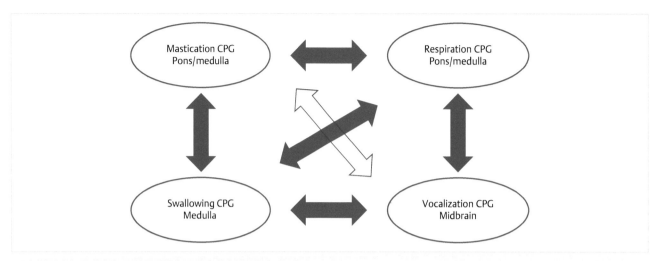

Fig. 22.5 Schematic of interactions between brainstem central pattern generators. The oromotor tasks of mastication, swallowing, and vocalization exhibit functional overlap, which requires several of oromotor muscle groups to work cooperatively. Central pattern generators that regulate oromotor behaviors appear to exhibit significant levels of interaction to coordinate the activity of the oromotor muscle groups and synchronize it with the process of respiration. The specific patterns of muscle activity for the oromotor muscles are controlled at different levels of the CNS and are task-dependent. Therefore, lesions in one region of the CNS may exhibit a more significant outcome than others. CPGs are capable of generating rhythmic motor activity in the absence of cortical and sensory input; however, there can be difficulty in executing and coordinating the movements of patterned responses, such as food manipulation and intraoral transport. Feedback from descending cortical pathways and sensory afferent fibers modulates CPG output to lower motor neurons. CNS, central nervous system; CPG, central pattern generator.

Table 22.4 Central pattern generators affecting oromotor activities

CPG	Predicted Location	Function
Masticatory	Reticular formation (pons/medulla)	Provides a rhythm and pattern of activity in jaw opening and closing and provides input to hypoglossal and facial nuclei to coordinate movement between tongue and jaw activity
Swallowing	Reticular formation (medulla)	Dorsal and ventral swallowing CPG which program the sequenced pattern of muscle contraction and relaxation
Vocalization	Reticular formation and PAG (midbrain/pons)	Nonverbal (emotive vocalization)
Respiratory	Pons and medulla	Dorsal and ventral respiratory CPG program breathing patterns and respond to signals from central and peripheral chemoreceptors (carotid sinus)

Abbreviations: CPG, central pattern generator; PAG, periaqueductal gray.
Note: *CPGs are groups of neurons that independently generate specific reflexive movements with a coordinated timing, pattern, and sequence.

Table 22.5 Summary of orofacial sensory receptors

Type of Sensory Receptor and Cranial Nerves	Location of Receptor	Sensory Information Provided
Nociceptive (ubiquitous) Thermoreceptors Mechanoreceptors (skin, oral mucosa) CNs V, IX, and X Primary afferent neuron in sensory ganglia	Skin Oral mucosa of oral cavity proper Periodontal ligament (PDL) Temporomandibular joint (TMJ) capsule and disk, Teeth and pulp Palatal, pharyngeal, and laryngeal mucosa	• Stereognostic input concerning food consistency, size, and texture of objects in oral cavity • Positional information about muscles, jaw, tongue, teeth, or position of food placement • Tactile input about bite force • Mediates protective pharyngeal, laryngeal, and masticatory reflexes • Stimulate salivary reflexes
Gustatory (chemoreceptors) CNs VII, IX, and X Primary afferent neuron in sensory ganglia	Dorsum of tongue Hard and soft palates Oropharynx Epiglottis	• Stimulate salivary reflexes to increase secretion due to gustatory input
Proprioceptive stretch receptors (muscle spindle) CNs V3, X, and XII Primary afferent neuron in mesencephalic nucleus of V of brainstem	Jaw-closing muscles Laryngeal muscles Tongue muscles	• Bite force and direction of occlusal forces • Monitor changes in muscle length based on the amount of stretch applied to muscle and assist in positional adjustments of jaw • Mediates jaw reflexes

Table 22.6 Jaw-closing reflex

Reflex	Trigger	Receptor	Path	Mechanism of Action
Jaw-closing reflex (jaw jerk reflex) Monosynaptic reflex Provides information concerning resting position of jaw Protects against dislocation; stabilizes jaw Partial tonus (sustained weak contraction) of jaw elevators prevents pull of gravity and maintains joint articulation	Increased stretch of jaw elevator muscles during jaw-closing phase May occur due to increased stretch of muscles following excessive opening due to size of food bolus, and increased resistance to food substance during power stroke	Proprioceptor—muscle spindles in jaw-closing muscle detect passive stretch of muscles Primary sensory neuron cell bodies found in **mesencephalic nucleus of V**	**Afferent path:** Primary afferent fibers (Type Ia) project from muscle spindle to cell body Central fibers project from mesencephalic nucleus and synapse on jaw-closing neurons in **trigeminal motor nucleus** **Efferent path:** Efferent fibers project from trigeminal motor nucleus to jaw elevator muscle to initiate reflexive jaw closing	Increase in stretch elicits an increase in excitatory efferent input to the jaw-closing muscles via α-motor neurons in trigeminal motor nucleus Passive stretching causes reactive contraction **During opening phase of the normal chewing cycle, the CPG inhibits jaw-closing muscle activity via** hyperpolarization of jaw-closing motor neurons

Abbreviation: CPG, central pattern generator.

Table 22.7 Jaw-opening reflex

Reflex	Trigger	Receptor	Path	Mechanism of Action
Jaw-opening reflex (nociceptive/withdrawal reflex in body) Polysynaptic reflex involving two or more synapses Function: Prevents overloading of teeth and muscles during chewing Protects teeth and soft tissue from damage caused by hard/sharp objects (i.e., pits, fish bones)	Painful or mechanical stimuli to the oral mucosa or teeth during occlusion leads to rapid jaw opening	Low-threshold mechanoreceptor Nociceptors Found in oral mucosa, tongue PDL Type II afferent of **CN V3** activated in the anterior part of masseter during occlusion Type II primary sensory neuron cell bodies found in **trigeminal ganglion**	**Afferent path:** Type II Aβ afferent fibers project to **chief sensory nucleus** Type III Aδ and unmyelinated C fibers project to **trigeminal spinal nucleus (nucleus caudalis)** Afferents synapse on inhibitory or excitatory interneurons that then project motor neurons into **trigeminal motor nucleus** **Efferent path:** Efferent fibers of V3 project to masticatory jaw muscles	Jaw-closing muscles are inhibited and jaw-opening muscles activated resulting in an open jaw During normal closing phase of the chewing cycle the CPG depresses the jaw-opening reflex by inhibiting the excitatory pathway from jaw-opening neurons, allowing for normal closure

Abbreviations: CPG, central pattern generator; PDL, periodontal ligament.

Table 22.8 Jaw unloading reflex

Reflex	Trigger	Receptor	Path	Mechanism of Action
Jaw unloading reflex Polysynaptic reflex A protective reflex to prevent the mandible from forcefully closing	Sudden breaking or collapse of hard object held statically between occlusal surfaces	Low-threshold mechanoreceptors transmit proprioceptive and tactile input from PDL and TMJ Primary sensory afferent neuron cell bodies in **trigeminal ganglion** **Mesencephalic nucleus**	**Afferent path:** Type II afferent fibers project to **mesencephalic nucleus** Type II afferent fibers project to **chief sensory nucleus** Fibers project to inhibitory interneuron which project to α-motor neurons into **trigeminal motor nucleus** **Efferent path:** Efferent fibers of V3 project from motor neurons in trigeminal nucleus to target muscles	Leads to inhibition of jaw elevators to prevent the mandible from forcefully closing Activation (excitation) of jaw opener

Abbreviations: PDL, periodontal ligament; TMJ, temporomandibular joint.

Table 22.9 Lingual reflex

Reflex	Trigger	Receptor	Path	Mechanism of Action
Lingual reflexes Polysynaptic protective reflex Protects tongue against damage during mastication; also serves as protective reflex of the airway leading to protrusion or retrusion during swallowing	Trigger tactile and nociceptive input from anterior or posterior tongue Elicits protrusive and retrusive tongue movements • Protrusive movement due to lingual nerve (CN V) • Retrusive due to glossopharyngeal (CN IX) or superior laryngeal (internal) of vagus (CN X)	Low-threshold mechanoreceptors of CNs V, IX, and X Primary afferent cell bodies in: **Trigeminal ganglion** **Superior ganglion** of CN IX **Superior ganglion** of CN X	**Afferent path:** Type II afferent fibers project to trigeminal sensory complex and **nucleus tract of solitarius (NTS)** Secondary afferents project from NTS to motor neurons of hypoglossal motor nucleus (CN XII) **Efferent path:** Efferent fibers of CN XII project to tongue muscles	CN XII mediated efferent response includes protrusive and retrusive tongue movements Type of movement depends on location of stimuli and afferent nerve

Table 22.10 Pharyngoglottal closure reflex

Reflex	Trigger	Afferent Receptor	Path	Efferent Mechanism of Action
Pharyngoglottal reflex Polysynaptic reflex Adduction of vocal cards provides protection of airway against aspiration during premature spill of oral contents	Mechanical or chemical stimuli of pharyngeal mucosa	Low-threshold mechanoreceptor, chemoreceptors, and nociceptors in pharyngeal and laryngeal mucosa Primary afferent cell bodies in: **Superior ganglion of CN IX** **Superior ganglion of CN X**	**Afferent path:** Type II afferent fibers carried by **CN IX (pharyngeal plexus)** and **CN X (internal laryngeal)** project to interneurons: • Nucleus tract of solitarius • Spinal trigeminal nucleus Interneurons synapse on **motor neurons in nucleus ambiguus** **Efferent path:** Efferent fibers of recurrent laryngeal nerve of CN X activate adductor laryngeal muscles	Bilateral stimulation of the lateral cricoarytenoid, (inter)arytenoid, and thyroarytenoid muscles Adduction of vocal cords and closure of laryngeal inlet during swallowing

Table 22.11 Swallow reflex

Reflex	Trigger	Afferent Receptor	Path	Efferent Mechanism of Action
Swallow reflex Initiates reflexive movement of the bolus to the pharynx by contraction of the tongue and palate Polysynaptic reflex involving two or more synapses	Tactile stimulation of oropharyngeal mucosa at tonsillar pillars, oropharyngeal isthmus, and tongue base	Low-threshold mechanoreceptor, chemoreceptors, and nociceptors in tonsillar pillars, oropharyngeal isthmus, base of tongue, and epiglottis Primary afferent cell bodies in: **Superior ganglion of CN X** **Superior ganglion of CN IX**	**Afferent path:** Type II afferent fibers transmit input via **CN IX** (lingual-tonsillar branches; afferent fibers of pharyngeal plexus) and **CN X (internal laryngeal)** Afferent fibers of interneurons project to **nucleus tract of solitarius** Afferents project to **spinal trigeminal** Interneurons synapse on efferent fibers project from **motor neurons in nucleus ambiguus** **Efferent path:** Efferent fibers of hypoglossal (**CN XII**), pharyngeal plexus, and **recurrent laryngeal nerve (CN X)** activate the tongue, palatal, pharyngeal, and suprahyoid muscle groups	Activation of tongue, palatal, pharyngeal, and suprahyoid muscle groups initiates swallow sequence Outcome: Rapid elevation of soft palate and closure of nasopharynx (velopharyngeal closure) and bilateral contraction of pharyngeal constrictors Elevation and anterior displacement of larynx

Table 22.12 Gag reflex

Reflex	Trigger	Afferent Receptor	Path	Efferent Mechanism of Action
Gag reflex (pharyngeal reflex /laryngeal spasm) Protective reflex response that prevents foreign objects or noxious material from entering pharynx, larynx, or trachea Not elicited during normal swallowing Polysynaptic involving more than one synapse	Tactile stimulation of mucosa lining of posterior pharyngeal wall of oropharynx	Low-threshold mechanoreceptors of CN IX	Type II afferent fibers transmitted by **glossopharyngeal CN IX** of pharyngeal plexus (GVA/GSA) **GVA fibers are main contributors to gag reflex. Primary afferent cell bodies in **inferior ganglia (petrous) of CN IX** GSA cell bodies in superior ganglion of CN IX Central afferent (GVA) fibers project to **nucleus tract of solitarius** Central afferent (GSA) fibers project to pars caudalis of spinal trigeminal nucleus Secondary afferent fibers project **bilaterally to nucleus ambiguous** Efferent fibers: SVE fibers of motor component of **pharyngeal plexus (CN X)**	Contraction of pharyngeal constrictors and soft palate musculature occurs both ipsilaterally as part of direct response and contralaterally as part of a consensual response to cause rapid bilateral elevation of the soft palate and contraction of pharyngeal muscles **Minor contribution of motor fibers of V3 and CN XII also involved; produce jaw opening and tongue thrust.

Abbreviations: GSA, general somatic afferent; GVA, general visceral afferent.

Table 22.13 Laryngeal adductor reflex

Reflex	Trigger	Afferent Receptor	Path	Efferent Mechanism of Action
Laryngeal adductor reflex (glottic closure reflex) Polysynaptic reflex Glottic closure prevents foreign material from entering airway Opening of upper esophageal sphincter concomitantly also occurs for swallowing	Tactile and chemical stimulation of laryngeal mucosa elicits glottic closure	Low-threshold mechanoreceptors and chemoreceptors transmit GVA and SVA input via internal laryngeal branch of superior laryngeal nerve of CN X *Some CN IX Primary afferent cell bodies in superior and inferior ganglion of CN X	**Afferent path:** Central afferent fibers of primary afferent neurons project to **NTS** Secondary afferent fibers project ipsilaterally **to nucleus ambiguus** **Efferent path:** Efferent fibers of the **recurrent laryngeal nerve of CN X** project from nucleus ambiguus and target laryngeal adductor muscles	Recurrent laryngeal nerve innervates thyroarytenoid, lateral cricoarytenoid, and transverse arytenoid Laryngeal muscles cause contraction and vocal folds adduction and glottic closure Opening of the upper esophageal sphincter (UES) also occurs due to recurrent laryngeal nerve stimulation Closure of glottis and vocal fold adduction tied with opening of esophagus

Abbreviations: GVA, general visceral afferent; NTS, nucleus tractus solitarius; SVA, special visceral afferent.

Table 22.14 Cough reflex

Reflex	Trigger	Afferent Receptor	Path	Efferent Mechanism of Action
Cough reflex Polysynaptic reflex Protection of airway against mucosal irritation Modifies breathing pattern with forced expiration to clear airway	Tactile and chemical stimulation of tracheal and laryngeal mucosa Stimulates modification of breathing pattern	Low-threshold mechanoreceptors; some polymodal nociceptors possible in trachea and larynx (pulmonary cough receptors) Primary afferent cell bodies in inferior ganglion (nodose) CN X	Afferent fibers: Type II afferent fibers transmitted by tracheal and laryngeal nerve fibers (of internal laryngeal and recurrent laryngeal nerve) Central afferents project to: **nucleus tract of solitarius (NTS)** and **spinal trigeminal nucleus** Secondary afferents project to CPG in respiratory centers of reticular formation of medulla Afferent fibers from reticular formation project to **nucleus ambiguus** and to motor neurons in **cervical spinal cord** **Efferent path:** Efferent fibers project from motor neurons in nucleus ambiguus for **vagal motor control** and from motor neurons of spinal cord as the **phrenic nerve**	Efferent fibers of **recurrent laryngeal nerve (CN X)** activate laryngeal muscles Cervical efferent fibers of **phrenic nerve** innervate the diaphragm Contraction of **posterior cricoarytenoid (abduction)** initiates rapid vocal folds abduction and inspiration followed by contraction of **lateral cricoarytenoid, interarytenoid, and thyroarytenoid** muscles for vocal cord adduction, then forceful expiration

Abbreviation: CPG, central pattern generator.

22.4 Mastication

- **Mastication**, or the act of **chewing**, is the process through which food in broken down into smaller particles for swallowing.
  - Mastication is a complex voluntary and reflexive process involving a series of bilateral rhythmic jaw movements occurring through the TMJ. The movements correlate with the coordinated manipulation and reduction of food by the structures of the **masticatory (stomatognathic) apparatus** (▶ Table 22.15).

22.4.1 Masticatory Movements

- The contraction of the primary and accessory masticatory muscles regulates the repetitive elevation and depression of the lower jaw. The muscles also control protrusive, retrusive, and lateral mandibular movements involved in mastication, and maintain the position of the condyle within the mandibular (glenoid) fossa.

- Each mandibular movement, known as an **excursive movement,** occurs through the TMJ and functions to move the mandibular dental arch relative to the maxillary dental arch. Most movements of the mandible that occur beyond the initial opening or closing involve both rotational, translational (gliding), and grinding actions (▶ Fig. 22.6a–d, ▶ Fig. 22.7a, b).
  - Proper positioning of the mandibular and maxillary dental arches depends on neuromuscular and reflexive control of the masticatory muscles, along with positional guidance provided by the condyle, the TMJ, and the **occlusal (biting)** tooth surfaces.
- The opening and closing of the mandible follow a repetitive cycle or chewing pattern, which may exhibit some variability based on individual occlusion and changes in food consistency.
  - The masticatory movement of a typical chewing pattern, when viewed from a frontal plane, is classically a "teardrop" shape. The masticatory movements of the TMJ involve rotation (opening/closing), translation (protrusion/retrusion), and grinding (lateral) motions that occur between the swinging and resting condyles.

Table 22.15 Structures of masticatory apparatus

Structure	General Function
Perioral muscles Buccinator Orbicularis oris	Lips and cheeks assist tongue to hold food between the occlusal surface; function cooperatively with tongue to manipulate, monitor, and select food for further reduction Motor activity depends on sensory feedback of tactile receptors
Primary masticatory muscles Masseter, temporalis, medial pterygoid, lateral pterygoid	Mediate positional changes in mandible through movement of condyle in glenoid fossa of TMJ Jaw closing (elevators) Jaw opening (depressor) Collective actions: Contraction mediates protrusive, retrusive, and lateral excursive movements necessary for mastication Most movements necessary for penetration of food by teeth are rotational, translational, and grinding motions Bilateral contraction stabilizes condyle in joint cavity
Accessory masticatory muscles Suprahyoid group Infrahyoid group	Assist in jaw opening via stabilization of the hyoid bone ****Both groups also involved in swallowing and speaking through movement of hyoid bone and larynx.
Tongue	Positioning of bolus; provide stereognostic information regarding size and location of bolus
Hard palate **Soft palate muscles**	Aid in bolus formation during mastication; cooperative movements between tongue and hard palate function during intraoral transport
Teeth and periodontium (structural tooth support)	Based on anatomical position and tooth morphology, different teeth perform different functions: • Incisors and canines initiate biting, tearing, and piercing foods • Premolar and molar teeth serve to crush and grind Mechanoreceptors in the periodontal ligaments (PDLs) provide feedback about bite force
Temporomandibular joint (TMJ)	Connects the lower jaw to the skull; permits movements of mandible relative to maxilla and assists in positioning mandible for occlusion of teeth Mastication occurs as a repetitive chewing cycle with an opening, closing, and intercuspal phase and involves vertical and lateral mandibular movements
Sensory receptors Proprioceptors Mechanoreceptors Nociceptors Thermoreceptors Chemoreceptors (taste)	Tactile, nociceptive, gustatory, and proprioceptive inputs from the oral mucosa and muscles provide reflexive jaw movements, salivary stimulation, ensure proper placement of bolus between the occlusal surfaces of the teeth, and detect the consistency and size of bolus which is necessary for safe swallowing Mechanoreceptors in the PDL and TMJ provide input regarding bite force and jaw position Proprioceptors in muscle, PDL, and TMJ provide sensory feedback about jaw movements and mediate protective jaw reflexes
Salivary glands Parotid Submandibular Sublingual Minor salivary glands	Reflexive production of saliva aids in lubrication of oral mucosa and bolus formation, swallowing, and taste detection

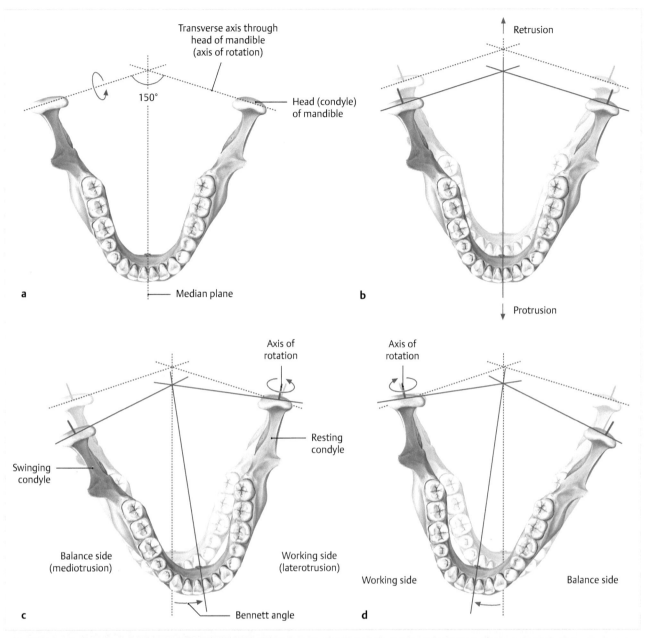

Fig. 22.6 (a–d) Movements of the mandible in the TMJ. Superior view. Most of the movements in the TMJ are complex motions that have three main components: Rotation (opening and closing of the mouth), translation (protrusion and retrusion of the mandible), and grinding movements during mastication. **(a)** Rotation. The axis for joint rotation runs transversely through both heads of the mandible. The two axes intersect at an angle of approximately 150 degrees (range of 110–180 degrees between individuals). During this movement the TMJ acts as a hinge joint (abduction/depression and adduction/elevation of the mandible). In humans, pure rotation in the TMJ usually occurs only during sleep with the mouth slightly open (aperture angle up to approximately 15 degrees). When the mouth is opened past 15 degrees, rotation is combined with translation (gliding) of the mandibular head. **(b)** Translation. In this movement the mandible is advanced (protruded) and retracted (retruded). The axes (condylar–hinge axes) for this movement are parallel to the median axes through the center of the mandibular heads. **(c)** Grinding movements in the left TMJ. In describing these lateral movements, a distinction is made between the "resting condyle" and the "swinging condyle." The resting condyle on the left working side rotates about an almost vertical axis through the head of the mandible (also a rotational axis), whereas the swinging condyle on the right balance side swings forward and inward in a translational movement. The lateral excursion of the mandible is measured in degrees and is called the Bennett angle. During this movement the mandible moves in laterotrusion on the working side and in mediotrusion on the balance side. **(d)** Grinding movements in the right TMJ. The right TMJ is the working side. The right resting condyle rotates about an almost vertical axis, and the left condyle on the balance side swings forward and inward. TMJ, temporomandibular joint. (Reproduced with permission from Schuenke M, Schulte E, Schumacher U. THIEME Atlas of Anatomy Third Edition, Vol 3. © Thieme 2020. Illustrations by Markus Voll and Karl Wesker.)

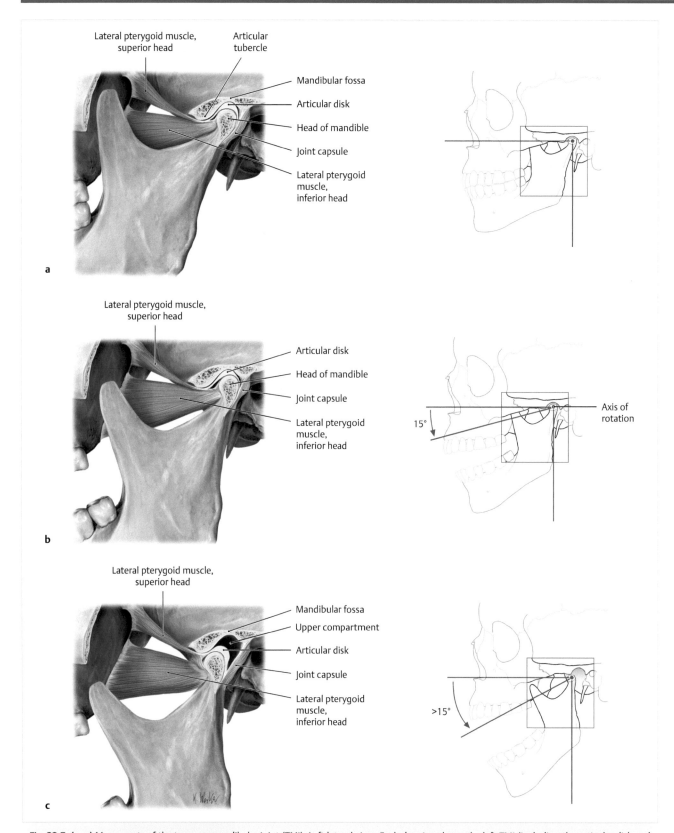

Fig. 22.7 (a–c) Movements of the temporomandibular joint (TMJ). Left lateral view. Each drawing shows the left TMJ (including the articular disk and capsule) and the lateral pterygoid muscle. Note: The gap between the heads of the lateral pterygoid is exaggerated. Each schematic diagram on the right shows the corresponding axis of joint movement. The muscle, capsule, and disk form a functionally coordinated musculo-disco-capsular system and work closely together when the mouth is opened and closed. **(a)** Mouth closed. When the mouth is in a closed position, the head of the mandible rests against the mandibular (glenoid) fossa of the temporal bone. **(b)** Mouth opened to 15 degrees. For up to 15 degrees of abduction, the head of the mandible remains in the mandibular fossa. **(c)** Mouth opened beyond 15 degrees. At this point, the head of the mandible glides forward onto the articular tubercle. The joint axis that runs transversely through the mandibular head is shifted forward. The articular disk is pulled forward by the superior part of the lateral pterygoid muscle, and the head (condyle) of the mandible is drawn forward by the inferior part of the muscle. (Reproduced with permission from Schuenke M, Schulte E, Schumacher U. THIEME Atlas of Anatomy Third Edition, Vol 3. © Thieme 2020. Illustrations by Markus Voll and Karl Wesker.)

Table 22.16 Stage I: Preparatory phase

Masticatory Cycle	Muscles Involved	Activity	Mandibular Movement

Stage I: Preparatory phase
Summary:
• Conscious voluntary control required to initiate opening movement
• Rapid initial opening
• Food placement in cavity
• Food placed on occlusal (bolus or working side) of dental arch; serves as chewing side
• Contralateral (opposing) side; stabilizing balance side
	• **Jaw opening muscles** depress mandible and lower jaw
	• **Lateral pterygoid** (inferior head) initiates opening
	• **Suprahyoid muscles** assist to stabilize hyoid bone and provide downward traction on the mandible
	  ○ **Anterior belly digastric**
	  ○ **Mylohyoid**
	  ○ **Geniohyoid**
	• **Tongue** positions food on working side
	• **Lips and cheeks** prepare and aid tongue in bolus formation
		• Jaw elevator muscles inhibited and undergo controlled relaxation
		• Jaw opens with gravity and isometric contraction of jaw openers
		• Mouth opens to receive food
		• Anterior teeth bite or tear if food piece too large for entry
		• Position food on posterior occlusal tooth surface (bolus/working side)
			• Resting position of mandible is typically open 2 to 4 mm (intercuspal freeway space)
			• Jaw opens further to initiate mastication
			• Initial 15 degrees of lower jaw opening involves **rotation of mandibular condyle** in **lower TMJ compartment (hinge movement)**
			• **Forward translational (sliding)** movement of the condyle occurs in the **upper TMJ compartment** as jaw continues to open
			At full opening (50–60 mm) the mandibular condyles and articular disks slide anteriorly to the articular eminence (see ▶ Fig. 22.7)

Abbreviation: TMJ, temporomandibular joint.

○ The chewing pattern involves a circular rotary movement, with jaw movement occurring downward, laterally, across the midline to the other side, and upward to close. The vertical and lateral mandibular movements may occur either clockwise or counterclockwise. Additionally, it may accompany the transfer of food from one side of the mouth across the midline to the other side of the mouth.
• Factors affecting jaw movement are discussed in Clinical Correlation Boxes 22.1 and 22.2.

22.4.2 Stages of Mastication

• The process of mastication consists of three stages, the **preparatory, masticatory (reduction),** and **intraoral transport stages,** which typically lead to swallowing as a functional outcome.
  ○ Since the processes of mastication and swallowing usually occur as a continuum, there is a degree of overlap when describing the stages of chewing and swallowing.
  ○ The duration of each of the three stages depends on whether the substance ingested is liquid or solid.
  ○ The three masticatory phases include the following. Additional factors that may influence the stages of mastication are highlighted in Clinical Correlation Box 22.3.
    – **Stage I: Preparatory stage (ingestion stage)** involves initial jaw opening, the placement of food into the oral cavity, and the positioning of the food by the tongue onto the occlusal surface of the posterior mandibular teeth. Chewing usually occurs on the occlusal surface of the first mandibular molars (▶ Table 22.16).
    – **Stage II: Masticatory (reduction) stage** consists of the **chewing cycle** and describes the path of the mandible as it moves through a repetitive sequence of opening and closing motions.
      ▪ The masticatory chewing cycle occurs as a continuous series but may be considered for descriptive purposes

as three phases: **(1) opening phase** (▶ **Table 22.17**), **(2) closing phase** (▶ Table 22.18, ▶ Table 22.19), and **(3) intercuspal phase** (▶ Table 22.20). The neural control of mastication is summarized in ▶ Table 22.21.
  – **Stage III: Pre-swallow (intraoral transport) stage** follows the completion of chewing and entails the movement of the prepared bolus toward the oropharynx (▶ Table 22.22). The remaining stages of swallowing are described in section 20.5.

Clinical Correlation Box 22.1: Limited Jaw Movement

Limitations in the range of jaw movement can occur due to variations in the cranioskeletal and TMJ morphology, alterations in dental occlusion, as well as anatomical variations in ligament and muscle attachments. Limited jaw opening (trismus) can also occur due to condylar fusion to the joint fossa (ankylosis) or can be limited by muscular pain or muscle spasms. Infections such as tetanus or neurological disease such as multiple sclerosis, dystonia, and muscular dystrophy may impact the opening and the masticatory functions.

Clinical Correlation Box 22.2: Abnormal Condylar Motion

Abnormal condylar motion in the mediolateral direction is noted in patients with unilateral crossbites when chewing on the affected side. Additionally, there is a difference in the cyclic chewing pattern; chewing often occurs in the reverse direction and may be characterized by unbalanced muscle activity.

Table 22.17 Stage II: Masticatory chew cycle: Rapid closing phase

Chew Cycle Phase	Muscles Involved	Activity	Mandibular Movement
Closing phase (rapid; initial) **Summary:** • Rapid isotonic contraction as the jaw elevator muscles contract with constant tension Process transitions to slower movement as teeth contact food and offer resistance	• **Tongue** • **Orbicularis oris**: Lips form anterior oral seal • **Buccinator** holds food on occlusal surface • **Mandibular elevators (jaw-closing muscles)** ○ Masseter (deep head) ○ Temporalis ○ Medial pterygoid Superior head lateral pterygoid—involved in power stroke of initial bite	Action: • Mandible elevates against gravity to close jaw • Posterior teeth brought into contact with food on occlusal (working) side with vertical alignment of opposing upper and lower teeth	**Condylar movement** • **Bolus (working) side**: Condyle upward, slightly posterior, and lateral • **Contralateral (nonworking) side** condyle moves upward, backward, and lateral on frontal plane **Outcome on mandibular movement** • **Bolus (working) side**: Mandible moves upward and outward (lateral) to bring the buccal cusps of the posterior mandibular and maxillary teeth into vertical alignment

Table 22.18 Stage II: Masticatory chew cycle: Slow closing phase

Chew Cycle Phase	Muscles Involved	Activity	Mandibular Movement
Closing phase (slow; power stroke) **Crushing movement** **Summary:** Part of slow closing phase hall-marked by vertical power stroke movement	• **Tongue** • **Orbicularis oris**: Lips form anterior oral seal • **Buccinator** holds food on occlusal surface • **Mandibular elevators (jaw-closing muscles)** ○ Masseter ○ Anterior temporalis ○ Medial pterygoid ○ Superior head lateral pterygoid—involved in power stroke of initial bite	Action: • Jaw elevator muscles gradually transition from an isotonic → isometric contraction as the teeth meet; increased resistance to push through the food ○ Crushing movements: Food is pierced with vertical force; teeth may not have occlusal contact	**Bolus (working) side**: Posterior mandibular teeth begin to inter-digitate with the maxillary teeth **Contralateral side**: Posterior teeth may or may not have occlusal contact

Table 22.19 Stage II: Masticatory chew cycle: Intercuspal phase

Chew Cycle Phase	Muscles Involved	Activity	Mandibular Movement
• **Intercuspal contact (tooth contact)** • **Grinding movement** **Summary:** • Part of slow closing; hallmarked by **intercuspal contact** and reduction of food by **side-to-side horizontal shearing force** movement across occlusal surface	• **Tongue** • **Orbicularis oris**: Lips form anterior oral seal • **Buccinator** holds food on occlusal surface • **Mandibular elevators** (jaw-closing muscles) **Lateral side-to-side movement** ○ Masseter ○ Anterior temporalis ○ Medial pterygoid ○ Superior head lateral pterygoid	• Muscle contraction creates side-to-side mandibular movement • Chewing occurs on the bolus (working) side through the cooperative action of the teeth in the upper and lower dental arches • Jaw **shifts** from **vertical motion** to a **side-to-side movement** • Food reduced through horizontal buccal-lingual shearing forces created by intercuspal contact • Softening of bolus and mixing with saliva to lubricate	• **Bolus (working) side mandible**: The condyle slides **upward** and **medial** into an **intercuspal position** to facilitate the interdigitation of mandibular and maxillary posterior teeth Following intercuspal contact: • **Bolus (working) side mandible**: ○ Mandible shifts slightly **downward** as the **mandibular teeth** move **medially** and **horizontally** as buccal cusps across the palatal cusps of the opposing maxillary teeth

Table 22.20 Stage II: Masticatory chew cycle: Opening phase

Chew Cycle Phase	Muscles Involved	Activity	Mandibular Movement
Opening phase **Summary:** • **Occurs slowly during cycle** • Slight depression of mandible—enough space for teeth to clear bolus and tongue to reposition bolus	• **Mandibular depressors** (jaw-closing muscles; act during opening phase) ○ **Lateral pterygoid** (inferior head) • **Suprahyoid muscles** ○ **Anterior belly digastric** ○ **Mylohyoid** ○ **Geniohyoid** **Tongue:** **Perioral** Orbicularis oris	The opening phase alternates repetitively with the closing phase during the chew cycle and in-volves depression of the mandible Tongue: Monitors consistency and size; may move bolus to opposite side During opening moves downward and forward Orbicularis oris releases and oral seal opens slightly	• **Bolus (working) side mandible**: Condyle moves downward and forward, slightly lateral toward bolus • **Contralateral (nonworking) side**: Condyle moves downward and forward, medially; the path of opening and closing phase overlap **Outcome of mandibular move-ment:** • **Bolus (working) side**: Mandible deviates **laterally** and slightly **posterior** toward the side where the food is positioned

Table 22.21 Neural control of mastication

Cortical Input	Function and Target
Frontal lobe (both hemispheres) • Primary motor cortex (M1) (UMN) Precentral gyrus: Orofacial motor area • Cortical masticatory motor area (CMA) • Supplementary motor area (SMA) • Premotor cortex (PMC) **Additional cortical areas:** Limbic—emotional reflex activity (cingulate gyrus) Insular (gustatory) cortex—integrates autonomic, viscerosensory, and visceromotor input including taste	Function: Plan, organize motor patterns, and execute movement • Voluntary control to initiate jaw opening and closing Ability to voluntarily alter chew cycle; reposition food and jaw Target: 1. Project directly: UMN → LMN in motor nuclei via corticobulbar path Target nuclei: V, VII, XII*, C1 cervical *Hypoglossal and facial (lower) receive contralateral input.* *Antagonistic excitatory and inhibitory input to jaw opening and closing muscles based on point in chew cycle.* 2. Cortical neurons project → to CPG interneurons to modulate motor response
Subcortical input (subcortical neurons) • Limbic system: Amygdala, hypothalamus, thalamus (relay station, sensory and motor tracts) • Basal ganglia: Inhibition of unwanted movements, planning to initiate movement • Cerebellum: Motor coordination based on environmental sensory input	Function: Feedback modulation • Indirectly provide feedback via extrapyramidal tract • Reciprocal input and output to cortical centers Targets: • LMNs • Masticatory CPG
Masticatory central pattern generators (CPGs) Predicted location: Pontomedullary region; between the facial and trigeminal motor, and chief sensory, possibly reticular, formation	Function: • Generate rhythmic activity of jaw and tongue movements via excitatory or inhibitory input to LMN controlling masticatory, tongue, and facial muscles • Regulates changes to masticatory chewing cycle based on sensorimotor feedback
Cranial motor nuclei (LMN) Location: • **Trigeminal motor** (CN V)—mid/caudal pons • **Facial motor** (SVE) (CN VII)—caudal pons • **Hypoglossal motor nucleus** (GSE) (CN XII)—medulla • **Spinal motor nuclei** (GSE)—cervical ventral horn (C1–C3)	Function: LMNs directly control masticatory, perioral and tongue, and suprahyoid and infrahyoid group muscle activity Cranial nerves involved SVE and GSE motor branches involved: • CN V3 • CN VII • CN XII • C1; ansa cervicalis
Afferent input source **Peripheral receptors:** Proprioceptors mechanoreceptors, nociceptors **Afferent primary neuron cell bodies** • Trigeminal ganglion (CN V) • Geniculate ganglion (CN VII) • Superior and inferior ganglion (CNs IX and X)	Functional role: Provide feedback about position of jaw tongue and perioral muscles and bite force Feedback about jaw pain, bolus consistency, hardness, size, position, and moisture content (saliva) • GSA fibers transmit: Tactile, pain, and temperature from PDL, TMJ, oral mucosa, and tongue; muscle spindles active during jaw closing • SVA fibers of CNs VII, IX, and X transmit gustatory input to NTS Cranial nerves involved: Palatal (CN V2), lingual (CN V3), pharyngeal plexus (CNs IX and X)
Secondary afferent neurons Trigeminal nuclear (sensory) complex • Main (chief) sensory (discriminative tactile) • Spinal trigeminal nucleus (pain, temperature, crude touch of CNs V, VII, IX, and X) • Mesencephalic nucleus (**exception includes primary afferent neurons for proprioceptive muscle spindles, jaw-closing muscles, tongue, and PDL mechanoreceptors) Nucleus tractus solitarius **Ascending pathways project to:** • CPG, subcortical areas, cerebellum • Somatosensory cortex and gustatory cortex via VPM of thalamus • Visceral reflex center, i.e., salivatory nuclei, respiratory centers	Functional role • Proprioceptive input from muscle spindles in jaw-closing muscles and tongue and PDL mechanoreceptors provide input about occlusal force to propagate jaw rhythm • Protective jaw reflex activity and lingual reflexes • Conscious perception about food status

Abbreviations: CPG, central pattern generator; GSE, general somatic efferent; LMN, lower motor neuron; NTS, nucleus tractus solitarius; PDL, periodontal ligament; SVE, special visceral efferent; TMJ, temporomandibular joint; UMN, upper motor neuron; VPM, ventral posteromedial.

Table 22.22 Stage III: Pre-swallow intraoral transport

Masticatory Cycle	Muscles Involved	Activity	Mandibular Movement
Pre-swallow (intraoral transport stage) **Summary:** Movement of the bolus from the oral cavity toward the oropharynx. Jaw chewing movements alternate with intermittent jaw cycles for swallowing	**Tongue** **Soft palate** **Infrahyoid group** **Suprahyoid muscles** • Anterior and posterior digastric • Mylohyoid • Geniohyoid **Jaw elevators** (jaw-closing muscles) • Masseter • Anterior temporalis • Medial pterygoid Superior head lateral pterygoid	Action: • Dorsum of tongue moves bolus toward oropharynx • Elevation and stabilization of hyoid bone through the suprahyoid and infrahyoid muscles • Jaw elevators help stabilize jaw during movement of tongue and soft palate	Teeth are not directly in contact. Condyle and jaw stabilized at point of intraoral transport

Note: Condylar movement is bilateral and should occur symmetrically; the bolus (working) side can be on the right or left side. For each table listed the right temporomandibular joint (TMJ) is the working side. Movement on the right side follows a clockwise pattern from opening to closing.

Clinical Correlation Box 22.3: Factors Influencing Mastication

- Food texture and size of food influence bite force—hard food requires more masticatory force, a longer chewing cycle, and stimulates rhythmic jaw activities. Soft foods decrease rhythmic activity and may potentiate an earlier swallowing phase.
- Decreased salivation due to neural, pharmacological, and physical blockage may lead to diminished taste, and difficulties in bolus formation and swallowing due to lack of lubrication.
- Alterations in tooth morphology and the contour of the occlusal surface due to dental attrition of the cuspal tips, a shallow fossa, or a steep occlusal inclination will alter chewing efficiency and may affect lateral load bearing of the tooth and periodontium. Lateral loading may, in turn, impact mechanosensory feedback to the central nervous system (CNS).
- The degree of occlusal contact, which is influenced by occlusal wear, malocclusion, tooth integrity, and tooth loss, may impact masticatory efficiency.
- The amount of masticatory bite force generated may be altered in neuromuscular diseases such as Parkinson's disease, cerebral palsy, and cerebellar disorders, or due to pain associated with temporomandibular disorders (TMD).
- Parafunctional habits such as bruxism, clenching, and jaw locking alter muscular activity patterns and can impair normal function.
- Craniofacial abnormalities including cleft lips and palates, or developmental anomalies affecting the first pharyngeal arch, impact jaw position and occlusion.

- TMD pain and trismus may influence the chewing side (see Chapter 23).
- Jaw movement disorders such as jaw stiffness, difficulties with jaw opening, painful movements, and unintentional movements will impact mastication. Many of these disorders are associated with systemic diseases such as multiple sclerosis, muscular dystrophy, tumors, tetanus, craniofacial pain, and Parkinson's disease.
- Intermittent, unintentional movements associated with Parkinson's disease result in alterations in the chewing cycle. The changes are associated with a decreased range of jaw motion and bite force, along with a longer and slower duration of the masticatory cycle.
- Dental prosthesis, including implants and dentures, may restore aesthetics and function; however, a change in masticatory efficiency will take time and depends on the adaptation of neural pathways.
- Neuromuscular diseases and stroke may affect the initiation and planning of motor control for the jaw and tongue.
- Elderly patients may exhibit chew cycles of longer and slower duration and possibly a decrease in bite force. Reduced mastication increases the risk of developing systemic diseases due to nutritional deficiencies and dysphasia (swallowing difficulties).

22.5 Swallowing

Swallowing is normally a rapid and continual process hallmarked by a series of bilateral, voluntary and involuntary (reflexive) muscular contractions that result in the transport of a food bolus from the mouth to the stomach.

- Anatomically and functionally, swallowing consists of several sequentially regulated phases, namely, the **oral preparatory,** **intraoral transport, pharyngeal transfer,** and **esophageal phases.**
  - Each phase is coordinated with respiratory activities and requires a sequential series of movements involving the masticatory apparatus and the muscles of the palate, pharynx, larynx, and esophagus.
- Difficulty in swallowing, is known as dysphagia and is discussed in Clinical Correlation Box 22.4.

22.5.1 Swallowing Process (▶ Fig. 22.8a, b)

- The **oral preparatory phase** of swallowing often begins with suckling or mastication (chewing) if the solid food requires breakdown (▶ Table 22.23).

- The **pharyngeal phase** of swallowing is a rapid and involuntary patterned **reflexive response** elicited by afferent stimulation of mechanoreceptors and chemoreceptors found in the mucosa covering the anterior faucial pillars, the soft palate, and posterior tongue, which comprise the structures of the oropharyngeal isthmus (▶ Table 22.24).

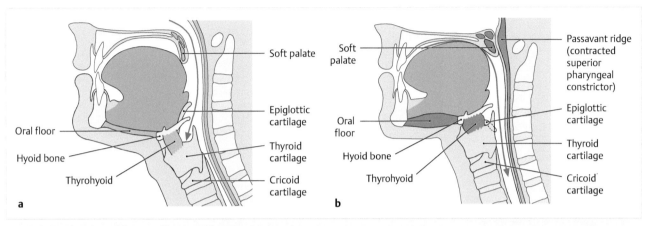

Fig. 22.8 Schematic depicting the structures involved in swallowing. Sagittal view of oral cavity and pharynx. The act of swallowing consists of three phases: (1) Voluntary initiation of swallowing, (2) reflex closure of the airway, and (3) reflex transport of the food bolus down the pharynx and esophagus. **(a)** As part of the airway, the larynx in the adult is located anterior to inlet to the digestive tract. **(b)** During the initial stages of swallowing the airway must be briefly occluded to keep food from entering the trachea. During the second phase of swallowing, the soft palate contracts and elevates, and presses against the posterior pharyngeal wall, sealing off the upper airway. Concomitantly, the oral floor muscles (mylohyoid and digastric) and the thyrohyoid muscles elevate the larynx, and the epiglottis covers the laryngeal inlet, sealing off the lower airway. The third phase involves the transport of food along the esophagus via peristalsis. (Reproduced with permission from Schuenke M, Schulte E, Schumacher U. THIEME Atlas of Anatomy. Second Edition, Vol 3. © Thieme 2016. Illustrations by Markus Voll and Karl Wesker.)

Table 22.23 Oral and intraoral transport phase of swallowing

Oral Preparatory Stage: Bolus preparation involves both volitional and reflexive control and occurs through the rhythmic chewing cycle and reflexive salivation.	
Movement	**Muscles and Action**
Orofacial movement	Contraction of the orbicularis oris and buccinator orofacial muscles seals the lips to prevent spillage and minimizes pocketing of food in the vestibule.
Masticatory movements	The muscles of mastication serve to move and stabilize the jaw during chewing as described in the previous mastication section.
Tongue movements	• Tongue movements coordinate with cyclic palatal and jaw movements • Once bolus formation is complete the **transverse intrinsic muscles** of the tongue, along with the **styloglossus** and **genioglossus** muscles, contract bilaterally to form a narrow trough on the dorsum of the tongue which holds the liquid or bolus in position for transport.
Palatal movement	• Elevation of posterior tongue occurs as the palatoglossus muscles bilaterally contract to depress the soft palate anteriorly toward the tongue. ○ The contact of the posterior tongue and soft palate form a transient **posterior oral seal.** • Closure between the oral cavity and oropharynx maintains the bolus in the oral cavity and allows the nasopharynx to initially remain open.
Respiratory movements	• The laryngeal inlet and nasopharynx remain open; nasal breathing may occur during the oral preparatory phase
Intraoral Transport Phase	
Movement	**Muscles and Action**
Tongue movement and palatal movement	• Intraoral transport begins as the **mylohyoid** and **superior longitudinal** muscles of the tongue contract causing the tip of the tongue to elevate from the floor of the mouth and contact the alveolar ridge of the hard palate. • As the tongue continues to push against the hard palate, the posterior (pharyngeal) tongue forms a chute, and contraction of the intrinsic and extrinsic tongue muscles along with soft palate pushes the bolus posteriorly toward the oropharynx.

Table 22.24 Pharyngeal phase of swallowing

Pharyngeal swallowing phase is a neural-mediated reflex triggered by tactile sensory input that results in a sequentially patterned motor response driven by CPGs found in the swallowing centers of the medulla. CPGs govern the motor output of LMNs in cranial motor nuclei.

Movements	Muscle and Action

Palatal movement
Key events:
• Velopharyngeal closure (soft palate–pharyngeal closure) occurs via soft palate elevation and soft palate and pharyngeal contraction
	• The coordinated action of the muscles comprising the soft palate and lateral and posterior pharyngeal walls function as valves to close the connection between the nasal and pharyngeal cavities during swallowing (**velopharyngeal closure**).
	  ○ Contraction of the **levator veli palatini, tensor veli palatini, and musculus uvulae** elevate the soft palate allowing the bolus to move into the oropharynx. The tensor veli palatini also functions to tense the palatal aponeurosis and open the auditory tube to equalize pressure between the middle ear and nasopharynx during swallowing.
	  ○ Contraction of **palatoglossus, palatopharyngeus, salpingopharyngeus, and the superior constrictor muscles** during swallowing raises the pharyngeal wall superiorly, anteriorly, and medially, and forms a small muscular projection in the posterior wall of the nasopharynx known as Passavant's ridge (palatopharyngeal sphincter).
	  ○ The elevated soft palate contacts Passavant's ridge on the posterior pharyngeal wall to **seal off the nasopharynx from the oropharynx** (▶ Fig. 22.8b).

Pharyngeal movements
Key events:
• Airway protection via hyoid bone elevation and upward and forward movement of larynx
• Relaxes UES
• Phasic contraction/ relaxation of pharyngeal wall
	• The inner longitudinally oriented muscles of the pharynx (**stylopharyngeus, salpingopharyngeus, palatopharyngeus**) function to widen the pharynx diameter while the superior constrictor muscle contracts to raise the pharyngeal wall over the bolus.
	• Contraction of **pharyngeal constrictor muscles** propels the bolus inferiorly and allows the posterior tongue to contact the posterior pharyngeal wall and seal off the region above the bolus.
	• As the bolus reaches the vallecula, contraction of the **suprahyoid muscles** and the **thyrohyoid (infrahyoid group)** along with **stylopharyngeus, salpingopharyngeus, and palatopharyngeus** elevates the larynx and hyoid bone superiorly and anteriorly to draw the larynx below the base of tongue and **provide airway protection.**
	  ○ **Elevation of the larynx** facilitates the relaxation of the **cricopharyngeus**, also known as the **upper esophageal sphincter (UES)**, and opening of esophagus.
	  ○ During normal resting conditions, the UES remains passively closed and exhibits tonic contraction resulting from myogenic activity.
	• The **pharyngeal constrictor** muscles contract and relax in a cranial to caudal sequence to produce a **pharyngeal stripping wave** of muscle contraction behind the bolus which propels it toward the esophagus.

Laryngeal movements
Key events:
• Protects airway via three laryngeal events:
  ○ Vocal fold closure
  ○ False vocal folds and the arytenoid cartilages adduct and pull forward to the epiglottis
  ○ Epiglottic inversion to close laryngeal inlet
	• Concomitant to **elevation of the larynx**, the laryngeal inlet reflexively closes to protect the airway via the movement of three laryngeal structures: **Vocal folds, ventricular (false) folds, and epiglottis.**
	• The **vocal fold adduct** via contraction of the **lateral cricoarytenoid, transverse interarytenoid, and thyroarytenoid muscles.**
	• False vocal folds and arytenoid cartilages adduct to close the vestibule.
	• **Epiglottis** tips inferiorly to **cover the laryngeal inlet** and protect the airway.
	  ○ The bolus laterally deviates as it passes over the inverted epiglottis forming two streams of food that follow along each side of the piriform fossae and then unite to enter the esophagus.
	• Following bolus passage through the UES, the vocal folds abduct (open), the epiglottis tips upward, the larynx and hyoid descend, the communication between the oropharynx and nasopharynx opens, and breathing resumes.

Respiratory movements Key event: • Swallow apnea	• **Respiration briefly ceases (swallowing apnea)** as food passes over the closed laryngeal inlet. Breathing resumes once bolus passes through UES. • Normal respiratory sequence: Exhale–swallow—exhale to clear passage of residual material • Pause in breathing during swallowing due to transient neural inhibition of respiratory CPG in brainstem and inhibition of diaphragm

Abbreviations: CPGs, central pattern generators; LMNs, lower motor neurons; UES, upper esophageal sphincter.

• The **esophageal phase** is an involuntary motor response involving rhythmic muscular contraction and relaxation (peristalsis) that moves the bolus through the esophagus and lower esophageal sphincter (LES) and into the stomach (▶ Table 22.25).
• Swallowing disorders due to neuromuscular deficits are discussed in Clinical Correlation Box 22.5.

Clinical Correlation Box 22.4: Dysphasia

• **Dysphagia** refers to difficulties in swallowing and can occur at any point during the swallowing sequence. Swallowing dysfunction may result from degenerative disorders, including dementia, and movement disorders or from nondegenerative changes resulting from strokes or motor neuron diseases such as **amyotrophic lateral sclerosis (ALS)**.

Table 22.25 Esophageal swallowing stage

Esophageal Phase	
Movement	**Muscle and Action**

Esophageal movements
 Key event:
 • Coordinated opening and closing of esophageal sphincters
 • Peristaltic activity
	• As the bolus moves past the cricopharyngeus (UES) muscle, relaxation of the UES terminates and the sphincter closes to prevent regurgitation and air from entering esophagus. Opening of sphincter is tied to glottic closure to prevent food from entering airway.
	 • Closure of the UES sphincter upon bolus entry into the esophagus correlates with relaxation of the esophageal muscular wall.
	 • **Esophageal peristaltic activity** occurs through the sequential inhibition (relaxation) and excitation (contraction) of the inner circular and outer longitudinal muscle layers of the muscularis externa in the esophageal wall.
	    ○ Relaxation distal to the bolus allows the food to move into the next segment while contraction proximal to the bolus propels it forward.
	    ○ As part of this peristaltic reflex the lower esophageal sphincter (LES) located at the cardiac esophageal junction relaxes allowing food to pass to the stomach. Following food passage, the LES contracts to prevent regurgitation of stomach contents.

Abbreviation: upper esophageal sphincter.

Table 22.26 Neural control of deglutition

Cortical Input	Function/Targets

Frontal lobe of both hemispheres
 • Primary motor cortex (M1) (UMN)
   Precentral gyrus: Orofacial motor area
    ○ Cortical masticatory motor area (CMA)
    ○ Cortical swallow area
    ○ Supplementary motor area (SMA)
 • Premotor cortex (PMC)
 Additional cortical areas:
 Limbic—emotional reflex activity
 (cingulate gyrus)
 Insular (gustatory) cortex integrates autonomic, viscerosensory, and visceromotor input including taste
	Function:
	 • Voluntary control during oral phase
	 • Cortical masticatory and swallowing areas work cooperatively to prevent premature trigger of swallow
	 • Provide cortical inhibition to prevent premature swallow reflex
	 Target:
	 1. Project directly:
	 UMN → LMN in motor nuclei via corticobulbar path
	 Target nuclei: V, VII, X, XII, C1 cervical
	 Hypoglossal and facial (lower) receive contralateral input.
	 2. Cortical neurons project → to CPG interneurons to modulate motor response

Subcortical input (subcortical neurons) • Limbic system: Amygdala, hypothalamus, thalamus (relay station, sensory and motor tracts) • Basal ganglia: Inhibition of unwanted movements, planning to initiate movement • Cerebellum: Motor coordination based on environmental sensory input	**Function:** • Indirectly provide feedback via extrapyramidal tract • Reciprocal input and output to cortical centers **Targets:** • Indirect LMNs • Swallowing CPG
Swallowing central pattern generators (CPGs) **CPG predicted location:** Ventral and dorsal swallowing center CPGs in medulla; interneurons located within and adjacent to NTS	**Function:** • CPGs provide the patterned and sequential control of the involuntary pharyngeal and esophageal swallowing phases • Following initiation of swallow reflex CPG can be modulated by afferent and cortical input • Coordinates respiratory swallow apnea reflex required during swallowing **Targets:** **Dorsal swallow group** in NTS (patterns activity) → stimulates **ventral swallow group** (sends sequence of motor activity) → project to LMNs controlling tongue, palatal, pharyngeal, laryngeal, and esophageal muscles

Cranial motor nuclei (LMN)
 • **Trigeminal motor** (CN V)—mid/caudal pons
 • **Facial motor** (SVE) (CN VII)—caudal pons
 • **Nucleus ambiguus** (SVE) (CN IX and CN X)—medulla
    ○ Pharyngeal motor neurons
    ○ Laryngeal motor neurons
 • **Dorsal motor nucleus** (GVE) (CN X)—medulla
 • **Hypoglossal motor nucleus** (GSE) (CN XII)—medulla
 • **Spinal motor nuclei** (GSE)
 • Cervical ventral horn (C1–C3)
	Function:
	 LMN in nuclei directly controls sequential contraction and relaxation of oropharyngeal muscles:
	 CN X mainly involved in swallowing; minor contributions from CNs IX, V, VII, and XII and C1–C3
	 Oral phase:
	 • Receive input directly from UMN cortical, subcortical, and CPG
	 Stimulation of LMNs directly controls masticatory, perioral, and tongue muscles necessary for bolus formation and transport
	 SVE and GSE branches involved:
	 • CN V3
	 • CN VII
	 • CN XII
	 • C1; ansa cervicalis
	 Pharyngeal phase:
	 LMNs primarily from CN X provide motor control of palatal, pharyngeal, and laryngeal reflex movements

Table 22.26 (*Continued*) Neural control of deglutition

Cortical Input	Function/Targets
	Innervation provided by SVE fibers via pharyngeal plexus and recurrent laryngeal nerve **Esophageal phase:** SVE and GVE of vagus (CN X from nucleus ambiguus and dorsal motor) innervate upper two-thirds of striated and lower one-third of smooth esophageal muscle (myenteric plexus—GVE)
Afferent input source **Peripheral receptors:** Mechanoreceptors, gustatory, nociceptor **Afferent primary neuron cell bodies** • Trigeminal ganglion (CN V) • Geniculate ganglion (CN VII) • Superior and inferior ganglion of CNs IX and X	**Functional role:** **Oral phase:** Provides feedback about bolus and moisture content **Pharyngeal phase:** Afferent input from CNs IX and X triggers CPG in swallowing center to initiate swallowing reflex Tactile, temperature, and taste trigger swallowing reflex GSA (CN V), SVA, and GVA (CNs IX and X) fibers transmit input to NTS * Internal laryngeal branch is key afferent branch. **Esophageal phase:** Sensory input modulates peristalsis and swallow intensity Cranial nerves involved: Pharyngeal plexus (CN IX) (GVA, GSA, SVA) Internal laryngeal branch of superior laryngeal nerve of CN X (SVA, GSA, GVA) Recurrent laryngeal of CN X (GVA, GSA)
Secondary afferent neurons • Trigeminal nuclear (sensory) complex • NTS **Ascending pathways project to:** • CPG, subcortical areas, cerebellum • Somatosensory cortex and gustatory cortex via VPM of thalamus • Visceral reflex centers, i.e., salivatory nuclei, respiratory centers	**Functional role** • Sensorimotor integration, sensory feedback to modulate function • Mediate protective oromotor reflexes • Mediate visceral reflexes, i.e., salivation; swallow apnea

Abbreviations: CPG, central pattern generator; GSE, general somatic efferent; GVE, general visceral efferent; LMN, lower motor neuron; NTS, nucleus tractus solitarius; SVE, special visceral efferent; UMN, upper motor neuron; VPM, ventral posteromedial.

Clinical Correlation Box 22.5: Outcomes of Neuromuscular Deficits during Swallowing

Neuromuscular deficits during oral preparatory and transfer stages
- Weak perioral muscles cause difficulty in maintaining bolus position.
- Weak masticatory muscles, malocclusion, or tooth loss cause inadequate chewing of food.
- Weak or paralyzed tongue (lingual) muscles may cause the bolus to spill back into the oral cavity, or the bolus may be aspirated into the airway, which remains open at this stage.
- Injury to UMNs in swallowing cortex or to descending fibers in the corticobulbar tract results in swallow apraxia, which is hallmarked by difficulty in programming the voluntary motor actions involved in bolus preparation.
- Loss of tactile and stereognostic input due to cerebral vascular accidents (stroke) affecting the somatosensory cortex may lead to difficulties in bolus formation and spillage.

Neuromuscular deficits during pharyngeal stages
- Reduced sensory input from afferent receptors in the oropharyngeal mucosa may lead to elevated threshold stimuli or a delayed swallow reflex.
- Nasal regurgitation of food can be caused by insufficiency in palatal elevation and velopharyngeal closure.
- Diminished pharyngeal constrictor activity or weakness leads to inadequate force, slower pharyngeal transit time, and possible accumulation of food in the vallecula or piriform recess.
- Failure to elevate the hyoid and larynx leads to inadequate airway protection and increased risk for aspiration.

- Topical anesthesia disrupts sensory input to the laryngeal mucosa and interferes with normal swallowing reflexes. May lead to accumulation of pharyngeal material and tracheal aspiration.

Neuromuscular deficits during esophageal stages
- Impaired opening of the upper esophageal sphincter (UES) may lead to retention of food in the piriform recess and laryngopharynx (hypopharynx). Failure to elevate the larynx by the suprahyoid muscle may also lead to the impaired opening of the UES. Both relaxation of the cricopharyngeus and inferior constrictor muscles and laryngeal elevation during the swallow sequence function to open the UES and allow bolus passage.
- Retention of food may also occur in the esophagus as a result of mechanical obstruction or motility disorders affecting peristaltic function. Achalasia is a well-characterized motility disorder associated with the failure of the LES to relax with swallowing, leading to tonic sphincter contraction. The obstruction leads to dysphagia. Parasympathetic innervation from the vagus controls peristaltic reflex activity and the sequential relaxation and contraction of the esophageal smooth muscle. In achalasia, the myenteric plexus degenerates with a loss of inhibitory neurons in the LES.
- Gastroesophageal reflux, also known as acid reflux, from the stomach into esophagus and pharynx can be due to impaired closure of the LES.

22.6 Speech Production

- Vocalization refers to any sound produced through the action of the respiratory system and larynx; and used for communication. Humans often use sounds to speak; however, sounds such as laughing, crying, or moaning, may also be produced in the absence of speech as non-verbal communication.
- Among oromotor behaviors, the process of verbal communication through speaking is one of the most complex human activities and encompasses three interrelated tasks:

(1) vocal sound production, (2) articulation of speech sounds, and **(3) language processing.**

- The anatomical components of the **vocal tract** that produce sound include the trachea, larynx, pharynx, and oral cavity.
- Vocal sound production involves three mechanisms, **respiration, phonation,** and **resonance**. The produced sound is then coupled to the process of **articulation** to form words. These four fundamental processes of vocalization occur synergistically to produce speech. The mechanisms of speech production are described in ▶ Table 22.27, ▶ Table 22.28, ▶ Table 22.29, ▶ Table 22.30.
- Speech disorders affecting articulation that may be associated with functional and structural causes are highlighted in Clinical Correlation Box 22.6.
- Neuromuscular disturbances that affect the sound production processes may lead to motor speech disorders. Two types of motor speech disorders, known as **dysarthria** and **apraxia**, are discussed in Clinical Correlation Box 22.7 and 22.8.

22.6.1 Mechanisms of Vocal Sound Production and Articulation

Respiration and Phonation

- The production of speech sounds (**phonation**) begins with the exhalation phase of respiration and the passage of air through the rima glottidis. As air pushes through the

opening, a pressure drop occurs, which causes vocal fold vibration and leads to the generation of a sound wave known as **voiced (laryngeal) sound** (▶ Table 22.27).
- Two types of voiced sound that may be produced are:
  - **Volitional (voluntary/learned) sound**
    - Characterized by a vocalized sound produced with the intent of verbal communication through speaking.
  - **Involuntary (innate/emotive) sound**
    - Describes a nonverbal vocalized sound produced to convey an innate response or emotion such as crying, laughing, shouting, screaming, and moaning.

Resonance

- Sound enters the **supraglottic vocal tract** that acts as a resonance chamber and functions to filter, amplify, and modulate the quality of the voiced sound.

Articulation

- **Articulation** is the process by which syllables and words are formed. As air enters the oral cavity, the movement of the lips, tongue, soft palate, and lower jaw work cooperatively with the hard palate, alveolar ridge, and teeth to form speech sounds (▶ Table 22.30).
- The oropharyngeal muscles and jaw movements alter the shape and size of the oral cavity and function to direct and constrict airflow. Coordinated orofacial movements permit the **articulation** of sounds as **consonants** and **vowels** that comprise the syllables of spoken words.
  - The assembly of syllables into words, phrases, and meaningful sentences occurs in the cerebral cortex as part of language processing.
- Two types of articulated sound, known as **voiced** and **unvoiced sound**, may be produced and are essential to produce vowels and consonants.
  - **Voiced sound** is produced in response to vocal cord vibration.
  - **Voiceless (unvoiced/breathed) sound** is produced without vocal cord vibration.

Table 22.27 Mechanism of vocal sound production: Respiration

Functional Mechanism: Respiration		
Anatomical Region	**Key Structural/Muscular Components**	**Functional Role in Speech Production**
Infraglottic vocal tract Describes the region below the level of vocal folds (cords) and rima glottis (laryngeal opening between the vocal folds) **Regions:** • Trachea • Bronchi • Lungs in thoracic cavity	**Inspiratory muscles** draw air into lungs as thoracic cavity increases in volume • Diaphragm • External intercostals • Vocal folds abducted via posterior cricoarytenoid **Expiratory muscles** • During quiet respiration muscles relax and passive recoil of alveoli releases air out of lungs • Lateral cricoarytenoid and thyroarytenoid adduct vocal folds and narrow the glottis to prevent lung collapse **Active expiration in phonation** force air out of lungs by decreasing thoracic volume using: • Diaphragm • Abdominal • Internal intercostals	• Pressure differences created through inhalation and exhalation generate **mechanical energy** in the form of **air pressure** to produce sound. • In the normal respiratory cycle, the phases of inspiration and expiration are of equal length. • Respiratory pattern is altered during speech. • During **phonation** inspiration is shorter and the **exhalation phase is prolonged.** • The change in respiratory rhythm and the long exhalation phase reflect the need for sustained and controlled air flow to maintain vocal fold vibration during sound production. **Clinical comments:** Insufficient air production due to respiratory disease (chronic obstructive pulmonary disease [COPD]) leads to a decrease in number of words produced in one expiratory cycle. Individuals tire easily when speaking and project with decreased voice volume.

Table 22.28 Mechanism of vocal sound production: Phonation

Functional Mechanism: Phonation		
Anatomical Region	**Key Structural/Muscular Components**	**Functional Role in Speech Production**
Larynx (voice box) **Intrinsic laryngeal muscles** function to move laryngeal cartilages and alter the position, length, tension, and thickness of the true vocal folds	**Key laryngeal cartilages** • Thyroid • Cricoid • Arytenoid **Intrinsic laryngeal muscles** **Adductors:** Close rima glottidis; medially compress vocal folds • Lateral cricoarytenoid • Thyroarytenoid • Interarytenoid **Abductors:** Open rima glottidis • Posterior cricoarytenoid **Vocal cord tension:** • Increase tension ○ Cricothyroid • Decrease tension ○ Vocalis	• The process of vocalization or phonation refers to the production of sound that results from vibration of the true vocal folds (cords) as air passes between the rima glottidis to generate a sound wave. • **Volitional sound** produced for speech • **Involuntary sound** produced to convey emotion (crying/laughing/shout/scream) • A key component in voiced phonation is vocal cord adduction (closure) mediated by the lateral cricoarytenoid, thyroarytenoid, and interarytenoid intrinsic laryngeal muscles. **Clinical comment:** Any disruption to voice production due to a physical disorder in the vocal tract is known as **dysphonia.** Dysphonia is characterized by a change in pitch, loudness, or voice quality, and may present as hoarseness, breathiness, or as a strained voice due to changes in vocal fold vibration and position.

Table 22.29 Mechanism of vocal sound production: Role of resonance

Functional Mechanism: Resonance		
Anatomical Region	**Key Structural/Muscular Components**	**Functional Role in Speech Production**
Supraglottic vocal tract: Series of interconnected, air-filled chambers /cavities through which sound passes: • Laryngeal vestibule • Pharynx • Nasal cavity • Oral cavity	**Pharyngeal muscles:** Longitudinal and constrictor muscles **Oral muscles:** • Masticatory muscles • Tongue extrinsic and intrinsic groups • Soft palatal group • Labial and buccal group	• The vocal tract chambers act as resonators to filter, amplify, and modulate the initial sound to produce a recognizable voice • Pharyngeal muscles that change length and diameter of pharyngeal tube serve as principal resonator • Pharyngeal muscles work in concert with soft palate to close nasopharynx and alter nasal resonance • Palatal elevation and depression change direction of air stream • Tongue muscles change shape and position to direct air stream • Masticatory muscles move jaw and work cooperatively with tongue, lips, and cheeks to alter degree of cavity opening

Table 22.30 Mechanism of vocal sound production: Articulation

Functional Mechanism: Articulation		
Anatomical Region	**Key Structural/Muscular Components**	**Functional Role in Speech Production**
Oral and nasal cavity Structures of oral/nasal cavity act as muscular valves to control the amount of airflow known as **oral articulators** (speech organs) Moveable (active) articulators • Lips • Tongue • Soft palate (velum) • Cheek • Jaw *Immovable (passive) articulators • Hard palate • Alveolar ridge of teeth • Incisors • Nasal cavity—minor role in altering sound depending on palatal seal **Modification of sound requires co-ordination of jaw movement and tongue and lips. Jaw movements can change the size and shape of the oral cavity.	**Primary oral articulators:** • **Tongue:** Most adaptable articulator due level of mobility; intrinsic and extrinsic muscles direct air streams for consonant formation; changes shape for vowel sounds; significant impact on articulation if damaged or mobility restricted • **Labial: Orbicularis oris** changes shape through rounding, protrusion, and retraction to produce vowel and consonant sounds • **Buccal: Buccinator** Control air pressure • **Soft palate:** Seals off nasopharynx (velopharyngeal closure) for all sounds except the nasal sounds (n/m/ng); damage or weakness causes significant impact on oral speech • **Mandible** Jaw movements can change the size and shape of the oral cavity to create resonance for vowels **Immovable articulators**	• Classification of sounds as voiced or unvoiced: ○ All vowels are voiced sounds ○ Consonants may be voiced or unvoiced sounds • The point of contact between two articulatory organs results in the constriction and direction of airflow and is used to produce consonant sounds. • Points of constriction may occur between the following anatomical structures ○ Both lips ○ Lips and teeth ○ Tongue and upper/lower incisors ○ Tongue and alveolar ridge ○ Tongue and hard palate ○ Tongue and soft palate • Consonants which are relevant to dentists and clinicians can be classified according to the anatomic structures involved in their production: ○ **Palato-lingual sounds**—produced by tongue, hard palate, or soft palate ○ **Labio-dental sounds**—produced by lips and teeth ○ **Linguo-dental sounds**—produced tongue and teeth ○ **Bilabial sounds**—produced by lips touching slightly • Pharyngeal muscles work in concert with soft palate to close nasopharynx and alter nasal resonance

(Continued)

Table 22.30 (*Continued*) Mechanism of vocal sound production: Articulation

Functional Mechanism: Articulation		
Anatomical Region	**Key Structural/Muscular Components**	**Functional Role in Speech Production**
	• **Alveolar ridge, incisors, hard palate** Serve as points of constriction; structural defects such as palatal clefts cause articulation problems	• Tongue muscles change shape and position to direct air stream • Masticatory muscles move jaw and work cooperatively with tongue, lips, and cheeks to alter degree of cavity opening **Clinical comment: Dysarthria** is characterized by difficulty in speech articulation. It may occur due to muscular weakness and/or abnormal muscle tone that affects the oral articulators, the laryngeal and pharyngeal muscles, or as a result of damage to the jaw and teeth.

Table 22.31 Neural control of vocalization and speech

Cortical Input	Function/Targets
Frontal lobe of both hemispheres • **Primary motor cortex (M1) (UMN)** Precentral gyrus: Orofacial motor area • **Speech (laryngeal) motor area (LMC)*** *Region localized near lateral sulcus • **Supplementary motor area (SMA)** • **Premotor cortex (PMC)** **Speech:** **Dominant hemisphere** (often left): Responsible for language and speech (semantic, syntax, grammar) Frontal cortex • Broca's area—language production Temporal/parietal lobe • Wernicke's area—language comprehension; word selection Temporal lobe • Primary auditory cortex—processing semantics Additional cortical areas: Limbic—emotional reflex activity (cingulate gyrus) Insular (gustatory) cortex—integrates autonomic, viscerosensory, and visceromotor input including taste	**Function:** • Voluntary control of verbal speech production requires input from higher cortical centers • Volitional control of expiration is required for vocalization; cortex changes rhythm and duration • Voluntary control is necessary to maintain vocal cord closure and vibration and to control articulator muscles • Voluntary control of voice intensity, pitch, and articulation ○ Language is primarily localized in the dominant hemisphere ○ Broca ○ Wernicke's area ○ Auditory To initiate spoken words: 1. Auditory input → Wernicke's area → via arcuate fasciculus → Broca's area → UMNs in orofacial and laryngeal motor cortex area project bilaterally and directly → to LMN via corticobulbar path Target nuclei: Nucleus Ambiguus, vagus (CN X), motor nuclei of CNs VII, XII, and V for articulation 2. Nonverbal emotive sounds (crying, laughing) involve projections from limbic cortical neurons → subcortical → to CPG interneurons to modulate laryngeal motor response
Subcortical input (subcortical neurons) • Limbic system: Amygdala, hypothalamus, thalamus (relay station, sensory and motor tracts) • Basal ganglia: Inhibition of unwanted movements, planning to initiate movement • Cerebellum: Motor coordination based on environmental sensory input	**Function:** • Indirectly provide feedback via extrapyramidal tract • Reciprocal input and output to cortical centers **Targets:** • Indirect LMNs • Swallowing CPG
Vocalization central pattern generators (CPGs) **CPG predicted location:** Midbrain lateral reticular formation, nucleus retroambiguus, and periaqueductal gray (PAG)	**Function:** CPGs provide inhibitory or excitatory input to laryngeal motor neurons in nucleus ambiguus; coordinate change in respiratory rhythm associated with vocalization Descending cortical pathways may influence the initiation of speech, pitch, and intensity (volume)
Cranial motor nuclei (LMN) • **Trigeminal motor** (CN V)—mid/caudal pons • **Facial motor** (SVE) (CN VII)—caudal pons • **Nucleus ambiguus** (SVE) (CN IX and CN X)—medulla ○ Pharyngeal motor neurons ○ Laryngeal motor neurons • **Hypoglossal motor nucleus** (GSE) (CN XII)—medulla • **Spinal motor nuclei** (GSE) • Cervical ventral horn (C1–C3)	**Function:** Vocalization and speech involve bilateral activation of LMN which directly control contraction of oropharyngeal muscles: • LMNs in nucleus ambiguus (CN X) project to laryngeal and pharyngeal muscles for phonation and resonance. • LMN and pharyngeal plexus (CN X) control velopharyngeal closure needed for articulation. • LMNs control adduction of glottis and regulate tension of vocal folds. All laryngeal muscles are innervated by recurrent laryngeal nerve (CN X) EXCEPT cricothyroid (external laryngeal). • Lower motor neurons (LMN) in ventral horn, at the level C2–C4 involved in respiratory control • LMNs from CNs V, VII, and XII for movable articulatory muscle in oral cavity SVE and GSE branches involved • CN X

(*Continued*)

Table 22.31 (*Continued*) Neural control of vocalization and speech

Cortical Input	Function/Targets
	• CN V3
	• CN VII
	• CN XII
	• C2–C4 cervical/phrenic (coordination of respiratory component)
Afferent input source **Peripheral receptors** **Afferent primary neuron cell bodies** • Trigeminal ganglion (CN V) • Geniculate ganglion (CN VII) • Superior and inferior ganglion of CNs IX and X	**Functional role:** GSA (CNs IX and X) and GVA (CNs IX and X) fibers transmit input from mechanoreceptors and nociceptors in vocal tract and provide feedback about laryngeal vocal fold position. GSA tactile input via CN V provides feedback about position of articulators within oral cavity to help coordinate movement; specifically helps guide tongue shape, and applied pressure and placement of tongue lips and jaw. Cranial nerves involved: Pharyngeal plexus (CNs IX and X) Internal laryngeal branch of superior laryngeal nerve of CN X Recurrent laryngeal of CN X Sensory of V2 and V3
Secondary afferent neurons • Trigeminal nuclear (sensory) complex • Nucleus tractus solitarius (NTS) **Ascending pathways project to:** • CPG, subcortical areas, cerebellum • Somatosensory cortex via VPM of thalamus • Visceral reflex center, i.e., respiratory centers	**Functional role** • Sensorimotor integration, sensory feedback to modulate function such as tongue placement during articulation; change pitch and intensity • Mediate protective oromotor reflexes

Abbreviations: GSE, general somatic efferent; LMN, lower motor neuron; SVE, special visceral efferent; UMN, upper motor neuron; VPM, ventral posteromedial.

Clinical Correlation Box 22.6: Articulation Disorders

Articulation disorders may result from the improper placement of the tongue, soft palate, and lips, which leads to difficulty in pronouncing vowels and consonants. Articulation errors can also result from neuromuscular deficits that affect the oral articulator muscles or due to structural deficits, such as malocclusion, jaw deformities, alteration in jaw position, and palatal clefts. Frequently these conditions are related issues due to abnormal craniofacial growth and development. Correction of palatal clefts and malocclusion through orthodontics or orthognathic surgery generally have positive outcomes on speech.

Palatal Clefts
• Speech problems resulting from palatal clefts and lips impact the formation of palatal-lingual, labio-dental, and linguo-dental sounds. Patients often exhibit nasality, and difficulty in producing consonants that require high intraoral pressure (i.e., p/d). These problems may be considered passive speech errors which may occur due to velopharyngeal insufficiency rather than improper placement of the oral articulators. Articulation errors may also develop as learned motor patterns to compensate for the anatomical defect and the inability to produce sounds correctly. These speech errors are often classified as active (compensatory) articulation errors and may involve positional changes in tongue placement.

Jaw Deformities
• Jaw deformities, malocclusion, misalignment, or spaces between the teeth can result in improper placement of the tongue and lips and the formation of labio-dental and linguo-dental consonants. Patients with different classes of malocclusion will exhibit different articulation errors. For instance, individuals with an anterior open bite exhibit a greater number of articulation errors due to lip incompetency and alterations in tongue placement. Additionally, patients with jaw deformities and associated malocclusion often exhibit issues with mastication and swallowing.

Tooth Loss
• The use of dentures to restore aesthetics and masticatory function following tooth loss may impact speech articulation due to position, placement, and size differences in the denture. Factors such as the thickness of the denture base, changes in the vertical dimension, as well as alterations in the size and position of the denture may lead to speech errors. Therefore, the placement of the lips and tongue and the production of speech sounds should be considered during the fabrication and positioning of fixed or removable dentures.

22.6.2 Vocal Sound Mechanics and Laryngeal Muscular Control

- The production of voiced sound occurs in response to the cyclic opening and closing of the vocal folds as air from the lungs passes between the folds and causes them to vibrate.
- The number vibratory (glottic) cycles occurring per second determines the frequency of voiced sounds and is under voluntary control. Based on somatosensory and auditory feedback an individual may change laryngeal muscle activation to produce changes in voice intensity and pitch.
  - The frequency of vocal fold vibration gives the quality known as **pitch.**
  - The **intensity** of sound or loudness (volume) varies based on the infraglottic pressure required to separate the vocal folds and the degree of adduction.

Clinical Correlation Box 22.7: Dysarthria

Neuromuscular (motor) speech disorders known as **dysarthrias** often manifest as a change in pitch, intensity (volume), and quality of voiced sound due to disruption of the vibratory cycle. Patients may also exhibit slurring and difficulty in articulating consonants. Dysarthrias are a group of sensorimotor speech disorders characterized by weakness and abnormal muscle tone of the laryngeal muscles, and/or the oral articulators (lips, tongue, soft palate). Dysarthrias can affect any of the four mechanisms of speech production, with phonation and articulation the most notable. Dysarthria classification is based on the region of the neural circuit that is damaged. Injury or stroke affecting the UMNs in the motor cortex may lead to **spastic dysarthria**, while damage to the LMNs in the motor nuclei of the brainstem, the cranial nerves, or damage to the neuromuscular junction may cause **flaccid dysarthria**. Additional forms of dysarthria may also arise from injury to the cerebellum or basal ganglia. Cerebellar damage may lead to **ataxic dysarthria**. Neurological damage to the basal ganglia may manifest as **hypokinetic** or **hyperkinetic dysarthria**. All types of dysarthria cause slurring of speech due difficulty in articulating consonants.

22.6.3 Language Processing (▶ Fig. 22.9)

- Language processing is an essential aspect of verbal communication and involves the ability to transform vocal sounds into words, build meaningful phrases, and comprehend spoken language within an emotional context.
- The perception and production of voluntary speech require the integration of information between the cortical language areas found in the dominant hemisphere.
- Disturbances in language processing may affect an individual's ability to express speech or comprehend written or spoken words. Language processing disorders that occur following neurological damage or trauma are known as aphasia and are discussed in Clinical Correlation Box 22.9.

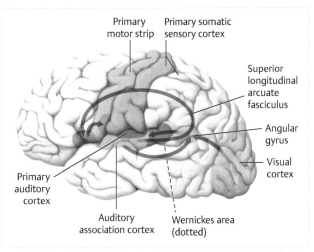

Fig. 22.9 Schematic depicting the language areas in the normal left dominant cerebral hemisphere. Left lateral view. The arrows indicate the proposed flow and sequence of language processing. Language processing involves the transmission of sensory input from the auditory and visual cortices to the angular gyrus in the parietal lobe. Sensory input is then passed from the angular gyrus to Wernicke's area in the temporal for the interpretation, processing, and comprehension of spoken language. Information passes from Wernicke's area to Broca's speech area in the frontal lobe through the arcuate fasciculus, an axonal tract that passes through the parietal, temporal, and frontal lobes. Broca's area, which serves to coordinate and program the vocalized response, communicates directly with upper motor neurons (UMNs) in the laryngeal motor cortex (LMC) and cortical masticatory area (CMA) to execute the motor response. The UMNs follow descending motor pathways to the brainstem where the LMNs involved in vocalization reside. (Reproduced with permission from Schuenke M, Schulte E, Schumacher U. THIEME Atlas of Anatomy Second Edition, Vol 3. © Thieme 2016. Illustrations by Markus Voll and Karl Wesker.)

- The principal regions involved include the **auditory cortex** and **Wernicke's area** of the **temporal lobe,** along with **Broca's area** and the **laryngeal motor cortex** (**LMC**) of the **frontal lobe.** Additional areas include the visual cortex in the occipital lobe and angular gyrus and somatosensory cortex in the parietal lobe (▶ Table 22.31).

Temporal (Posterior) Lobe

- **Primary auditory cortex** and **auditory association cortex** receive auditory input and interprets sound.
- **Wernicke's speech area** serves as the receptive component of language processing.
  - Wernicke's area receives sensory input from the auditory and visual cortex, and serves to interpret, comprehend, assign meaning, and recall the auditory form of spoken words.
- Wernicke's area transmits the information to **Broca's area** in the inferior frontal lobe through a bidirectional axonal tract known as the **arcuate fasciculus,** which interconnects the two language areas.

Frontal (Inferior) Lobe

- **Broca's area** in the inferior frontal cortex serves an integration point between Wernicke's area and the **LMC** of the precentral gyrus.
- Broca's area functions as the expressive component for language production. Neurons in the region plan, organize, and formulate which words to speak and develop programs for speech articulation.
- The LMC and cortical masticatory area (CMA) in the primary motor strip receive motor commands from Broca's area and control the execution of laryngeal movements necessary for phonation and articulation through direct projections to the LMNs in the cranial nerve nuclei.
- Comparable to other oromotor activities, the production, processing, and modulation of speech also involve the premotor and supplementary motor areas, the cerebellum, basal ganglia, and brainstem, as well as sensory feedback to help coordinate the sequence of motor movements.
- In the nondominant hemisphere, the corresponding speech areas of the frontal and temporal lobes are involved in conveying and comprehending the emotional aspects of speech, such as the intonations produced in response to feelings of happiness, depression, or anger.

Clinical Correlation Box 22.8: Apraxia

Apraxia is defined as an inability to plan and execute purposeful movements. Apraxia of speech (verbal apraxia) is a neurogenic communication disorder characterized by an impaired capacity to program, plan, and coordinate the sequence of movements necessary for speech. Patients with verbal apraxia exhibit normal language comprehension of both spoken and written words, and also have intact motor function of the musculature involved in phonation and articulation. However, damage to the regions of the motor cortex involved in planning and coordinating the sequence of speech leads to an inability to communicate effectively. Due to these differences, verbal apraxia may be distinguished from aphasia, which is associated with the formulation and comprehension of language, and dysarthrias, which are motor disturbances in the muscles controlling speech production.

Clinical Correlation Box 22.9: Aphasia

- **Aphasia** refers to language impairment affecting the production or comprehension of speech and the ability to read or write. Aphasia results from trauma or injury to the cortex and is most often associated with strokes occurring to the language areas in the dominant hemisphere. In most individuals, the dominant hemisphere is on the left side. The type of aphasia depends on extent of damage and the cortical region involved. Two forms are discussed below.
  - **Broca's aphasia** is an expressive or motor aphasia characterized as nonfluent. It most often occurs from a lesion in left inferior frontal gyrus. Individual can read and understand language, but have difficulty in word selection and formation of complete sentences. Sentences are short, articulation is poor, and there is a prolonged output of words when speaking. Writing is also difficult. Due to the proximity of Broca's area with the motor cortex, larger lesions in this region may affect the supplementary motor areas and cause difficulty in planning and coordinating motor activities **(apraxia)**. Damage to the primary motor cortex may result in paralysis of the lower face and contralateral upper limb.
  - **Wernicke's aphasia** is a receptive or sensory aphasia characterized as fluent. Individuals with this form of aphasia have difficulty in comprehending all forms of language and often cannot write. Individuals typically speak in long sentences that have no meaning or create new words. Due to issues in language comprehension, they are unable to recognize their mistakes.
- Lesions occurring in the right frontal lobe (nondominant hemisphere) lead to loss of prosody (aprosody), which is an impairment in producing or understanding speech intonations associated with emotions. In comparison, lesions in the right temporal lobe result in difficulties in acoustic processing and loss of ability to understand the inflections in speech produced by others.

22.6.4 Nonverbal (Emotive) Sound Production

- Speech and emotive sounds are both forms of expression that convey meaning and require language-processing skills for interpretation and comprehension.
- The areas of the brain involved in eliciting voluntary and involuntary sounds exhibit functional overlap within the brainstem, cerebellum, and basal ganglia; however, the cortical regions which control sound production differ and represent a fundamental distinction between these forms of vocalization.
  - In comparison to voluntary speech production, nonverbal communication involving emotive or innate vocal patterns such as moaning, crying, or laughing does not require direct cortical input from the LMC.
  - Mediation of innate (emotional) sounds appears to involve the anterior cingulate cortex of the limbic lobe. Cortical fibers from the limbic system project to interneurons of CPGs which reside near the periaqueductal gray and reticular formation of midbrain.
  - The CPGs provide inhibitory and excitatory input to laryngeal motor neurons in the nucleus ambiguus to elicit emotive sound.
  - Afferent fibers are predicted to project to vocalization CPGs and mediate unconditioned (innate) reflex responses, such as shrieking in pain.

Questions and Answers

1. A 68-year-old patient presents with a 6-month history of dysphasia of solids and liquids. A barium radiograph and esophageal swallowing study (esophageal manometry) demonstrate aperistalsis with the swallowing of liquids in the lower one-third of esophagus. The patient has no history of gastric reflux, heart burn, or dysphonia, and a tentative diagnosis of achalasia is made. Which of the following structures is most likely damaged?
   a) GVE fibers of CN X
   b) Cortical swallowing area
   c) Nucleus ambiguus
   d) Dorsal motor nucleus

Level 3: Difficult

Answer A: Achalasia results in the failure of the lower esophageal sphincter (LES) to relax. The postganglionic parasympathetic (GVE) fibers are most likely damaged in the myenteric plexus, along with the inhibitory neurons that innervate the LES. A loss of inhibitory neurons prevents the relaxation of LES during peristaltic activity. (**B**) The cortical swallowing area in the primary motor cortex is most likely not affected since swallowing may be initiated and executed by the patient. (**C**). The nucleus ambiguus contains (SVE) lower motor neurons of CN IX and CN X that innervate branchiomeric derived skeletal muscles of the pharynx, larynx, and upper one-third of the esophagus. Damage of the LMNs and the SVE fibers would cause difficulties in swallowing but would also impact speech and airway regulation. These mechanisms are still intact in the patient. The wall of the lower one-third of the esophagus and the LES contains two layers of smooth muscle that is innervated by parasympathetic and enteric nerves (**D**). The dorsal motor nucleus contains preganglionic autonomic neurons of the vagus and provides GVE parasympathetic innervation to the respiratory, heart, and gastrointestinal (GI) tract, so damage to the GVE neurons in the nucleus would most likely result in widespread autonomic dysfunction of several organ systems and not just an isolated issue.

2. To protect the airway during swallowing, the relaxation of the upper esophageal sphincter (UES) is coordinated with vocal cord adduction and glottic closure. The nerve branch that mediates the efferent limb of the reflex is the

   _____.

   a) External laryngeal nerve
   b) Recurrent laryngeal nerve
   c) Internal laryngeal nerve
   d) Anterior vagal branch

Level 2: Moderate

Answer B: The recurrent laryngeal nerve carries SVE fibers and innervates the cricopharyngeus of the UES and all laryngeal muscles, except the cricothyroid muscle. Vocal cord adduction occurs through the action of the lateral cricoarytenoid, thyroarytenoid, and transverse interarytenoid muscles. The innervation of both muscle groups by the recurrent laryngeal nerve allows for the coordinated movement of vocal cord adduction and the concomitant relaxation of the UES. The combined movement prevents refluxed material from entering the airway and protects against choking and aspiration pneumonia. The external laryngeal nerve (**A**) innervates the crico-

thyroid, which tightens the vocal cords, but doesn't affect adduction. The internal laryngeal nerve (**C**) transmits only sensory innervation from the laryngeal mucosa in the region above the true vocal fold and does not mediate muscle movement. The anterior vagal branch (**D**) does not innervate the vocal cords; it carries GVE fibers and provides secretomotor function to the glands of the GI tract.

3. A 38-year-old female patient was recently diagnosed with myasthenia gravis, an autoimmune disease that damages the neuromuscular junctions associated with skeletal muscles. The patient is experiencing difficulty in chewing hard due to a decreased capability in generating bite force. She requires a longer duration to chew, and her jaw is rapidly fatigued halfway through a meal. Each of the following clinical problems may also occur in the patient due to her condition EXCEPT one. Which one is the exception?
   a) Dysphasia
   b) Apraxia
   c) Ptosis
   d) Dysarthria

Level 3: Difficult

Answer B: Apraxia is the exception and is not associated with myasthenia gravis (MG). Speech apraxia is characterized by difficulty in planning and coordinating the movements associated with speaking. Patients with apraxia are unable to perform a movement correctly in response to verbal or written requests, even though they understand the request. All motor function remains intact and patients with apraxia do not exhibit muscular weakness. MG is characterized by skeletal muscle weakness due to autoantibodies binding the acetylcholine receptor at the neuromuscular junction and disrupting the mechanism of skeletal muscle contraction. Bulbar and ocular weakness of the skeletal muscles controlling chewing, swallowing, speaking, and eye movements are affected. Weakened masticatory muscles leads to decreased biting force with a longer chew cycle. Choices (**A**), (**C**), and (**D**) will also occur due to muscular weakness. Disturbances in swallowing (**A**. Dysphasia) and difficulty in articulation of speech (**D**. Dysarthria) will occur due to weakness of the tongue, lips, palatal, pharyngeal, and laryngeal musculature. Ptosis (**C**) is a drooping eyelid that will occur if the levator palpebrae superioris muscle is weak or if the oculomotor nerve (CN III) is damaged.

Use the following scenario to answer questions 4 and 5

A 78-year-old patient suffers a stroke that primarily affects the region of the inferior frontal gyrus of the left frontal cortex. The area of the primary motor cortex, including the orofacial motor area, and parts of the premotor area are also impacted. Evaluation of the patient's speech and language skills reveal the patient can understand what is said but is unable to formulate intelligible words or sentences. A diagnosis of nonfluent (motor) speech is submitted, and the patient is scheduled to begin speech and physical therapy.

4. Which of the following is the most likely diagnosis involving the language deficit?
   a) Broca's aphasia
   b) Dysarthria
   c) Aprosodia
   d) Wernicke's aphasia

Level 2: Moderate

Answer A: Broca's aphasia is the most likely diagnosis based on the location of the lesion in the left frontal gyrus. Language function primarily involves the frontal, temporal, and parietal lobes and is usually associated with one hemisphere known as the dominant hemisphere. In most individuals, this is the left hemisphere. The dominant hemisphere of the brain is on the side opposite the dominant hand. Dysarthria (**B**) is a motor disorder characterized by slurred speech due to difficulty in articulation. It is associated with muscle weakness of the lips, soft palate, pharynx, and larynx, and can be caused by damage to the LMNs or due to peripheral nerve damage. Fluency of speech and comprehension of the spoken and written word is not affected in patients with dysarthria. In this patient, however, it is difficult to assess articulation because Broca's aphasia leads to an inability to formulate words and may mask the signs of dysarthria. A loss of prosody, known as aprosodia (**C**), is the result of lesions occurring in the *nondominant* hemisphere. Aprosodia interferes with the patient's capacity to produce intonations and inflections in speech (right frontal lobe lesion) or the ability to understand and sense changes in the tonality of speech. Wernicke's aphasia (**D**) is considered a receptive language deficit, hallmarked by a difficulty in comprehending spoken and written language. The fluency of speech is not affected; however, sentences often have no meaning. The inferior region of the premotor cortex and the oromotor area of the primary motor cortex lie in proximity to Broca's area and can be affected to varying degrees, depending on the size of the lesion. Lesions in these areas may manifest as motor and speech apraxia, characterized by the inability to plan and coordinate movements, as well as contralateral paralysis (hemiplegia) of muscles of the body, the lower facial muscles, and tongue.

5. Based on the location of the infarct presented in the scenarios above, which of the following clinical findings may be observed upon assessment of the patient's oromotor function?
   a) Complete facial paralysis is noted on the left side of the face
   b) The jaw deviates to left upon opening
   c) An increased gag reflex and hyperactive jaw jerk reflex are noted
   d) The tongue deviates to the right side upon protrusion
   e) The tongue exhibits atrophy and fasciculations on the left side

Level 2: Moderate

Answer D: The extrinsic genioglossus muscles of the tongue receive contralateral input from UMNs in the oromotor cortex. Therefore, in this scenario, the tongue will deviate to the contralateral (right) side when the patient is asked to protrude the tongue. Choice (**A**) is incorrect and complete paralysis of the facial muscles on the side of the lesion will not occur. The facial motor nucleus contains a dorsal and ventral group of motor neurons. The dorsal group receives bilateral innervation from cortical UMNs, whereas the ventral groups receive only contralateral (crossed) fibers from the UMNs. As a result, a left-side unilateral supranuclear lesion should only impact the right ventral facial motor nucleus. The outcome in this scenario should be facial paralysis of the contralateral (right-side) lower facial muscles, with sparing of the forehead and eye muscles. (**B**) The jaw will not deviate to the left upon opening. This is a characteristic of unilateral damage to the LMNs or a peripheral injury of the trigeminal. (**C**) Hyperactive reflexes, an increase in muscle tone, and spastic paralysis are not associated with unilateral cortical lesions but are observed in bilateral supranuclear lesions. The trigeminal motor nucleus (CN V), nucleus ambiguus (CNs IX and X), and dorsal region of the facial motor nucleus (CN VII) each receive bilateral innervation from the UMNs in the oromotor area of the primary motor cortex. Therefore, unilateral lesions of the cortex or the corticobulbar tracts occurring *above* the level (supranuclear) of these cranial motor nuclei may not produce significant weakness of motor function. (**E**) The tongue should not exhibit atrophy or fasciculations, since these signs are characteristic of LMN lesions, and not UMN lesions. Atrophy and fasciculations occur due to the loss of synaptic contact to the skeletal muscle following axonal (Wallerian) degeneration.

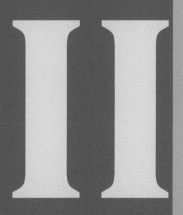

II

23 Temporomandibular Joint

Gilbert M. Willett

Learning Objectives

1. Describe the gross anatomy of the temporomandibular joint.
2. Explain the sensory innervation of the temporomandibular joint.
3. Describe the neuromuscular contributions of temporomandibular joint movement.
4. Given a clinical example, provide an appropriate anatomical explanation.

23.1 Overview of the Temporomandibular Joint

The temporomandibular joints (TMJs) and related structures play an essential role in mastication (chewing). The act of chewing is resultant from coordinated neuromuscular interaction between cranial nerves of the central nervous system, muscles of mastication, tongue, teeth, and the paired TMJs. The TMJ complex is also involved to some degree in speaking and swallowing.

23.2 Anatomy Overview

- The TMJ is classified as a ginglymoarthrodial joint (displays both hinge and sliding capabilities).
  - Movements at the joints are referred to as rotational (hingelike) and translational (sliding).
  - Bony components of the TMJ (bilateral on the skull).
    - Superior: the concave mandibular fossa (also known as the glenoid fossa) and articular eminence of the temporal bone.
      - During mastication, joint contact/compression occurs along the slope of the articular eminence due to translational/sliding movement of the joint, not at the concave roof of the mandibular fossa (common misconception).
    - Inferior: the convex mandibular condyles.
      - The articular surfaces are covered with dense fibrous connective tissue in adults.
- Dental (teeth) occlusion and TMJ positioning (location of the mandibular condyles) are interrelated (▶ Fig. 23.1).
  - Connective tissues:
    - A dense fibrous articular disk sits between the bony components of the TMJ. This oval disk is shaped to fit optimally between the mandibular condyle and the articular eminence of the temporal bone.
      - The disk is thicker anteriorly and posteriorly, which helps it maintain position over the mandibular condyle.
      - Only the disk periphery is innervated and vascularized (▶ Fig. 23.2).
      - Circumferential disk attachment to the surrounding joint capsule creates superior and inferior joint cavities (▶ Fig. 23.2).
        - Synovial cells line the inner layer of the TMJ capsule and produce fluid for each cavity.
        - Anterior/posterior translational or "sliding" joint movements occur in the superior cavity.
          - ✓ Superior cavity is the space between the disk and the temporal bone articular eminence.
        - Rotational/hinge movement occurs in the inferior joint cavity.
          - ✓ Inferior joint cavity is the space between the mandibular condyle and the disk.
      - A retrodiskal tissue (pad) is attached to the posterior aspect of the disk/capsule.
        - It has two layers, an elastic superior retrodiskal lamina (SRL) and nonelastic inferior retrodiskal lamina (IRL; see ▶ Fig. 23.3).
      - Anteriorly, the capsule and disk fuse.
        - The superior portion of the lateral pterygoid muscle also has fibers inserting into this area.

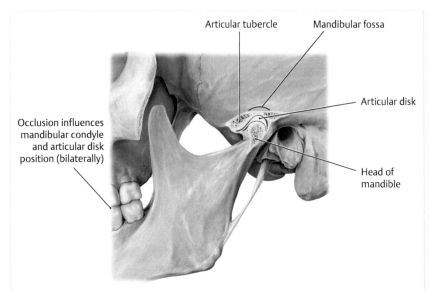

Articular tubercle   Mandibular fossa

Articular disk

Occlusion influences mandibular condyle and articular disk position (bilaterally)

Head of mandible

Fig. 23.1 Occlusion influences positioning of the mandibular condyle and disk. (Reproduced with permission from Schuenke M, Schulte E, Schumacher U. THIEME Atlas of Anatomy Third Edition, Vol 3. © Thieme 2020. Illustrations by Markus Voll and Karl Wesker.)

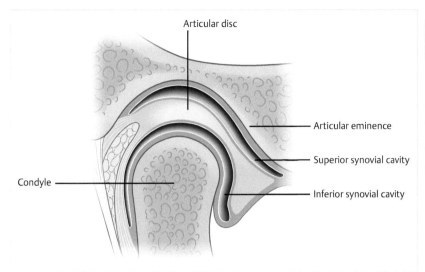

Fig. 23.2 Anatomy of the temporomandibular joint (TMJ). The intra-articular disk creates a superior and inferior joint space.

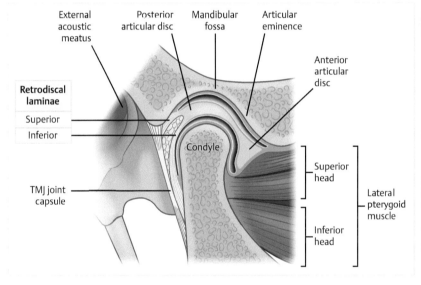

Fig. 23.3 Posterior attachments of the temporomandibular joint (TMJ) disk.

- Medial and lateral aspects of the joint capsule and disk are attached to their respective condyle poles via lateral collateral and medial collateral ligaments.
  - Two accessory TMJ ligaments (sphenomandibular and stylomandibular) help suspend the mandible from the skull. They are located medial to the joint and oriented in an anterior and inferior direction from the skull base (▶ Fig. 23.4).
    - The sphenomandibular ligament may also help limit lateral mandibular movement.
    - The stylomandibular ligament may help limit end range mandibular protrusion.
    - Overall, accessory ligament contributions to typical masticatory function appear to be limited.
- Vascular supply of the TMJ.
  ○ Provided by branches of the external carotid artery found near the joint.
    - Most commonly cited vascular contributions to the TMJ include:
      ▪ Superficial temporal.
      ▪ Maxillary.

▪ Anterior tympanic.
▪ Deep auricular.
  – Additional potential contributions, less commonly noted:
    ▪ Transverse facial.
    ▪ Middle meningeal.
    ▪ Ascending pharyngeal.
- A key consideration for mandibular surgery and trauma management: the primary blood supply to the condylar heads of the mandible is the inferior alveolar artery on each side (▶ Fig. 23.5).
  ○ The inferior alveolar artery enters the bone at the mandibular foramen and supplies the bone marrow and the cortical bone of the entire mandible.

23.3 TMJ Sensory (Afferent) Innervation

Hilton's law is an excellent tool for understanding joint innervation. It states that a joint will receive sensory innervation from the nerves that supply the muscles that cross and act on the joint.

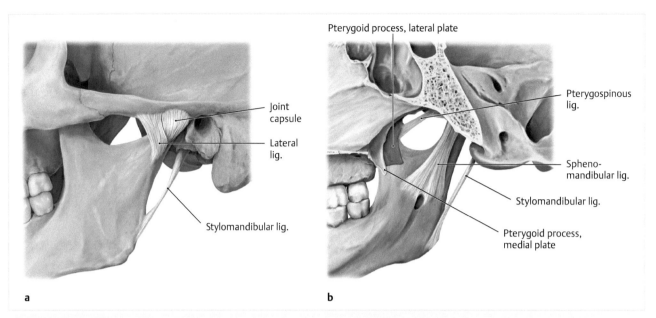

Fig. 23.4 (a,b) Ligamentous structures contributing to the temporomandibular joint (TMJ) stability. (Reproduced with permission from Schuenke M, Schulte E, Schumacher U. THIEME Atlas of Anatomy Third Edition, Vol 3. © Thieme 2020. Illustrations by Markus Voll and Karl Wesker.)

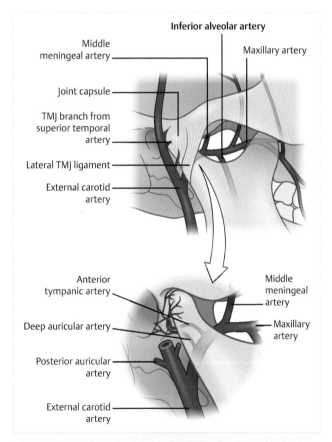

Fig. 23.5 Arterial supply of the temporomandibular joint (TMJ).

- The primary source for sensory innervation of the TMJ capsule (see ▶ Table 23.1) is branches of the mandibular division of the trigeminal nerve (V_3).
  ○ Auriculotemporal nerve is the most commonly cited source of sensory innervation.

Table 23.1 Sensory innervation of the temporomandibular joint (TMJ)

Sensory Nerve	Anatomical Description
Auriculotemporal	Branch off the posterior division of V_3 Supplies the entire TMJ capsule, especially the medial and posterior aspects
Masseteric	Branch off the anterior division of V_3 May supply anterolateral TMJ capsule
Posterior deep temporal	Branch off the anterior division of V3 May supply posteromedial TMJ capsule
Great auricular	Branch off the cervical plexus, C2–C3 ventral rami contributions May supply lateral TMJ capsule

○ Additional branches of V_3 that may also provide afferent TMJ innervation:
- Masseteric nerve.
- Deep posterior temporal nerves.
- Great auricular nerve from the cervical plexus (C2–C3):
  ▪ May also innervate part of the TMJ and surrounding anatomy due to proximity of the dermatome and potential for sensory overlap between this nerve and V_3.
○ Sensory receptors/nerve endings in the TMJ:
- Primarily free nerve endings.
- •Some Ruffini's nerve endings, Golgi–Mazzoni corpuscles, and Pacinian corpuscles are also present (▶ Fig. 23.6).

23.4 TMJ Neuromuscular Control

- Many muscles contribute directly or indirectly to mandibular movement (see ▶ Table 23.2). Those which directly affect mandibular movement are the muscles of mastication (see ▶ Fig. 23.7, ▶ Fig. 23.8, ▶ Fig. 23.9):
  ○ Masseter.
  ○ Temporalis.
  ○ Medial pterygoid and lateral pterygoid.

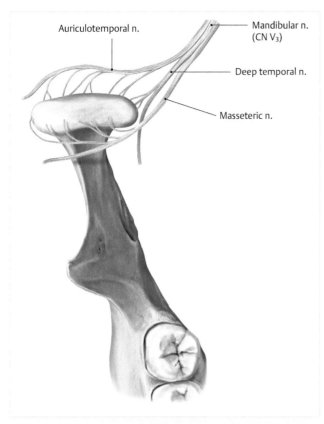

Auriculotemporal n.

Mandibular n. (CN V₃)

Deep temporal n.

Masseteric n.

Fig. 23.6 Sensory innervation of the temporomandibular joint (TMJ). (Reproduced with permission from Gilroy AM, MacPherson BR. Atlas of Anatomy. Third Edition. © Thieme 2016. Illustrations by Markus Voll and Karl Wesker.)

○ Additional muscles that influence mandibular movement include:
  – Suprahyoid muscle group.
  – Infrahyoid muscle group.
  – Platysma (considered muscle of facial expression).

23.5 Common Temporomandibular Joint–Related Disorders and Differential Diagnosis Clinical Correlation Examples

Temporomandibular joint–related disorders (TMD) are disorders of the musculoskeletal system and represent the most common cause of chronic pain in the orofacial region. The signs and symptoms of TMD commonly include:
- Pain in and around the TMJs and muscles of mastication.
- Muscle and joint tenderness on palpation.
- Joint sounds (clicking/crepitus).
- Limitation and/or incoordination of mandibular movement.
- Headaches.
- Otalgia (pain within the ear).

Table 23.2 Neuromuscular contributions to mandibular movement

Muscles	Innervation	Action on mandible
Masticatory muscles		
Masseter	masseteric nerve of V₃[a]	Elevation, protrusion,[a] retrusion,[b] lateral movements (ipsilateral side)[b]
Temporalis	deep temporal nerve branches of V₃[a]	Elevation, retrusion (posterior fibers), and lateral movements (ipsilateral side)[b]
Medial pterygoid	medial pterygoid nerve of V₃[a]	Elevation, protrusion,[b] and lateral movements (contralateral side)
Lateral pterygoid	lateral pterygoid nerve of V₃[a]	Protrusion (bilateral action), depression, and lateral movements (contralateral side)
Suprahyoid muscles		
Digastric (anterior belly)	mylohyoid nerve (inferior alveolar nerve branch) of V₃	Depression (when infrahyoid muscles stabilize or depress hyoid)
Digastric (posterior belly)	digastric branch of the facial nerve (CN VII)	Depression (when infrahyoid muscles stabilize or depress hyoid)
Geniohyoid	C1 ventral rami (travels with hypoglossal nerve [CN XII])	Depression[c] (via hyoid stabilization)
Mylohyoid	mylohyoid nerve (inferior alveolar nerve branch) of V₃	Depression[c] (via hyoid stabilization)
Stylohyoid	Stylohyoid branch of the facial nerve (CN VII)	Depression[c] (via hyoid stabilization)
Infrahyoid muscles		
Sternothyroid	C2 and C3 ventral rami (ansa cervicalis branch)	Depression[c] (via hyoid stabilization)
Sternohyoid	C1–C3 ventral rami (ansa cervicalis branch)	Depression[c] (via hyoid stabilization)
Thyrohyoid	C1 ventral rami (travels with the hypoglossal nerve [CN XII])	Depression[c] (via hyoid stabilization)
Omohyoid	C1–C3 ventral rami (ansa cervicalis branch)	Depression[c] (via hyoid stabilization)
Facial expression muscle		
Platysma	Facial nerve (CN VII), cervical branch(s)	Depression[b]

[a]Anterior trunk of the mandibular division of the fifth cranial nerve (trigeminal nerve).
[b]Plays a secondary role (agonist) in the movement.
[c]Plays an indirect role (stabilization) in the movement.

23.5.1 Common TMD Diagnoses

- **Myogenous pain:** spasm involving one or more of the muscles of mastication. Mandibular opening may or may not be limited.
- TMJ disk:
  ○ **Disk displacement with reduction** characterized by clicking late on closing of the mandible.

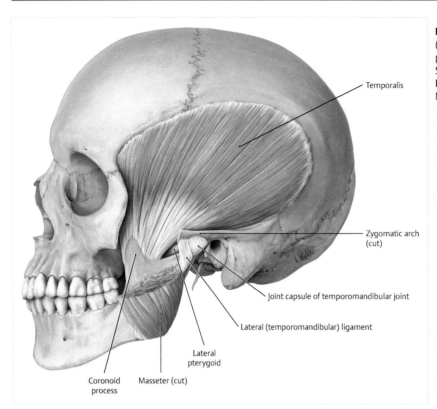

Fig. 23.7 Superficial muscles of mastication (temporalis and masseter). (Reproduced with permission from Schuenke M, Schulte E, Schumacher U. THIEME Atlas of Anatomy Third Edition, Vol 3. © Thieme 2020. Illustrations by Markus Voll and Karl Wesker.)

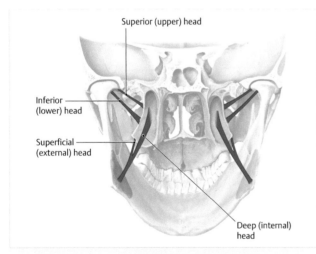

Fig. 23.8 Deep muscles of mastication (medial and lateral pterygoids). (Reproduced with permission from Schuenke M, Schulte E, Schumacher U. THIEME Atlas of Anatomy Third Edition, Vol 3. © Thieme 2020. Illustrations by Markus Voll and Karl Wesker.)

○ **Disk displacement without reduction with limited opening** characterized by "closed lock" (limited opening due to the displaced disk blocking the anterior glide of the mandibular condyles).

• **Hypermobility:** excessive opening of the mandible accompanied by anterior subluxation of the mandibular condyles.

• **Inflammation:** difficulty identifying the primary tissue involved (e.g., synovitis, capsulitis, retrodiskitis) often results in the label of "arthralgia."

• **Osteoarthritis** - signs and symptoms include TMJ-related degeneration, pain, and crepitus.

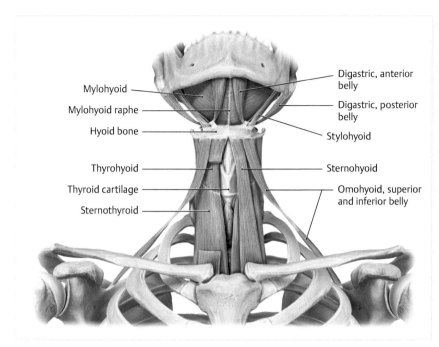

Mylohyoid

Mylohyoid raphe

Hyoid bone

Thyrohyoid

Thyroid cartilage

Sternothyroid

Digastric, anterior belly

Digastric, posterior belly

Stylohyoid

Sternohyoid

Omohyoid, superior and inferior belly

Fig. 23.9 Additional muscles that influence movement of the mandible (suprahyoid, infrahyoid, and platysma). (Reproduced with permission from Schuenke M, Schulte E, Schumacher U. THIEME Atlas of Anatomy Third Edition, Vol 3. © Thieme 2020. Illustrations by Markus Voll and Karl Wesker.)

Clinical Correlation Box 23.1: Trigeminal Neuralgia ("Tic Douloureux")

Trigeminal neuralgia (TN), also known as "tic douloureux," is a neuropathic pain condition that can be mistaken for a TMJ disorder. TN involves the fifth cranial nerve (trigeminal nerve). This disorder is most commonly characterized by episodes of intense, stabbing pain along the sensory distribution of the trigeminal nerve. It can include any number of the three divisions (ophthalmic, maxillary, and mandibular) of the nerve. It is most commonly unilateral, but can be bilateral. In some cases, TN may also manifest as a less intense, more constant dull aching or burning pain.

Potential causes of TN may include pressure on the nerve (e.g., blood vessel aneurysm or tumor) or possibly due to a neural disease such as multiple sclerosis. Dental care–related trauma to the nerve is another potential source of origin. In some cases, no underlying cause can be identified (idiopathic). The cause of symptom variation (intense stabbing vs. dull ache) is also unknown. TN is managed pharmacologically and/or by surgery or injection of neurotoxic agents.

Clinical Correlate Box 23.2: Dental Pathology (Periapical Abscess of a Maxillary Molar)

A maxillary molar infection can result in severe, persistent, throbbing aching in the molar area as well as radiation to the ear, mandible, or neck. Dental caries or bacterial entrapment related, this infection can progress from the space between the tooth and the alveolar bone to abscess formation around the apex region of the involved tooth root. If untreated, the abscess could erode into the surrounding areas (all near the TMJ). Potential routes include the maxillary sinus, nasal cavity, surrounding bone (osteomyelitis), or surrounding soft tissues (cellulitis and facial swelling). Significant problems or even death are likely to occur if the infection spreads into the retropharyngeal, mediastinal, intracranial, or the intraorbital spaces.

The maxillary molars are innervated by the posterior superior alveolar branch of the maxillary division of the trigeminal nerve. Sensory overlap with the primary source of TMJ sensory innervation (auriculotemporal branch of the mandibular division of the trigeminal nerve) is likely in this area. Dental periapical abscess signs and symptoms include fever, tooth pain, facial swelling, dysphagia, trismus, and possibly dyspnea. Radiological imaging is the most common tool used to diagnose this condition. Management includes abscess drainage, root canal or extraction of the involved tooth, and appropriate antibiotic therapy.

Cluster headaches (CH) are an uncommon, severe form of primary neurovascular headaches, diagnostically classified as a trigeminal autonomic cephalgia. Unilateral, severe (searing, burning, and stabbing) headache pain behind or above the eye or at the temple are commonly described symptoms of a CH. In addition, unilateral autonomic signs and symptoms are associated with CH. They are ipsilateral and only occur during the painful stage of a CH; they include ptosis, miosis, lacrimation, conjunctival injection, rhinorrhea, and nasal congestion.

The pathogenesis of CH is complex and has not been fully confirmed. The two most widely accepted theories of pathogenesis are the following: (1) primary CH is characterized by hypothalamic activation with secondary activation of the trigeminal autonomic reflex, probably via a trigeminal-hypothalamic pathway, and (2) neurogenic inflammation of the walls of the cavernous sinus obliterates venous outflow and thus injures the traversing sympathetic fibers of the intracranial internal carotid artery and its branches. For patients with suspected CH, neuroimaging with a cranial computed tomography (CT) scan or a cranial magnetic resonance imaging (MRI) study is recommended to exclude abnormalities of the brain and pituitary gland. Initial treatment recommendations include pharmacological management with triptans or oxygen therapy. There are several promising but unproven neurostimulation-based approaches being used to treat unresponsive CH. However, these interventions remain investigational with unproven long-term benefit and safety.

Questions and Answers

1. Which of the following signs or symptoms is least likely to occur with TMJ dysfunction?
   a) Tinnitus
   b) Preauricular pain
   c) Pain in the external auditory meatus area
   d) Swelling of the TMJ

Level 1: Easy
Answer C: The auricular branch of the vagus nerve innervates the concha and most of the area around the auditory meatus. Thus, it should not be affected by TMJ related problems. **(A)** tinnitus or "ringing" in the ears is a common symptom reported by individuals with TMJ dysfunction; **(B)** the auriculotemporal branch of V_3 innervates this area as well as the TMJ, therefore pain in the TMJ may be referred to this area; **(D)** swelling is a common sign which occurs in conjunction with TMJ dysfunction.

2. Which of the following tissues is not innervated, thus a patient would **not** feel pain if the tissue was damaged?
   a) Central region of the TMJ articular disc
   b) Lamina of the retrodiscal tissue
   c) Lateral aspect of the TMJ capsule
   d) Tendon of the lateral pterygoid muscle

Level 1: Easy
Answer A: Only the disc periphery is innervated and vascularized. **(B)** This area is innervated the auriculotemporal branch of V_3 and sensitive to irritation/injury. **(C)** This area is commonly innervated by V_3 and sometimes the great auricular branch of the cervical plexus. **(D)** The nerve to the lateral pterygoid muscle provides both motor and sensory innervation to the muscle and tendon.

3. A teenager fell forward onto a concrete surface making initial contact with his chin. This resulted in a fracture of the neck of the mandibular condyle on one side. Blood supply to the mandibular condyle must remain intact to promote proper healing of the condylar region and prevent subsequent deformity of the condyle due to boney necrosis. Which artery (located in the bone marrow) supplies this area, thus placing it at risk in a fracture such as the one described above?
   a) Superficial temporal
   b) Anterior tympanic
   c) Ascending pharyngeal
   d) Inferior alveolar

Level 2: Moderate
Answer D: The main source of condylar head vascularization is the inferior alveolar artery. The artery enters the bone at the mandibular foramen and supplies the bone marrow of the whole mandible as well as its cortical layer. This is a key consideration for mandibular surgery and trauma management. **(A)** This artery may supply the TMJ area, but not condylar head specifically. **(B)** This artery may supply the TMJ area, but not condylar head specifically. **(C)** This artery may supply the TMJ area, but not condylar head specifically.

4. When you ask your patient to protrude their mandible, their mandible protrudes slightly, but primarily deviates to the left. Injury of which nerve is most likely to cause this?
   a) Left CN VII
   b) Right ansa cervicalis
   c) Left CN V3
   d) Right CN V_3

Level 2: Moderate
Answer C: The left lateral pterygoid is not functioning in this example. It is innervated by the left CN V_3. **(A)** Injury to the left facial nerve would not affect mandibular movement, but it would affect the muscles of facial expression on the left side of the face. **(B)** The ansa cervicalis does not innervate any of the muscles of mastication, but does innervate some muscles that assist with mandibular movement—however damage to this nerve would not significantly affect mandibular protrusion. **(D)** Injury to the right CN V_3 would affect function of the R lateral pterygoid muscle. This loss would result in mandibular movement towards the right when protrusion is attempted.

24 Salivary Glands

Learning Objectives

1. Describe the function of the structural components associated with major and minor salivary glands.
2. Explain the function of saliva and the mechanism of production.
3. Explain how alterations in flow rate may impact the composition of saliva and the physiological significance of a low flow rate.
4. Explain the neural mediated reflex pathway that controls stimulated salivary secretion.
5. Describe the types of afferent stimuli involved in eliciting salivation. Include the types of sensory receptors and the afferent path followed.
6. Describe the efferent outflow path for the major salivary glands. Include both parasympathetic and sympathetic fibers.
7. Explain how medications may affect the efferent signaling pathway and alter secretion.

24.1 Overview of the Salivary Glands

Salivary glands associated with the oral cavity produce a complex, slightly alkaline watery secretion that contains various proteins, ions, and enzymes. Salivary secretion occurs continuously, at low levels, with intermittent increases occurring in response to eating and oral stimulation through autonomic innervation. The composition and continual secretion of saliva function to maintain oral cavity homeostasis. Saliva serves to cleanse and protect the oral mucosa, provide antimicrobial protection, maintain a neutral pH, and preserve tooth integrity. The lubrication and moisture produced by saliva facilitates speaking and mediates digestive functions, including the process of chewing, taste, bolus formation, and swallowing. Salivary gland dysfunction has a significant impact on oral health and quality of life. This chapter discusses the anatomical structure, location, and neural mechanisms that control the secretion of the major and minor salivary glands.

24.1.1 General Development of Salivary Glands

- Salivary glands develop concomitantly with the formation of the orofacial complex during the 6 to 12 weeks of embryonic development and arise from the oral epithelium.
- Each gland undergoes extensive branching within the underlying connective tissue to form clusters of **salivary secretory cells**, known as **acinar units**, and **excretory ducts**, which open onto the epithelial surface to release saliva into the oral cavity.
  - **Secretory acinar units** function to produce saliva and may consist of two types of **secretory acinar cells: serous** and **mucous cells**.
    - Salivary glands may contain just serous cells, only mucous cells, or both. The predominant type of acinar unit present in a gland defines the type of saliva produced. Glands that contain predominantly serous cells produce a thin watery enzyme-rich secretion, whereas glands comprised mainly of mucous cells secrete a thick, viscous, mucin-rich secretion.
  - The duct system serves to collect and then modify the ionic composition of the saliva produced by the secretory acinar cells. The smaller collecting ducts found within the gland eventually coalesce to form larger excretory ducts that transport saliva to the oral mucosal surface.

24.1.2 Gland Classification

- Salivary glands are primarily classified into two groups based on size and location, as **major** and **minor salivary glands**. Alternatively, salivary gland classification may be based on the type of saliva produced and include serous glands, mucous glands, and seromucous (mixed) glands (▶ Fig. 24.1).
  - Major salivary glands include the parotid, submandibular, and sublingual glands.
    - The three major salivary glands are large, bilateral, paired structures that reside outside the oral cavity (extraoral) and empty salivary secretions into the oral cavity via long excretory ducts. The excretory ducts open onto either side of the dental arch and serve to saturate the food bolus with saliva during chewing.
    - The three major salivary glands collectively produce **90%** of the **total salivary output**.

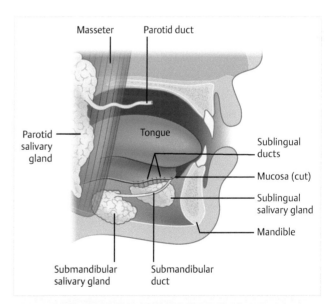

Fig. 24.1 Location of the three major salivary glands. Right lateral view: mandible and mylohyoid removed. The parotid, submandibular, and sublingual gland represent the major salivary glands and produce 90% of the total salivary output. The major glands are bilateral paired structures, located outside the oral cavity proper. Each gland empties into the oral cavity via a long excretory duct.

- **Minor salivary glands**, which are named based on their anatomical location within the oral cavity, include **labial, buccal, lingual, palatal**, and **pharyngeal glands**.
  - Minor salivary glands are small, nonencapsulated structures found within the submucosal layer of the oral cavity (intraoral) and release saliva through short excretory ducts onto the oral mucosa.
  - Minor salivary glands contribute the remaining **10%** of the **total salivary output**.

24.2 Anatomical Overview of Major and Minor Salivary Glands

24.2.1 Parotid Glands

- The paired **parotid glands**, which are the largest of the three major glands consist of serous acinar cells, and produce a thin, low-viscosity, enzyme-rich secretion (▷ Fig. 24.2).
- Each parotid gland resides in a triangular space, the **parotid fossa**, in the preauricular region, just anterior to the ear and along the posterior border of the mandibular ramus.
  - The facial nerve (cranial nerve [CN] VII), the external carotid artery, and the retromandibular vein also lie within the parotid fossa and should be considered during surgery involving the parotid gland.
- The stylomandibular ligament and facial nerve (CN VII) pass through the parotid gland, dividing each gland into a superficial lobe and a deep lobe.
- The large excretory duct of the parotid gland, known as **Stensen's (parotid) duct**, emerges from the deep lobe along the anterior border of the parotid gland, crosses the masseter muscle, and pierces the buccinator muscle to enter the oral cavity.
  - The duct opens at the **parotid papilla** onto the buccal mucosa that lines the vestibule of the mouth in the region opposite the **second maxillary molar**.
- Nerve structures anatomically associated with the parotid gland include the **facial nerve (CN VII), greater auricular nerves (C2–C3)**, and **auriculotemporal nerves (CN V3)**.
  - The **facial nerve (CN VII)**, which passes through the parotid gland, *does not* provide innervation to the gland.
    - The motor (SVE) division of the facial nerve exits the base of the skull and immediately gives rise to three branches that innervate the stylohyoid, posterior digastric, and auricularis muscles.
    - The facial nerve enters the gland, bifurcates into two main trunks, and then divides into five terminal branches to form the **parotid nerve plexus**. The five terminal branches of the plexus include the **temporal, zygomatic, buccal, marginal mandibular**, and **cervical nerve branches**, which innervate the **muscles of facial expression**.

- The **greater auricular nerve**, which originates from C2–C3 of the cervical plexus, and the **auriculotemporal** branch of V3 nerve, both transmit **general sensation (general somatic afferent [GSA] fiber)** from the region of the skin covering the parotid gland.
- **Secretomotor (general visceral efferent [GVE] fiber)** innervation originates from both parasympathetic and sympathetic divisions. The parotid glands produce approximately 25% of total salivary output under unstimulated (basal) conditions. However, during autonomic stimulation, the parotid secretes 60% of the total salivary flow.
  - Parasympathetic innervation arises from the inferior salivatory nuclei and travels to the parotid gland via the **tympanic branch of CN IX** and the **lesser petrosal** nerve (CN IX). Postganglionic fibers originate from the **otic ganglion** and accompany the **auriculotemporal** branch (V3) for secretomotor distribution to the parotid gland.
  - Sympathetic innervation arises from neurons in the lateral horn of the thoracic spinal (T1–T4) cord and synapse in the **superior cervical ganglion**. Postganglionic fibers follow the vascular supply.

Clinical Correlation Box 24.1: Frey's Syndrome

Frey's syndrome is a relatively rare disorder associated with **gustatory sweating**, which occurs shortly after eliciting a salivary reflex in response to chewing. It is characterized by unilateral flushing and sweating of the skin in the region supplied by the auriculotemporal nerve. The segmental distribution pattern of innervation includes the frontotemporal region (forehead), check, anterior ear, and parotid region. Frey's syndrome occurs most often following parotid surgery and is presumably associated with damage to the GSA and GVE fibers associated with the auriculotemporal nerve. It is predicted that following surgery, the GVE parasympathetic fibers join the sympathetic fibers as the auriculotemporal nerve fibers regenerate. The intermingling of fibers results in flushing and sweating during salivation due to sympathetic innervation.

Clinical Correlation Box 24.2: Parotidectomy

Neoplasms arising in the parotid gland, which may be benign (80%) or malignant (20%), occur in the superficial or deep lobe, respectively. A key consideration for any parotidectomy is the isolation of the facial nerve at the level of the main trunk as it exits the stylomastoid foramen. Benign tumors are most often associated with the superficial lobe and removed through a superficial parotidectomy. Tumors occurring in the deep lobe must be resected from the stylomandibular ligament, which separates the superficial and deep lobes. Deep parotid tumors may push the facial nerve (CN VII) superficially and increase the risk of injury.

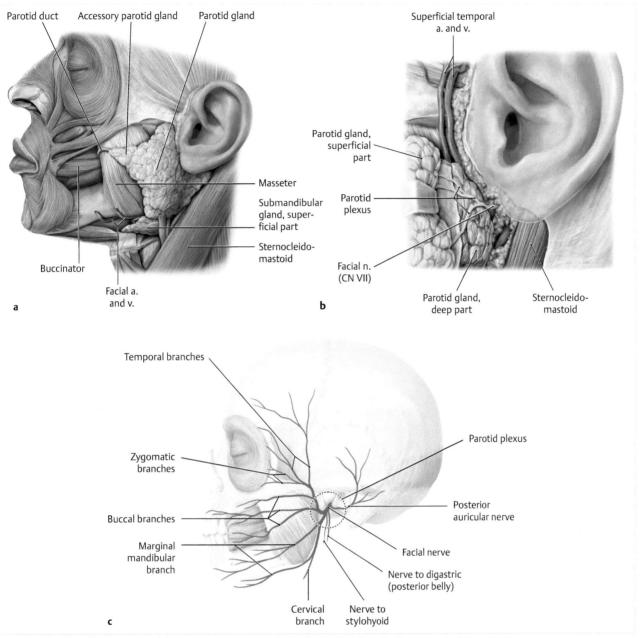

Fig. 24.2 Left lateral view of the anatomical location of the parotid gland in the parotid fossa. **(a)** The parotid gland, which consists of a superficial and deep lobe, sits anterior to the ear and along the posterior border of the mandibular ramus. The parotid duct arises from the deep lobe, crosses the face superficial to the masseter muscle, and pierces the buccinator to enter the oral cavity. The parotid duct opens into the buccal vestibule of the mouth opposite the second maxillary molar. The parotid produces a pure serous, watery secretion. **(b)** Magnified image of the parotid gland demonstrating the position of the facial nerve. The facial nerve passes through the parotid gland, splitting the gland into a superficial lobe and a deep lobe, but does provide innervation to the gland. The facial nerve emerges from the stylomastoid foramen, enters the parotid gland, and divides into five terminal branches, to form the parotid nerve plexus. **(c)** Schematic of the terminal motor branches of the facial nerve. (Reproduced with permission from Schuenke M, Schulte E, Schumacher U. THIEME Atlas of Anatomy. Third Edition, Vol 3. © Thieme 2020. Illustrations by Markus Voll and Karl Wesker.)

Parotitis refers to inflammation of the parotid gland or duct that may be caused by bacterial or viral infections. Other diseases associated with inflammation such as the mumps, tuberculosis, the autoimmune disease, Sjogren's syndrome, or the human immunodeficiency virus (HIV) may also cause parotitis. Inflammation of the gland leads to decreased salivary flow and, in some cases, scarring and obstruction of the ducts, which allow for bacteria and viruses to infect the secretory portions of the gland. Clinical manifestations include localized ear pain, tenderness anterior to the ear, and difficulty or pain with chewing and swallowing. Neurological complications are rare but may include meningitis (inflammation of meninges), deafness, and facial nerve inflammation (facial neuritis).

24.2.2 Submandibular Glands

- The paired submandibular glands, which are smaller than the parotid, are mixed salivary glands containing primarily serous cells with some mucous acinar cells.
- Each submandibular gland sits just below the angle of the mandible, in the **submandibular (digastric) triangle**, an anatomic region formed by the anterior and posterior digastric muscles and the inferior border of the mandible. The submandibular gland creates a **C**-shaped ring around the posterolateral edge of the mylohyoid muscle to form a superficial lobe and a deep lobe (▶ Fig. 24.3).
- The **main excretory duct** of the submandibular gland, known as **Wharton's duct**, exits the medial side of the gland and passes between the hyoglossus and mylohyoid muscles to enter the floor of the oral cavity.
  - The submandibular duct exhibits a long, convoluted path in comparison to the ducts of other major glands. The long route may serve as a contributing factor to the formation of salivary calculus (**sialolithiasis**) and lead to the obstruction of saliva released into the oral cavity.
  - Each duct empties just lateral to the midline, behind the mandibular incisors at the **sublingual papillae (caruncle)**, which is near the base of the lingual frenulum (▶ Fig. 24.3).
- Nerve structures associated with the submandibular gland include the **marginal mandibular branch of VII**, the **lingual nerve (CN V3)**, and the **hypoglossal nerve (CN XII)**.
  - Each of these nerves exhibits a close association with the submandibular gland and **Wharton's duct** as the duct passes along the floor of the oral cavity. The nerves may be at risk of injury with the removal of the submandibular gland or surgical intervention to dislodge salivary stones (**sialolith**).
- The **lingual nerve**, a branch of the mandibular (V3) division of the trigeminal, enters the posterior portion of the oral cavity through the infratemporal fossa and travels with the chorda tympani (VII) along the floor of the oral cavity.
  - The **submandibular parasympathetic ganglion** lies on the lateral surface of the hyoglossus muscle, near the deep lobe of the submandibular gland, and attaches to the lingual nerve. The ganglion serves as the synaptic connection for

the preganglionic (GVE) fibers of the chorda tympani nerve (▶ Fig. 24.4).
  - The lingual nerve crosses the submandibular (Wharton's) duct passing from the lateral side, inferiorly, and then medial to the submandibular duct, to supply GSA fibers to the oral mucosa and submandibular glands (▶ Fig. 24.3 and ▶ Fig. 24.4).
- The **hypoglossal nerve (CN XII)** enters the posterior portion of the oral cavity through the submandibular triangle and runs inferior to **Wharton's duct**, the **submandibular gland**, and the **lingual nerve**. The hypoglossal nerve does not innervate the submandibular gland; it provides **GSE** fibers to all intrinsic and extrinsic muscles of the tongue, except for the palatoglossus muscle (▶ Fig. 24.5).
- The submandibular gland, which produces approximately 50% of the total salivary output during resting conditions, receives neural stimulation from both parasympathetic and sympathetic innervation. During autonomic stimulation, salivary secretions constitute only 30% of the total salivary output.
  - Parasympathetic (GVE) innervation originates from the **superior salivatory nuclei** and travels to the submandibular gland via the **chorda tympani** branch of the facial nerve (CN VII). Postganglionic (GVE) fibers arise from the **submandibular ganglion** and continue to travel with the **lingual nerve (V3)** for secretomotor distribution to the **submandibular** and **sublingual glands**.
  - Sympathetic innervation arises as preganglionic fibers from the intermediolateral cell column (IMLC) of the spinal cord (T1–T4), which then synapse in the superior cervical ganglion of the sympathetic trunk. Postganglionic fibers follow the vascular supply to reach the gland.

Salivary gland inflammation, known as **sialadenitis**, may be associated with pain, tenderness, redness, and swelling in the region of the gland. Bacterial and viral infections of the parotid or submandibular gland are often associated with acute onset of sialadenitis. In cases of infection, fever, malaise, and inflammation of the ductal papillae are often associated with symptoms. Chronic and recurring forms of sialadenitis also exist. Obstruction due to salivary calculi (sialoliths) or stricture in the duct often leads to pain, inflammation, and swelling. Obstructive sialadenitis due to a sialolith is referred to as sialolithiasis and most often occurs in the submandibular duct (Wharton's duct). The increased incidence of sialoliths in Wharton's duct is attributed to the length, position, and path of the duct. Patients often complain of tenderness, sudden swelling, and increased pain that is associated with salivation during eating. Dehydration, anticholinergics, and conditions related to xerostomia (dry mouth), including the autoimmune disease, Sjogren's disease, may increase the incidence of sialolithiasis (stone formation) and possible infection due to decreased salivary flow. Long-term complications of chronic sialadenitis and untreated sialolithiasis can lead to scarring and glandular atrophy.

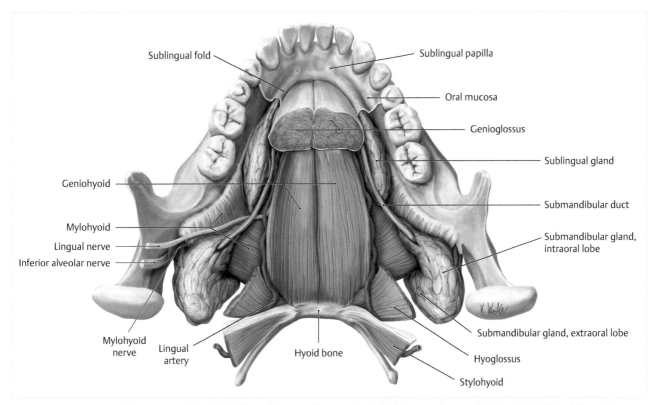

Fig. 24.3 Anatomical location of the submandibular and sublingual glands in the floor of the mouth. Superior view of the floor of the oral cavity, with the tongue removed. The submandibular glands are mixed salivary glands producing both mucous and serous secretions. The glands sit below the angle of the mandible in the floor of the oral cavity. The glands wrap as a **C**-shaped ring around the posterolateral edge of the mylohyoid to form a superficial lope and a deep lobe. The submandibular duct (Wharton's duct) emerges from the medial surface of the gland, crosses over the lingual nerve, and passes anteriorly to open on to the sublingual papilla. Note the submandibular duct cross over the lingual nerve. the **sublingual glands** are predominantly mucous-secreting salivary glands, located anteriorly in the floor of the oral cavity, between the oral mucosa and the mylohyoid muscle. The sublingual gland drains through several smaller excretory ducts that open on the sublingual fold. Alternatively, the sublingual glands may have a main duct that opens into the submandibular duct at the sublingual papillae. (Reproduced with permission from Schuenke M, Schulte E, Schumacher U. THIEME Atlas of Anatomy Third Edition, Vol 3. © Thieme 2020. Illustrations by Markus Voll and Karl Wesker.)

Clinical Correlation Box 24.5: Clinical Considerations with Submandibular Gland Surgery

Based on the anatomical relationship of the submandibular duct and submandibular gland to the vessels and nerves that pass through the submandibular triangle, several structures should be considered during the excision of the submandibular gland, or during the removal of salivary duct stones. The superficially located marginal mandibular and cervical branches of VII, as well as the medially positioned hypoglossal nerve (CN XII), and the lingual nerve (CN V3), should be considered during the excision of the submandibular gland, or during the removal of salivary duct stones. The facial artery passes deep to the gland, whereas the facial vein lies superficially. Among structures at risk, the marginal mandibular branch (VII) is the most likely structure damaged or bruised during submandibular gland removal. However, the hypoglossal and lingual nerves, along with the secretomotor fibers carried by the chorda tympani nerve, are also potentially at risk. During surgery, the submandibular duct should also be identified and dissected to avoid damage to the lingual nerve, or the submandibular ganglion.

24.2.3 Sublingual Glands

- The paired sublingual glands (▶ Fig. 24.6), which are the smallest of the three major salivary glands, lack a definitive connective capsule and lie below the oral mucosa, anteriorly in the region of the floor of the oral cavity.
- The sublingual glands are **mixed**, consisting mainly of mucous acinar cells with only a few serous cells.
- The sublingual glands, which contribute only 5 to 10% of the total salivary output during resting conditions, receive neural stimulation from both parasympathetic and sympathetic innervation.
  - The parasympathetic and sympathetic secretomotor (GVE) fibers that innervate the submandibular gland also provide innervation to the sublingual glands.
- The main duct, **Bartholin's duct**, opens into the submandibular duct at the **sublingual papillae (caruncle)**.
  - Several small sublingual ducts, also known as the **ducts of Rivinus**, may also be present and open along the sublingual fold on the floor of the oral cavity.
  - Both the sublingual glands and the minor salivary glands exhibit a limited excretory duct system, with striated ducts often absent. The short ducts reduce the occurrence of salivary duct stone formation.

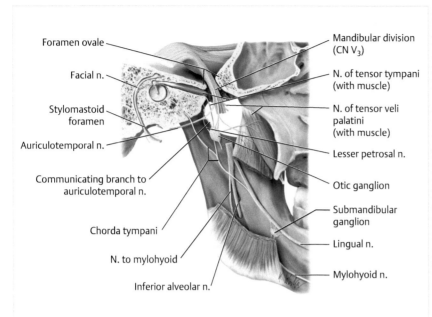

Fig. 24.4 The location of the submandibular parasympathetic ganglion in the submandibular triangle. Right lateral view of the medial surface of the mandible, with the medial pterygoid muscle cut. The ganglion is suspended inferiorly from the lingual nerve and lies on the lateral surface of the hyoglossus muscle, near the deep lobe of the submandibular gland. The preganglionic parasympathetic fibers from the superior salivatory nucleus in the central nervous system (CNS) accompany the nervus intermedius and the chorda tympani nerve (CN VII). The chorda tympani nerve joins the pathway of the lingual nerve in the infratemporal fossa and travels with the lingual nerve to reach the submandibular ganglion. Postganglionic secretomotor fibers pass to the submandibular, sublingual, and minor lingual and labial glands in the anterior floor of the mouth and lower lip. (Reproduced with permission from Schuenke M, Schulte E, Schumacher U. THIEME Atlas of Anatomy Third Edition, Vol 3. © Thieme 2020. Illustrations by Markus Voll and Karl Wesker.)

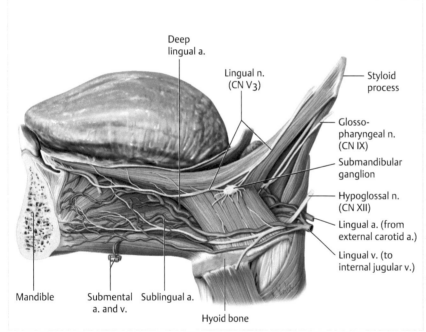

Fig. 24.5 Left lateral view of the anatomical relationship between the submandibular duct, submandibular ganglion, hypoglossal nerve, and lingual nerve, with the submandibular gland and the mylohyoid muscle removed. The lingual nerve and the submandibular ganglion lie on the lateral surface of the hyoglossus muscle, near the deep lobe of the submandibular ganglion. The duct runs superior to the hypoglossal nerve (CN XII) and inferior to the lingual nerve as it passes between the hyoglossus and mylohyoid muscle. The lingual nerve crosses the duct laterally at the anterior border of the hyoglossus muscle, and then loops beneath the submandibular duct, and continues medially to the duct as the nerve passes anteriorly toward the tip of the tongue. The hypoglossal nerve (CN XII) lies inferior and deep to the submandibular gland and passes superficial to the hyoglossus muscle. (Reproduced with permission from Schuenke M, Schulte E, Schumacher U. THIEME Atlas of Anatomy Third Edition, Vol 3. © Thieme 2020. Illustrations by Markus Voll and Karl Wesker.)

24.2.4 Minor Salivary Glands

- Approximately 600 to 1,000 minor salivary glands reside in the submucosal connective tissue within the oral cavity and the oropharynx (▶ Fig. 24.7).
- The glands are nonencapsulated, consisting of small aggregates of mucous and serous acinar cells, which produce approximately 5 to 10% of total salivary output (see ▶ Table 24.1 and ▶ Table 24.2).
- Minor glands secrete saliva continuously through constitutive exocytosis; however, feedback from the parasympathetic and sympathetic system, as well as physiological and pharmacological input, may modify secretory activity.

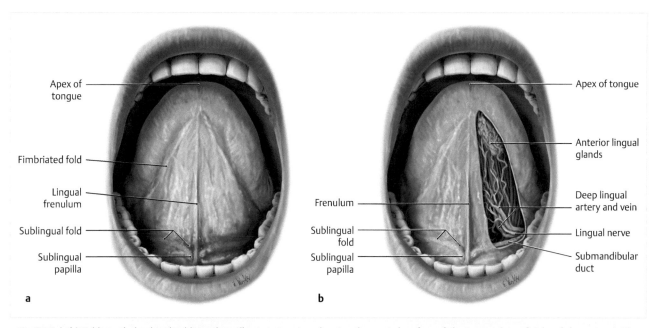

Fig. 24.6 (a,b) Sublingual gland and sublingual papilla. Anterior view showing the ventral surface of the tongue (superficial and deep views). The paired sublingual glands lie below the oral mucosa in the floor of the oral cavity. The main duct (Bartholin's duct) empties into sublingual papilla. (Reproduced with permission from Schuenke M, Schulte E, Schumacher U. THIEME Atlas of Anatomy Third Edition, Vol 3. © Thieme 2020. Illustrations by Markus Voll and Karl Wesker.)

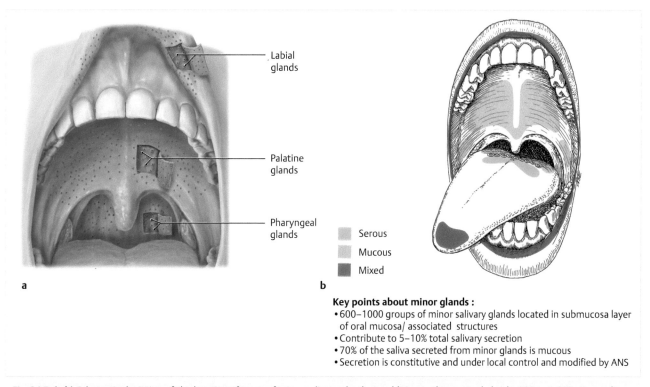

Key points about minor glands :
- 600–1000 groups of minor salivary glands located in submucosa layer of oral mucosa/ associated structures
- Contribute to 5–10% total salivary secretion
- 70% of the saliva secreted from minor glands is mucous
- Secretion is constitutive and under local control and modified by ANS

Fig. 24.7 (a,b) Schematic depiction of the location of types of minor salivary glands. In addition to three paired glands, 600 to 1,000 minor salivary glands secrete pure mucous, pure serous, or a mixed salivary secretion into the oral cavity. Minor glands only produce 5 to 8% of the total saliva output, but this amount suffices to keep the oral cavity lubricated when the major glands are at rest. (Fig. 24.7a: Reproduced with permission from Schuenke M, Schulte E, Schumacher U. THIEME Atlas of Anatomy Third Edition, Vol 3. © Thieme 2020. Illustrations by Markus Voll and Karl Wesker.)

Table 24.1 Overview of salivary glands

Component	Parotid	Submandibular	Sublingual	Minor glands
Location	Anterior to the preauricular region of the ear, the parotid fossa	Angel of mandible, submandibular triangle	Floor of the anterior mouth	Variable: • palatal • buccal • oropharynx • lingual • labial
CT capsule	Thick; divides the gland into superficial and deep lobes	Thick; divides the gland into superficial and deep lobes	Not well developed	Absent, due to intraoral location
Main excretory duct	Stensen's duct, opens at the parotid papillae; opposite the second maxillary molar	Wharton's duct, opens at the sublingual papillae; opposite the mandibular incisors	Bartholin's duct and the ducts of Rivinus open at the sublingual papillae	Absent, product released onto the local mucosa surface
Type of secretory acinar cell	Only serous	Mixed: mainly serous, some mucous	Mixed: mainly mucous, some serous	Varies based on location
Properties of product released	Low viscosity; enzyme-rich solution	Slightly higher viscosity; mucin-rich solution	High viscosity; mucin-rich solution	Collectively saliva produced is high viscosity; mucin-rich
Principal method of saliva release: • Constitutive • Regulated	Both, mainly regulated exocytosis	Both, mainly constitutive exocytosis	Both, mainly constitutive exocytosis	Constitutive, modified by ANS
Salivary flow rate % contribution: • Unstimulated • Stimulated	25% 60%	50% 30%	5–8% 5–8%	5–10% 5–10%
ANS (GVE) nerve supply	ANS-stimulated neural reflex: • Inferior salivatory nuclei of CN IX (parasympathetic) • Superior cervical (sympathetic)	ANS-stimulated neural reflex • Superior salivatory nuclei of CN VII (parasympathetic) • Superior cervical (sympathetic)	ANS-stimulated neural reflex • Superior salivatory nuclei of CN VII (parasympathetic) • Superior cervical (sympathetic)	Constitutive activity modified by ANS nerve supply depends on location
Sensory (GSA) nerve supply	Auriculotemporal branch of V3 C2–C3 greater auricular	Lingual nerve (V3)	Lingual nerve (V3)	Varies based on location; may be branches of CN V2, CN V3, or CN IX

Abbreviation: ANS, autonomic nervous system (includes parasympathetic and sympathetic); CN, cranial nerve; GSA, general somatic afferent; GVE, general visceral efferent.

Table 24.2 Summary of minor salivary glands

Minor Gland	Location	Type of Acinar Cell Secretion Serous vs. Mucous	Parasympathetic Innervation
Palatal glands	Submucosa Posterior third hard palate	Mucous few serous	Greater petrosal (VII) → pterygopalatine ganglion → via greater palatine (V2) nerve
	Submucosa Soft palate and uvula	Mucous few serous	Greater petrosal (VII) → pterygopalatine ganglion → via lesser palatine (V2) nerve
Labial	Labial surface (inner lip mucosa)	Mixed; mainly mucous > some serous	Chorda tympani (VII)/lingual nerve → submandibular ganglion → via lingual nerve (V3)
Lingual (tongue)	Anterior tip of the tongue (ventral)	Mixed; mainly mucous > some serous	Chorda tympani (VII)/lingual nerve submandibular ganglion → via lingual nerve (V3)
	Anterolateral to circumvallate papillae and foliate papillae *Glands of von Ebner*	Serous only	Lesser petrosal (IX) → otic ganglion → via glossopharyngeal nerve
	Posterior one-third of the tongue (oropharynx) region of lingual tonsils[a]	Mucous few serous	Lesser petrosal (IX) → otic ganglion → glossopharyngeal nerve
Palatoglossal (glossopalatine)	Submucosa Oropharynx fauces	Mucous only	Lesser petrosal → otic ganglion → auriculotemporal nerve (V3)
Buccal	Submucosa buccal	Mixed; mucous some serous	Lesser petrosal → otic ganglion → buccal nerve

[a]Minor glands constitutively secrete but may be modified by the autonomic nervous system (ANS).

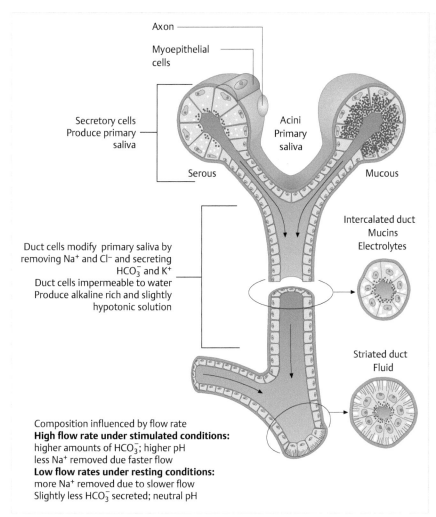

Fig. 24.8 Schematic of salivary gland acinar and duct cells. Primary saliva produced from the major salivary glands is ionically modified by the duct cells, leading to the production of an alkaline-rich, slightly hypotonic solution. (Modified with permission from Probst R, Grevers G, Iro H. Basic Otorhinolaryngology: A Step-by-Step Learning Guide. Second Edition. © Thieme; 2017)

Labels in figure:
Axon
Myoepithelial cells
Secretory cells Produce primary saliva
Serous
Acini Primary saliva
Mucous
Duct cells modify primary saliva by removing Na^+ and Cl^- and secreting HCO_3^- and K^+
Duct cells impermeable to water
Produce alkaline rich and slightly hypotonic solution
Intercalated duct Mucins Electrolytes
Striated duct Fluid
Composition influenced by flow rate
High flow rate under stimulated conditions:
higher amounts of HCO_3^-; higher pH
less Na^+ removed due faster flow
Low flow rates under resting conditions:
more Na^+ removed due to slower flow
Slightly less HCO_3^- secreted; neutral pH

- Secretomotor fibers that innervate the minor glands follow preganglionic fibers of the glossopharyngeal or facial nerves. Postganglionic fibers are distributed through branches of CNs V2 and V3.
- Most of the saliva (70%) secreted from the minor glands is a thick, viscous, mucin-rich secretion that is essential for the lubrication and hydration of the oral mucosa in the palatal, oropharyngeal, labial and buccal regions.
  - Minor glands that contain primarily mucous cells are found in the submucosa of the **oropharyngeal isthmus**, **the posterior hard and soft palates**, and **the posterior one-third of the tongue**.
  - Minor **mixed** glands reside in the **tip of the anterior tongue** and the **labial** and **buccal regions**.
  - Minor glands containing only **serous** acinar cells are situated anterior to the sulcus terminalis in association with taste buds of the circumvallate and foliate papillae.
- The duct system in minor glands is less extensive than the major glands. Small collecting ducts serve to release unmodified, isotonic saliva constitutively onto the mucosal lining of the oral cavity.

24.3 Saliva Production, Composition, and Flow Rates

24.3.1 Saliva Production and Composition

- The synthesis and release of saliva into the oral cavity is a two-step process influenced by parasympathetic and sympathetic input (▶ Fig. 24.8).
  - The first step involves the synthesis of **primary saliva**, an **isotonic** solution produced by the acinar cells, that consists of water, electrolytes, salivary enzymes, and mucin proteins.
    - The secretion of primary saliva from the acinar cells may occur **constitutively** or through **regulated exocytosis** as an outcome of autonomic stimulation.
  - The second step involves **ionic modification** of the primary secretion as it flows through the duct system. The rate of flow through the duct system is subject to change due to autonomic stimulation and leads to an altered ionic composition of the final product.

Table 24.3 Overview of impact of flow rate on salivary composition

Properties	Unstimulated Slow Flow Rate (Constitutive Release)	Stimulated Fast Flow Rate (Regulated Release)
Flow rate	0.3–0.5 mL/min	1.5–4.0 mL/min
Tonicity (relative to plasma)	Hypotonic: remove more ions	Isotonic: remove fewer ions
pH (6.3–7.4 is neutral)	6.4: neutral buffering capacity	6.9–7.3: higher buffering capacity
Salivary protein content	Low: mucin mainly	High: type of protein varies based on nerve stimuli
Fluid transport	Low	Variable: depends on type of nerve stimuli

Table 24.4 Positive and negative influences on salivary flow rates

Increased Salivary Flow	Decrease Salivary Flow
Nausea	Dehydration
Oral manipulation: duration	Sleep: levels lowest at night
Chewing: duration and force	Stress/anxiety
Tasting: sour vs. sweet	Hemorrhage
Inflammation/infection of oral mucosa	Radiotherapy: head/neck cancer Systemic and local disease

- The duct cells of the major salivary glands, which are impermeable to water, secrete potassium (K^+), bicarbonate (HCO_3^-), and reabsorb sodium (Na^+) and chloride (Cl^-) ions from the primary saliva. The modification in the ionic composition creates an alkaline-rich solution that is slightly hypotonic relative to plasma.
    - This bicarbonate-rich saliva serves to neutralize the acids produced by oral bacteria, facilitate gustatory activity, and aid in protecting the teeth and mucosa.
- Approximately 600 to 1,000 mL of saliva is produced daily from the combined secretions of the major and minor glands.
- The collective contribution of primary saliva from each gland, along with desquamated oral epithelial cells, white blood cells, and microorganisms from the oral cavity, constitutes **whole saliva (oral fluid)**.
    - The volume and composition of whole saliva vary based on circadian secretion patterns, neural stimulation, and flow rates. Diseases and medication, which alter flow rates, or modify neural input, may also alter the volume and composition of salivary secretions.

24.3.2 Salivary Flow Rates

- Salivary secretion occurs in the absence and presence of external stimuli. Saliva secreted intrinsically is classified as **unstimulated saliva**, whereas saliva produced in response to external input is known as **stimulated saliva**.
- Secretion of primary saliva into the oral cavity occurs continuously, at low levels, without exogenous stimuli through the process of **constitutive exocytosis**.
    - The **basal** or **resting rate** of constitutive exocytosis reflects the **unstimulated flow rate** and varies for each gland. Under resting conditions, unstimulated saliva is hypotonic

relative to plasma and enters the oral cavity at a rate of 0.3 to 0.5 mL/min.
    - Unstimulated saliva serves to protect the teeth and lubricate the oral mucosa in the oral cavity and oropharynx. The sublingual, submandibular, and minor glands contribute significantly to resting levels of salvia.
- **Stimulated flow rates** represent transient surges in salivary flow due to an increase in fluid volume and the stimulated release of salivary proteins through the process of **regulated exocytosis**.
    - **Stimulated flow** occurs in response to **neural stimulation** as part of a salivary reflex and may increase the rate of saliva production and delivery by 10-fold.
    - The volume and composition of saliva secreted is dependent on the intensity and type of stimuli. Stimulated saliva, which enters the oral cavity at a rate of 1.5 to 4 mL/min is more isotonic than unstimulated saliva, contains higher levels of bicarbonate (HCO_3^-), sodium (Na^+), and chloride (Cl^-), and is at a slightly higher pH (6.9–7.3) due to acinar cell stimulation and faster flow rates.
        - The increased levels of salivary proteins and fluid delivered during neural stimulation facilitate taste, chewing, bolus formation, and swallowing.
        - The increased buffering capacity of stimulated saliva serves to counteract the elevated levels of acid produced by oral bacteria during eating and protects against enamel demineralization.
- The relative amount of saliva produced by the major and minor glands varies between stimulated (neural-mediated) and unstimulated (basal/resting) states (▶ Table 24.3).
- Several physiological factors including stress, individual hydration levels, the time of day, duration, and force of mastication, as well as the smell, taste, size, and texture of food may influence flow rates (▶ Table 24.4).
- Changes in the amount of saliva produced may also result from systemic and local diseases, neurological disorders, medication side effects, and salivary gland dysfunction (▶ Table 24.4).

The composition of whole saliva is essential for oral health and serves as an important layer of protection for the oral cavity. Saliva contains numerous antimicrobial components, salivary proteins, electrolytes, and buffering agents that protect the teeth and oral mucosa. A reduction in the quantity of saliva or its biochemical properties may lead to dental caries, erosion, halitosis, abrasive mucosal lesions, candidiasis, and infections. The loss of secretory acinar cells following disease or radiation therapy for head and neck cancer often leads to salivary hypofunction and increases the patient's risk of dental-related issues. Whole saliva is currently used as a diagnostic tool due to the noninvasive approach of collection. Unstimulated and stimulated salvia may be collected by draining methods and expectoration (spitting), respectively, and then analyzed for biological markers. To date, changes in specific biomarkers and bacteria may be detected in saliva and used in the diagnosis of dental caries, periodontal disease, oral cancer, and diabetes.

Dry mouth or **xerostomia** refers to the oral sensation of dryness and is a common symptom frequently associated with salivary gland hypofunction. In general, unstimulated flow rates of less than 0.1 mL/min and a stimulated flow rate of less than 0.7 mL/min suggest salivary gland hypofunction.

Oral dryness compromises the process of chewing, swallowing, and speaking, and over time may lead to diminished taste. Patients with xerostomia may experience discomfort and oral pain while wearing dentures due to the formation of mucosal ulcerations. Additionally, patients may exhibit difficulty in retaining the position of full dentures due to loss of lubrication and adherence of the denture to the mucosal surface. Salivary hypofunction may also lead to increased susceptibility to oral infections, candidiasis, periodontal disease, salivary stone formation, and an increased risk of dental caries, tooth demineralization, and sensitivity.

Several conditions may lead to reduced salivary output including over-the-counter medication, drugs, head and neck radiation, and the autoimmune disease Sjogren's syndrome. Sjogren's syndrome is an autoimmune disease characterized by the formation of autoantibodies against the glandular acinar cells of the lacrimal and salivary glands. A dry mouth and dry eyes are hallmark symptoms; however, the disease is often accompanied by other autoimmune disorders, such as rheumatoid arthritis or lupus.

Salivary hypersecretion, known as **sialorrhea**, is defined as an increased amount of saliva accumulating in the oral cavity and may be attributed to increased production or decreased clearance of saliva. Oral lesions, mild inflammation of oral tissue, dental caries, malocclusion, and side effects from medications may lead to hypersecretion. Patients with Parkinson's disease, cerebral palsy, and macroglossia often exhibit excess salvia and pooling within the oral cavity due to oromotor difficulties in swallowing **(dysphagia)** and salivary clearance. **Ptyalism**, or drooling, is often present as an associated outcome of dysphagia.

24.4 Neural Mediated Salivary Reflex Pathways

Salivary secretion is an innate, neural reflex **(salivary reflex)** induced by afferent (sensory) input and mediated by efferent (motor) output of the parasympathetic and sympathetic nervous system. A simplified path is highlighted below:

- **Afferent stimuli → brainstem salivatory nuclei → efferent ANS →salivary gland target.**
- The neural link between the afferent and efferent paths occurs through several multisynaptic ascending and descending pathways and may be modulated by higher brain centers (▶ Fig. 24.9).

24.4.1 Afferent Input

- Peripheral receptor activation leads to the secretion of large volumes of saliva via several known salivary reflexes including the **gustatory-salivary reflex, masticatory-salivary reflex, oral nociceptive-salivary reflex, olfactory-salivary reflex**, and **esophageal-salivary reflex** (▶ Table 24.5).
- The principal mechanism for inducing a salivary reflex occurs through the direct stimulation of sensory receptors found within the oral cavity.
  - The activation of gustatory, thermal, nociceptive, and tactile receptors, located in the mucosa, tongue, and periodontal ligament, typically produces an increase in salivary flow. Among the types of stimuli, taste and masticatory activity during eating elicit the most significant increases in salivary flow rates above resting levels.
- Salivary reflexes may also occur in the absence of direct oral stimulation. Changes in salivary flow may be induced

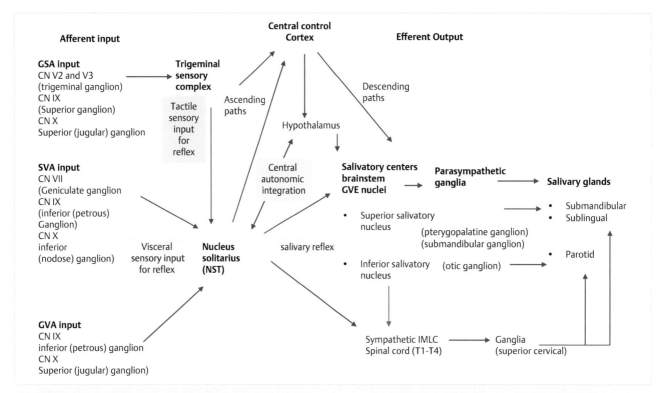

Fig. 24.9 Overview of the salivary gland reflex pathways. Salivary secretion is a neural reflex induced by afferent input and mediated by parasympathetic and sympathetic output. The process involves several ascending and descending pathways and may be modulated by higher brain centers

through odors, visceral input caused by esophageal and gastric distention, acid reflux into the oropharynx, and the sensation of nausea.
- Salivary reflexes are modifiable by central afferent input arising from higher brain centers and include psychogenic influence, such fear or anxiety due to psychological or emotional stress. Salivary reflexes are also subject to input from circadian rhythms.
- **CNs V**, **VII**, **IX**, and **X** transmit somatic, gustatory, and visceral input from peripheral sensory receptors to second-order neurons located in the **trigeminal nuclear complex** and **nucleus solitarius (nucleus tract of solitarius [NTS];** ▶ Fig. 24.10).
  - The NTS, which receives input directly from special visceral afferent (SVA) and general visceral afferent (GVA) receptors and indirectly from the trigeminal nuclear complex, plays a critical role in the modulation and integration of autonomic visceral reflexes.
    - The nucleus solitarius may indirectly influence salivation through ascending fiber projections to higher brain centers.
    - The nucleus solitarius may also project directly to preganglionic parasympathetic and sympathetic neurons found in the cranial nerve brainstem nuclei and IMLC, respectively.

24.4.2 Central Control

- Ascending afferent tracts project to several higher brain centers, which include the following:

- The **primary sensory cortex** for conscious perception and to aid in the coordination of oromotor behaviors involved in salivary clearance through swallowing.
- The cortical **somatosensory association areas** for the integration of visceral sensory input and to determine the size and texture of the stimulus.
- The **gustatory insular cortex** for the processing taste.
- Areas of the **limbic system**, including the **hypothalamus**, **hippocampus**, and **amygdala**, for the integration and modification of afferent stimuli including olfaction.
- Descending tracts project from these higher brain centers to salivatory nuclei in the brainstem and function to coordinate and mediate efferent outflow of the parasympathetic system. Additionally, higher brain centers exert excitatory or inhibitory influences on salivation by coupling to the salivatory centers that control salivary gland secretion.
- Descending pathways originating from the salivatory nuclei control parasympathetic and sympathetic output.

24.4.3 Efferent Outflow

- The efferent component of the salivary reflex path occurs through the cooperative integration of **parasympathetic** and **sympathetic stimulation**.
- Efferent outflow originates from the **salivatory centers** in the brainstem:
  - **preganglionic parasympathetic neurons** in the **superior salivatory (VII)** and **inferior salivatory (IX) nuclei**.

Table 24.5 Afferent stimuli initiating salivary reflex

Stimuli Fiber Type and Receptor	Cranial Nerve	Locus Primary Afferent Neuron	Locus Second-Order Neurons	Ascending Tracts and Termination	Descending Tracts and Targets
Gustatory (taste) **SVA fibers** Originate from gustatory chemoreceptors of taste buds	• Facial (VII): chorda tympani branch to taste buds on anterior two-thirds of the tongue • Glossopharyngeal: lingual-tonsillar branch from the taste buds on the posterior one-third tongue and the circumvallate papillae	• Geniculate (VII) • Inferior (petrosal) ganglion (IX) •	Rostral nucleus solitarius (rNTS) rNTS projects → Gustatory insular cortex, limbic, or salivatory centers	Gustatory insular cortex via thalamus Limbic (amygdala; hippocampus, hypothalamus) Intersects olfactory pathway to modulate salivation Interprets emotional aspects of eating	Cortical input → salivatory nuclei →Salivatory nuclei and IMLC of spinal cord
	• Vagus: internal laryngeal branch of the superior laryngeal nerve (X) from the taste buds on the epiglottis	• Inferior (nodose) ganglion (X)		rNTS → direct reflex to salivatory centers	→Directly to salivatory nuclei center in brainstem and IML of spinal cord
General visceral sensory (GVA) **GVA fibers** Visceral input from mucosa of oropharynx and viscera Originates from: • mechanoreceptors • chemoreceptors • nociceptors	• Facial: chorda tympani nerve from anterior two-thirds of the tongue • Glossopharyngeal: lingual-tonsillar branch to posterior one-third of the tongue and circumvallate papillae • Vagus: internal laryngeal branch of the superior laryngeal nerve (X) to the epiglottis and the root of the tongue • Vagal fibers: esophageal plexus related to swallowing/esophageal distention	• Geniculate ganglion (VII) • Inferior (petrosal) ganglion (IX) • Inferior (nodose) ganglion (X)	Caudal nucleus solitarius (cNTS) cNTS projects →Viscerosensory cortex, salivatory centers, or hypothalamus	Viscerosensory cortex → somatosensory association cortex cNTS → direct reflex to salivatory centers NTS → hypothalamus → reflex centers → Vomiting centers of NTS	→ directly to salivatory nuclei center → salivatory nuclei center
Somatic (GSA) Mechanosensory thermal and nociceptive input due to masticatory activity **GSA fibers** Originate from: • Orosensory pain/temperature • Nociceptors • Thermoreceptors • Orotactile: fine touch/pressure • Mechanoreceptors • Proprioceptors • Proprioception from PDL	Trigeminal V2/V3: • lingual branch of V3 oral mucosa anterior two-thirds of the tongue/floor of the mouth • Inferior alveolar V3 branch: mandibular dental arch of the teeth • Palatal branch of V2: hard/soft palate oral mucosa • Superior alveolar branch of the maxillary dental arch	• Trigeminal ganglion • Mesencephalic nucleus (proprioception)	• Trigeminal nuclear complex • Spinal trigeminal (V) nucleus (pain/temperature) • Chief sensory (touch/pressure)	Trigeminal nuclear complex → Primary somatosensory cortex and somatosensory association to interpret size and texture of food/item Trigeminal nuclear complexprojects → NTS	→ cortical oromotor areas to coordinate swallowing and chewing Cortical input → salivatory nuclei in the brainstem NTS → salivatory nuclei in the brainstem
	• Lingual-tonsillar branches of the glossopharyngeal nerve from the posterior one-third tongue and oropharynx • Vagus: internal laryngeal branch of the superior laryngeal nerve (X) from the epiglottis; laryngopharynx	• Superior ganglion of (IX) • Superior (jugular) ganglion (X)	Spinal trigeminal nucleus (V)	Spinal trigeminal nucleus and chief sensory projects → NTS	NTS → salivatory nuclei in the brainstem

Abbreviations: NTS, nucleus tract of solitarius; IMLC, intermediolateral cell column; PDL, periodontal ligament; SVA, special visceral afferent.

○ **preganglionic sympathetic neurons** in the **IMLC** in the **lateral horn of the spinal cord** at the upper thoracic levels (T1–T4).

• Preganglionic axons synapse with neurons in the peripheral autonomic ganglia, which then send postganglionic parasympathetic and sympathetic fibers to provide secretomotor innervation to the secretory acinar cells and duct cells of the major and minor salivary glands.

○ In general, the GVE fibers originating from superior salivatory nucleus follow CN VII and provide secretomotor activity to all major and minor salivary glands, except the parotid, minor buccal, and minor posterior lingual glands. The inferior salivatory nucleus provides GVE innervation to parotid and buccal glands through branches of the glossopharyngeal nerve (CN IX).

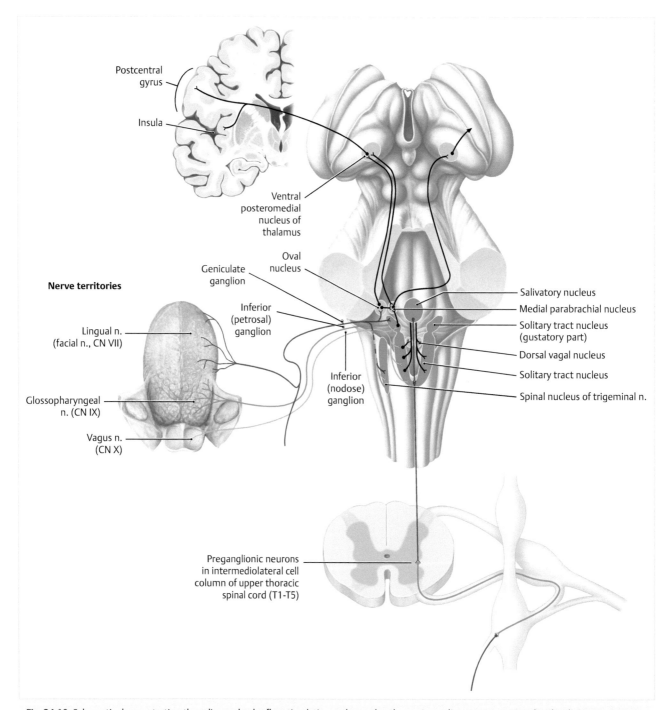

Fig. 24.10 Schematic demonstrating the salivary gland reflex stimulation and neural pathway. Ascending tracts associated with salivary input project to several higher brain centers including the somatosensory cortex, gustatory insular cortex, and parts of the limbic system. (Modified with permission from Gilroy AM, MacPherson BR, Ross LM. Atlas of Anatomy. Second Edition. © Thieme 2012. Illustrations by Markus Voll and Karl Wesker.)

- Specific efferent pathways for the major and minor pathways are outlined in ▸ Table 24.6, ▸ Table 24.7, ▸ Table 24.8 and shown in ▸ Fig. 24.11, ▸ Fig. 24.12, ▸ Fig. 24.13.

24.4.4 Neurotransmitter Release

- Parasympathetic and sympathetic stimulation of salivary gland secretion occurs through the release and binding of **neurotransmitters** to specific receptors expressed on salivary acinar and duct cells (▸ Fig. 24.8).
  - All **preganglionic parasympathetic** and **sympathetic neurons** release **acetylcholine**, which binds to **nicotinic receptors** on **postganglionic cells**, causing membrane depolarization and excitation of postsynaptic neurons (see chapter 18 for review).

- All **postganglionic parasympathetic neurons** are **cholinergic** and release the neurotransmitter **acetylcholine**. Depending on the organ system, acetylcholine binds to nicotinic or muscarinic receptors (see chapter 18 for review).
  - In salivary glands, **acetylcholine** binds to specific **muscarinic receptor subtypes** found on the surface of the acinar and duct cells.
  - Most **postganglionic sympathetic neurons**, including those which innervate salivary glands, are **adrenergic neurons** that release **norepinephrine**.
    – In salivary glands, norepinephrine may bind to β_1 **adrenergic receptors** or α_1 **adrenergic receptors**.
- The binding of cholinergic and adrenergic neurotransmitters to specific receptors activates second messenger cascades

Table 24.6 Efferent parasympathetic outflow from superior salivatory nucleus

General visceral efferent (GVE) nuclei	Path of preganglionic fibers	Autonomic ganglion	Path of postganglionic fibers	Target glands
• The **superior salivatory nucleus** contains the cell bodies of the GVE preganglionic parasympathetic neurons associated with the **facial nerve (CN VII)**	• Preganglionic parasympathetic axons emerge from the brainstem via the **nervus intermedius** (sensory root facial nerve [CN VII]) and travel with: ○ **Greater petrosal branch of VII** ○ **chorda tympani branch of VII**	• **Greater petrosal** fibers join the **nerve of the pterygoid canal** and then synapse on the postganglionic neurons in the **pterygopalatine (sphenopalatine) ganglion** located in the pterygopalatine fossa	• Secretomotor fibers of the postganglionic neurons travel with the **greater** and **lesser palatine nerve**s of the maxillary (V2) division through the greater palatine canal to supply secretomotor innervation to nasal and **minor palatal glands**	**Minor glands:** Postganglionic fibers carried by the palatine nerves terminate on: • Palatal glands • Glossopalatine glands
		• The **chorda tympani nerve** of VII transmits the GVE and SVA fibers and joins the **lingual branch of the mandibular (V3) division** of the **trigeminal** nerve in the infratemporal fossa • The GVE fibers from the chorda tympani synapse with the postganglionic parasympathetic neurons in the **submandibular ganglion**	• Secretomotor fibers of the postganglionic neurons accompany the **lingual branch** of the mandibular (V3) division of the **trigeminal nerve**	**Major gland** Postganglionic fibers travel with lingual nerve: • Submandibular • Sublingual **Minor glands**[a] Postganglionic fibers travel with the lingual nerve, which innervate the: • labial salivary glands • anterior lingual glands

[a]Secretomotor (GVE) fibers to minor glands modulates constitutive secretion.

Table 24.7 Efferent parasympathetic outflow from inferior salivatory nucleus

Nuclei	Path of Preganglionic Fibers	Autonomic Ganglion	Path of Postganglionic Fibers	Target Glands
• The **inferior salivatory nucleus** found in the medulla contains the cell bodies of the **preganglionic parasympathetic neurons** (GVE) associated with **glossopharyngeal nerve (CN IX)**	• Preganglionic parasympathetic fibers emerging from the inferior salivatory nucleus travels with the **glossopharyngeal nerve (IX)**, which exits the jugular foramen to give rise to the **tympanic nerve** and the **tympanic plexus**	• Preganglionic fibers pass through the plexus to form the **lesser petrosal** nerve and synapse on postganglionic parasympathetic cell bodies in the **otic ganglion**	• Secretomotor fiber of postganglionic neurons travel with the **auriculotemporal branch** of the **mandibular (V3) division** of the **trigeminal nerve**	**Major gland:** • Parotid **Minor glands:** • Lingual (von Ebner's gland/ posterior one-third) • Buccal

Abbreviation: GVE, general visceral efferent.
Note: Secretomotor (GVE) fibers to minor glands modulates constitutive secretion.

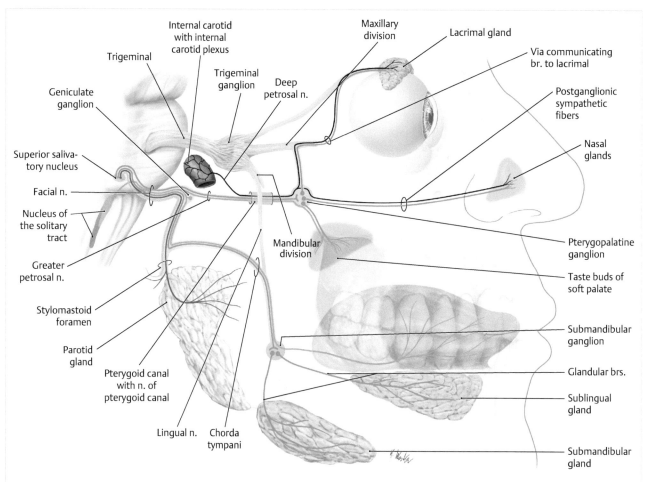

Two paths of GVE fibers from superior salivatory nucleus:
Superior salivatory nucleus → Greater petrosal of VII → nerve of pterygoid canal → synapse in pterygopalatine ganglion in the pterygopalatine fossa → target glands (palatal and glossopalatine glands) via greater and lesser palatine N of V2

Superior salivatory nucleus of VII → chorda tympani of VII → synapse in submandibular ganglion in floor of oral cavity → target glands (submandibular, sublingual, labial, and anterior lingual glands) via lingual N of V3

Fig. 24.11 Schematic of the general visceral efferent pathway of the facial nerve. The visceral motor (parasympathetic) is shown as *black fibers*. Preganglionic fibers originate from the superior salivatory nucleus. Postganglionic parasympathetic and sympathetic fibers follow branches of maxillary (CN V2) and mandibular (CN V3) nerves to reach their target organs. (Reproduced with permission from Schuenke M, Schulte E, Schumacher U. THIEME Atlas of Anatomy Third Edition, Vol 3. © Thieme 2020. Illustrations by Markus Voll and Karl Wesker.)

Table 24.8 Efferent outflow: sympathetic fiber path of salivary glands

Nuclei	Path of Preganglionic Fibers	Autonomic Ganglion	Path of Postganglionic Fibers	Target Glands
• Intermediolateral cell column (IMLC) of the spinal cord at T1–T4	• Enter the sympathetic trunk • Ascend to the superior cervical ganglion	• Preganglionic sympathetic fibers synapse in the **superior cervical ganglion (C2)**	• Follow the internal carotid artery plexus → to deep petrosal nerve → nerve of pterygoid canal → pterygopalatine ganglion[a] → maxillary (V2) branch • Follow the branch of the facial arterial plexus • Follow the branch of the external carotid artery plexus to gland	• Minor palatal salivary • Submandibular sublingual • Minor labial and anterior lingual • Parotid • Minor buccal and posterior lingual/von Ebner's gland

Note: Postganglionic fibers pass without synapse and continues with greater and lesser palatine branches of maxillary V2 branch.

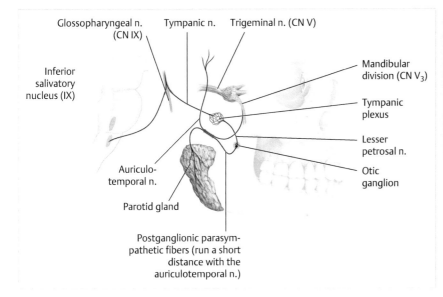

Fig. 24.12 Schematic of the general visceral efferent pathway of the glossopharyngeal nerve. Preganglionic fibers arise from inferior salivatory nucleus. Postganglionic parasympathetic and sympathetic fibers follow the auriculotemporal branch of the mandibular (CN V3) nerves to reach their target organs. (Reproduced with permission from Schuenke M, Schulte E, Schumacher U. THIEME Atlas of Anatomy Third Edition, Vol 3. © Thieme 2020. Illustrations by Markus Voll and Karl Wesker.)

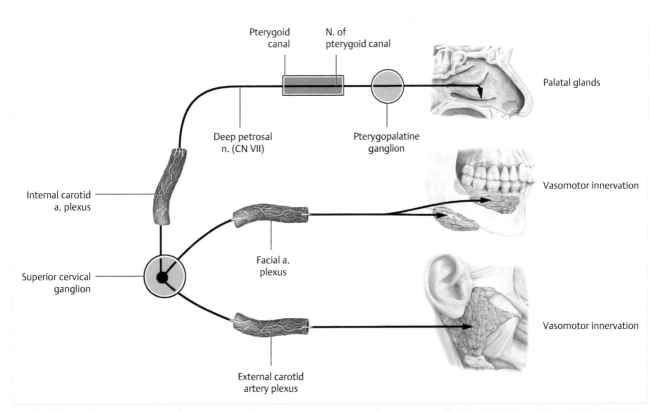

Fig. 24.13 Schematic demonstrating the path of sympathetic innervation to the salivary glands. Preganglionic sympathetic fibers originate from the intermediolateral cell column in the lateral horn of the spinal cord and synapse in the superior cervical ganglion. Postganglionic sympathetic fibers follow arterial plexuses and are distributed along the same path as parasympathetic fibers to target organs. (Reproduced with permission from Schuenke M, Schulte E, Schumacher U. THIEME Atlas of Anatomy Third Edition, Vol 3. © Thieme 2020. Illustrations by Markus Voll and Karl Wesker.)

Table 24.9 Impact of neurotransmitter binding

Type of ANS Neuron	Neurotransmitter	Receptor	Second Messenger System and Effect	Outcome on Gland	Effect on Flow Rate	Effect on Saliva Composition
Postganglionic parasympathetic (cholinergic neuron)	Acetylcholine	Muscarinic (M_1)	PLC/IP3 increase → elevated Ca^{2+}	Open water channels in acinar cell Electrolyte transport acinar and duct cells Some protein exocytosis	Increase release from acinar cells and increase flow rate through duct Increased flow rate leads to increased volume of release	Thin, watery secretion; low-viscosity protein content Increased flow rate may result in isotonic saliva due to limited ion transport occurring in duct
		Muscarinic (M_3)	PLC/IP3 increase → elevated Ca^{2+}			
Postganglionic sympathetic (adrenergic neurons)	Norepinephrine	β_1	cAMP induces elevated Ca^{2+}	Regulated exocytosis of acinar cell proteins	Negligible change in flow rate	Low fluid; Thick viscous saliva; Enzyme rich
	Norepinephrine	α_1	PLC/IP3 increase → elevated Ca^{2+}	Open water channels in acinar cell Electrolyte transport acinar and duct cells	Increased flow rate leads to increased volume of release	Thin, watery secretion; lower-viscosity protein content Increased flow rate may result in isotonic saliva due to limited ion transport occurring in duct

Abbreviations: cAMP, cyclic adenosine monophosphate; IP3, inositol triphosphate; PLC, phospholipase C.
Note: Most exocrine protein secretion occurs in response to β adrenergic activation, whereas fluid secretion follows muscarinic activation. Sympathetic stimulation works cooperatively with parasympathetic stimulation and has a synergistic effect.

that result in the subsequent elevation of intracellular Ca^{2+}. Elevation of Ca^{2+} stimulates electrolyte transport involved in fluid secretion and regulated exocytosis of salivary proteins (▶ Table 24.9).

- In general, the release of **acetylcholine** from **postganglionic parasympathetic nerve fibers** results in fluid secretion and active transport of electrolytes.
- **Sympathetic nerve fibers** release **norepinephrine** to activate **β_1-adrenergic receptors** leading to exocytosis of protein and a small-volume response.
- **Norepinephrine** released from **postganglionic sympathetic fibers** may also stimulate fluid secretion through activation of **α_1-adrenergic receptors**.
- Hormonal and other noncholinergic and nonadrenergic stimuli may also stimulate or modulate salivary secretion (▶ Fig. 24.14).
  - Additionally, noncholinergic and nonadrenergic stimuli act on capillary beds associated with acinar cells to cause vasoconstriction and vasodilation.
  - Blood flow to the capillaries surrounding the acinar units impacts the amount of saliva produced. In general, increased blood flow correlates with an increase in salivation.

24.4.5 Outcomes of Salivary Gland Stimulation

- The parasympathetic and sympathetic innervation mediates **regulated exocytosis** of saliva from acinar cells and regulates the amount of ion and fluid transport in the duct cells by influencing the flow rate of **major salivary glands**.
- **Minor salivary glands** release saliva continuously without exogenous stimuli. Parasympathetic and sympathetic secretomotor (GVE) fibers supply the minor glands and modulate the **constitutive** release of salivary proteins.
- **Salivary gland stimulation leads to:**
  - Increased release of salivary proteins via regulated exocytosis.
  - Increased fluid and ion transport from acinar cells.
  - Increased flow rates through ducts and increased volume delivery to the oral cavity.
- Salivary composition depends on the flow rate, type of nerve stimulated, frequency of nerve firing, type of neurotransmitter released, and physiological status of the individual including factors such as hydration levels, stress, and medication use.

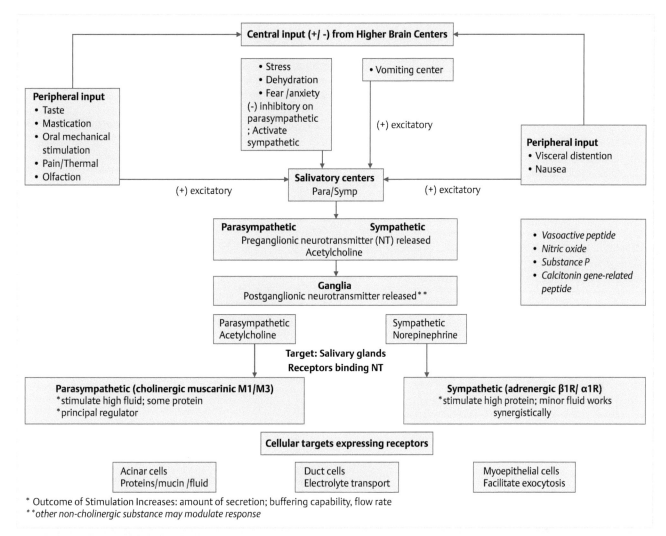

Fig. 24.14 Summary of the neural pathway control of salivation.

Control of salivary gland secretion occurs through the autonomic nervous system (ANS) and therefore salivary gland function may be modulated by a variety of drugs. Clinically, prescription and over-the-counter medications prescribed for other conditions may alter salivary gland flow and composition as an unwanted side effect. In general, drugs that target the parasympathetic or sympathetic system alter salivary secretion by disrupting neural mediated salivary reflex pathways. Prescribed medications, if they can pass through the blood–brain barrier, may act on premotor autonomic neurons in higher brain centers or on preganglionic brain stem nuclei. Other drugs may exert local effects at postganglionic neurons within the ganglion, act on receptors on the postsynaptic membrane, or modulate neurotransmitter release. Additionally, drugs that act as vasoconstrictors will decrease salivary outflow due to changes in blood flow to the acinar cell. Drugs that have anticholinergic action (antidepressants, anxiolytics, antipsychotics, antihistamines, and antihypertensives) may cause a reduction in salivary flow rate and alter saliva composition. Drugs with sympathomimetic properties act on beta-receptors to stimulate the production of thick viscous saliva, with little fluid production. Alternatively, a muscarinic agonist, such as pilocarpine, may bind to neurotransmitter receptors to induce an increase in salivary flow (**sialorrhea**). Pilocarpine is prescribed for some patients with Sjogren's disease or following head and neck radiation therapy due to its effect of increasing salivation.

Clinical Correlation Box 24.10: Salivary Flow and Dental Procedures

Peripheral and central inputs trigger neural mediated salivary reflexes associated with alterations in salivary flow rates and composition. Understanding potential causes for modifications in salivary flow rates should be considered during dental treatment planning and procedures. Peripheral input such as direct mechanical manipulation in and around the mouth during dental procedures stimulates salivary flow rates and should be considered when taking impressions for dental prosthesis, fitting dentures, and performing restorations. Patients suffering from neurological disorders such as Parkinson's disease and cerebral palsy may exhibit excessive salivation (**sialorrhea**) due to impaired swallowing, whereas elderly patients or those taking certain medications, as well as those patients who experience dental-related anxiety, may exhibit oral dryness that may impact dental procedures.

Questions and Answers

1. Your 45-year-old patient complains of an ipsilateral loss of taste, diminished salivary flow, and loss of sensation in the anterior two-thirds of the tongue. Your patient does not exhibit any facial droop and her corneal reflex is still intact. You suspect nerve damage following a recent surgery. Which of the following is the most likely structure damaged?
   a) Inferior salivatory nucleus.
   b) Chorda tympani.
   c) Lingual nerve.
   d) Facial nerve.

Level 2: Moderate.

Answer (C): The lingual nerve of V3 is most likely damaged given the symptoms involving loss of taste *and* loss of sensation to the ipsilateral tongue. The lingual nerve provides only general somatic afferent (GSA) sensation to the anterior two-thirds of the tongue; however, the postganglionic fibers of the chorda tympani (CN VII) accompany the lingual nerve to the anterior part of the tongue. The chorda tympani nerve **(B)** transmits both taste (special visceral afferent [SVA]) and secretomotor fibers (general visceral efferent [GVE]), but not GSA. A loss of only taste and secretion would suggest damage to the chorda tympani nerve. The point of damage to the chorda tympani would most likely occur in the facial canal, or during its course through the tympanic cavity or the infratemporal fossa, proximal to where it joins the lingual nerve. Damage to the chorda tympani nerve in the facial canal would most likely result in concomitant damage to the facial nerve **(D)**. Damage to the facial nerve would lead to complete ipsilateral facial paralysis, including a loss of the efferent limb of the corneal reflex. The patient is not exhibiting signs of facial nerve damage. Damage to the facial nerve, distal to where the chorda tympani branches from the facial nerve, would spare taste and secretomotor function and only impact motor function. The inferior salivatory nucleus **(A)** is not involved. It contains the preganglionic GVE parasympathetic neurons for glossophar-

yngeal nerve (CN IX), not CN VII. The superior salivary nucleus contains the preganglionic cell bodies of CN VII. Damage to the superior salivatory nucleus would produce a greater loss of salivation along with ipsilateral corneal dryness due to the accompanying loss of lacrimation.

2. Which of the following is **CORRECT** regarding striated ducts?
   a) Ions are actively transported from the duct lumen.
   b) Striated ducts are also classified as interlobular ducts.
   c) Primary saliva is synthesized by striated ducts.
   d) Water resorption occurs in the striated ducts.

Level 1: Easy

Answer (A): All other answers are incorrect. **(B)** The striated duct is found within the lobule, so it is considered an intralobular duct. Interlobular ducts are the larger collecting ducts that receive saliva from the striated ducts. **(C)** Primary saliva is synthesized by the acinar cell, not by a striated duct. **(D)** The striated duct modifies the saliva by removing ions, but because the duct is impermeable to water, the resulting saliva is hypotonic. The slower the flow rate, the more ions may be transported from the duct. A faster flow rate will result in a more isotonic solution due to the decreased time for transport.

3. Parasympathetic nerve fibers innervating the sublingual gland will _____.
   a) synapse in the otic ganglion
   b) release the neurotransmitter norepinephrine
   c) decrease salivary fluid volume
   d) activate water and electrolyte secretion from the acinar cells

Level 2: Moderate

Answer (D): Parasympathetic fibers when stimulated will release acetylcholine, which leads to water and electrolyte secretions from the acinar cell. **(A)** The parasympathetic fibers of the sublingual gland synapse in the submandibular ganglion, not the otic ganglion. Parasympathetic fibers from the glossopharyngeal nerve synapse in the otic ganglion and innervate the parotid gland. **(B)** Sympathetic fibers release norepinephrine, whereas parasympathetic release acetylcholine. Sympathetic stimulation usually results in a thick viscous solution with little fluid volume **(C)**.

4. Within the last 2 hours, your patient has taken an antihistamine and is now complaining of a "dry mouth" and decreased saliva production. Based on this information, which of the following receptors is most likely blocked?
   a) β-adrenergic.
   b) nicotinic.
   c) α-adrenergic.
   d) muscarinic.

Level 2: Moderate

Answer (D): Muscarinic receptors (subtypes M1 and M3) are classified as cholinergic receptors and respond to parasympathetic stimulation that results from acetylcholine binding to the muscarinic receptor. The β-adrenergic **(A)** and α-adrenergic receptors **(C)** mediate sympathetic stimulation via norepinephrine **(A and C)**. Nicotinic receptors **(B)** are found on postganglionic neurons in the ganglion associated with the salivary glands, but they are not found on acinar cells. Because the receptors are only found in the salivary ganglion, they are indirectly involved in the stimulation of the acinar cell. Acetylcholine is the neurotransmitter that binds to nicotinic receptors in the ganglion, and stimulation of the nicotinic receptor in the ganglion will lead to postganglionic parasympathetic and sympathetic activation. Postganglionic fibers will elicit a response in the peripheral tissue when they release a neurotransmitter, and it binds to an appropriate receptor. The postganglionic fibers of the salivary gland release acetylcholine or norepinephrine. Antihistamines are considered antagonists to parasympathetic function and classified as an anticholinergic. Antihistamines may bind to both histamine receptors and muscarinic receptors. Because of their ability to also bind to muscarinic receptors, the use of antihistamines in the treatment of allergies often results in the unwanted side effect of decreased fluid and salivary flow. The action of the antihistamine may act as an antagonistic and bind to muscarinic m1 and M3 subtypes to block parasympathetic activity.

5. Each of the following outcomes may occur if the diminished flow rate continues EXCEPT one. Which one is the exception?
a) Increase in dental caries.
b) Decrease in salivary pH.
c) Decrease in mucosal inflammation.
d) Increase in Na^+ resorption by the duct cells.

Level 2: Moderate
Answer (C). A decrease in mucosal inflammation is the exception. Mucosal inflammation and possible infection will increase as an outcome of a decreased flow rate due to the loss of lubrication, buffering, and immunoprotection. At a slower flow rate, there is a decrease in salivary pH (**B**) and a decreased buffering capacity, due to the decrease in bicarbonate secretion from the acinar cells. The change in pH can lead to an increase in dental caries (**A**). Diminished flow rates also lead to an increase in Na^+ resorption by the duct cells (**D**).

25 Teeth

25.1 Anatomical and Structural Components of Teeth

Knowledge of the specific distribution of the nerves supplying the dental arches and oral cavity is important for understanding the basis of orofacial pain, assessing nerve damage of the oral tissues, and determining the appropriate nerve to anesthetize for different dental procedures. The following chapter describes the anatomical and structural components of the teeth along with the innervation to the pulp and periodontium. The trigeminal pathway for pain, temperature, mechanosensory, and proprioceptive input is briefly reviewed. A detailed description of central trigeminal pathways is covered in Chapter 13.

25.1.1 Overview of Teeth and Dental Arch

- Humans have two sets of teeth: the primary (**deciduous**) dentition and secondary (**permanent; succedaneous**) dentition.
  - A total of 20 deciduous teeth develop prenatally within the bony sockets (**alveoli**) of the mandibular and maxillary dental arches. The eruption of the primary teeth begins postnatally in the sixth month and is complete by 3 years of age.
  - The complete primary dentition consists of 10 teeth in each dental arch, with each side of the arch (quadrant) containing 3 basic tooth forms: **2 incisiform (incisors), 1 caniniform (canines), and 2 molariform (molars)**. The incisors, canines, and molars function in biting, tearing, and grinding, respectively.
  - The primary teeth that function between ages 2 through 6 years are gradually shed (**exfoliated**) and replaced by the permanent teeth between 6 and 12 years of age (▶ Fig. 25.1).

- The complete permanent dentition contains 32 teeth in total, with 16 in each jaw. The teeth are sequentially numbered, 1 to 32, in a clockwise direction, beginning with the upper right third maxillary molar as tooth 1 and continuing to the lower right third mandibular as tooth 32 (▶ Fig. 25.2).

- Each quadrant contains a similar arrangement of the incisors, canines, and molars as the primary dentition with two notable exceptions (▶ Fig. 25.3).
  - Each half of the maxillary and mandibular dental arch contains two **premolar (bicuspids)** teeth that function in piercing foods. The premolars are unique to the permanent dentition and replace the two deciduous molars.
  - There are three permanent molars in each quadrant. The permanent molars are considered accessional teeth that lack deciduous predecessors and develop distal to the primary dentition.

- For reference, several terms are used to describe the external surface of the tooth and the regions of the tooth relative to the arch (▶ Fig. 25.4 and ▶ Table 25.1).

25.1.2 Anatomical and Structural Components of the Tooth

- All teeth consist of two anatomical regions, a **crown** and **root**, and are anchored similarly within the dental arch by the supportive structures of the **periodontium** (▶ Fig. 25.5; ▶ Table 25.2 and ▶ Table 25.3).

- The **crown** is the portion of the tooth visible in the oral cavity and may be subdivided into three regions: an **incisal one-third (anterior teeth)** or **occlusal one-third (posterior teeth)**, a **middle one-third**, and a **cervical one-third**.
  - **Enamel**, a highly mineralized layer comprised of tightly packed, inorganic hydroxyapatite crystals, covers and protects the external surface of the crown.

- The **root** lies below the oral surface, within a bony socket (alveolus) of the maxillary and mandibular jawbones. The root also contains three subdivisions, the **cervix**, the **body**, and the **root apex**.
  - **Cementum**, a mineralized layer similar in composition to bone tissue, covers the external surface of the root.

- The **cervix (neck)** of the tooth refers to the junction between the crown and the root of the tooth. The body of the tooth contains **dentin**, a mineralized tissue layer composed of numerous fluid-filled **dentinal tubules**. Dentin provides structural support to the overlying enamel and cementum and surrounds the pulp cavity.

- The mineralized regions of the crown and the root surround and protect an inner core of richly innervated and well-vascularized loose connective tissue (CT), known as the **dental pulp**. The pulp tissue extends from the crown to the root and resides within an anatomical space known as the **pulp chamber** and **root canal**, respectively.

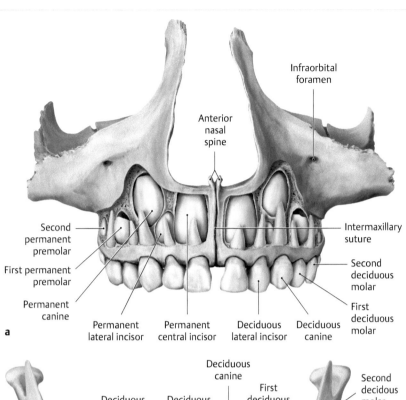

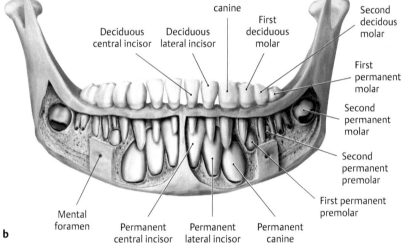

Fig. 25.1 Deciduous and permanent teeth of a 6-year-old child. The anterior bone was removed above the roots of deciduous teeth. Frontal view of the **(a)** maxillary and **(b)** mandibular arch illustrating the erupted deciduous teeth and the position of the developing crowns of the anterior permanent teeth and permanent premolars. The permanent incisors and canines are positioned palatal and lingual to the primary teeth. Note the crowns of the two permanent premolars in both arches are visible in the mandibular arch between the roots of the primary molars. By 6 years of age, all deciduous teeth have erupted and are present, along with the first permanent tooth, the first permanent molar. Note the erupted permanent mandibular molar (6-year molar) with a portion of the root developed is visible. Root formation continues after tooth eruption and growth of the jaw. (Reproduced with permission from Schuenke M, Schulte E, Schumacher U. THIEME Atlas of Anatomy. Second Edition, Vol 3. © Thieme 2016. Illustrations by Markus Voll and Karl Wesker.)

Fig. 25.2 Universal numbering system of adult teeth; numbering shown from the perspective of the viewer. The universal numbering system is commonly used in the United States to designate the position of the permanent teeth within the dental arch. Teeth in both arches are numbered sequentially, 1 to 32, in a clockwise direction, beginning with the upper right maxillary third molar as number 1 and continuing to the left maxillary molar (tooth 16). The numbering of the lower arch continues clockwise from 17 to 32. (Reproduced with permission from Schuenke M, Schulte E, Schumacher U. THIEME Atlas of Anatomy. Second Edition, Vol 3. © Thieme 2016. Illustrations by Markus Voll and Karl Wesker.)

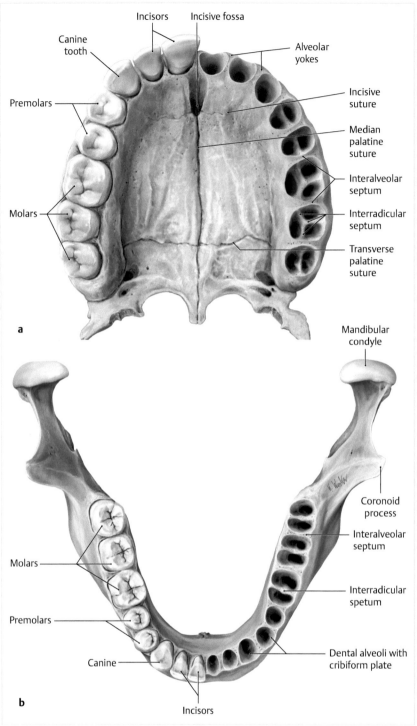

Fig. 25.3 Arrangement of permanent teeth within the maxillary (upper) and mandibular (lower) dental arches. **(a)** Inferior view of the maxilla. **(b)** Superior view of the mandible. Chewing surfaces are shown on the right side. Each arch contains 16 teeth arranged bilateral and symmetrical within two quadrants. Each quadrant contains 2 incisors, 1 canine, 2 premolars, and 3 molars. The alveolar process after removal of teeth can be seen on the left side. Support for the tooth is provided by the periodontal ligament and the components of the alveolar process, which include an outer cortical plate, intervening spongy bone, and the alveolar bone proper, which lines the dental alveoli (tooth sockets). The interalveolar septum lies between the adjacent alveoli, and an inter-radicular septum is present in the alveoli anchoring multirooted teeth. (Reproduced with permission from Schuenke M, Schulte E, Schumacher U. THIEME Atlas of Anatomy. Second Edition, Vol 3. © Thieme 2016. Illustrations by Markus Voll and Karl Wesker.)

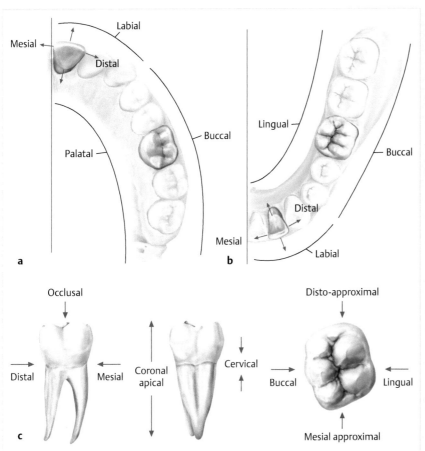

Fig. 25.4 Designation of tooth surfaces and directions of the dental arches. **(a)** Inferior view of the maxillary dental arch. **(b)** Superior view of the mandibular dental arch. Buccal, distal, and occlusal views of the left mandibular first molar (tooth 19). **(c)** The coronal, apical, and cervical directions of a tooth and the approximal surfaces, which contact, or face, the adjacent teeth are also depicted. These designations are used to describe the precise location of small carious lesions. (Reproduced with permission from Schuenke M, Schulte E, Schumacher U. THIEME Atlas of Anatomy Third Edition, Vol 3. © Thieme 2020. Illustrations by Markus Voll and Karl Wesker.)

Table 25.1 Surfaces of tooth and regions of dental arch

Surface of tooth within jaw	Description of region
Occlusal	Part of tooth that is in contact with tooth of the opposite jaw; serves as the chewing/grinding surface In proper occlusion, every tooth contacts two opposing teeth Teeth are offset from each other so that the cusp of one posterior tooth fits into the fissures of the two opposing teeth
Incisal	The cutting edge of the anterior teeth
Lingual	Tooth surface adjacent or closest to the tongue
Palatal	Region adjacent to the palate of the maxillary arch
Buccal	Adjacent closest to the cheek (vestibule); term used for posterior teeth (premolar and molars)
Labial/facial	Adjacent or closest to the mucosal surface of the lip used for anterior teeth (canines and incisors)
Distal and mesial	Side of the adjacent teeth within the same jaw The mesial surface of the tooth is oriented anteriorly toward the midline of the arch; distal surface is farthest from the midline of the arch

Table 25.2 Summary of anatomical regions of the tooth

Anatomical regions of tooth	
Crown	**Anatomic crown:** portion of the tooth covered by enamel; extends from the occlusal or incisal surface to the cervix of the tooth: • Divided into three regions: incisal one-third (anterior) or occlusal one-third (posterior), middle one-third, and cervical one-third **Clinical crown:** portion of the crown that is visible in the oral cavity
Root	**Clinical root:** portion of the tooth that lies below the oral surface, within a bony socket (alveolus) of the maxillary and mandibular jaw bones **Anatomic root:** the portion of the tooth covered externally with cementum: • Divided into three regions: the cervix, the body, and the root apex • **Apical foramen** located at the root apex transmits the neurovascular structures into pulp cavity; forms open communication between pulp cavity and periodontal connective tissue
Cervix (cervical line)	Represents the anatomical boundary between the crown and the root Cervical line demarcates the **cementoenamel junction (CEJ)**, a point where the enamel and the cementum meet. Areas in the tooth cervix may be devoid of cementum, resulting in the exposure of the underlying dentin and may cause dentin sensitivity, and increased risk of caries

Table 25.3 Structural components of the tooth

Structural components: external coverings of the tooth	
Enamel	• Hardest mineralized tissue in body covers the external surface of tooth crown • Thin, translucent layer comprised of 95% inorganic hydroxyapatite crystals; crystals arranged parallel to each other and perpendicular to tooth surface • Produced during crown stage of tooth development prior to tooth eruption • Cellular layer of formative ameloblast cells which synthesize enamel degenerate following crown formation • Devoid of neurovascular and cellular structures • Enamel is incapable of repair • Remineralization possible due to ionic composition and buffering capacity of saliva
Cementum	• Mineralized tissue covering the external surface of the root • Principal function is to connect the alveolar bone with tooth via the gingival and periodontal ligament • Similar in composition to bone tissue; comprised of (45–55%) inorganic hydroxyapatite crystals • Produced initially during root formation (prefunctional eruption); continued deposition over life of tooth to maintain tooth position; cellular layer of formative **cementoblasts** that lines the external root surface • Devoid of neurovascular structures • Limited repair; no remodeling

Structural components: body of the tooth	
Dentin	• Mineralized layer of tissue that forms the bulk of the tooth; provides structural support to the overlaying enamel and cementum • Surrounds and protects the centrally located pulp tissue; defines the boundary of pulp cavity • Dentin production starts in the crown stage, continues throughout the life of the tooth; a cellular layer of formative **odontoblasts** remains along the pulpal border throughout the life of the tooth and contributes to the dentin–pulp complex • Comprised of 70% inorganic hydroxyapatite crystals; characterized by numerous fluid-filled **dentinal tubules** that run through the entire thickness of the dentin • Dentinal tubules contain dentinal fluid and the cellular part of odontoblast known as the odontoblastic process. Aδ afferent nerve fibers extend into the initial portion of the dentin tubules • Odontoblasts may deposit dentin in response to dental caries or other potentially damaging insult to the pulp • Exposed dentin caused by loss of the overlying enamel or cementum leads to dentin sensitivity

Pulp cavity	• Central space of the tooth containing neurovascular loose connective tissue (CT) known as dental pulp tissue
	• Pulp follows the contour of tooth and consists of two regions: a **pulp chamber** located in the crown and a **root (pulp) canal** located in the root
	  ○ Areas of pulp tissue within pulp chamber extend into cusps to form **pulp horns**
	  ○ The number of root (pulp) canals varies based on tooth type
	  ○ **Apical foramen** is the distal opening of pulp cavity at the root apex; permits passage of neurovascular structures from the periodontium to the pulp

Dental pulp	• Neurovascular loose CT) required to maintain vitality of the tooth; fibroblasts are the primary cell type; pulpal stem cells present; odontoblasts present in the periphery of the pulp and comprise the pulpal border • Pulp tissue in the region of the crown or the pulp chamber is known as the coronal pulp; pulp tissue in the root or root canal is known as the radicular pulp • Intradental nerve fibers include myelinated low-threshold mechanoreceptors (type IIAβ, and type IIIAδ fibers), nociceptors (myelinated type IIIAδ fibers and unmyelinated type IVC fibers), postganglionic unmyelinated sympathetic C fibers • Communicates with the periodontal ligament (PDL) in the periodontal space through the apical foramen; potential mechanism for spread of infection

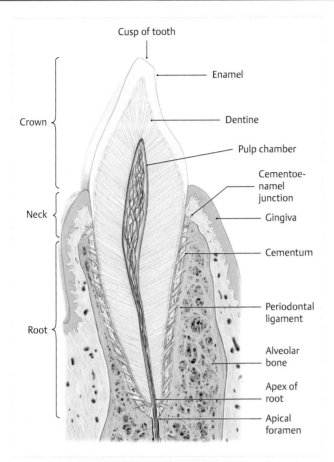

Cusp of tooth

Enamel

Crown

Dentine

Pulp chamber

Cementoe-
namel
junction

Neck

Gingiva

Cementum

Periodontal
ligament

Root

Alveolar
bone

Apex of
root

Apical
foramen

Fig. 25.5 Structures and anatomical regions of the tooth. The longitudinal section of the mandibular incisor. Enamel covers the crown of the tooth from the cusp to the cervix (neck). The cementum covers the external surface of the root and anchors the tooth to the alveolus via the periodontal ligament. The dentin, which supports the overlying enamel and cementum, and surrounds the pulp cavity, forms the body of the tooth. The apical foramen is the opening at the tooth apex that permits the passage of the neurovascular structures from the periodontal tissue to the pulp cavity. (Reproduced with permission from Schuenke M, Schulte E, Schumacher U. THIEME Atlas of Anatomy. Second Edition, Vol 3. © Thieme 2016. Illustrations by Markus Voll and Karl Wesker.)

25.2 Periodontium

The periodontium refers to the tissue that supports the teeth in the upper and lower dental arches. The structures of the periodontium include **cementum**, **periodontal ligament (PDL)**, **alveolar bone**, and **gingiva** (▶ Table 25.4).

25.2.1 Gingiva

- The gingiva, which is comprised primarily of the masticatory mucosa, functions to protect the root surface and alveolar bone from the external environment. Distinct bundles of CT fibers comprise the **dentogingival**, **transseptal**, and **circular fiber groups** that connect the gingiva to the tooth and alveolar bone and hold the gingiva in place.
- The gingiva may be further subdivided into two regions: **free (marginal) gingiva** and **attached gingiva** (▶ Fig. 25.6).

- The **attached gingiva** consists of the masticatory mucosa that is tightly bound to the periosteum of the alveolar bone, whereas the free gingiva forms an unattached cuff around the cervix (neck) of the tooth.
- The **marginal gingiva** is located approximately 1 mm above (coronal) the **cementoenamel junction (CEJ)**.
- The **gingival sulcus** is a space between the medial wall of the free gingiva and the enamel of the tooth. The **sulcular epithelium** lines the gingival sulcus and attaches to the tooth via the **junctional epithelium** at the base of the sulcus. The **junctional epithelium** forms the epithelial attachment between the tooth and gingival tissue and plays a critical role in maintaining oral health.
- The distribution and types of sensory receptors found in the gingiva are comparable to those found in other regions of the oral mucosa. The gingival mucosa contains a high density of mechanoreceptors, thermoreceptors, and nociceptors, which provide afferent feedback concerning gingival displacement, inflammation, and tissue damage.
- Transmission of sensory innervation occurs by the same terminal branches of V2 and V3 that supply the alveolar mucosa and palatal mucosa (▶ Table 25.5 and ▶ Table 25.6).

25.2.2 Periodontal Ligament

- The PDL is dense fibrous CT that occupies the space between the external layer of the cementum covering the root and the compact layer of bone comprising the alveolus (alveolar bone proper; ▶ Fig. 25.7).
- The PDL consists of distinct bundles of CT fibers, known as the **principal (dentoalveolar) fiber groups**, which are embedded within the cementum and extend into the alveolus.
  - Each fiber group is oriented in a specific direction along the root surface to aid in transmitting occlusal loads based on the direction of forces applied to the crown of the tooth.
- Neurovascular structures run between the CT fiber bundles and communicate with the vessels and nerves found in the gingiva, the alveolar bone, and the pulp of adjacent teeth.
- The types of sensory receptors found in the PDL include **interdental nociceptors** and **Ruffini-like, low-threshold mechanoreceptors** (▶ Table 25.5 and ▶ Table 25.6).
  - Typically, when an occlusal force of a certain magnitude is applied to a tooth, the tooth moves in the tooth socket, which induces stress (tension) on the PDL. Depending on tooth position within the arch, the anterior and posterior teeth respond differently to occlusal loads:
    - Anterior teeth are more sensitive at low tooth loads and play a role in performing specific tasks involving the manipulation and holding of food.
    - Posterior teeth respond to higher occlusal loads and provide feedback involved in regulating chewing patterns based on food resistance.
  - The Ruffini-like nerve endings of the PDL are nonencapsulated, low-threshold mechanoreceptors found along the length of PDL that respond to deformation (increased tension/stretch) and exhibit directional sensitivity based on the occlusal forces applied to the crown of the tooth.

Table 25.4 Overview of periodontium

Periodontium	
Periodontal ligament (PDL)	• Dense connective tissue (CT) organized as distinct fiber bundles that are embedded in the cementum matrix and the portion of the alveolar bone forming the osseous tooth socket • Prevents force applied to the tooth from being directly transmitted to the alveolar process • Provides mechanosensory input concerning masticatory bite force, jaw position, along with the direction, intensity, and velocity of the occlusal forces applied to the crown of the tooth. • Comprised primarily of fibroblasts that continually remodel the PDL; abundant neurovascular structures run through the PDL: ○ Interdental nerves fibers and receptors include myelinated type IIAβ (mechanoreceptors) and type IIIAδ (nociceptors) fibers and unmyelinated type IVC (nociceptors) and C (postganglionic sympathetic) fibers
Cementum	• Mineralized tissue covering the external root surface. Cementum matrix embeds bundles of collagen fibers (Sharpey's fibers) of the PDL and anchors the tooth
Alveolar process (alveolus)	• Components of the alveolar process include an **outer cortical plate**, intervening spongy bone, and the **alveolar bone proper (alveolus)**, which is a region of compact bone lining the tooth socket • The alveolus (osseous tooth socket) is the portion of the mandible and maxilla in which the dental roots are embedded. Socket lined with periosteal CT (periosteum) containing neurovascular structures and stem cells • Fibers of the PDL extend from the cementum of the root and insert into the alveolus via **Sharpey's fibers** to anchor the tooth • It contains neurovascular structures that anastomose with PDL, gingiva and pulp • Bone capable of extensive repair and remodeling, and functions to maintain the tooth in the occlusal position • The presence of a tooth is necessary to maintain the alveolar process

Gingiva (gums)	• A region of oral mucosa that surrounds and protects the tooth. Subdivided into an **attached gingiva** and **free gingiva**.
	  ○ Free (marginal) gingiva comprises a 1-mm cuff of unattached tissue surrounding the tooth. The medial surface of the free gingiva is anchored to the cervical enamel through the **junctional epithelium**
	  ○ Attached gingiva binds the underlying alveolar periosteum and supports the crown of the tooth
	• Neurovascular structures similar to PDL; extensive anastomoses with vessels of PDL, and alveolar bone and pulp
	• Gingival nerve fibers and receptors similar to oral mucosa and include:
	  ○ myelinated type IIAβ (low-threshold mechanoreceptors) and type IIIAδ fibers (nociceptors) and unmyelinated type IVC fibers (nociceptors) and type C fibers (postganglionic sympathetic)
	• **Gingival sulcus**: space between the enamel of the tooth and gingival margin. The depth of the sulcus varies, but it is normally 0.5 to 1.5 mm above the base of the sulcus

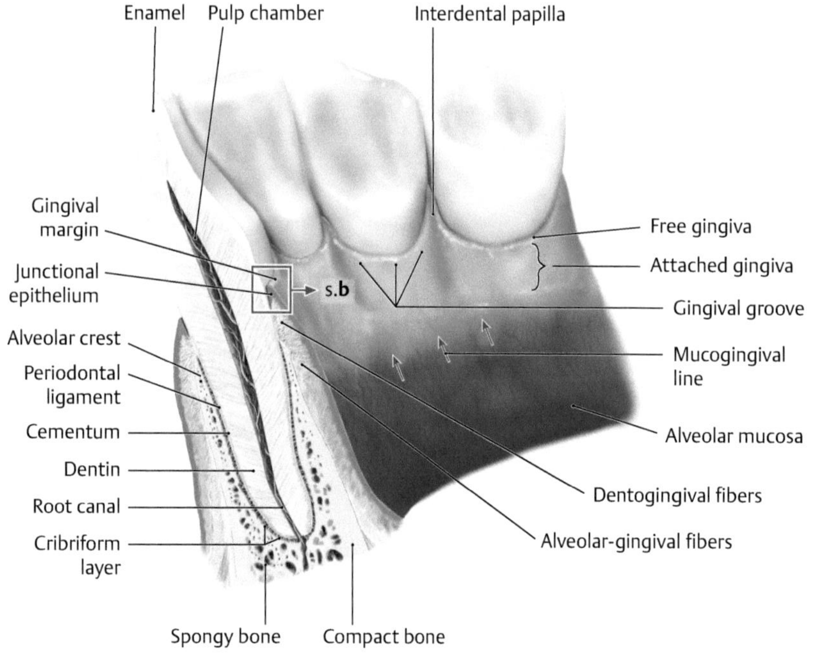

Fig. 25.6 Regions of the periodontium and gingiva. The longitudinal section of the tooth shown within the dental arch. The gingiva includes regions of the free (marginal) and attached gingiva. The free gingiva surrounds the neck of the tooth, forming a cuff that is attached by the junctional epithelium to the cervical enamel. The attached gingiva extends to the mucogingival line and adheres tightly to the alveolar bone. Collagenous connective tissue fibers course through the gingiva to form the gingival fiber group that works functionally as a unit to reinforce the junctional epithelium. The gingival fiber group includes fiber bundles that extend from the gingiva to the alveolar bone or cementum, and function to resist gingival displacement. Additional fiber bundles also contribute to this supra-alveolar group; some encircle the tooth and others serve to link adjacent teeth together or connect the oral and vestibular interdental papilla. (Reproduced with permission from Schuenke M, Schulte E, Schumacher U. THIEME Atlas of Anatomy. Second Edition, Vol 3. © Thieme 2016. Illustrations by Markus Voll and Karl Wesker.)

Table 25.5 Sensory distribution of maxillary (V2) nerve to teeth and mucosa

Maxillary arch	Anterior arch (incisors/canines)	Middle arch (premolar)	Posterior arch (molar regions)
• **Facial/vestibular surface** Innervation of alveolar mucosa and buccal gingiva	**Anterior superior alveolar (ASA) nerve of V2** Branch of infraorbital nerve of V2	**Middle superior alveolar (MSA) nerves of V2** Branch of infraorbital nerve of V2	**Posterior superior alveolar (PSA) of V2** Branch of maxillary nerve of V2
• **Palatal surface** Innervation of palatal gingiva, alveolar mucosa absent	Nasopalatine nerve of V2	Greater palatine nerve of V2	Greater palatine nerve of V2
• **Teeth** Pulp, periodontal ligament (PDL), alveolar process (bone)	Anterior superior alveolar (ASA)	**Middle superior alveolar (MSA)** Innervates the mesiobuccal root of the first maxillary molar	**Posterior superior alveolar (PSA)** Except the mesiobuccal root of the first maxillary molar

Table 25.6 Sensory distribution of the mandibular (V3) to the mandibular teeth and mucosa

Mandibular arch region	Anterior arch (incisors/canines)	Middle arch (premolar)	Posterior arch (molar regions)
• **Facial/vestibular/buccal surface** Innervation of alveolar mucosa and buccal gingiva	**Mental nerve** Branch of inferior alveolar of V3	**Mental and incisive nerves** Branch of inferior alveolar nerve of V3	**Long buccal nerve of V3** Contribution from inferior alveolar nerve
• **Lingual surface** Innervation of alveolar mucosa and gingiva	**Lingual nerve of V3**	**Lingual nerve of V3**	**Lingual nerve** and minor contribution from inferior alveolar nerve of V3
Teeth Pulp, periodontal ligament (PDL), alveolar process (bone)	**Incisive branch V3** Branch of inferior alveolar nerve of V3	**Inferior alveolar**	**Inferior alveolar**

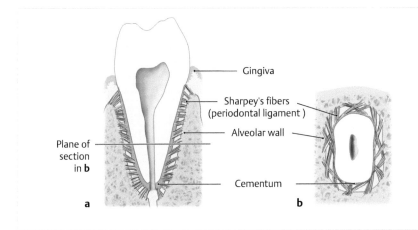

Gingiva

Sharpey's fibers (periodontal ligament)

Alveolar wall

Plane of section in **b**

Cementum

a

b

Fig. 25.7 Periodontal ligament (PDL): **(a)** longitudinal and **(b)** cross-section of a tooth. The PDL consists of several collagenous fiber bundles known as the dentoalveolar fiber group, which serve as the principal anchor of the tooth to the alveolus. Sharpey's fibers are the bundles of connective tissue that pass obliquely downward from the alveolar bone and insert into the cementum. Fiber bundle orientation serves to resist vertical and intrusive occlusal forces and transmits the masticatory forces acting on the tooth to the PDL and bone. (Reproduced with permission from Schuenke M, Schulte E, Schumacher U. THIEME Atlas of Anatomy. Second Edition, Vol 3. ©Thieme 2016. Illustrations by Markus Voll and Karl Wesker.)

○ The Ruffini-like receptors respond differently to occlusal loads based on their location within the ligament.
  – Receptors close to the middle third of the root, which acts as a fulcrum for occlusal forces, respond rapidly, whereas those near the root apex respond slowly and fire continually during the duration of the stimulus.
  – Variations in the response from receptors at different locations along the root surface provide feedback about the direction, intensity, and velocity of the initial stimulus, along with input about the duration of the stimulus.
○ Ruffini-like receptors of the PDL provide the mechanosensory and proprioceptive feedback involved in controlling bite force, modulation of jaw position, and tooth position, based on sensory input about the direction,

intensity, and duration of the occlusal forces applied to the tooth. The information concerning tooth position and mechanical loading is necessary to alter the bite force and masticatory rhythm during the chewing cycle. Afferent input from PDL receptors, along with proprioceptive input from muscle spindles in jaw-closing muscles, mediate reflex behaviors that protect the teeth and jaw (see Chapter 22).
• Terminal branches of maxillary and mandibular nerves that carry both myelinated and unmyelinated nerve fibers enter the PDL through the foramina in the alveolar bone and along the root apex. These terminal branches are identical to those providing innervation to the alveolar bone and dental pulp (► Table 25.7 and ► Table 25.8).

Table 25.7 Overview of mechanoreceptors in the gingiva, the periodontal ligament (PDL), and the pulp

Location	Receptor characteristics and stimuli	Afferent fiber type	Function
Oral mucosa Gingiva	**Merkel cell** Nonencapsulated mechanoreceptor Merkel cell–neurite complex: • Low threshold • Slowly adapting type I (SAI) receptor Stimuli: superficial pressure/touch	Myelinated type IIAβ fiber Large diameter Fast transmission	Provide mechanosensory feedback about gingival fiber displacement and position of the gingiva
Oral mucosa Gingiva	**Meissner's** Encapsulated mechanoreceptor: • Low threshold • Rapidly adapting type I (RAI) receptor Stimuli: fine touch	Myelinated type IIAβ fiber Large diameter Fast transmission	Fine discriminative touch Provide mechanosensory feedback about gingival fiber displacement and position of the gingiva
Oral mucosa Gingiva	**Ruffini endings** Encapsulated mechanoreceptor • Low-threshold mechanoreceptor (LTM) • Slowly adapting type II (SAII) receptor Stimuli: stretch, deformation	Myelinated type IIAβ fiber Large diameter Fast transmission	Provides mechanosensory feedback about gingival fiber displacement and position of the gingiva
PDL	**Ruffini-like ending** nonencapsulated mechanoreceptor unique to PDL[a]: • Low threshold • Overall (SAII) properties • Stimuli: stretch, deformation of the PDL due to occlusal load	Myelinated type IIAβ fiber Large diameter Fast transmission	• Provides mechanosensory input about the direction, intensity, and duration of applied force (stimuli) • Provide tooth proprioceptive feedback about tooth position and bite force
Pulp	**Mechanoreceptor** • LTM Stimuli: light touch, pressure, mechanical vibration	Myelinated type II Aβ fiber Large diameter Fast transmission	• Similar to Aδ LTM • Evokes pain when stimulated in pulp
Oral mucosa Gingiva PDL Pulp	**Free nerve ending** **Mechanoreceptor** • LTM Stimuli: light touch, pressure	Lightly myelinated type IIIAδ fiber Small diameter Fast transmission	• Crude, nondiscriminative touch • Evokes sharp, fast pain when stimulated in pulp
Oral mucosa Gingiva PDL	**Free nerve ending** **Thermoreceptor** • Low-threshold thermoreceptor • Large receptive field Stimuli: innocuous temperature change cool range	Lightly myelinated type IIIAδ fiber Small diameter Fast transmission	Cool
Oral mucosa Gingiva PDL	**Free nerve ending** **Thermoreceptor** • Low threshold • Large receptive field Stimuli: innocuous temperature change, warm range and cool	Unmyelinated type IVC fibers Thin diameter Slow transmission	Warm and cool

[a]See chapter 11 for a complete list of sensory receptors associated with the oral cavity, including chemoreceptors and proprioceptors

25.3 Dental Pulp

- The **dental pulp** is a highly vascularized loose CT forming the central core of the crown and root of the tooth. The pulp contains numerous cells including fibroblasts, immune cells, stem cells, and odontoblasts, which respond to damage and aid in maintaining the vitality of the pulp. The mineralized dentin matrix, which is characterized by numerous **fluid-filled dentinal tubules** passing through the entire thickness of dentin, encloses and protects the dental pulp. The serum transudate produced from pulpal blood vessels fills the dentinal tubules and serves as a nutritive source for the dentin.
  - Small apical extensions from the odontoblast, known as the **odontoblastic process**, project into the dentinal tubule.
  - **Odontoblast cells**, located along the peripheral border of the pulp, function to synthesize and maintain the integrity of the dentin matrix. The viability of the dentin–pulp complex determines both the vitality and the ability of the tooth to respond to injury.
  - Pulpal injury resulting from tooth trauma, caries, periodontal disease, restorative dental procedures, or periapical infections may cause pulpal inflammation (**pulpitis**) and the release of inflammatory mediators that stimulate an immune response and activate nociceptive nerve fibers in the pulp.

Table 25.8 Summary of nociceptive and sympathetic input from gingiva, periodontal ligament (PDL), and pulp

Location	Receptor Characteristics and Stimuli	Afferent Fiber Type	Function
Oral mucosa Gingiva PDL Pulp	Free nerve ending mechanothermal nociceptor • High-threshold nociceptive specific • Small receptive field Stimuli: responsive to intense mechanical or mechanothermal stimuli	Lightly myelinated type IIIAδ fiber Small diameter Fast transmission	Fast, sharp localized pain
Oral mucosa Gingiva PDL Pulp	Free nerve ending polymodal nociceptor • High-threshold nociceptive-wide dynamic range • Large receptive field Stimuli: responsive to intense stimuli; includes heat, mechanical and chemical mediators released during inflammation	Unmyelinated type IVC fibers (polymodal nociceptor) Thin diameter Slow transmission	Slow, dull, diffuse pain
Oral mucosa Gingiva PDL Pulp	Free nerve ending silent nociceptor • High-threshold nociceptive Stimuli: normally unresponsive to noxious mechanical stimuli	Unmyelinated silent nociceptors Type IVC fibers Thin diameter Slow transmission	Becomes sensitized; activated and responsive following inflammation

Postganglionic sympathetic			
Location	Receptor characteristics and stimuli	Afferent fiber type	Function
Oral mucosa Gingiva PDL Pulp	Free nerve ending **Autonomic** Autoregulatory control: Stimuli: neurotransmitter release, response altered during inflammation	Unmyelinated postganglionic sympathetic C fibers Thin diameter Slow transmission	• Vasomotor control of blood flow to pulp, gingiva, and periodontal region • Release of inflammatory mediators

○ Depending on the extent of the injury and the inflammatory response, any resulting collateral tissue damage may be repaired.

– Mild injury and acute inflammation may stimulate existing odontoblasts to synthesize reactionary dentin, whereas significant tissue injury or chronic inflammation inhibits tissue repair and may cause odontoblast death, loss of dentin, and pulp exposure.

– The repair of dental tissues following odontoblast destruction occurs through the recruitment of stem cell–derived odontoblastlike cells to form a bridge of reparative dentin over the exposed pulp. Stem cell differentiation may lead to regeneration of the pulpal CT.

25.3.1 Pulp Innervation

• The dentin pulp is richly innervated by myelinated type IIAβ and IIIAδ fibers and unmyelinated C fibers (▶ Fig. 25.8).

○ There are five types of receptors associated with these fibers, which include low-threshold mechanoreceptors and high-threshold nociceptors (▶ Table 25.5 and ▶ Table 25.6).

○ Small, unmyelinated postganglionic sympathetic C fibers also reside in the pulp and control vasomotor activity of pulpal blood vessels and the release of inflammatory mediators. Parasympathetic nerve fibers have not been detected in the pulp.

• The myelinated and unmyelinated nerve fibers that innervate the dental pulp are the terminal nerve fibers from the superior and inferior dental plexuses of the maxillary (V2) and mandibular (V3) divisions.

• Nerve fibers enter the **radicular (root) pulp** as part of a neurovascular bundle through the apical foramen located at the root apex. The majority the nerve fibers innervating the

dentin–pulp complex enter as myelinated axons, but gradually lose their myelin sheath in the crown.

○ A few collateral branches supply the root, and then the myelinated and unmyelinated nerve fibers ascend toward the crown to form an extensive nerve plexus in the **coronal pulp**.

○ Type IIAβ and IIIAδ fibers are found primarily along the dentin–pulpal border, whereas unmyelinated type IVC fibers are located deeper in the central regions of the pulp.

• Several notable features of the coronal pulp include:

○ A large number of primary afferent fibers in the pulp correspond to low-threshold mechanoreceptors that, when stimulated, evokes the sensation of dental (odontogenic) pain. This response is different from the oral mucosa or skin, in which a stimulus, such as thermal, mechanical, or chemical input, produces a distinct type of sensation.

○ The coronal pulp is extensively innervated in comparison to the radicular pulp. Each crown contains a coronal nerve plexus, known as the **plexus of Raschkow**, which is located subjacent to the peripheral odontoblasts, in an area known as the **subodontoblastic region**.

○ Terminal ends of type Aδ fibers emerge from the nerve plexus, as unmyelinated fibers, and project a short distance (150 μm) into the fluid-filled dentinal tubules to terminate near the odontoblastic process of each cell.

– In general, the dentinal tubules found in the regions of the pulp that project into cusps (**pulp horns**) contain a higher percentage of intratubular unmyelinated type Aδ fibers than the tubules in other regions of the crown or root. The pulp horns and coronal plexus represent the pulpal areas with the highest nerve density. The difference in distribution is presumably associated with regional variations in tooth sensitivity.

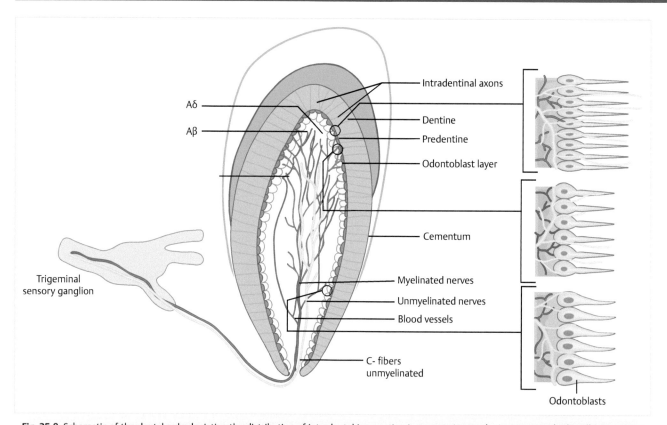

Fig. 25.8 Schematic of the dental pulp depicting the distribution of intradental innervation in an anterior tooth. A neurovascular bundle containing unmyelinated C fibers and myelinated afferent A fibers of the trigeminal maxillary (V2) and mandibular (V3) divisions enters the root via the apical foramen. A few collaterals of the neurovascular bundle supply the root before ascending and branching extensively in the coronal pulp. Unmyelinated C fibers reside in the central pulp. Postganglionic sympathetic fibers provide vasomotor control to pulpal blood vessels. Myelinated Aβ and lightly myelinated Aδ fibers project peripherally toward the dentin–pulpal border. The myelinated nerve fibers gradually lose their myelin sheath as the fibers move peripherally. Odontoblasts, which maintain the integrity of dentin matrix, reside along the peripheral border and send small apical extensions, known as an odontoblastic process, into the dentinal tubules. The Aδ nerve fibers, which pass from the coronal nerve plexus as unmyelinated fibers, extend into the dentinal tubules. The nerve endings of the A and C fibers respond to thermal, mechanical, and nociceptive stimuli, which are perceived as sharp and dull pain.

- The fluid in the dentinal tubules may be induced to move through thermal, osmotic, and tactile stimuli, and serves as the basis for the proposed mechanotransduction mechanism leading to the activation of low-threshold mechanoreceptors nerve fibers (Aδ and Aβ) and the perception of dental pain. This mechanism is known as the **hydrodynamic theory** (see Chapter 26).
- Stimulation of the dentin pulp by noxious thermal, chemical, and mechanical input results in the activation of myelinated Aβ and Aδ fiber and unmyelinated C fibers and the perception of pain (see Chapter 26).

25.4 Trigeminal Pathway

25.4.1 Innervation Patterns to Dental Arches

- Terminal nerve branches of the maxillary (V2) and mandibular (V3) divisions of the trigeminal nerve transmit somatic sensations from the specific regions of each arch that contain the teeth, gingiva, and alveolar mucosa (▶ Fig. 25.9 and ▶ Fig. 25.10; ▶ Table 25.7 and ▶ Table 25.8).

- The specific path of maxillary and mandibular nerve branches that supply the teeth and supportive periodontium may be found in Chapter 20.

25.4.2 Central Ascending Trigeminal Path

- As discussed in Chapter 13, the primary afferent neurons that transmit the protopathic and epicritic sensations from the teeth and periodontium reside in the trigeminal ganglion. In contrast, the primary afferent cell bodies for proprioceptive fibers arising from the PDL are found in the mesencephalic nucleus.
- Central axonal processes of the primary afferent neurons will enter the pons through the sensory root and project to specific nuclei in the trigeminal nuclear complex. The type of input transmitted from the first-order neuron determines the point of termination within the trigeminal nuclear complex (▶ Fig. 25.11; see Chapters 13 and 20 for details).
  - **Protopathic sensations** originate from the teeth (pulp) and periodontium and follow Aβ, Aδ, and C fibers to synapse on second-order neurons in the pars oralis (Vo),

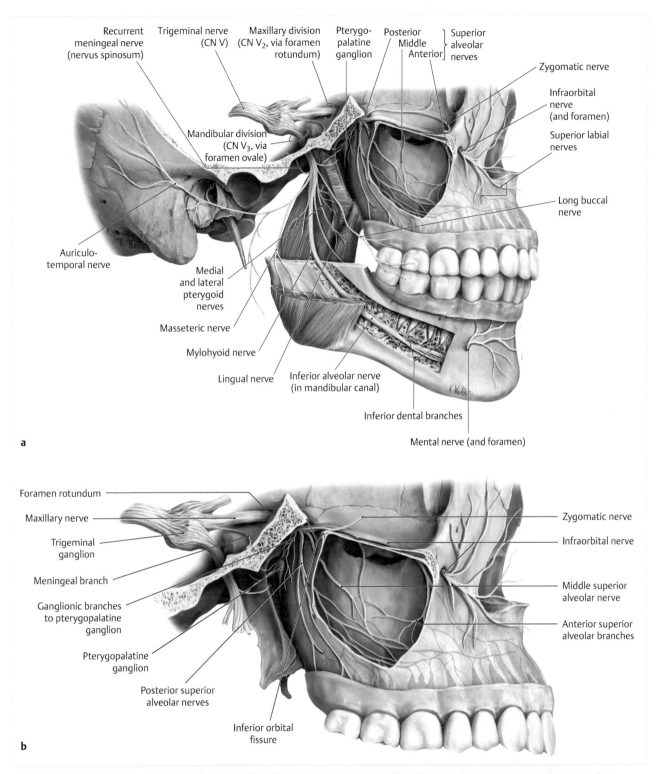

a

b

Fig. 25.9 Right lateral view of peripheral distribution of the trigeminal nerve. The maxillary division of the trigeminal nerve (CN V2) and the mandibular division of the trigeminal nerve (CN V3) innervate the structures of the oral cavity via their many branches. (a) Note the inferior alveolar nerve passes through the mandibular canal, and terminally branches into the inferior dental and incisive branches. **(b)** Note the terminal branches of the infraorbital nerve (V2) form the superior dental plexus and provide sensory innervation to the maxillary teeth. (Reproduced with permission from Schuenke M, Schulte E, Schumacher U. THIEME Atlas of Anatomy Third Edition, Vol 3. © Thieme 2020. Illustrations by Markus Voll and Karl Wesker.)

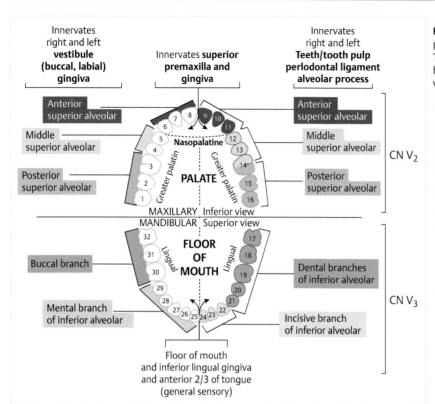

Fig. 25.10 Schematic showing the innervation pattern of the maxillary and mandibular arches. The peripheral distribution of the terminal branches of the trigeminal nerve to the lips, vestibular mucosa, gingiva, and teeth is shown.

the interface between the pars interpolaris and pars caudalis Vi/Vc, or the pars caudalis (Vc) of the spinal trigeminal nucleus (STN).

- In general, the type of primary afferent fiber (Aβ, Aδ, and C fibers) determines the type of second-order neuron on which the fiber synapses (nociceptive specific [NS] or wide dynamic range [WDR]) and the ascending pathway followed. The perceived sensation is also influenced by the neurotransmitters released and the extent of inhibitory or excitatory modulation provided from other interneurons within the STN.
  - Ascending secondary afferents cross the midline and follow the ventral trigeminothalamic tract (VTT) to the contralateral ventral posteromedial (VPM) nucleus. Thalamocortical third-order neurons project directly to the orofacial region of the somatosensory cortex for conscious perception. This pathway is associated with the perception of fast, sharp, and specifically localized pain transmitted from the periphery by Aδ fibers.
  - Some secondary afferent fibers ascend bilaterally in the trigeminoreticular tract and project to the reticular formation, intralaminar thalamic nuclei, and limbic system for the unconscious processing of pain. This pathway is primarily associated with the perception of slow, dull, and diffuse pain transmitted from the periphery by unmyelinated C fibers.
    - Ascending secondary fibers, which project to the reticular formation and limbic regions, are involved in pain modulation and the emotional processing of nociceptive input (see Chapters 14 and 26).

- Central axonal processes carrying **epicritic sensations** from the periodontium and gingival mucosa will synapse on second-order neurons in the chief (principal/main) sensory nucleus. Ascending secondary afferent fibers from the teeth and oral cavity remain ipsilateral and follow the dorsal trigeminothalamic tract (DTT) to the ipsilateral VPM and then the cortex. Mechanosensory input from the face crosses the midline at the level of the pons to follow the VTT pathway to the cortex.
- **Proprioceptive input** from primary afferent fibers originating from the PDL pass through the mesencephalic nucleus of V and projects to second-order neurons in the chief sensory and spinal trigeminal nuclei. Secondary afferent fibers ascend via the trigeminocerebellar tract to the cerebellum for unconscious proprioceptive feedback.

25.4.3 Summary of Trigeminal Orofacial Sensory Pathways

Protopathic Sensations

Pain, temperature, crude nondiscriminative touch of pulp, gingiva, oral mucosa, and the periodontium carried by V2 and V3.
- Conscious pain:
  - Trigeminal ganglion → STN → contralateral VTT→VPM→ sensory cortex.
- Unconscious pain:
  - Trigeminal ganglion → STN →trigeminoreticular tract →reticular formation→ limbic system.

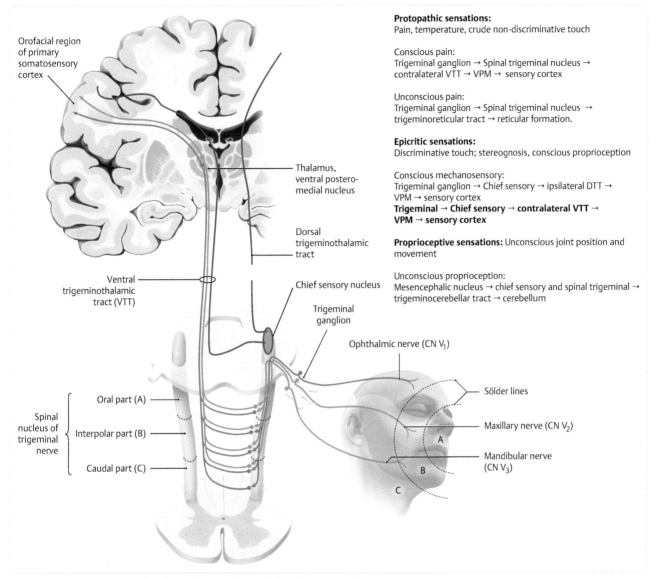

Protopathic sensations:
Pain, temperature, crude non-discriminative touch

Conscious pain:
Trigeminal ganglion → Spinal trigeminal nucleus → contralateral VTT → VPM → sensory cortex

Unconscious pain:
Trigeminal ganglion → Spinal trigeminal nucleus → trigeminoreticular tract → reticular formation.

Epicritic sensations:
Discriminative touch; stereognosis, conscious proprioception

Conscious mechanosensory:
Trigeminal ganglion → Chief sensory → ipsilateral DTT → VPM → sensory cortex
Trigeminal → Chief sensory → contralateral VTT → VPM → sensory cortex

Proprioceptive sensations: Unconscious joint position and movement

Unconscious proprioception:
Mesencephalic nucleus → chief sensory and spinal trigeminal → trigeminocerebellar tract → cerebellum

Fig. 25.11 Protopathic and epicritic central ascending trigeminal pathways. (Reproduced with permission from Schuenke M, Schulte E, Schumacher U. THIEME Atlas of Anatomy Third Edition, Vol 3. © Thieme 2020. Illustrations by Markus Voll and Karl Wesker.)

Epicritic Sensations

Discriminative touch, stereognosis, conscious proprioception of pulp, gingiva, oral mucosa, and the periodontium carried by V2 and V3.
- Conscious mechanosensory:
  ○ Oral cavity:
    – Trigeminal ganglion → chief sensory→ ipsilateral DTT → VPM→ sensory cortex.
  ○ Face:
    – Trigeminal ganglion→ chief sensory → contralateral VTT →VPM→ sensory cortex.

Proprioceptive Sensations

Unconscious movements and tooth position of PDL carried by V2 and V3.
- Unconscious proprioception:
  ○ Mesencephalic nucleus →chief sensory and spinal trigeminal → trigeminocerebellar tract → cerebellum.

Clinical Correlation Box 25.1: Impact of Dental Procedures on Sensory Input

Changes in mechanosensory and nociceptive input in the orofacial region may result from several mechanisms including oral infections, inflammation, dental procedures, or parafunctional habits. The altered input to peripheral receptors will impact central afferent inputs to the trigeminal sensory nuclear complex and may lead to adaptive changes in the central nervous system (CNS) that influence cortical motor output or influence sensory perception.

- Dental procedures and parafunctional habits that affect tooth occlusion, such as orthodontically induced tooth movements, dentures, oral appliances, and TMD, will alter mechanosensory input.
- Nociceptive input to the CNS may be increased or decreased in response to peripheral nerve injuries that occur as a complication from dental extractions, oral surgery, or placement of dental implants.
- Oral infections and inflammation may also cause an increase in nociceptive input in response to sensitization of peripheral nociceptors (peripheral sensitization) or due to changes in the excitability of the primary afferent neuron (peripheral sensitization). Over time, the prolonged increase in nociceptive activity to the CNS can lead to central sensitization (see Chapter 14).
- Tooth extractions and dental implants will decrease proprioceptive and nociceptive input due to the loss of the PDL.
- Endodontic therapy (root canal), which involves the removal of the neurovascular structures, will lead to a complete loss of nociceptive input from the treated tooth. The removal of the neurovascular structures following a root canal or tooth extraction leads to dental deafferentation and a significant alteration in afferent input to the CNS due to the physical connections of the teeth by the PDL and dental nerve plexuses. Given the overlapping pattern of innervation of adjacent teeth, the treatment of one tooth may impact sensory input and feedback from other teeth. As a result, persistent pain following endodontic treatment may occur (see Chapter 26).

Clinical Correlation Box 25.2: Osseointegrated Implants

The loss of the PDL results in difficulty in controlling oromotor activities involved in mastication and mediating protective reflexes. Patients often exhibit difficulty in determining positional information concerning food placement on the teeth, controlling bite force, and changing the chewing cycle in response to mechanical differences in food properties. To address this deficit, the use of osseointegrated implants, which are believed to provide a level of tactile sensibility known as osseoperception, is often the preferred treatment option over a removable prosthesis. Osseoperception refers to the mechanoreception provided, in the absence of PDL, by the masticatory muscles, TMJ, oral mucosa, and periosteal mechanoreceptors. The exact mechanism of osseoperception is unknown; however, neuroplasticity of the CNS may play a role. Additionally, the role of using engineered bioimplants of living PDL tissue during the osseointegrated restoration is currently being investigated.

Questions and Answers

Use the following clinical scenario for questions 1 to 5.

A 50-year-old man complains of dull, throbbing pain in one of his teeth in his lower jaw, on the right side. An examination of the patient reveals multiple teeth in the mandibular region have visible caries. Radiographs of the painful area show carious lesions on teeth nos. 27, 29, and 30 and a lesion at the root tip of tooth no. 30. It appears that the lesion on tooth no. 30 has progressed to the pulp of the tooth.

1. The pain from tooth no. 30 is relayed in the:
    a) Inferior alveolar nerve.
    b) Lingual nerve.
    c) Mental nerve.
    d) Auriculotemporal nerve.

Level 1: Easy

Answer (A): The inferior alveolar nerve provides innervation to all the teeth in the lower arch. Anesthetizing the inferior alveolar nerve will block transmission from all mandibular teeth including the anterior teeth, which receive innervation from the incisive branch. The mental nerve (**C**) is also a terminal branch of the inferior alveolar but primarily innervates soft-tissue structures in the labial region. The lingual nerve (**B**) provides general sensory afferent (GSA) innervation to the oral mucosa of the floor and the alveolar and gingival mucosa on the lingual side of the lower arch. The auriculotemporal nerve (**D**) provides innervation to the area of the skin in the vicinity of the parotid gland.

2. The cell that deposits dentin along the pulp border in response to the carious lesion is the:
   a) Ameloblast.
   b) Cementoblast.
   c) Odontoblast.
   d) Fibroblast.

Level 1: Easy

Answer (C): Odontoblasts produce dentin. In response to a carious lesion, odontoblasts may produce a type of dentin, known as tertiary (reactionary) dentin, as a mechanism to protect the pulp. The other cells listed deposit cementum (**B**), enamel (**A**) is deposited by ameloblasts, and (**D**) connective tissue fibers are synthesized by fibroblasts. Ameloblasts are not present in a mature erupted tooth. Cementoblasts lie on the external root surface and synthesize the cementum matrix. Fibroblasts reside in both the periodontal ligament (PDL) and pulp; however, stimulation of fibroblasts will not cause dentin deposition. Stem cells in the pulp may be induced to differentiate into an odontoblastlike cell under the appropriate conditions; however, the resulting dentin lacks dentinal tubules and differs structurally.

3. The type of afferent nerve fiber found in the dental pulp of tooth no. 30 that transmits slow, dull pain is the ___fiber.
   a) Aβ
   b) Aγ
   c) Aδ
   d) C

Level 1: Easy

Answer (D): Unmyelinated type IVC fibers transmit slow dull pain from nociceptors. Aβ (**A**) and (**C**) Aδ fibers may act as low-threshold mechanoreceptors and transmit crude, nondiscriminative touch, and/or sharp pain. In the pulp, most mechanosensory input is perceived as sharp pain. The specific reason why it is perceived as pain is not completely understood. (**B**) Aγ fibers transmit efferent impulse from gamma motor neurons to muscle spindles. Muscle spindles are found in some orofacial skeletal muscles.

4. The ascending tract followed by the nerve fiber that is causing the dull, diffuse pain is _____.
   a) Ventral trigeminothalamic tract (VTT)
   b) Trigeminoreticular tract
   c) Trigeminocerebellar tract
   d) Dorsal trigeminothalamic tract

Level 2: Moderate

Answer (B): The trigeminoreticular path transmits nociceptive signals primarily from unmyelinated C fibers to the reticular formation for unconscious processing and to diffuse areas of the cortex. As a result, the input is often interpreted as diffuse, poorly localized pain. (**A**) The VTT is associated with the transmission of conscious, sharp localized pain from Aδ. The pain occurs rapidly at the onset of damage or stimulation. Fast, sharp pain follows the VTT. At the level of the mid-pons, secondary afferent fibers carrying epicritic sensations from the main sensory nucleus join the VTT and ascend together as the trigeminal lemniscus. The trigeminocerebellar (**C**) and dorsal trigeminothalamic (**D**) tracts carry unconscious and conscious proprioceptive and tactile input from the mechanoreceptors in the PDL and the mucosa.

5. Which of the following nerve branches doesn't need to be anesthetized in order to block the sensation of pain to the pulp and all surrounding bone and gingiva of tooth no. 27 prior to preforming a restoration?
   a) Long buccal nerve
   b) Mental nerve
   c) Incisive nerve
   d) Inferior alveolar nerve

Level 2: Moderate

Answer (A): The long buccal nerve is correct. All other nerves transmit sensory input from the gingiva, periodontium, or the tooth pulp in the region of tooth no. 27. The long buccal nerve transmits GSA input from the gingiva in the molar region. Innervation usually does not extend as far forward as the first premolar (tooth no. 27). An injection of the mental nerve (**B**) will block innervation to soft tissue in the region of premolar, and with a slight variation may also anesthetize the incisive branch (**C**) within the mandible. The inferior alveolar nerve (**D**) divides into the mental and incisive nerves, so an injection of the inferior alveolar nerve will also anesthetize these two terminal branches.

Unit VII

Orofacial Pain and Dental Anesthesia

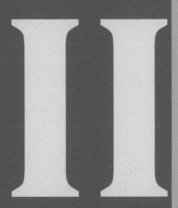

26 Orofacial Pain

26.1 Overview of Orofacial Pain Pathways

Pain information for the head and oral cavity is largely carried on the trigeminal nerve (CN V). The first-order cell bodies for the trigeminal system are located in the trigeminal ganglion. Nociceptive information is transmitted from the periphery into the central nervous system (CNS) via sensory receptors that communicate with the first-order neurons. The peripheral process of the first-order neuron travels in the three divisions of CN V: ophthalmic (V1), maxillary (V2), and mandibular (V3). The central processes of the first-order neurons project to the trigeminal nuclear complex, specifically the spinal trigeminal nucleus (STN), where the second-order neurons reside. In general, pain information from the face will synapse in the pars caudalis nucleus. Nociceptive input from the oral cavity (teeth, periodontal ligament [PDL], and oral mucosa) will terminate in the pars oralis nucleus. Although it is less well characterized, it is generally accepted that some oral pain information will also travel to the pars interpolaris nucleus. Secondary afferents from the STN decussate to form the ventral trigeminothalamic tract, which then ascends and synapses in the contralateral ventral posteromedial (VPM) nucleus of the thalamus (third-order neurons). Fibers from the third-order neurons of the thalamus project toward the sensory strip of the cortex (postcentral gyrus) where they synapse in their respective somatotropic-specific area (▶ Fig. 26.1; see Chapter 13).

26.2 Nociceptive Orofacial Pain

Nociceptive pain is evoked as a result of the stimulation of pain receptors. This is the most common type of pain and results from trauma/injury or local inflammation. The sensation of pain is initiated by the stimulation of nociceptors. Dental pain originating from hot and cold stimuli is perceived quite differently, with heat producing dull, long-lasting pain and cold producing short, sharp pain. It has been proposed that pain from hot and cold temperatures is the result of dentinal fluid movement within microtubules present in the dentin of sensory neurons expressing nociceptors (**hydrodynamic theory**). Another theory on pain resulting from thermal stimuli is the **neural theory**, which suggests that temperature changes at the surface of the tooth are conducted through the enamel and dentin to the nociceptors located at the **dentin–enamel junction** (**DEJ**). The nerve fibers that transmit noxious stimuli are lightly myelinated alpha δ or unmyelinated C fibers. The major categories of nociceptive orofacial pain include **odontogenic**, **mucosal**, **musculoskeletal**, and **referred**.

26.2.1 Odontogenic Pain

Odontogenic pain refers to pain that initiates from teeth or the periodontium, the maxilla or the mandible. A "*toothache*" is caused by inflammation of the **dental pulp**, often due to **dental caries** (tooth decay). **Periodontal disease** is a common cause of infection that can produce odontogenic pain (▶ Table 26.1). The source of odontogenic pain is the **pulpo-dentin complex** and **periapical tissue**. In healthy pulp, thermal stimuli produce short, sharp pain that lasts approximately 1 to 2 seconds (▶ Table 26.2). This indicates that the nerve fibers are functioning. A response to cold indicates vital pulp, whereas an increased response to heat suggests a pulpal or periapical pathology that may require endodontic treatment.

- **Dental pulpitis** (inflammation of the pulp) can be due to caries present near the pulp. It is classified as **reversible** or **irreversible**.
  ○ In **reversible pulpitis**, the pulp can remain viable if treated, which typically requires removal of the caries followed by restoration. It is characterized by short, quick bursts of pain induced by a cold stimulus that ceases immediately upon its removal.
  ○ **Irreversible pulpitis** occurs when the pulp is damaged beyond repair. It is characterized by intense pain and is one of the most common reasons for emergency dental visits. As the inflammation spreads, the cellular organization of the pulp breaks down. It is typically associated with tooth decay, a cracked tooth, or trauma. Management for irreversible pulpitis is either **pulpectomy** (root canal treatment) or **tooth extraction**. Pain symptoms with irreversible pulpitis include:
  – Intense persisting pain with warm stimulus. After removal of the stimulus, the pain becomes dull and pulsating. Early pain information is carried on both A-δ and C fibers; however, as the inflammation progresses, C fibers become the predominant carriers for pain transmission.
  – Pain subsides with cold stimulus, likely due to vasoconstriction and a decrease in intrapulpal pressure. This symptom is highly indicative of necrotic pulp.
  – When C fibers become the predominant mode of transmission, the pain becomes more diffuse and is more difficult to localize.

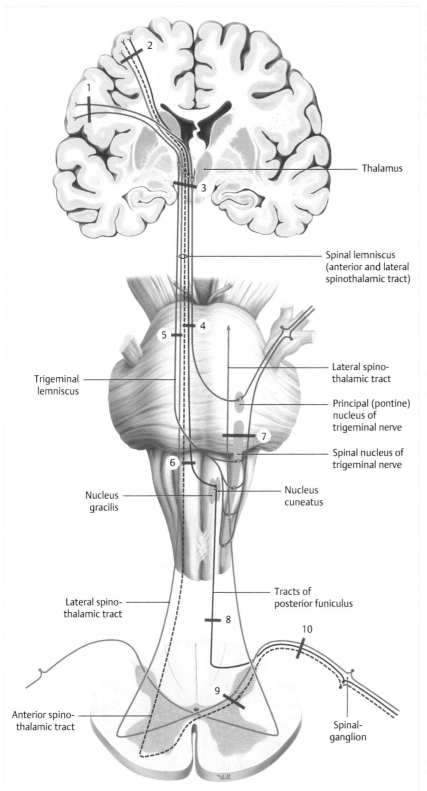

Fig. 26.1 Pain information from the face and oral cavity is carried on the trigeminal nerve and ascends to the somatosensory cortex via the trigeminothalamic tract. (Reproduced with permission from Schuenke M, Schulte E, Schumacher U. THIEME Atlas of Anatomy. Second Edition, Vol 3. © Thieme 2016. Illustrations by Markus Voll and Karl Wesker.)

Thalamus

Spinal lemniscus (anterior and lateral spinothalamic tract)

Trigeminal lemniscus

Lateral spino-thalamic tract

Principal (pontine) nucleus of trigeminal nerve

Spinal nucleus of trigeminal nerve

Nucleus gracilis

Nucleus cuneatus

Tracts of posterior funiculus

Lateral spino-thalamic tract

Anterior spino-thalamic tract

Spinal-ganglion

- Intense and prolonged pain can refer to the ear, temporal area, and the cheek.
- Once the **periapical tissue** becomes involved, the tooth becomes sensitive to **percussion**.
○ **Necrotic pulp** results from continued degeneration of inflamed pulp. There is no reparative potential. In addition to the moderate to severe spontaneous pain, the patient may experience swelling in the jaw and lymphadenopathy. Pain receptors in necrotic pulp often become damaged and may not respond to thermal stimuli. If the pulp is only partially affected, there may be some response present.

Table 26.1 Diagnostic tests for dental pain

Pulp sensitivity test	Ice is applied on the neck of the tooth. Pain indicates pulp is vital. No response indicates pulp necrosis
Percussion test	Tooth is tapped on longitudinal angle with instrument. Pain response indicates potential periapical inflammation (abscess)
Probing	A blunt probe placed into the gingival sulcus around the tooth can provide information regarding the health of the tissue. Bleeding and/or depths greater than 3–4 mm indicates gum disease
Mobility test	Visible movement with manipulation indicates bone loss
Palpation	Palpation of the area in question can demonstrate tenderness and swelling
Mucosal sinuses	Dental abscesses often drain to the buccal surface creating sinuses that extend through the mucosa
Radiology	Radiographs will show apical and periapical structures of the tooth in question and those adjacent as well as caries

Source: Adapted from Renton 2011.[1]

Table 26.2 Differential diagnoses of endodontic conditions

Reversible pulpitis	Short duration of pain Reacts to cold and heat stimuli No reaction to percussion Not evident on radiograph
Irreversible pulpitis	Lingering pain in response to heat and cold Typically does not react to percussion Pain initially sharp, then dull, throbbing Pain poorly localized
Pulp necrosis	May or may not be painful Lingering pain to heat, sometimes relieved by cold
Acute apical periodontitis	Tenderness to percussion Pain with chewing May have pulp symptoms
Chronic apical periodontitis	None to minimal symptoms Periapical radiolucency
Acute abscess	Pus in periapical tissues Tenderness to percussion and palpation Pain when chewing Intraoral swelling may be present
Cellulitis	Facial swelling, red, diffuse Often not painful Fever may be present

Source: Adapted from Linn et al., 2007.[2]

- **Periapical pain** can be caused by an infection spreading through the **apical foramen** of the tooth into the periodontal region. The infection can transform into a dental abscess if left untreated.
- **Exposed cementum** and **dentin** on teeth can produce pain. Under ordinary circumstances, tooth sensitivity can be present with healthy pulp. If gingival recession is present, the patient underwent recent scaling, or they suffer from gastric reflux, there can be dentin sensitivity. The pain is described as sharp and short in duration. It is thought that the pain is due to movement of fluids in and out of the dentin tubules in response to osmotic or temperature changes.
- **Incomplete fractures** of a tooth may cause pain. Patients often complain of sharp pain when they bite or release from biting. Symptoms may also include sensitivity to cold temperatures. Cracks are often difficult to see in the oral cavity and may not show up on radiographs.
- **Periodontal disease** is a chronic inflammatory disorder initiated by oral microbes that can eventually affect

supporting structures of the tooth and the surrounding bone. In general, it is not considered a chronic pain disorder, as initial symptoms are gingival sensitivity and bleeding. However, **periodontal abscesses** can develop. This type of acute infection does not develop from the pulp but typically arises in a preexisting periodontal pocket. In this situation, the most common symptom is pain. Other symptoms include swelling of the gingiva and oral mucosa surrounding the affected tooth. Lymphadenopathy and fever may be present.

- **Alveolar osteitis** or "*dry socket*" is one of the most common complications following a tooth extraction. In this condition, the clot that developed post extraction fails, leaving an empty socket and exposed alveolar bone. Bone pain can result from noxious stimulation of the periosteum. Additionally, food and debris can get trapped and become necrotic, further irritating the nerve endings. Pain from a dry socket is typically described as dull and throbbing. Smoking is a major factor in the development of a dry socket, most likely due to the reduction in blood supply. Alveolar osteitis rarely occurs in the maxilla and generally develops 3 to 5 days following a mandibular tooth extraction.

26.2.2 Mucosal Pain

Pain in the oral mucosa is typically associated with mucosal lesions caused by local or systemic diseases. Mucosal pain can be localized or diffused. Local pain is often associated with breaks in the mucosa such as an **ulcer** or **erosion**. Diffuse pain can be caused by an infection or other factors such as a systemic condition. **Acute mucosal pain** is usually related to tissue damage; thus, it typically responds to treatment and/or heals in a relatively short period. Chronic mucosal pain can last from months to years after healing and in the absence of obvious stimuli (lesions) (see Section 26.3).

A significant amount of oral mucosal disorders causing pain is due to the formation of ulcers or erosions. A mucosal erosion is a superficial break in the mucus membrane. A **mucosal ulcer** is defined as loss of surface tissue and degeneration of both the **epithelium** and the **lamina propria**. It involves the **submucosa** and can even run as deep as the muscle or the periosteum. Mouth ulcerations can develop from a number of situations including poorly fitting dentures, systemic disease, and **iatrogenic** or treatment-related causes.

- Lesions of **odontogenic** origin:
  - Dental and periodontal issues primarily affect the **gingiva** and adjacent **alveolar mucosa. Dental abscesses**

originating from necrotic pulp often produce swelling in the mucosa.

- ○ **Gingivitis** or inflammation of the gingiva is commonly the result of dental plaque and can cause discomfort in individuals. Factors other than dental plaque that are related to gingivitis are orthodontic brackets, mouth breathing, and pregnancy.
- Lesions caused by poorly fitting **dentures:**
  - ○ Irritation from dentures affects the **alveolar ridge** and **palate**.
  - ○ Acute and severe irritation can produce significant ulcerations.
  - ○ Chronic irritation results in a proliferative response that mimics the shape of the denture.
  - ○ As the alveolar bone is continuously resorbed, the denture sits more deeply in the sulcus, exacerbating the ulcerative condition.
  - ○ Maxillary dentures that are poorly adapted to the palate can produce **papillary hyperplasia** (**polyps**).
- Lesions caused by **trauma:**
  - ○ Trauma to the oral mucosa from biting, rubbing on sharp edges of teeth, or restorations can result in the formation of ulcers.
    - – These types of ulcerations can appear very similar to carcinomatous lesions so care must be taken to rule out malignancy.
  - ○ Milder trauma can produce **hyperkeratinization** or **fibroepithelial hyperplasia**, which can become an irritant resulting in pain.
  - ○ Thermal and chemical burns to the oral mucosal can also cause pain.
- **Recurrent aphthous ulcers** (*canker sores*) in the oral mucosa are fairly common. The incidence has been reported as high as 20% of the general population.
  - ○ Lesions are sharply demarcated, round to ovoid with **erythematous halos**.
  - ○ These lesions will typically heal within 1 week. Ulcers lasting longer than 3 weeks should be evaluated for possible malignancy or other underlying diseases.
  - ○ Although there are some cases where there appears to be a genetic basis, most individuals develop ulcers randomly. Factors associated with the development of **aphthae** include stress, menstruation, pregnancy, and food allergies. Aphthae are also common in HIV, Crohn's disease, and celiac disease, among others.
- Mucocutaneous pain:
  - ○ Oral lesions are very common in mucocutaneous diseases such as lichen planus, pemphigus vulgaris, erythema multiforme, and chronic ulcerative stomatitis (▶ Table 26.3).
  - ○ These diseases produce erosive and ulcerative lesions that are extremely painful.

26.2.3 Musculoskeletal Pain

Temporomandibular disorders (**TMD**) are the most common *nondental* cause of orofacial pain. **Musculoskeletal pain** from TMD is primarily extra oral and typically localizes around the TMJ and muscles of mastication. It can also produce headaches and pain within the ear (**otalgia**; see Chapter 23).

Table 26.3 Systemic and iatrogenic origins of oral ulcers

Microbial diseases	Herpes simplex
	Varicella zoster
	Herpes zoster
	Hand, foot, and mouth disease
	Tuberculosis
	Syphilis
	Fungal infections
Cutaneous diseases	Lichen planus
	Pemphigus
	Erythema multiforme
	Chronic ulcerative stomatitis
Neoplasms	
Blood disorders	Anemia
	Leukemia
	Neutropenia
Gastrointestinal disorders	Celiac disease
	Ulcerative colitis
	Crohn's disease
Pharmacologic	Cytotoxic drugs
	Chemotherapies
Radiotherapy	Radiation burns

Source: Adapted from Scully et al 2005.[3]

- **Myalgia** is defined as pain caused by jaw movement or palpation of the masseter or temporalis. Myalgia typically presents as dull aching pain. It is commonly seen as acute, but with continued muscle strain, it can last for long periods of time.
- If pain radiates to adjacent structures, it is termed **myofascial pain**.
- Myofascial pain also presents as dull, aching, continuous pain that may refer to other sites upon palpation. Myofascial pain tends to be chronic and may have **trigger points** that, when stimulated, will elicit pain.
- **Myositis** (inflammatory myopathy) refers to any condition that results in inflammation of muscles. In dentistry, it refers to localized, transient swelling that involves facial muscles and tissues. Myositis can occur following dental anesthesia or trauma. Pain may be increased with mandibular movement.
- Acute **articular disk displacement** is often associated with pain, whereas chronic disk dislocation is more likely to be nonpainful. Disorders of the disk often produce clicking or **crepitus**. Osteoarthritis of the articular disk often results in deterioration of the articular surface. This condition can result in intense pain that is exacerbated by mandibular movement.

Treatment of Temporomandibular Disorders

- Patients typically seek medical attention when they experience pain and/or limited function such as inability to open, joint locking, pain when chewing, facial pain, or headache.
- Treatment goals include elimination of decreasing pain and restoring normal range of motion as well as jaw function and chewing.
- TMD is often self-limiting with extended periods of remission.

- Nonsurgical medical treatment involves physical therapy and pharmacotherapy.
  - Physical therapy is helpful for restoring normal function of the joint and muscles of mastication.
  - Common pharmacological agents include nonsteroidal anti-inflammatory drugs (NSAIDS), analgesics, local anesthetics, muscle relaxants, botulinum toxin, and antidepressants.

26.2.4 Referred Pain

Referred pain is a phenomenon whereby pain is felt in an area that is remote from the actual location where the nociceptors were stimulated. Although the mechanisms behind referred pain are not entirely understood, there are several theories that have been proposed to explain how it occurs. They include the **convergence theory** and **central centralization** (see Chapter 14).

- Dental patients often have difficulty identifying the source of their pain including which tooth is affected. Additionally, they often experience referred orofacial pain and seek medical or dental attention for the referred pain rather than the dental pain.
- Most referred orofacial pain is of odontogenic origin; however, it can be caused by other disorders. The following conditions have been shown to produce referred pain in teeth:
  - TMD.
  - Myofascial pain.
  - Sinusitis.
  - Otitis media.
  - Muscle tension headaches.
  - Chronic neck problems.
  - Fibromyalgia.
  - Trigeminal neuralgia.
  - Cardiac disorders.

26.3 Neuropathic Orofacial Pain

Neuropathic pain results from abnormal signaling due to injury or dysfunction of peripheral nociceptive neurons (see Chapter 14). The defining characteristic is that pain can be produced without nociceptive activity. In orofacial pain, hallmark symptoms include **hyperalgesia** (**nociceptive sensitization**) and **allodynia** (**central sensitization**), paroxysmal shooting pain, or constant burning. Patients may also experience **constant aching** or **pressure pain**. There is a subset of patients that may present without pain but complain about altered taste or **paresthesia**. Neuropathic pain commonly has an inflammatory component, which must also be addressed in order to effectively correct the condition. Neuropathic pain is typically chronic and can escalate over time, which is quite different from nociceptive pain that decreases with time and healing. Neuropathic pain does not respond well to traditional pain treatment regimens.

26.3.1 Neurovascular Origins of Orofacial Pain

Neurovascular disorders involving dilation or constriction of blood vessels can cause orofacial pain. These disorders usually affect the face rather than the oral cavity but can cause pain in both areas in certain circumstances. They are a heterogeneous group of disorders that share a common anatomic location (head) however; the etiologies are different and possibly multifactorial. In general, it is thought that in these disorders, the nociceptors associated with vessels in the head and dura become activated. Historically, they were described as "vascular pains" but is now fairly well accepted that it involves central and peripheral sensitization, at least in part.

- **Migraines** are severe, debilitating, typically unilateral, headaches thought to be caused by vasodilation of extracranial arteries or compression of the carotid or temporal arteries on the affected side. Symptoms can include auras, nausea, and photophobia. **Ocular migraine** sufferers may or may not display pain as seen in classic migraines. Both ocular and classical migraine sufferers with auras report seeing lights, zigzag lines, and stars or experience blind spots. Patients are commonly dysfunctional from their symptoms that can last for a period of minutes or hours to days.
- **Migrainous neuralgias** (**cluster headaches**) are less common than migraines but are more likely to cause orofacial pain. Males are more likely to be affected and generally present in middle age. Pain is unilateral, and occurs in "attacks," often described as "burning." The attacks can be very precise in intervals, occurring at the same time of day or night. Cluster headaches often localize around the eyes, sometimes causing **conjunctivitis** and **rhinorrhea** on the affected side. The etiology is not completely understood although vascular causes and the hypothalamus have been implicated.
- **Temporal arteritis** is an uncommon condition that produces severe headaches as well as myofascial pain. It is a systemic inflammatory **vasculitis** of unknown etiology. It most commonly involves the temple but can also present with a pattern following the facial or lingual artery. Symptoms include visual disturbances, headache, neck pain, facial pain, and fatigue. It is important to diagnose and treat this condition early as it can cause permanent blindness.

26.3.2 Neuralgias

- **Neuralgias** are a group of disorders that are caused by irritation or damage to a nerve. It is typically described as burning and/or stabbing pain that can occur anywhere in the body.
  - **Trigeminal neuralgia** is a chronic **paroxysmal** neuropathic disorder that produces intense and sometimes debilitating unilateral pain. Most often, it localizes to V2 and V3 of the trigeminal nerve (CN V), intraorally or extraorally or to both sites simultaneously. Trigeminal neuralgias are associated with trigger zones usually within the trigeminal nerve distribution pattern that sets off the attack. The length of the attack varies and can occur several times a day. There is often a period of remission that may last for extended periods of time.
    - The etiology is typically related to **vascular compression**; however, there are cases reported of nonvascular origins such as neoplasms (meningiomas and neuromas). If vascular compression has been

identified as the cause, surgical decompression is usually very successful. More recently, ablative procedures such as the use of a **gamma knife** have shown some efficacy. Other than surgery, anticonvulsants are the treatment of choice.

○ **Glossopharyngeal neuralgia** is a fairly rare orofacial condition that follows the innervation pattern of the glossopharyngeal nerve (CN IX). Sites involved include nasopharynx, posterior aspect of the tongue, throat, tonsil, larynx, and ear. Glossopharyngeal neuralgia is a paroxysmal neuropathic disorder that can be triggered by mechanical stimulation of the trigger zone (oropharyngeal region) by swallowing, coughing, talking, and head movements.

– Painful episodes may continue for months. There can also be periods of remission. Due to the close proximity of the glossopharyngeal and vagus nerves, episodic attacks may be associated with **cardiac dysrhythmias**.

– Pharmacological treatment is similar to trigeminal neuralgias. Surgical intervention would involve decompression of the glossopharyngeal nerve.

○ **Herpetic neuralgia** is caused by reactivation of the herpes zoster virus (**shingles**) that can remain latent in the dorsal root ganglia of individuals who have previously contracted chicken pox.

– The characteristic rash and ulcerations may be accompanied by neuralgia. The neuralgia may persist after the rash resolves.

– Treatment includes antivirals, acetaminophen, ibuprofen, and topical antibiotics.

26.3.3 Atypical Orofacial Pain

Atypical orofacial pain is a persistent pain that does not fit any of the diagnostic criteria associated with specific disorders. Additionally, there is often no identifiable cause. It is characterized by aching, burning, or nagging pain that is difficult for patients to describe or localize and does not follow any anatomic distribution for sensory nerves. It can be unilateral or bilateral. Typically, it is constant although there may be periods of exacerbation. There are no trigger points generally reported with this group of disorders.

• **Burning mouth syndrome** (**BMS**) is defined as burning or painful sensations of the oral mucosa without clinical signs of pathology or identifiable medical or dental causes.

○ Burning pain in the oral mucosa is the defining characteristic of BMS. The most commons sites are the anterior tongue, anterior hard palate, and the lips.

○ BMS is categorized as primary and secondary. Primary BMS occurs without underlying medical/dental condition. Secondary BMS is associated with medical/dental issues.

– A significant number of patients experience **xerostomia** (dry mouth) and/or disruption in taste.

○ Pain associated with BMS is mild to severe. Symptoms are often negligible in the morning and increase in intensity over the course of the day with the most severe occurring at night. Pain is usually bilateral and symmetrical. Eating or drinking sometimes relieves the pain.

○ Although the etiology is unclear, some studies have shown that small fiber–related neuropathies are common in this disorder. There are also cases where it has been shown that the patients suffer from trigeminal lesions or chorda tympani dysfunction. More recently, central sensitization involving the somatosensory/trigeminal, gustatory, and olfactory pathways has been implicated.

○ Current treatment includes the use of antidepressants, vitamins, or in the case of secondary BMS, treatment of the underlying condition may alleviate symptoms. Behavioral group therapy has also been shown to be somewhat effective.

26.3.4 Orofacial Pain and Cancer

Orofacial pain from **cancer** can be symptomatic of local, regional, or distant cancer. It can also be the result of cancer treatment. The pain can mimic that of many disorders and is described as dull, aching, stabbing, shooting, and throbbing. It can also refer to local craniofacial structures or to distant sites.

• Cancer pain may be the result of primary or metastatic disease and can involve the central and peripheral nervous systems.

• Cancer cells can infiltrate the epineural, perineural, and endoneural spaces, thereby inducing tissue inflammation and possible nerve damage. Not all cancers result in **perineural invasion**, but it has been reported to be as high as 80% in head and neck cancers.

• Around 90% of head and neck cancers are squamous cell carcinomas. Oral squamous cell carcinomas commonly occur in the tongue and are reported to be extremely painful. Spontaneous facial pain is also a prevalent complaint in this condition.

• Orofacial pain is not only spontaneous but also exacerbated by normal function such as in eating, drinking, and talking.

• The onset of orofacial pain is associated with the transition from oral precancer to cancer.

• Pain as a consequence of cancer therapy is a very common problem.

○ Chemotherapy can result in severe peripheral neurotoxicity leading to neuropathic pain.

○ Neuropathic pain can also result from surgery and radiotherapy.

○ Many patients receiving radio and chemotherapy develop **oral mucositis**, which is reported to be extremely painful. Additionally, xerostomia commonly develops, making them susceptible to the development of **caries**, **candidiasis**, and **herpetic infections**.

• Pain management for orofacial cancer pain includes opioids, anticonvulsants, antidepressants, cannabinoids, topical agents, and local anesthesia.

References

1. Renton T. Dental (odontogenic) pain. Reviews in Pain. 2011; 5(1): 1-7.
2. Linn J, Trantor I, Teo N, Thanigaivel R, Goss A. the differential diagnosis of toothache from other orofacial pains in clinical practice. 2007; 52(1): S100-S104.
3. Scully C, Felix D. Oral medicine – update for the dental practitioner-orofacial pain. BDJ. 2006;200(2):75-83.

Suggested Readings

Abd-Elmeguid A, Yu D. Dental pulp neurophysiology: Part 1. Clinical and diagnostic implications. JCDA. 2009; 75(1): 55-59

Bradley G. Disease of the oral mucosa. Can Fam Physician. 1988; 34:1443-1451

Bubteina N, Garoushi S. Dentine hypersensitivity: a review. Dentistry. 2015;5(9). doi: 10.4172/2161-1122.1000330

Gopikrishna V, Pradeep G, Venkateshbabu N. Assessment of pulp vitality: a review. IJPD. 2009; 19:3-15

Gupta R, Mohan V, Mahay P, Yadav K. Orofacial pain: A review. Dentistry. 2016;6(3)1-6

Kumar K, Elavarsi P. Definition of pain and classification of pain disorders. J Advanced Clinical & Research Insights. 2016;3 (3): 87-90

Lin M, Luo Z, Bai B, Xu F, Lu T. Fluid mechanics in dentinal microtubules provides mechanistic insights into the difference between hot and cold dental pain. Plos ONE. 2011;6(3): e18068. doi: 10.1371/journalpone.0018068

Lin M, Genin G, lu T. Thermal pain in teeth: electrophysiology governed by thermomechanics. https://www.ncbi.nim.gov/pmc/articles/PMC4240033. 2017:1-24

Liu X, Ross T. Neuroplasticity, central sensitization and odontogenic referred orofacial pain. J Pain and Relief. 2015;4(6): 1-5. doi:10.4172/2167-0846.1000206

Ossipov M, Dussor G, Porreca F. Cental modulation of pain. J Clinical Investigation. 2010:120(11): 3779-378

Osterweis M.The anatomy and physiology of pain. In: Osterweis M, Kleinman A. and Mechanic D. ed. Pain and disability: clinical, behavioral and public policy. Washington DC. National Academic Press; 1987: 1-17

Ray A. Neuroplasticity, sensitization and pain. In: Treatment of Chronic Pain by Integrative Approaches. American Academy of Pain Medicine. 2015. doi: 10.1007/978-1-4939-1821-8_2

Romero-Reyes M, Uyanik J. Orofacial pain management: current perspectives. J of Pain Research. 2014; 7:99-115

Romero-Reyes M, Salvemini D. Cancer and orofacial pain. Med Oral Pathol Oral Cir Bucal. 2016; 21(6):665-671. doi:10.4172/2161-1122.1000367

Scully C, Shotts R. Mouth ulcers and other causes of orofacial soreness and pain. BJM. 2000:321: 162-165

Steeds C. The anatomy and physiology of pain. Surgery. 2009;27(12): 507-511

Yang Y, Zhang P, Li W. Comparison of orofacial pain of patients with different stages of precancer and oral cancer. www.nature.com/scientificreports . 2017; 7(203):1-5. doi:10.1038/s41598-017-00370-x

Zakrzewska J. Multi-dimensionality of chronic pain and the oral cavity and face. J of Headache and Pain. 2013; 14(37): 1-10. http://www.thejournalofheadacheandpain.com/content/14-1-37

Questions and Answers

1. Oral examination of Patient A shows a fistula on the anterior mandibular labial gingiva. The patient denies any pain or temperature sensitivity in the area. Thermal pulp testing did not elicit a response nor did percussion. Which of the following diagnoses do you suspect is most likely?
   a) Reversible pulpitis
   b) Irreversible pulpitis
   c) Necrotic pulp
   d) Periradicular abscess

Level 3: Difficult

Answer C: Necrotic pulp is correct because there is no thermal or percussive response. This is because the pain receptors are not viable due to the necrosis; (**A**) reversible pulpitis would respond to cold stimulus; (**B**) irreversible pulpitis would respond to warm stimuli; (**D**) periodontal abscess would respond to percussion.

2. Which of the following statements is **CORRECT**?
   a) TMD pain is typically intraoral.
   b) TMD pain is always neuropathic.
   c) TMD pain can become myofacial pain.
   d) TMD pain is always sharp and intense.

Level 2: Medium

Answer C: TMD is called myofacial pain if it radiates to adjacent structures; (**A**) TMD is rarely intraoral; (**B**) TMD can be both neuropathic and nociceptive; (**D**) TMD pain is usually dull and aching unless there is degeneration of the articular disc.

3. Patient B comes into the doctor's office complaining of sharp cutaneous pain along the right mandible. Physical examination reveals a rash with ulcerations along the mandible with a very specific linear pattern. Which of the following conditions do you suspect?
   a) Trigeminal neuralgia
   b) Herpetic neuralgia
   c) Glossopharyngeal neuralgia
   d) Atypical facial pain

Level 3: Difficult

Answer B: Herpetic neuralgia associated with varicella zoster which produces rash with ulcerations. (**A**) Trigeminal neuralgias do not produce rashes or ulcerations. (**C**) Glossopharyngeal neuralgias is not associated with the mandible. (**D**) Atypical facial pain is associated with dull chronic pain and does not produce ulcerations.

4. A patient comes into your office complaining of a burning sensation on the anterior aspect of the tongue. Oral examination revealed no ulcerations or lacerations in the area. The patient also complained of having a dry mouth and stated that eating seemed to relieve the pain for short periods of time. Which of the following conditions do you consider as the cause for the symptoms?
   a) Burning mouth syndrome
   b) Glossopharyngeal neuralgia
   c) Trigeminal neuralgia
   d) Referred Pain

Level 3: Difficult

Answer A: Burning mouth syndrome. The lack of any evidence of a dental or medical issue, along with the localization to the tongue and the dry mouth are symptoms of this condition. (**B**) Symptoms and location of pain is not consistent with glossopharyngeal neuralgia. (**C**) Symptoms and location of pain is not consistent with trigeminal neuralgia. (**D**) No evidence of medical or dental disease. Also, xerostomia is indicative of an issue in the oral cavity.

5. A male patient is seen in the acute care clinic for severe headache. The patient indicates that the pain is most intense around his left eye and that it occurs with some frequency in the evening. Patient also indicates that the attack is often accompanied by a runny nose. Which of the following conditions is most likely to be the diagnosis?
a) Migraine
b) Temporal arteritis
c) Trigeminal neuralgia
d) Cluster headache

Level 3: Difficult

Answer D: Cluster headaches are often associated with conjunctivitis or rhinorrhea and localize to the eyes. **(A)** Migraines do not commonly localize around eyes or cause rhinorrhea, **(B)** Temporal arteritis often produces visual disturbances as well as facial pain, **(C)** Trigeminal neuralgia most often localizes to V2 and V3 and are associated with trigger zones.

27 Local Anesthesia: Intraoral Injections

Margaret A. Jergenson

Learning Objectives

1. Describe the action of local anesthetic on nerve cell membranes.
2. Explain the branches of the trigeminal nerve that are anesthetized to perform dental procedures.
3. Describe, in general, the anatomic landmarks important in the administration of local anesthetics.

27.1 Overview of Dental Local Anesthesia

Local anesthetic solution is injected to block the production of nerve impulses that relay sensory information. This is accomplished by decreasing the permeability of the ion channels to sodium ions. The decrease in the sodium conductance causes a failure to reach the threshold level of depolarization for the production and propagation of an action potential.

- Local anesthetic is delivered in two types of injections. In both types, the local anesthetic prevents the nerve impulse from traveling centrally from the site of anesthetic deposition.
  - Local infiltration (supraperiosteal injection) is the injection of local anesthetic into a relatively small area with the aim of anesthetizing the terminal nerve branches in the area of the planned procedure. This is most effective for procedures of limited scope.
  - A nerve block requires the deposition of anesthetic in proximity to the trunk of a nerve usually at a site somewhat distant from the area of the procedure. This usually results in a larger area of anesthesia and is useful for multiple or more extensive procedures.
- Basic instrumentation in both types of injection includes a syringe, disposable needle, and anesthetic cartridge.
  - Commonly used syringe is a metallic, breech loading cartridge type. These can be of an aspirating or self-aspirating type. Alternatives include various disposable plastic syringes that accommodate the cartridge and computer-controlled local anesthetic delivery systems.
  - The disposable needle that delivers the solution into the tissues from the cartridge is usually made of stainless steel.
    - Needles are beveled to form the point. The gauge or diameter of the lumen used is 30, 27, or 25. Thirty gauge is the smallest diameter of these and 25 gauge the largest.
    - Needles come in short and long lengths, with average lengths being 20 mm for the short and 32 mm for the long.
  - The dental cartridge is a glass cylinder containing 1.8 mL of the selected anesthetic solution.
    - The smaller end of the cartridge has an aluminum cap that holds a diaphragm of semipermeable latex rubber membrane for the blunt end of the needle to penetrate.
    - The open end of the cartridge has a stopper, slightly inset, to allow the harpoon of an aspirating syringe to embed for applying back pressure on the plunger.

27.2 Mandibular Local Anesthesia

Sensory innervation to the mandibular arch, including teeth, supporting structures, and soft tissue, is derived from the mandibular division of the trigeminal nerve (V_3). The specific branches of V_3 involved are the inferior alveolar, the lingual, and the buccal. The inferior alveolar further divides into the mental and incisive branches. Block injections are usually chosen due to the anatomy and thickness of the bone of the mandible. The specific dental procedure planned determines which block injection is used.

27.2.1 Inferior Alveolar Nerve Block

The most commonly used block for restorative and surgical procedures in the mandibular arch, this injection is also the most challenging in oral anesthesia.

- Nerves targeted: the inferior alveolar before it enters the mandible at the mandibular foramen, which will include the mental and incisive branches of the inferior alveolar, and the lingual, which is just anterior and medial to the inferior alveolar when it enters the foramen (▶ Fig. 27.1a-1).
- Anesthetizes: all the teeth and supporting structures to the midline; buccal soft tissues anterior to the mandibular first molar, the lower lip, and chin to midline; and lingual soft tissues, floor of oral cavity, and the anterior two-thirds of the tongue (▶ Fig. 27.1a-2).
- Anatomic landmarks: coronoid notch, the greatest concavity on the anterior border of the ramus of the mandible; pterygomandibular raphe, a mucosal fold spanning from posterior of the mandibular dental arch toward the maxilla; and the occlusal plane of the mandibular dental arch.
- Technique:
  - The operator's thumb in the coronoid notch stabilizes the tissue and indicates the vertical position of the injection because the deepest part of the notch is at the level of the mandibular foramen.
  - The syringe should approach the injection site parallel to the occlusal plane of the mandibular teeth from the opposite premolar area (▶ Fig. 27.1a-1).
  - The needle should penetrate the tissue lateral to the pterygomandibular raphe at a level that will be above the mandibular foramen (▶ Fig. 27.1a-3).
  - The needle is advanced about 20 to 25 mm until it is stopped by contact with bone. At this point, it is withdrawn slightly, about 1 mm (▶ Fig. 27.1a-4).
  - Aspiration is important to assure against intravascular administration of the anesthetic.
  - If the aspiration is negative, inject the cartridge of anesthetic slowly over 60 seconds.
  - Slowly withdraw the needle and allow time for the anesthetic to bathe and penetrate the nerve.
- Successful block is indicated by numbness and tingling in the lower lip, which indicates the mental nerve, the terminal branch of the inferior alveolar, has been anesthetized.
- Failure of successful block:

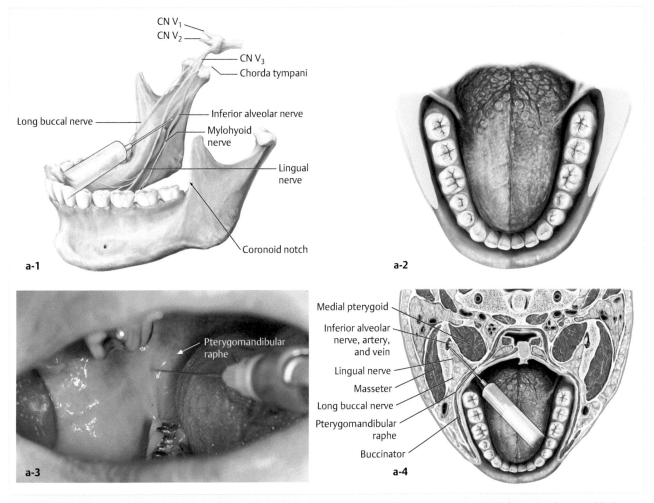

Fig. 27.1 (a-1) Syringe position for the inferior alveolar nerve block, left lateral view. **(a-2)** Areas anesthetized by inferior alveolar nerve block, superior view. **(a-3)** Intraoral injection site for inferior alveolar nerve block. **(a-4)** Transverse section just above the occlusal plane of the mandibular teeth, superior view.

(Continued)

- Penetration of the needle is inadequate, the lingual nerve may be anesthetized but not the inferior alveolar.
- The injection is too low, anesthetic will be below the foramen where the nerve enters the bone and will not be effective.
- The needle is advanced beyond the posterior border of the mandible, it enters the parotid gland space, and injection will affect the facial nerve (VII) to cause paralysis of the muscles of facial expression (Bell's palsy).
- Clinical considerations:
  - If a bony stop is encountered too early, the needle has contacted the mandible too far anterior and must be partially withdrawn and repositioned to reach the proper depth for the injection.

- If no bony stop is encountered, the angle of the injection should be increased so the syringe is positioned over the contralateral first molar and advanced until a stop is met.
- Inferior alveolar or lingual nerves may be contacted by the needle during the injection, resulting in a "shock" sensation to the patient. This usually results in rapid and profound anesthesia. This seldom results in nerve damage.
- Anatomic variations that should be considered effect the position of the mandibular foramen. In children, it is relatively farther posterior on the ramus of the mandible. In adults with a protrusive mandible, it is relatively higher on the ramus.

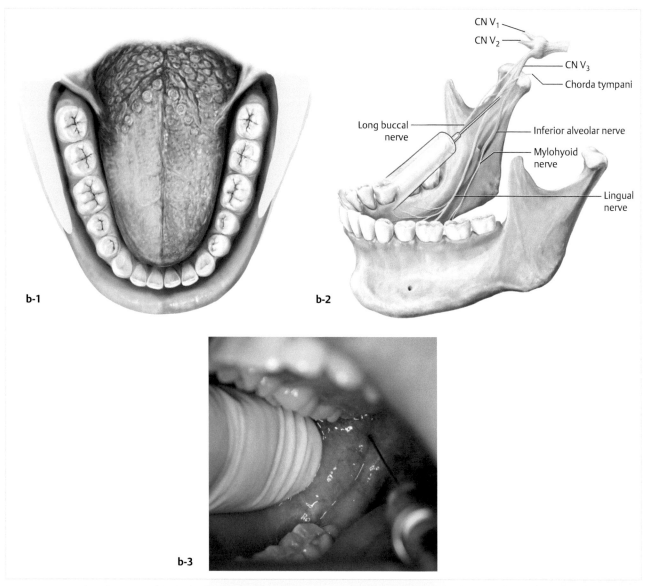

Fig. 27.1 (*Continued*) **(b-1)** Areas anesthetized by Gow-Gates block, superior view. **(b-2)** Intraoral injection site for Gow-Gates block. **(b-3)** Syringe position for the Gow-Gates block, left lateral view.

(Continued)

27.2.2 Gow-Gates Block

Considered to be a true mandibular nerve block, this injection is a variation of the inferior alveolar nerve block in which the anesthetic deposition is very high in the pterygomandibular space and should affect all branches of the mandibular nerve (V$_3$).

- Nerves targeted: the inferior alveolar with its mental and incisive branches, the lingual, mylohyoid, auriculotemporal, and buccal (long buccal).
- Anesthetizes: all the teeth and supporting structures to the midline; buccal soft tissues of the same side of the mandibular arch; lingual soft tissues, floor of oral cavity, and the anterior two-thirds of the tongue; skin of the cheek and anterior temporal region (▶ Fig. 27.1b-1).
- Anatomic landmarks: lower border of the tragus of the ear and the corner of the mouth extraorally and the maxillary second molar intraorally.
- Technique:
  ○ The patient must open their mouth as wide as possible and maintain that position.
  ○ The operator should retract the cheek with the thumb in the coronoid notch of the mandible.

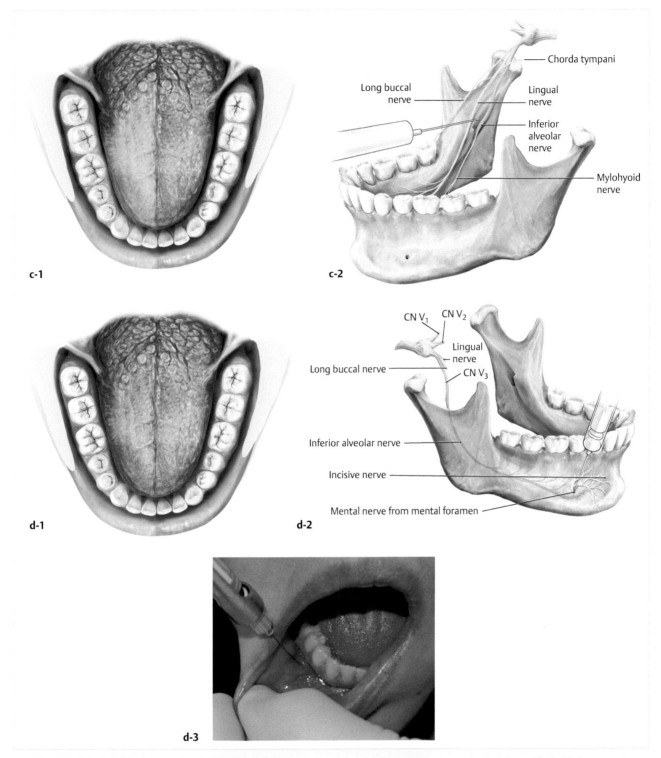

c-2

Chorda tympani

Long buccal nerve

Lingual nerve

Inferior alveolar nerve

Mylohyoid nerve

c-1

d-1

d-2

CN V₁

CN V₂

Lingual nerve

Long buccal nerve

CN V₃

Inferior alveolar nerve

Incisive nerve

Mental nerve from mental foramen

d-3

Fig. 27.1 (*Continued*) **(c-1)** Areas anesthetized by the Akinosi block, superior view. **(c-2)** Syringe position for the Akinosi block. **(d-1)** Area anesthetized by the mental nerve block. **(d-2)** Syringe position for the mental nerve block. **(d-3)** Intraoral injection site for the mental nerve block.

(*Continued*)

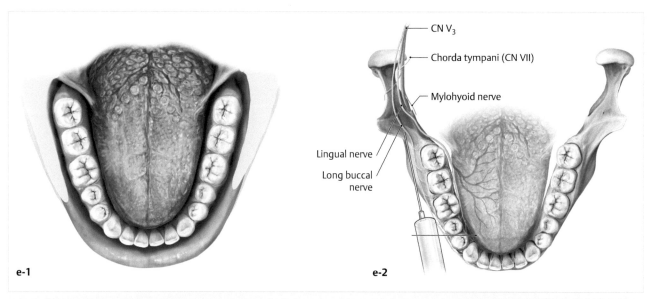

Fig. 27.1 (*Continued*) **(e-1)** Area anesthetized by the long buccal nerve block. **(e-2)** Syringe position for the long buccal nerve block. (Reproduced with permission from Baker EW. Anatomy for Dental Medicine. Second Edition. © Thieme 2015. Illustrations by Markus Voll and Karl Wesker.)

○ The syringe barrel should be positioned toward the injection site from the corner of the mouth on the opposite side. The syringe must be parallel to a line from the angle of the mouth to the lower edge of the tragus of the ear on the side of the injection.

○ The needle should penetrate the tissue just posterior and lateral to the maxillary second molar at the level of the mesiolingual cusp (▶ Fig. 27.1b-2).

○ The needle is advanced to about 25 mm and should make contact with the bone of the neck of the mandible (▶ Fig. 27.1b-3). At this point, it is withdrawn slightly, about 1 mm.

○ Aspiration is important to assure against intravascular administration of the anesthetic.

○ If the aspiration is negative, inject the cartridge of anesthetic slowly over 60 to 90 seconds.

○ Slowly withdraw the needle. The patient will need to remain in the maximally open position for another 1 to 2 minutes.

• Successful block is indicated by numbness and tingling in the lower lip, which indicates the mental nerve, the terminal branch of the inferior alveolar, has been anesthetized.

• Failure of successful block:

○ Failure of this block is rare after the operator has become accustomed to the procedure.

○ The larger diameter of the nerve at this level may require that a larger volume of anesthetic be used. If anesthesia is incomplete, inject additional solution.

• Clinical considerations:

○ If no bony stop is encountered, do not inject anesthetic. Needle should be withdrawn and redirected laterally.

○ Some patients have difficulty maintaining the wide open position for a long period.

27.2.3 Akinosi Block

This closed-mouth inferior alveolar block is a variation of the inferior alveolar nerve block. It can be used when the patient has a restricted ability to open the mouth.

• Nerves targeted: the inferior alveolar with its mental and incisive branches before it enters the mandible at the mandibular foramen and the lingual just anterior and medial to the inferior alveolar.

• Anesthetizes: all the teeth and supporting structures to the midline; buccal soft tissues anterior to the mandibular first molar, the lower lip, and chin to midline; lingual soft tissues, floor of oral cavity, and the anterior two-thirds of the tongue (▶ Fig. 27.1c-1).

• Anatomic landmarks: junction of the gingiva and mucosa superior to the maxillary third (or second) molar, the maxillary tuberosity, and the coronoid notch on the anterior border of the ramus of the mandible.

• Technique:

○ The patient should have their teeth gently touching and the muscles of mastication relaxed.

○ The operator should retract the cheek as much as possible with their thumb or index finger resting in the coronoid notch.

○ The syringe is held parallel to the occlusal plane of the maxillary teeth at the level of the mucogingival junction of the third molar (second molar if the third molar is not present).

○ The needle should penetrate the buccal mucosa and be oriented slightly laterally to a depth of about 25 mm from the maxillary tuberosity (▶ Fig. 27.1c-2). No bony contact should be expected. At this point, the tip of the needle should be in the middle of the pterygomandibular space.

○ Aspiration is important to assure against intravascular administration of the anesthetic.

○ If the aspiration is negative, inject the cartridge of anesthetic slowly over 60 seconds.

○ Slowly withdraw the needle.

• Successful block is indicated by numbness and tingling in the lower lip, which indicates the mental nerve, the terminal branch of the inferior alveolar, has been affected.

• Failure of successful block:

○ The needle is directed too far medially, medial to the sphenomandibular ligament, if the lateral flare of the mandible is underestimated. The path of the needle should parallel the ramus of the mandible.

○ The needle inserted too low will not produce anesthesia. Retry at a higher insertion level.

○ Inserting the needle too far or not far enough. There is no bony contact to help judge the depth of penetration. The 25-mm recommendation if for average patients. It has to be adjusted for larger or smaller individuals.

• Clinical considerations:

○ Transient facial nerve (VII) paralysis will result if the needle is over-inserted and the needle enters the parotid gland space and injection of anesthetic occurs.

27.2.4 Mental Nerve Block with Incisive Nerve Block Variation

The mental nerve should be anesthetized to perform soft-tissue procedures anterior to the mental foramen. With a relatively simple variation, this injection can be effective in anesthetizing the incisive branch of the inferior alveolar as well. Use of this sometimes can eliminate the need for bilateral inferior alveolar blocks, which are very uncomfortable for the patient.

• Nerves targeted: mental nerve just outside the mental foramen, and with a modification of the technique, the incisive branch within the bone of the mandible.

• Anesthetizes: all buccal and labial soft tissue of the mandibular arch anterior to the mental foramen, and with modification, the mandibular incisors, canine, and first premolar along with the supporting structures to the midline (▶ Fig. 27.1d-1).

• Anatomic landmarks: the mental foramen and the mandibular second premolar.

• Technique:

○ The patient's mouth should be in a partially closed position so the cheek is loose.

○ If there is a radiograph of the area, the mental foramen should be visible in the area of the apex of the second premolar. It may be slightly anterior or posterior to that tooth.

○ The operator should palpate the mandible in the buccal vestibule from the first molar region anteriorly. With practice, the mental foramen can be discerned (▶ Fig. 27.1d-2).

○ The needle is inserted into the buccal mucosa at the level of the first premolar and directed toward the mental foramen (▶ Fig. 27.1d-3).

○ Aspiration is important to assure against intravascular administration of the anesthetic.

○ If the aspiration is negative, inject about a third of the cartridge of anesthetic slowly.

○ Slowly withdraw the needle.

• Technique variation for incisive nerve anesthesia:

○ The process is the same as above except for the application of gentle finger pressure over the mental foramen during the injection of the anesthetic. The finger pressure will facilitate the flow of anesthetic solution into the mental foramen.

○ The finger pressure over the foramen must be maintained for 1 to 2 minutes after the needle has been withdrawn.

• Successful block is indicated by numbness and tingling in the lower lip and lack of pain during dental treatment.

• Failure of successful block:

○ Failure is rare but may be due to inadequate amount of anesthetic.

○ If there is inadequate pulpal anesthesia of the incisive nerve, the duration of the pressure applied after injection was not long enough.

• Clinical considerations:

○ Anesthesia of the mental branch alone is sufficient for only soft-tissue procedures.

○ In varying the injection to encompass the incisive nerve, the pulpal anesthesia is assured from the first premolar to the midline. The second premolar may have adequate coverage for restorative procedures, but more extensive work or extraction will require an inferior alveolar block.

27.2.5 Buccal Nerve Block

Commonly called the long buccal nerve block, this injection targets the soft tissue on the buccal side of the mandibular molars. This area is not anesthetized by any of the previous injections except the Gow-Gates Block.

• Nerves targeted: the buccal branch of V_3, commonly called the long buccal nerve/

• Anesthetizes: the buccal mucosa and gingiva overlying the mandibular molars (▶ Fig. 27.1e-1).

• Anatomic landmarks: anterior border of the ramus as it flattens lateral to the third molar.

• Technique:

○ The operator retracts the patient's cheek to expose the buccal aspect of the mandibular arch.

○ The syringe is advanced so the needle penetrates the buccal mucosa just posterior to the last molar tooth present (▶ Fig. 27.1e-2).

○ The bevel of the needle should be facing the bone. The depth of penetration of the tissue is minimal, 2 to 3 mm. After aspiration, about a quarter of the cartridge is injected slowly.

• The success of this block is reflected in the absence of discomfort for the patient. If this is supplementing another injection, the patient may not be aware of any obvious effect.

• Clinical consideration:

○ A separate injection for this tissue is only necessary when there will be direct impact on the tissues as in an extraction.

- Care should be taken to assure that the bevel is totally covered by tissue so that the anesthetic is not spilled into oral cavity.

27.3 Maxillary Local Anesthesia

Sensory innervation to the maxillary arch is derived from the maxillary division of the trigeminal nerve (V_2). The three superior alveolar nerves supply the teeth and supporting structures. The posterior superior alveolar (PSA) nerve consistently innervates the molars with the exception of the mesiobuccal root of the first molar, which is more variable. The middle superior alveolar (MSA), which is absent in some individuals, innervates the mesiobuccal root of the first molar and the two premolars. The anterior superior alveolar (ASA) nerve innervates the canine and incisors. In addition, the greater palatine and nasopalatine nerves are the sensory nerves of the hard palate.

The nature of the bone of the maxilla is very different than the mandible. The bone is very thin and is easily penetrated by the anesthetic. This facilitates the administration of acceptable clinical anesthesia. The specific dental procedure planned determines the placement of the injection.

27.3.1 Local Infiltration (Supraperiosteal Injection)

This is the most commonly used injection for anesthesia of the maxillary teeth. It is more properly called a supraperiosteal injection and is performed successfully with ease. It is used when treating individual teeth or multiple teeth that are not adjacent to each other.

- Nerves targeted: terminal nerve branches of the tooth to be treated.
- Anesthetizes: the tooth targeted along with the supporting structures, buccal mucosa, and overlying lip or cheek of that tooth. Anesthesia of the tooth on either side of targeted tooth may also be adequate for operative procedures (▶ Fig. 27.1a-1).
- Anatomic landmarks: the mucobuccal fold apical to the crown of the tooth targeted. Understanding of the root anatomy of the various teeth is also required.
- Technique:
  - The operator lifts the lip of the patient to expose the desired teeth and to tighten the tissue.
  - The syringe is advanced parallel to the crown of the tooth being targeted. The needle should penetrate the tissue at the height of the mucobuccal fold to the approximate depth of the root apex of the tooth (▶ Fig. 27.2a-2 and a-3).
  - After aspiration, about one-third of the anesthetic cartridge should be slowly injected.
  - Slowly withdraw the syringe and allow the anesthetic to work for 3 minutes before proceeding.
- Successful injection should cause a feeling of numbness in the area.
- Clinical consideration:
  - Very effective anesthesia for limited area when pulpal and/or soft-tissue coverage is necessary.

- When care is used in administration, this injection is atraumatic.
- Insertion of the needle too close to the bone can cause discomfort if the needle tip is on the periosteum. The syringe should be parallel to the tooth, slightly away from the bone.
- If a dental procedure is going to involve the palatal tissue, it must be injected separately. For isolated teeth, this can be accomplished with a local infiltration of the palatal mucosa over the specific tooth.

27.3.2 Posterior Superior Alveolar Nerve Block

This block is used when there is a need to anesthetize multiple maxillary molars. It is a very atraumatic and effective injection.

- Nerves targeted: the PSA nerve as it enters the bone of the maxilla.
- Anesthetizes: the maxillary molars, EXCEPT the mesiobuccal root of the first molar in some individuals, along with the supporting structures of the teeth and the buccal soft tissues (▶ Fig. 27.2b-1).
- Anatomic landmarks: the zygomatic process of the maxilla, the maxillary second molar, and the mucobuccal fold.
- Technique:
  - The patient should be in a partially open position. A wide open position brings the coronoid process of the mandible forward to block the buccal vestibule.
  - The operator retracts the cheek to pull the tissue taut while placing a finger on the zygomatic process of the maxilla.
  - The syringe is oriented on a line that is angled posteriorly, superiorly, and medially (▶ Fig. 27.2b-2).
  - The needle should penetrate the tissue at the height of the mucobuccal fold superior to the maxillary second molar (▶ Fig. 27.2b-3).
  - The needle is advanced to about one-half the length of a long needle though this should be varied according to the size of the patient.
  - Aspiration is important to assure against intravascular administration of the anesthetic.
  - If the aspiration is negative, inject the anesthetic slowly over 60 seconds.
  - Slowly withdraw the needle and allow time for the anesthetic to act.
- Success rate of this block is very high, but because of the loose nature of the cheek tissue, the patient may not have awareness of anesthesia.
- Clinical consideration:
  - There is no bony stop in this injection to verify depth of needle placement. Over-insertion can intrude into the area of the pterygoid plexus of veins. If this happens, the needle can injure vessels and cause bleeding into the tissue, a hematoma. Although it is not generally a problem, it can be unsightly and cause minor discomfort.
  - Because of the thin and porous bone of the maxilla, under-insertion of the needle usually still results in adequate anesthesia.

27.3.3 Middle Superior Alveolar Nerve Block

Since the MSA nerve is not present in some individuals, this injection may have limited clinical use. However, due to the porosity of the maxilla, effective pulpal anesthesia can still be achieved for the desired teeth.

- Nerve targeted: MSA as it descends in the lateral wall of the maxillary sinus.
- Anesthetizes: both maxillary premolars and the mesiobuccal root of the first molar along with their supporting structures and buccal soft tissue (▶ Fig. 27.2c-1).
- Anatomic landmark: maxillary second premolar.
- Technique:
  - The operator lifts the lip of the patient to expose the second premolar and to tighten the tissue.

- The syringe is advanced parallel to the crown of the second premolar. The needle should penetrate the tissue at the height of the mucobuccal fold and advance to a depth above the root apex of the tooth (▶ Fig. 27.2c-2 and c-3).
- After aspiration, about one-half of the anesthetic cartridge should be slowly injected.
- Slowly withdraw the syringe and allow the anesthetic to act before proceeding.
- Success rate of this block is very high and the patient will have a numb lip in the area.
- Clinical consideration:
  - When care is used in administration, this injection is atraumatic.
  - Insertion of the needle too close to the bone can cause discomfort if the needle tip is on the periosteum. The syringe should be parallel to the tooth, slightly away from the bone.

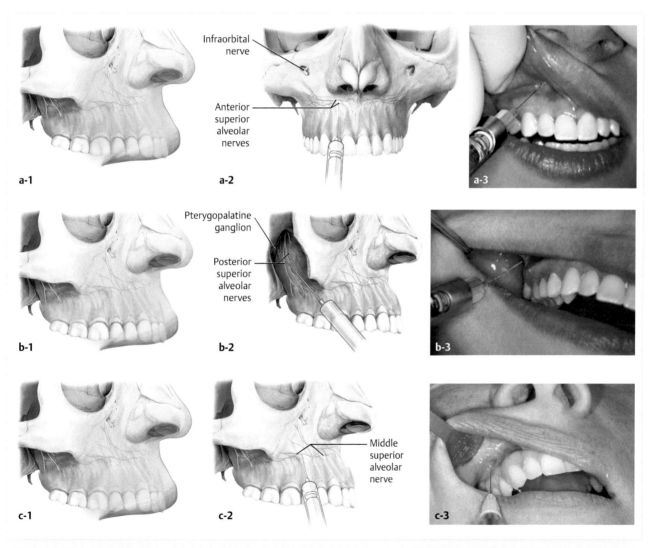

Fig. 27.2 (a-1) Area anesthetized by a local infiltration injection to a maxillary lateral incisor. **(a-2)** Syringe position for a local infiltration injection to a maxillary lateral incisor. **(a-3)** Intraoral injection site for a local infiltration injection to a maxillary lateral incisor. **(c-1)** Area anesthetized by a middle superior alveolar (MSA) nerve block. **(c-2)** Syringe position for an MSA nerve block. **(b-1)** Area anesthetized by a posterior superior alveolar (PSA) nerve block. **(b-2)** Syringe position for a PSA nerve block. **(b-3)** Intraoral injection site for a PSA nerve block. **(c-3)** Intraoral injection site for an MSA nerve block.

(Continued)

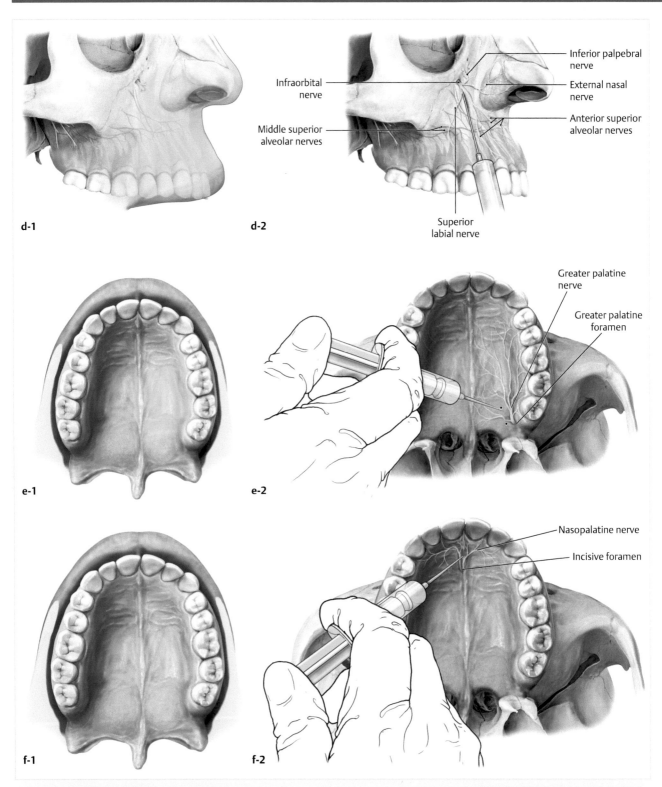

d-1

d-2

Inferior palpebral nerve

Infraorbital nerve

External nasal nerve

Middle superior alveolar nerves

Anterior superior alveolar nerves

Superior labial nerve

e-1

e-2

Greater palatine nerve

Greater palatine foramen

f-1

f-2

Nasopalatine nerve

Incisive foramen

Fig. 27.2 *(Continued)* **(d-1)** Area anesthetized by an anterior superior alveolar (ASA) nerve block. **(d-2)** Syringe position for an ASA nerve block. **(d-3)** Intraoral injection site for an ASA nerve block. **(e-1)** Area anesthetized by a greater palatine nerve block. **(e-2)** Syringe position for a greater palatine nerve block. **(f-1)** Area anesthetized by a nasopalatine nerve block. **(f-2)** Syringe position for a nasopalatine nerve block.

(Continued)

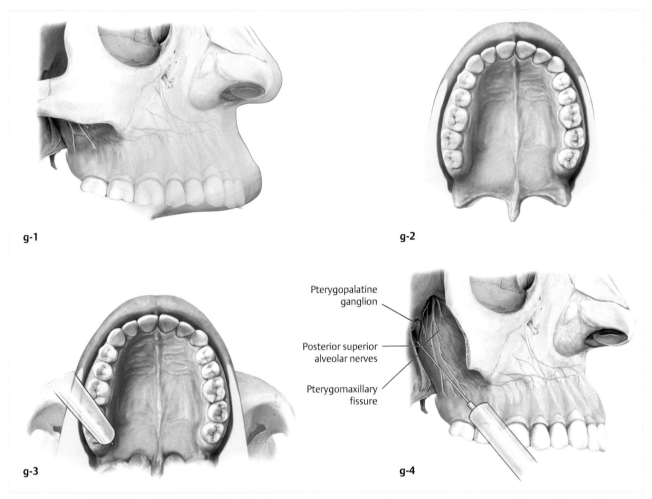

Fig. 27.2 *(Continued)* **(g-1)** Area anesthetized by a maxillary nerve block, lateral view. **(g-2)** Area anesthetized by a maxillary nerve block, palatal view. **(g-3)** Syringe position for a maxillary block by the greater palatine approach. **(g-4)** Syringe position for a maxillary block by the high tuberosity approach. (Reproduced with permission from Baker EW. Anatomy for Dental Medicine. Second Edition. © Thieme 2015. Illustrations by Markus Voll and Karl Wesker.)

27.3.4 Anterior Superior Alveolar Nerve Block

Often called the infraorbital nerve block, this injection anesthetizes a large area with one injection and can be very useful in clinical application. Many dentists are reluctant to use this block, feeling that the risk of injury is high due to the proximity of the infraorbital foramen to the eye. However, correctly administered, this is a very safe and effective procedure.

- Nerves targeted: the infraorbital nerve terminal branches, the ASA nerve, and the MSA nerve.
- Anesthetizes: the maxillary incisors and canine in all individuals and the premolars and mesiobuccal root of the first molar in about three-fourths of the population; the supporting structures of the teeth and the buccal soft tissues; and the lower eyelid, side of the nose, and the upper lip (▶ Fig. 27.2d-1).

- Anatomic landmarks: infraorbital foramen, inferior margin of the orbit, and maxillary premolars.
- Technique:
  ○ Locating the infraorbital foramen is important in this injection. This can be done by palpating the inferior margin of the orbit directly below the patient's pupil when they are gazing straight ahead. You may feel a slight notch in the rim. Then move your finger inferiorly into the concavity below the margin. You will feel the outline of the foramen. This should be directly superior to the second maxillary premolar. The patient may report a mild discomfort when pressure is placed on the infraorbital nerve. Your finger should remain in place over the foramen for the injection.
  ○ The upper lip is then lifted and the tissue is held taut.
  ○ The syringe should be oriented in a line parallel to the long axis of the premolar teeth (▶ Fig. 27.2d-2).
  ○ The needle should penetrate the tissue at the height of the mucobuccal fold superior to the first premolar. It is then

advanced toward the infraorbital foramen staying parallel to the bone of the maxilla until a bony stop is reached. This is the roof of the foramen. At this point, it is withdrawn slightly, about 1 mm.
  - Aspiration is important to assure against intravascular administration of the anesthetic.
  - If the aspiration is negative, inject half to three-fourths of the cartridge of anesthetic slowly over 60 seconds while maintaining gentle finger pressure over the foramen.
  - Slowly withdraw the needle. Maintain finger pressure over the foramen for 1 to 2 minutes after the needle is removed to facilitate the diffusion of the anesthetic into the canal.
- Successful block is indicated by numbness and/or tingling of the upper lip, the side of the nose, and the lower eyelid. The absence of discomfort for the patient during the procedure should be present in the distribution of the ASA nerve and usually the MSA nerve.
- Failure of successful block:
  - Most commonly due to inadequate depth of injection. The operator should estimate the depth before inserting the needle. If a stop is reached too soon, reposition the needle farther from bone.
- Clinical considerations:
  - Hematoma in this area is possible but if finger pressure is consistently applied, it is not likely.
  - If finger pressure is not maintained over the foramen, the infraorbital branches will be anesthetized but possibly not the ASA and MSA. This may be adequate for certain soft-tissue procedures.

27.3.5 Greater Palatine Nerve Block

None of the preceding maxillary injections will have any effect on the palatal soft tissue or bone. If a dental procedure is going to involve these tissues, the palatal tissue must be injected separately. For procedures that involve the palatal tissue and are more extensive than a single tooth, the greater palatine block is utilized for the area posterior to the canine tooth.
- Nerve targeted: greater palatine.
- Anesthetizes: the hard palate and overlying tissue from the point of injection anteriorly to the first premolar and medially to the midline (▶ Fig. 27.2e-1).
- Anatomic landmarks: greater palatine foramen.
- Technique:
  - The greater palatine foramen should be located by palpating the palate superior to the maxillary molars. If the operator begins at the first molar area and moves posteriorly, a depression will be felt just posterior to the second molar. This can be performed with a cotton swab.
  - The syringe should be advanced from the opposite side of the arch with the needle penetrating the mucosa anterior to the foramen (▶ Fig. 27.2e-2).
  - The needle will only penetrate approximately 10 mm before bone is contacted. The needle should be retracted 1 mm.
  - Aspiration is important to assure against intravascular administration of the anesthetic.
  - If the aspiration is negative, inject one-fourth of the cartridge of anesthetic slowly over 30 seconds while maintaining gentle pressure over the foramen.

  - Slowly withdraw the needle.
- Successful anesthesia is routine and results in numb and tingling sensation in posterior palate.
- Clinical considerations:
  - The soft tissue of the palate is tightly adherent to the bone and not very thick. It is a very uncomfortable area to receive an injection. Careful technique along with the use of topical and pressure anesthesia can help minimize discomfort.
  - Blanching of the tissue will be seen as anesthetic is deposited in tissue and ischemia spreads.

27.3.6 Nasopalatine Nerve Block

The nasopalatine block is very important in maxillary anesthesia as it is the only place to anesthetize the anterior hard palate. But it is an extremely uncomfortable area for an injection due to the thin and very tightly adherent tissue. Great care should be used in administering this injection.
- Nerves targeted: the nasopalatine nerves emerging at the incisive foramen.
- Anesthetizes: the hard palate and overlying soft tissue from canine to canine (▶ Fig. 27.2f-1).
- Anatomic landmark: incisive papilla.
- Technique:
  - The incisive papilla is a tear-shaped elevation in the midline directly posterior to the central incisors. It lies directly over the incisive foramen.
  - The syringe should be oriented toward the papilla from one side with the needle penetrating the tissue at the lateral base of the papilla. The needle is advanced toward the midline (▶ Fig. 27.2f-2).
  - The tissue in this area is very thin, so penetration is shallow. Bone will be lightly contacted, then withdrawn slightly.
  - Aspirate and then inject up to about one-fourth of the cartridge over 30 seconds. The injection requires some force to infuse the anesthetic due to the very tight tissue.
  - Slowly withdraw the needle.
- Successful anesthesia is routine and results in a numb and tingling sensation in the anterior palate.
- Clinical considerations:
  - The soft tissue of the palate in this area is the thinnest and most tightly adherent to the bone. It is an extremely uncomfortable area to receive an injection. Careful technique along with the use of topical and pressure anesthesia should be utilized to minimize discomfort as much as possible.
  - Blanching of the tissue will be seen as anesthetic is deposited in tissue and ischemia spreads.

27.3.7 Maxillary Nerve Block

The entire maxillary division of the trigeminal nerve (V_2) can be anesthetized by a single injection. This requires some skill and experience, so it is not advisable for a predoctoral student. But because all local anesthesia is heavily dependent on an understanding of the anatomy of the oral region, it does offer a valuable concept lesson in anesthesia.

- Nerves targeted: the maxillary division of the trigeminal nerve in the pterygopalatine fossa.
- Anesthetizes: the entire maxillary nerve distribution on the side of the injection, which includes all maxillary teeth, supporting structures, and soft tissues (▶ Fig. 27.2g-1 and ▶ Fig. 27.2g-2).
- Landmarks: requires thorough knowledge of the pterygopalatine fossa anatomy, the infratemporal fossa, and the greater palatine foremen.
- Technique: two intraoral approaches to nerve.
  - The greater palatine foramen on the hard palate is the opening to the palatine canal. This is a direct passage to the pterygopalatine fossa in which the trunk of the maxillary nerve (V_2) is located. After initial anesthesia of the tissue of the hard palate, the needle can be carefully advanced into the greater palatine foramen and deeper into the palatine canal until the fossa is reached. Deposition of a single cartridge of anesthetic will cause numbness of the entire distribution of the maxillary nerve (V_2; ▶ Fig. 27.2g-3).
  - Similarly, at the posterior wall of the maxilla, the pterygomaxillary fissure is a gap that opens into the pterygopalatine fossa. If a needle is introduced in a similar manner as the PSA block but advanced to a deeper level, the tip will be near the fissure. Anesthetic deposited at the opening of the fissure will also enter the fossa and anesthetize the maxillary nerve (V_2; ▶ Fig. 27.2g-4).
- Clinical considerations:
  - A block of the entire maxillary division is desirable for extensive procedures of the maxillary arch, particularly surgical procedures. With a single injection and minimal volume of solution, profound and broad anesthesia can be obtained.
  - The deep position of the pterygopalatine fossa requires skill and care in introducing the needle. Complications of overextension, misplacement of the needle, bleeding, or introduction of infection have serious consequences in this area.

Questions and Answers

1. Local anesthetics inhibit the production of nerve impulses by decreasing the permeability of ion channels to:
   a) Potassium ions.
   b) Sodium ions.
   c) Chloride ions.
   d) Calcium ions.

Level 1: Easy
Answer B: The local anesthetic blocks the influx of sodium ions that causes depolarization of the nerve membrane. **(A)** Potassium ions cross the membrane during repolarization. **(C)** There is no net diffusion of chloride ions during the depolarization/repolarization process. **(D)** Calcium is not involved in the depolarization/repolarization process.

2. To perform dental procedures on multiple teeth on one side of the mandibular arch in a single session, the nerve that should be anesthetized is the:
   a) Mental nerve.
   b) Incisive nerve.

   c) Inferior alveolar.
   d) Long buccal.

Level 1: Easy
Answer C: Pulpal innervation of the mandibular teeth is by the inferior alveolar. The anterior teeth are specifically innervated by the incisive branch but since it is a terminal branch of the inferior alveolar, anesthesia of the parent nerve will be effective for the anterior teeth as well. **(A)** The mental nerve innervates only soft tissue anterior to the mental foramen. **(B)** The incisive nerve innervates only the first premolar to the central incisor so any posterior teeth involved would not be anesthetized. **(D)** The long buccal nerve innervates only the buccal soft tissue of the molars.

3. Local anesthesia for dental procedures in the maxillary arch is most frequently accomplished by use of a local infiltration injection because
   a) The bone of the maxilla is very thin and allows penetration of the local anesthetic.
   b) The nerves of the maxillary teeth are found very superficially.
   c) The small diameter of the maxillary division branches allows easier penetration.
   d) The cortical plate of the maxilla is easily penetrated by the anesthetic.

Level 1: Easy
Answer A: The maxilla is made up of porous, cancellous bone. **(B)** The sensory nerves of the maxillary teeth are found within the bone of the maxilla. **(C)** The size of the nerve does affect the rapidity of action but access to the nerve through bone is the more important factor. **(D)** The maxilla does not have a cortical plate.

4. In general, nerve block injections could have an advantage over local infiltration injections when
   a) A larger area of anesthesia is needed.
   b) Multiple procedures are planned in a given area.
   c) It is desirable for the injection to be given at a distance from the site of the procedure.
   d) The location of the nerve endings precludes the anesthetic from reaching them.
   e) All of the above.

Level 2: Moderate
E. is correct. All options could be reasons for using a block injection depending on the site and condition of the planned procedure.

5. A dentist plans to extract a maxillary third molar. The dentist decides to use a posterior superior alveolar block injection. What additional nerve block would be necessary for the patient's comfort?
   a) Middle superior alveolar
   b) Maxillary
   c) Greater palatine
   d) Nasopalatine
   e) Lesser palatine

Level 2: Moderate
Answer C: The superior alveolar nerves provide sensory innervation to the pulp of the teeth and the supporting

structures, as well as buccal soft tissues. The palatal bone and soft tissue are innervated by the greater palatine nerve and must be injected separately if that tissue is effected by the procedure. **(A)** The middle superior alveolar innervation is too far anterior for the third molar. **(B)** A maxillary nerve block would effectively anesthetize the whole area but would not be needed in addition to a PSA block. For a single extraction, it would be an excessive treatment. **(D)** The nasopalatine nerve innervates the anterior palate only. **(E)** The lesser palatine nerve innervates the soft palate and usually does not need to be anesthetized for dental procedures.

Appendix: Compilation of Muscles Involved in Chapter 22

Appendix A

Reference Table A: Muscles of Mastication

Muscle Group	Action		
Primary muscles of mastication—Stabilize TMJ and move mandible relative to maxilla via elevation, depression, protrusive, retrusive, and lateral excursive movements to mediate chewing, swallowing, and speaking behaviors			
Jaw elevators	Functional role	**Motor innervation:** LMNs in motor nucleus of V	**Sensory innervation** Primary afferent neurons in mesencephalic and trigeminal ganglion
Masseter muscle (contains superficial and deep heads)	Bilateral action: Primarily elevates mandible Protrusion of mandible (posterior fibers superficial head)—secondary action Retrusion of mandible (deep head) —secondary action Unilateral action: Lateral excursion to ipsilateral side Aids in side-to-side movements/Grinding movements	Masseteric N. of anterior division of V3	Muscle spindle receptors present in muscle—provide GSA proprioceptive feedback Mechanoreceptors, nociceptors GSA
Medial pterygoid muscle (contains superficial and deep heads)	Bilateral action: Elevates mandible Assists to protrude mandible (acts as agonist) Side-to-side excursion (lateral excursion) Unilateral contraction acts to deviate mandible to contralateral side	Nerve to medial pterygoid Branch from main trunk of V3	Muscle spindle receptors present in muscle provide GSA proprioceptive feedback Mechanoreceptors, nociceptors GSA
Temporalis muscle (contains vertical and horizontal fibers)	Bilateral action: Vertical (anterior) fibers: Elevate mandible Horizontal (posterior) fibers: Retract mandible (retrusion) Unilateral action: Lateral excursion of mandible to ipsilateral side Aids in side-to-side movement	Anterior deep temporal n. and Posterior deep temporal n. (terminal branches of anterior division of V3)	Muscle spindle receptors present in muscle provide GSA proprioceptive feedback Mechanoreceptors, nociceptors GSA
Lateral pterygoid—superior head (contains superior and inferior heads)	Bilateral function: Superior head: Activated during mandibular retrusion and clenching Elevation of mandible Power stroke during jaw closing	**Nerve to lateral pterygoid** (terminal branches of anterior division of V3)	Muscle spindle receptors present in muscle provide GSA proprioceptive feedback Mechanoreceptors, nociceptors GSA associated with mucosa, skin, TMJ
Primary muscles of mastication			
Jaw depressors	Action	Motor innervation	Sensory innervation
Lateral pterygoid—inferior head	Inferior head: • Depresses mandible—initiates opening of jaw; provides rotational movement in lower TMJ compartment *Aided by gravity and digastric muscles • Protrudes mandible • Side-to-side movement (lateral excursion) during chewing Unilateral action: Side-to-side movement causes mandible to laterally deviate the contralateral side *Muscle most commonly involved in myofascial pain syndrome due to masticatory muscle spasm, often associated with chronic pain or TMJ disorders	**Nerve to lateral pterygoid** (terminal branches of anterior division of V3)	Muscle spindle receptors present in muscle provide GSA proprioceptive feedback Mechanoreceptors, nociceptors GSA associated with mucosa, skin, TMJ

Abbreviations: GSA, general somatic afferent; TMJ, temporomandibular joint

Appendix B

Reference Table B: Tongue musculature

Muscle Group	Functional role
Tongue—food placement and bolus formation during mastication and bolus transfer during swallowing; positional changes and tooth/palatal contact facilitate articulation of vowels, consonants, and alter pitch of sound; tongue pushed against hard palate/alveolar ridge creates consonants t/d	
Intrinsic group functions to alter the shape of the tongue; extrinsic group functions to change the (bodily) position of the tongue	

Intrinsic muscles	Action	Motor innervation: LMNs in hypoglossal motor nucleus	Sensory innervation
Superior longitudinal	Shortens and curls apex and lateral margins of tongue upward	Hypoglossal nerve—GSE	Muscle spindle receptors present in muscle provide GSA proprioceptive feedback
Inferior longitudinal	Shortens and curls tongue downward		Travel via ansa cervicalis
Vertical	Flatten/compress and widen tongue		
Transverse	Narrows and elongates tongue		

Extrinsic muscles	Functional role	Motor innervation	Sensory innervation
Genioglossus	Protrusion of tongue; depress center (forms groove)	Hypoglossal nerve—GSE	Muscle spindle receptors present in muscle provide GSA proprioceptive feedback
Hyoglossus	Depresses tongue/retrusion		Travel via ansa cervicalis
Styloglossus	Retrusion of tongue Elevation of tongue		
Palatoglossus	Elevation of the root of tongue Narrow the entrance of oropharynx isthmus for swallowing by pulling palatoglossal folds to midline	SVE fibers; pharyngeal nerve of X; motor branch of pharyngeal plexus LMNs in nucleus ambiguus	

Abbreviations: GSA, general somatic afferent; GSE, general somatic efferent; LMN, lower motor neuron; SVE, special visceral efferent

Appendix C

Reference Table C: Suprahyoid and infrahyoid muscles

Muscle Group		Functional role	

Suprahyoid group—functions as accessory jaw opening muscles during mastication**; stabilizes and elevates hyoid bone; facilitates airway protection by elevating larynx during oropharyngeal phase of swallowing; positional changes in laryngeal elevation (high pitch) and depression (decrease pitch) alter pitch of vibration

Accessory muscle of mastication	Action	Innervation	Sensory innervation
Mylohyoid**	Elevates the floor of the oral cavity Assists in elevating the hyoid bone during swallowing If hyoid fixed: Assists in mandible depression during mastication	N. to mylohyoid of V3 (br. from inferior alveolar) (CN VII)	Muscle spindles absent
Geniohyoid**	If mandible fixed: Moves tongue and hyoid bone anteriorly during swallowing If hyoid fixed: Assists in mandible depression during mastication	C1 ventral rami (travels with hypoglossal nerve)	Muscle spindles few
Anterior digastric**	During mastication depress and retract mandible (via hyoid stabilization)	N. to mylohyoid of V3 (br. from inferior alveolar)	Muscle spindles absent
Posterior digastric**	If mandible fixed: Works with anterior belly to elevate hyoid bone during swallowing If hyoid fixed: Depress mandible and retract mandible during mastication	Digastric br. of facial n.	Muscle spindles absent
Stylohyoid	Elevates and retracts hyoid bone and lifts base of tongue during swallowing*	Stylohyoid br. of facial n. (CN VII)	Muscle spindles—few

Muscle Group	Functional role		

Infrahyoid group——acts as accessory muscles in mastication; serves as accessory laryngeal muscles during swallowing and speech; depresses larynx; alters resonance frequency (lowers pitch of vibration)

Accessory muscle for mastication	Action	Motor innervation (GSE)	Sensory innervation (GSA)
Sternothyroid	Depress mandible via stabilization of hyoid Pulls larynx inferiorly during swallowing; lengthens vocal tract; lowers vibration pitch during speech	C2 and C3 ventral rami (ansa cervicalis)	Muscle spindles—few
Sternohyoid	Depress mandible via stabilization of hyoid; pulls larynx inferiorly during swallowing; lengthens vocal tract; lowers vibration pitch during speech	C1–C3 ventral rami (ansa cervicalis)	Muscle spindles—few
Omohyoid	Depress mandible via stabilization of hyoid; pulls larynx inferiorly during swallowing; lengthens vocal tract; lowers vibration pitch during speech	C1–C3 ventral rami (ansa cervicalis)	Muscle spindles—few
Thyrohyoid	Depress mandible via stabilization of hyoid; decreases distance between hyoid bone and thyroid cartilage	C1 ventral rami (travels with hypoglossal nerve)	Muscle spindles—few

Abbreviations: GSA, general somatic afferent; GSE, general somatic efferent

Appendix D

Reference Table D: Palatal muscles

Muscle Group	Functional role		

Palatal group—aids in bolus formation during mastication; mediates palatal elevation and closure of nasopharynx; velopharyngeal closure during pharyngeal swallowing phase; palatal elevation assists in articulation of all consonant sounds except m/.n/ng which form with relaxed soft palate

Soft palate	Action	Motor innervation: Nerve branches	Sensory innervation
Levator veli palatini	Elevate soft palate during swallowing	Pharyngeal br. of CN X—motor of pharyngeal plexus	Lesser palatine (V2) of maxillary
Palatopharyngeus	Elevates pharynx and larynx Assists in closure of nasopharynx		
Musculus uvulae	Retracts uvulae in posterior superior direction		
Palatoglossus* also considered a tongue muscle	Elevates base of tongue Narrows inlet of oropharynx		
Tensor veli palatini**	Tense palate; open auditory tube laterally during swallowing/yawning	SVE motor fibers Tensor branch from trunk of mandibular division trigeminal V3	

Appendix E

Reference Table E: Perioral facial muscles

Muscle Group	Action
Perioral group—buccolabial muscles of facial expression which include the circumferentially arranged orbicularis oris muscles, several muscles that are radially arranged from the orbicularis oris, along with the buccinator of the cheek and the risorius that extend from the corners of the mouth Functions in food placement and bolus formation during mastication and oral phase of swallowing, along with positional and shape changes, the group facilitates articulation of vowels, consonants; aids in forced expiration	

Lips	Functional role	Motor innervation; nerve branches	Sensory innervation
Orbicularis oris	Perioral sphincter of mouth; controls shape and degree of opening oral orifice; purses and protrudes lips Aids in mastication, bolus preparation for swallowing and facilitates articulation	SVE fibers; Buccal/mandibular br. of facial (CN VII)	Cutaneous sensation (GSA) via trigeminal N V2 and V3
Levator labi superioris	Elevates upper lip	Zygomatic and buccal br. of facial (CN VII)	Cutaneous sensation (GSA) via trigeminal N V2
Depressor anguli oris	Depress corner of mouth inferiorly and laterally	Buccal/Mandibular br. of facial (CN VII)	Cutaneous sensation (GSA) via trigeminal N V3
Depressor labii inferioris	Depresses lower lip	Mandibular br. of facial (CN VII)	Cutaneous sensation (GSA) via trigeminal N V3
Cheek/facial	**Functional role**	**Motor innervation: Nerve branch**	**Sensory innervation**
Buccinator	Maintains tension of cheek to hold bolus in vestibule; during contraction pushes against dental arch; works with tongue to place bolus onto occlusal surface Retracts modiolus** Aids in forced expiration and sucking actions Aids in articulation Retraction of modiolus	Buccal br. of facial (CN VII)	Cutaneous sensation (GSA) via trigeminal N V3 (long buccal)
Zygomaticus major	Moves angle of mouth superiorly, laterally Retraction and elevation of modiolus**	Zygomatic and buccal br. of facial (CN VII)	Cutaneous sensation (GSA) via trigeminal N V2
Zygomaticus minor	Helps elevate lip	Zygomatic and buccal br. of facial (CN VII)	Cutaneous sensation (GSA) via trigeminal N V2 and V3
Levator anguli oris	Elevates angle of mouth; deepens nasiolabial furrow	Zygomatic/buccal br. of facial (CN VII)	Cutaneous sensation (GSA) via trigeminal N V2 and V3
Risorius	Elevates corners of mouth laterally—smiling	Buccal/mandibular br. of facial (CN VII)	Cutaneous sensation (GSA) via trigeminal N V2 and V3

Note: **The facial modiolus is an area of fibromuscular tissue **that lies 10 to 12 mm lateral to the angle of the mouth** and represents the point of intersection for the perioral musculature. The modiolus functions to maintain constriction during mastication, aids in bolus positioning, to prevent spillage during chewing and swallowing, and serves a functional role in articulation.*
Muscle spindle few to absent.

Appendix F

Reference Table F: Laryngeal muscles

Muscle Group	Functional role		
Laryngeal group—principal role in **phonation**; protects airway during **swallowing** and maintains airway patency and conduit for **respiration** Adductor group* functions to adduct the laryngeal inlet, acting as sphincter to close airway during swallowing and coughing; adduction of vocal cords causes medial compression (force) at point of vocal cord contact necessary for vocal intensity changes Abductor group facilitates movement of air during respiration and mediates air passage			
Intrinsic	**Action**	**Motor innervation: Nerve branches**	**Sensory innervation**
Lateral cricoarytenoid*	Powerful adductor vocal cords; increases medial compression (force) at point of vocal cord contact Close rima glottidis	Recurrent laryngeal nerve of vagus (CN X) (inferior laryngeal nerve)	Muscle spindles few to absent Mechanoreceptors provide feedback for voice control GSA—internal laryngeal br. of X above vocal folds GSA—recurrent laryngeal br. of X below vocal folds
Transverse (arytenoid) interarytenoid (unpaired)	Assist in adduction of vocal cords Close rima glottidis	Recurrent laryngeal nerve of vagus (CN X) (inferior laryngeal nerve)	
Oblique (arytenoid) interarytenoid*	Assist in adduction of vocal cords Close rima glottidis	Recurrent laryngeal nerve of vagus (CN X) (inferior laryngeal nerve)	
Thyroarytenoid	Assist in adduction of vocal cords Close rima glottidis	Recurrent laryngeal nerve of vagus (CN X) (inferior laryngeal nerve)	
Vocalis *Inferior fibers of thyroarytenoid	Decrease (shorten) tension of vocal cords No action on rima glottidis	Recurrent laryngeal nerve of vagus (CN X) (inferior laryngeal nerve)	Muscle spindle present
Posterior cricoarytenoid	Abductor of vocal folds; antagonists to lateral cricoarytenoid Opens rima glottidis Works cooperatively with cricothyroid to increase diameter of larynx during inspiration	Recurrent laryngeal nerve of vagus (CN X) (inferior laryngeal nerve)	Muscle spindle present
Laryngeal group			
Extrinsic	**Action**	**Innervation**	**Sensory innervation**
Cricothyroid	Increase tension (lengthen) of vocal ligament No action on rima glottidis	External br. Of superior laryngeal of vagus (CN X)	Superior laryngeal br. (X) GSA

Note: *Presence of muscle spindles variable.
Abbreviations: GSA, general somatic afferent

Appendix G

Reference Chart G: Pharyngeal muscles

Muscle Group	Functional role		
Pharyngeal group—involved in pharyngeal phase of swallowing including phasic contractions/relaxation; assists in velopharyngeal closure between soft palate and pharynx during swallowing and speech; functions as resonance chamber for speech by changing luminal diameter and length of pharyngeal space			
Longitudinal	**Action**	**Motor innervation: Nerve branches**	**Sensory innervation**
Salpingopharyngeus	Elevates the upper and lateral parts of pharyngeal wall	Pharyngeal motor br. of vagus (CN X) (pharyngeal plexus)	Pharyngeal plexus GSA fibers from CN IX
Palatopharyngeus	Elevates the oropharynx and aids in closing the nasopharynx		
Stylopharyngeus	Elevates the pharynx and expands the sides of the pharynx	Glossopharyngeal N (CN IX)	
Pharyngeal group			
Constrictors	**Functional role**	**Motor innervation**	**Sensory innervation**
Superior constrictor	Constricts the upper portion of the pharynx	Pharyngeal motor br. of vagus (CN X) (pharyngeal plexus)	Pharyngeal plexus GSA fibers from CN IX
Middle constrictor	Constricts the middle portion of the pharynx		
Inferior constrictor Cricopharyngeus Lower division of inferior constrictor at esophageal boundary	Constricts inferior portion of the pharynx Upper esophageal sphincter—normally constricted; relaxes as part of swallowing reflex	Recurrent laryngeal br. of vagus (CN X)	Recurrent laryngeal br. of vagus (CN X)

Index

Note: Page numbers set **bold** or *italic* indicate headings or figures, respectively.